Good Dialysis Practice
Edited by Jörg Vienken
Volume 5

Good Dialysis Practice

Understanding Membranes and Dialysers

I. Uhlenbusch-Körwer, E. Bonnie-Schorn, A. Grassmann, J. Vienken

PABST SCIENCE PUBLISHERS
Lengerich, Berlin, Bremen, Miami,
Riga, Viernheim, Wien, Zagreb

Library of Congress Cataloging-in-Publication Data

Bibliographic information published by Die Deutsche Bibliothek
Die Deutsche Bibliothek lists this publication in the Deutsche Nationalbibliografie; detailed bibliographic data is available in the Internet at <http://dnb.ddb.de>.

(Good Dialysis Practice ; Vol. 5)
ISBN 3-89967-005-1 (Europe), ISBN 1-59326-058-X (USA)

For further comments and correspondence:
Prof. Dr. Ing. Jörg Vienken
Vice President "BioScience Department"
Fresenius Medical Care
Else-Kroener-Straße 1
61352 Bad Homburg

Tel.: xx49 - 6172 - 609 2463
Fax.: xx49 - 6172 - 609 2468
E-mail: joerg.vienken@fmc-ag.com

Typesetting: Armin Vahrenhorst
Printing: Krips bv, NL-7944 HV Meppel

Illustrations: Jana Roth, Kronberg, Germany

ISBN 3-89967-005-1 (Europe), ISBN 1-59326-058-X (USA)

Preface

Haemodialysis therapy is still associated with side effects and long-term problems which the attending physicians and staff strive to minimise through the therapy and care they give. The dialyser and the membrane included therein constitute the centrepiece of renal replacement therapy, and the medical device industry continuously endeavours to improve the quality of these, adapting them according to the latest scientific findings and modern therapy concepts.

In a given treatment modality, the performance characteristics of the dialyser determine the quantity and nature of the uraemic toxins removed from the patient's blood, provided that an adequate treatment time and flow conditions were prescribed. The optimal dose of dialysis to be targeted, as well as the exact nature of those toxins that should be removed, have long been subjects of discussion and ongoing research. There is a clear trend towards the use of high-flux membranes rather than low-flux membranes, as the former facilitate the removal of those larger uraemic toxins involved in chronic dialysis-related diseases (e.g. ß2-microglobulin in amyloidosis). Besides toxin removal, efficient and gentle removal of excess fluid is another fundamental goal of dialysis therapy. This can be achieved with all dialysers currently available on the market.

The most frequently investigated but also most controversially discussed feature of dialysers and their membranes is their biocompatibility. For several hours, three times a week, patient blood is exposed to an artificial surface which is recognised by the immune system as being foreign. The consequent immune stimulation can be detected using a variety of parameters, such as complement activation and cytokine induction. If and how these observable effects influence clinical outcome is still one of the most disputed issues in the dialysis community. However, the market has already responded to the open discussion in that synthetic, biocompatible membranes have long replaced less biocompatible membranes made from regenerated cellulose as market leaders.

More than 1000 different types of dialysers are currently available on the market. The abundance of literature describing these is overwhelming. This book provides the reader with an overview of the basic topics discussed in association with dialysers and, consequently, offers valuable assistance in judging which dialyser is best for the individual patient in the sense of "Good Dialysis Practice".

The authors extend their heartfelt thanks to Sabine Borst, Sudhir Bowry, Bernd Breuer, Christian Busse, Jörg Hoffmann, Carsten Hornig, Anne Mayer, Bernd Nederlof, Thomas Pohl and Hans-Joachim Wörz for their valuable suggestions and contributions, and the time and effort they invested in a critical reading of the manuscript. They also gratefully acknowledge the indispensable organising support of Sabine Sochan.

Bad Homburg, December 2003

Jörg Vienken
Fresenius Medical Care
BioScience Department

Table of contents

Section A.
Dialyser components and aspects of dialyser construction

Section B.
Dialyser performance

Section C.
Dialyser biocompatibility

Section D.
Clinical experience

Section E.
Dialyser reuse

Section A.
Dialyser components and aspects of dialyser construction

1. Historical overview

Membrane and dialyser development has always closely followed trends in dialysis therapy and advances in scientific cognition (**figure 1.1**). Therefore, the choice of membrane polymer, the membrane form and its physical and biological properties have changed over time, having to adapt to various clinical demands. Following a period of basic research in the field of dialysis, which started as early as 1861, one can identify three major phases in which fundamental scientific discoveries in renal replacement therapy particularly influenced membrane and dialyser development. In phase I, 1945-1965, the major concern was simply to sustain life and to make treatment available for a larger group of patients (**table 1.1**). Dialysers were more or less "hand-made", being manufactured only in small quantities. Removal of uraemic toxins was mainly achieved by diffusion and limited to low molecular weight substances. Phase II (1966-1985) was characterised by increasing patient numbers and the availability and widespread application of industrially manufactured, disposable dialysers. Scientists and physicians turned their attention to device compatibility and treatment tolerance parameters. In the beginning, mainly only acute side effects were considered, but later parameters of the body's humoral and cellular defence systems, which could not always be directly linked to patient reactions, also received much attention. Furthermore, removal of middle molecules came to be considered important, so that the contribution of convection to toxin removal was increased by developing membranes that were more open. Phase III (1986 to the present) can be considered a phase of quality considerations. Dialyser and membrane development became directed towards improving survival and quality of life for the patients. The ultimate aim is a symptom-free treatment that should result, in the long-term, in a reduction of morbidity and mortality in chronic haemodialysis patients.

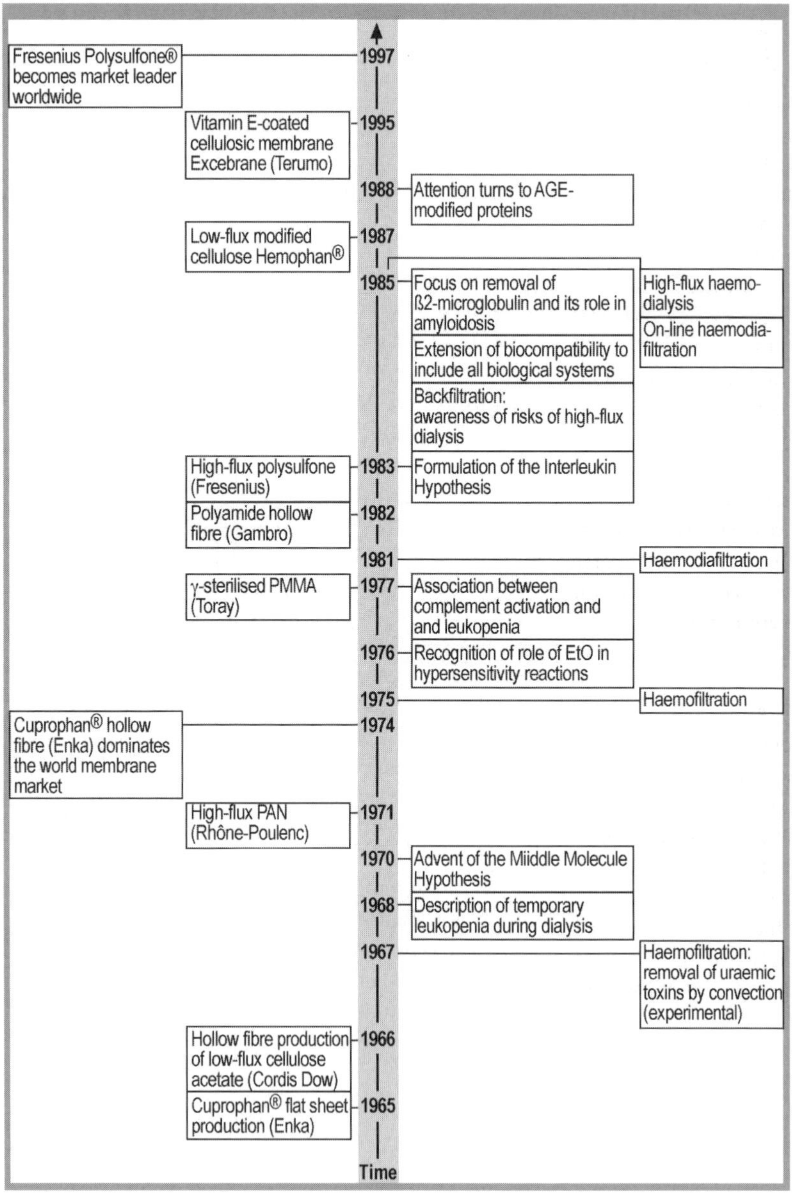

Figure 1.1: Scientific discoveries and key steps in the development of membranes and dialysers.

Phase I: Establishment of haemodialysis as a standard therapy – development of affordable cellulosic membranes and disposable dialysers of adequate performance (1945-1965)

In 1913, Abel and Rountree produced the first "dialysis membrane" from collodium, a cellulose nitrate derivative (**figure 1.2**) [2], and dialysis membranes were made exclusively from cellulose until 1970 (**table 1.1**). During this time, dialysis therapy evolved into a standard treatment and, parallel to this, industrial manufacturing of large quantities of dialysis membranes became possible. These developments included improvements in the geometry of the membrane: a process which went from tubes (dialyser in **figure 1.3** and **1.4**) to coils (dialyser in **figure 1.5** and **1.6**), to flat sheets (**figure 1.7**) and, finally, to hollow fibres (**figure 1.8**). Hollow fibres can be manufactured at high velocities and with a high degree of reproducibility. Advances in production technology permitted a reduction in filter dimensions and blood compartment volume, and allowed the application of higher transmembrane pressures (compare figures **1.6** and **1.8**). In hollow-fibre dialysers, flow conditions are significantly more uniform for blood and dialysis fluid, reducing performance loss due to fluid stagnation. The pioneers in membrane and dialyser development are listed in **table 1.1,** together with their respective landmark inventions that established haemodialysis treatment as a standard therapy.

As in most other technologies, the apparatus used for the treatment has become less elaborate (smaller in size, easier to handle). Particularly the size of dialysers and filters has decreased considerably over time; in fact, this development is still ongoing. A comparison of dialysers from 1970 with present dialysers of equal performance illustrates this point. Miniaturisation can only be accomplished by increasing the performance characteristics of the dialyser or haemofilter and the membrane. With cellulosic membranes, this goal was achieved by reducing the diffusive barrier, i.e. the wall thickness. The strong physical strength of cellulosic membranes, based on their unique chemical structure, allowed considerable wall thickness reductions over time.

Year	Inventor, company	Device, membrane polymer	Development
1861	T. Graham (Glasgow and London, GB)	Vegetable pergament (parchment paper)	Diffusion of cristalloids, not colloids, between separated aqueous solutions: dialysis [1]
1913	J. Abel, L. Rowntree, B. Turner (Baltimore, USA)	*Vivi-diffusion apparatus:* device with cellulose trinitrate (collodion) tubes (figure 1.2)	First artificial kidney used on nephrectomised dogs [2]
1924	G. Haas (Giessen, Germany)	Tubular device Cellulose trinitrate (collodion) (figure 1.3)	First human dialysis [3]
1932	R. Weingand (Bornlitz, Germany)	Tubes from cellulose solutions	First continuous cellulose tube manufacturing [4]
1937	W. Thalheimer (New York, USA)	Cellulose-hydrate (cellophane) (normally used as protective film in the sausage industry)	First flat haemodialysis membrane produced [5]
1944	W. Kolff, H. Berk (Kampen, NL)	*Rotating drum:* wooden, later stainless steal drum, wound by a cellophane tube (sausage casing) and immersed in a dialysis fluid bath (figure 1.4)	First recovery of an acute renal failure patient [6]
1947	N. Alwall (Lund, Sweden)	*Alwall kidney:* stainless steal drum, wound by membrane coils and immersed in a dialysis fluid bath (figure 1.5)	Ultrafiltration using hydrostatic pressure [7, 8]
1956	W. Kolff, B. Watschinger (Cleveland, USA)	*Coil dialyser:* tubular membrane, sandwiched between woven fibreglass and wrapped around a solid core (figure 1.6)	First employed in the late sixties with a single-pass dialysis fluid delivery system [9]

Year	Inventor, company	Device, membrane polymer	Development
	Travenol (USA)	Twin Coil dialyser: twin blood pathways	First disposable haemodialyser
1960	F. Kiil (Oslo, Norway)	Kiil dialyser: plate dialyser which could be reassembled; contained grooved polypropylene boards which supported the cellulosic flat sheet membrane (sausage packaging industry) (figure 1.7)	Parallel-flow artificial kidney which could be used without a blood pump [10]
1966	R. Stewart et al. Cordis Dow (USA)	Cellulose acetate hollow fibre** (used for desalination) (figure 1.8)	First capillary hollow-fibre production [11]
1966	Enka AG* (Wuppertal, Germany)	Cuprophan® (regenerated cellulose) flat sheets	First standardised industrial production of flat sheet membranes
1967	L.W. Bluemle, L.W. Henderson (USA)	Polyelectrolyte membrane "Diaflo" (figure 1.9)	First investigations with haemofiltration [12]
1969	Enka AG* (Wuppertal, Germany)	Cuprophan® capillary fibres	
1969	Hospal (Meyzien, France)	AN69® polyacrylonitrile (figure 1.10)	First synthetic membrane with an ultrafiltration coefficient suitable for high-flux dialysis [13]
1970	Gambro (Lund, Sweden)	*Alwall dialyser:* multiple stacked membrane layers separated by thinner membrane support plates (figure 1.11)	First disposable parallel-plate dialyser, presterilised [14]

**Enka later became Akzo Faser, then Akzo Nobel and is now Membrana*
***Functionally regenerated cellulose rather than cellulose acetate because of a de-esterification step in the manufacturing process [15]*

Table 1.1: Pioneers in dialyser and membrane development and their inventions during the evolution of haemodialysis to a standard therapy.

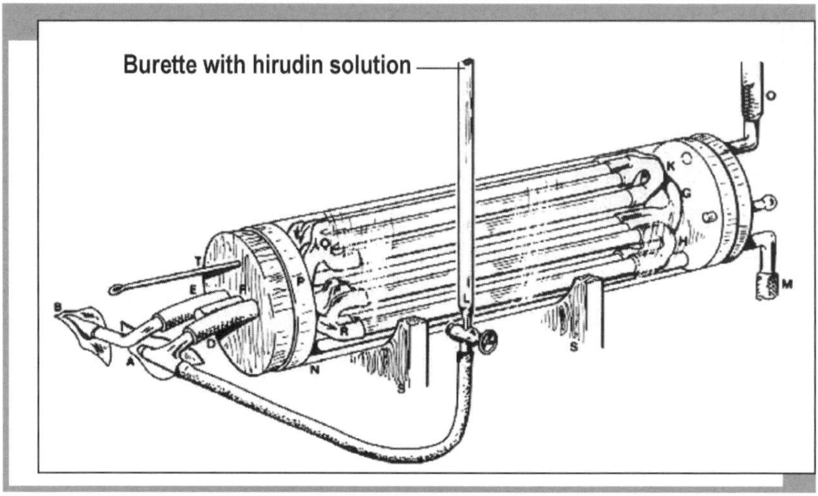

Figure 1.2: Vivi-diffusion apparatus from Abel and Rountree, which was used for dialysis on nephrectomised dogs in 1913.

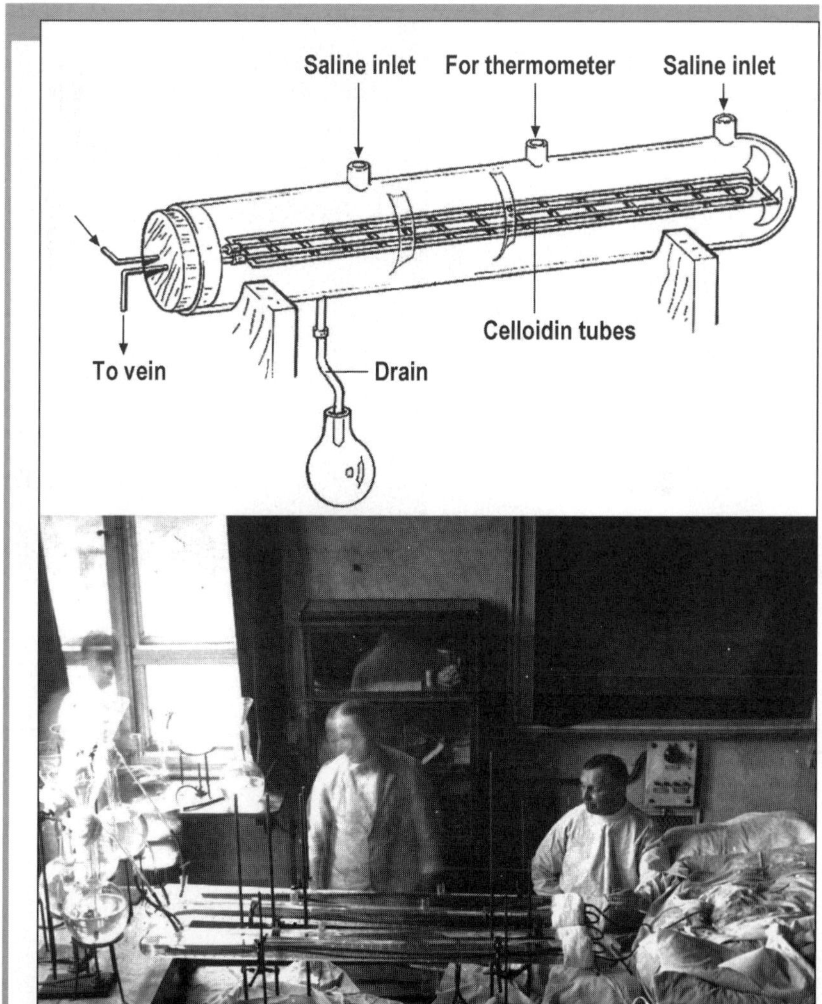

Figure 1.3: Schematic drawing of the "Haas dialyser" and photograph of one of the first human dialysis in 1924.

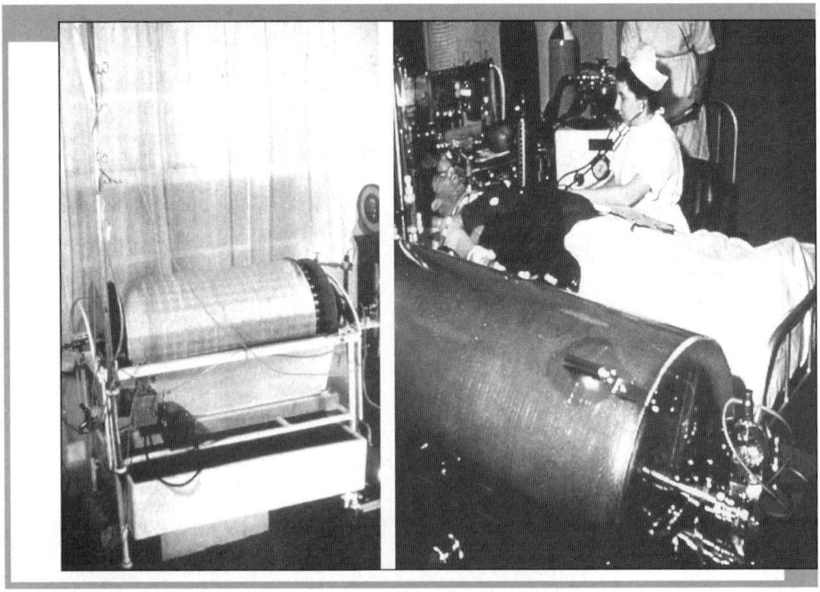

Figure 1.4: Kolff's rotating drum in 1944 (on the left) and dialysis with this device in Glasgow in 1965 (on the right).

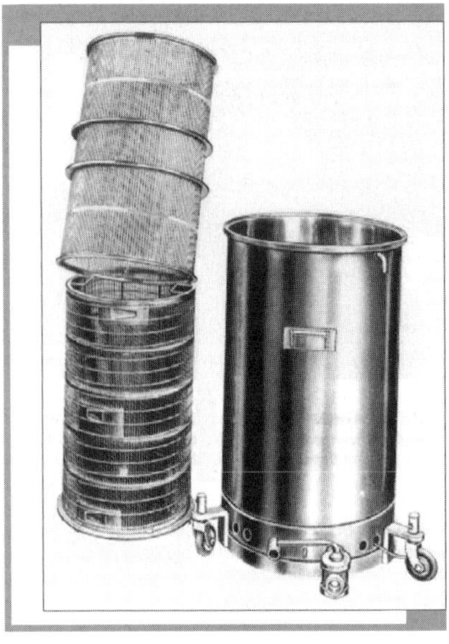

Figure 1.5: Alwall kidney, consisting of a stainless steel drum, wound by membrane coils and immersed in a dialysis fluid bath (1947).

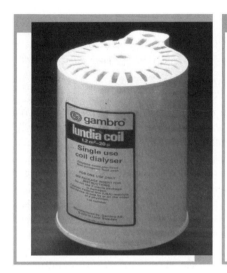

Figure 1.6: Coil dialyser, Lundia 1.2 m², from 1956.

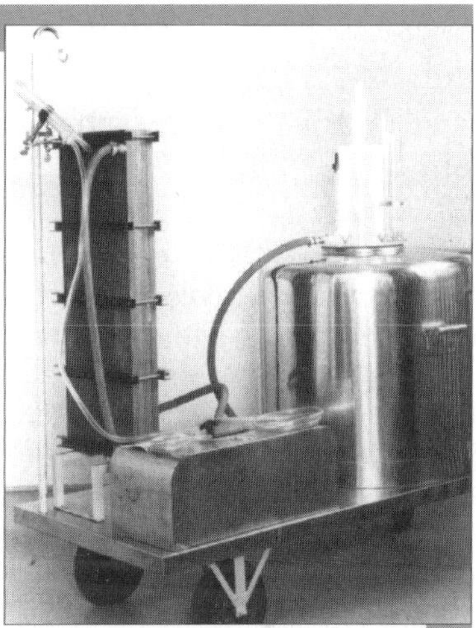

Figure 1.7: Kiil Dialyser from 1960, which could be used without a blood pump.

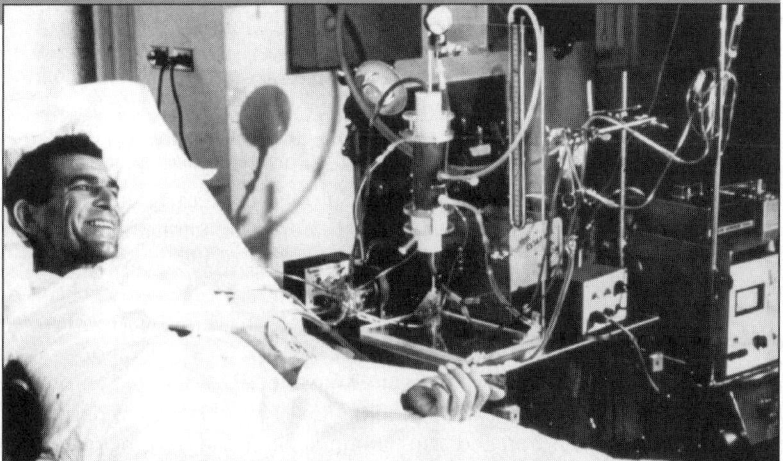

Figure 1.8: Capillary hollow-fibre dialyser from Stewart, CDAK 1.3 (1966).

Phase II: The middle molecule hypothesis, start of the debate on biocompatibility – development of synthetic membranes with greater permeabilities and higher degrees of biocompatibility (1966- 1985)

All early dialysis membranes were of low hydraulic permeability and removed only low molecular weight molecules. Elimination of small uraemic toxins was accomplished predominantly by diffusion. Convection was only employed to remove the interdialytic fluid gain. This concept changed when Bluemle and Henderson published their first results on haemofiltration using a highly permeable "polyelectrolyte" membrane (sodium polystyrene sulfonate and polyvinylbenzyltrimethyl ammonium chlorid, called "Diaflo") in 1967 [12] (**figure 1.9**). The aim of their experiments was to relate the rate of solute removal to the applied pressure gradient (which could be adjusted to the particular clinical situation) and not, as it is the case in diffusion, to the concentration gradient [12]. Although their Diaflo membrane failed to become a successful product commercially, the results initiated a change in direction in membrane development towards the production of membranes with higher permeabilities for larger solutes. The theoretical basis for the use of such highly permeable membranes was supplied in the beginning of the nineteen seventies by the so-called "Middle Molecule Hypothesis": the retention of higher molecular weight uraemic toxins (here molecular weight > 300 up to 2000) was believed to be responsible for a number of clinical manifestations of the uraemic status, and their removal was clearly desirable [16]. The first commercial membrane of high hydraulic permeability was developed in 1969 and introduced into the market in 1971; it was made from an acrylonitrile sodium methallylsulfonate copolymer, better known under the brand name AN69® (Rhône-Poulonc, France) [13] (**figure 1.10**). With this polymer, a new class of dialysis membranes was born: the synthetic membranes. Use of such membranes with increased ultrafiltration properties demanded the development of appropriate dialysis machines with automatic ultrafiltration control, a fact that probably hindered the widespread usage of high-flux dialysis in the years that followed.

Parallel to the introduction of high-flux dialysis, haemofiltration was gaining popularity for some special patient groups. In 1974, the first chronic renal failure patient was treated by haemofiltration [17]. Although widespread application of haemofiltration and also haemodiafiltration [18] is hindered by the greater costs involved compared to standard haemodialysis, the number of patients treated with these methods is still growing, albeit slowly. Almost all dialyser manufacturers have developed a filter containing a synthetic mem-

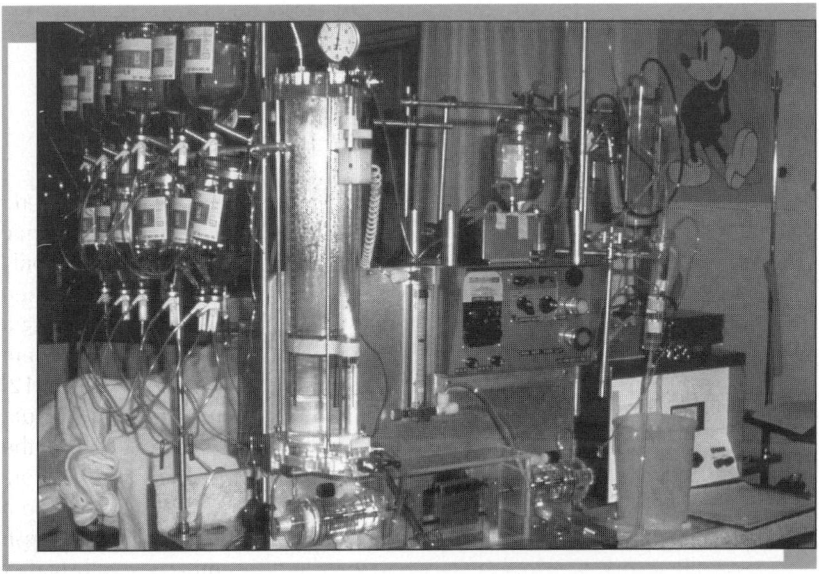

Figure 1.9: Early haemofiltration set-up by Hendersen et al. (approx. 1970).

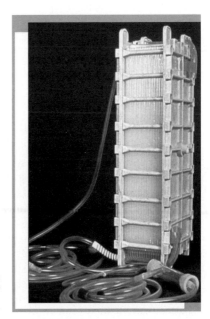

Figure 1.10: First high-flux dialyser from Rhône Poulenc, RP6 with the AN69® membrane (1969).

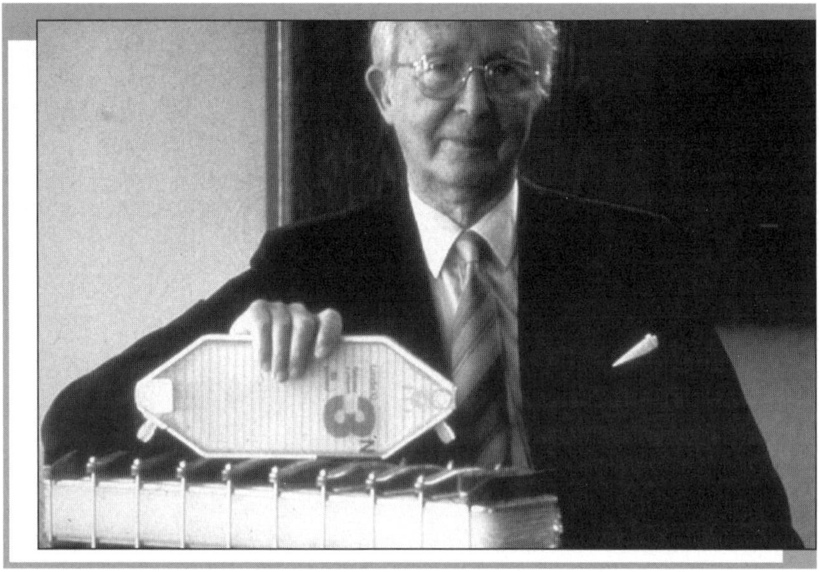

Figure 1.11: Nils Alwall with the "Alwall dialyser" from 1970 and a modern plate dialyser that was commercially available until the early nineties.

brane of sufficiently high hydraulic permeability for these particular applications.

The development of other synthetic membranes, such as polymethylmethacrylate (PMMA in 1977 by Toray, Japan), polyamide (in 1982 by Gambro, Sweden) and polysulfone (in 1983 by Fresenius, Germany), started in the late seventies and is still ongoing. This development process was further stimulated by the findings that synthetic membranes are generally better accepted by the patient's defence systems than membranes made of regenerated cellulose (e.g. Cuprophan®). In 1968, Kaplow and Goffinet were the first to report a transient decrease of leukocytes in the peripheral blood of patients during dialysis with membranes made from regenerated cellulose [19]. Craddock explained the basic mechanism behind these observations was an activation of the complement cascade by artificial surfaces [20, 21]. The hydroxyl groups on cellulosic membranes were thought to be responsible for this activation because they react with the C3 complement protein, thereby triggering the complement cascade (the concept has since been extended, and is explained in chapter 7 in more detail). The leukopenia and complement activation observed with the original cellulose membrane provided the platform for the introduction of the biocompatibility concept into membrane development. Since then, each new membrane is not only judged on the basis of its performance characteristics and observable incompatibilities, such as clotting of the fibres, but is also assessed according to its interaction with biological systems (e.g. the complement system); this interaction should be as low as possible or, according to another definition, be considered "appropriate" [22].

Phase III: ß2-microglobulin, ultrapure dialysis fluid, morbidity and mortality of haemodialysis patients – state-of-the-art membranes are highly permeable, biocompatible and synthetic (1986 to now)

In response to the biocompatibility debate, chemical modifications of the cellulose polymer were undertaken with the aim of blunting its immune system activating potential. Hemophan® (di-ethyl-amino-ethyl, or DEAE cellulose), introduced to the market in 1987, is one result of such a modification [23].

Extensive clinical experience has made basic biomaterial researchers, membrane manufacturers and medical scientists aware that no dialysis membrane can be absolutely inert. Based on the experimental work of Lyman et al., Okano et al. and Matsuda et al., a "domain structure" in which hydrophobic and hydrophilic structures are balanced on the membrane surface was accepted as being a beneficial feature regarding membrane biocompatibility; this structure is typical of nearly all biocompatible membranes presently available [24-30]. Adsorption of proteins onto the membrane surface depends on the particular hydrogen bonds, electrical charges and hydrophilic-hydrophobic forces present. The absence of surface nucleophils, such as hydroxyl-groups (as present in regenerated cellulose), a low surface charge and a balanced distribution of hydrophilic and hydrophobic domains appear to characterise more biocompatible membranes [28-30]. Hydrophobic surfaces adsorb proteins and cells, leading to platelet adhesion, whereas hydrophilic surfaces interact with blood cells and activate complement [27]. If an artificial surface exhibits alternating hydrophilic and hydrophobic domains on a nanometer scale (i.e. so that stable interactions with microdomains on cell membranes are not possible), cell activation can successfully be avoided [28-31].

The discovery of ß2-microglobulin (ß2-m) in amyloid deposits of long-term haemodialysis patients, published in 1986 by Geyjo and colleagues, brought another important factor into the discussion on the optimal function of a dialysis membrane [32]. As a protein with a molecular weight of 11,818, ß2-m is removed by high-flux membranes and normally retained with low-flux membranes. Furthermore, some evidence appeared that bioincompatible membranes stimulate ß2-m production [33]. Although the clinical relevance of dialytic ß2-m removal remained a subject of debate, low-flux membranes made from regenerated cellulose came under increasing pressure. Today, evidence exists from clinical data that convective treatment modes involving highly permeable membranes (i.e. haemofiltration and haemodiafiltration) [34, 35] and ultrapure dialysis fluid [36] have a positive impact on the development of dialysis-related amyloidosis: clinical manifestations of the illness are attenuated or delayed by these treatment modes.

In the early eighties, attention began to be focussed on the microbial quality of the dialysis fluid. Henderson, Koch, Dinarello and Shaldon postulated in their "Interleukin Hypothesis" that bacterial products from contaminated dialysis fluid may induce cytokine release in haemodialysis patients, and that this release may be responsible for a number of dialysis-related side effects (e.g. hypotension) [37, 38]. Later, it was proven that the dialysis membrane is not a safe barrier against bacterial degradation products [39, 40]. Transfer of bacterial products from dialysis fluid into blood is particularly easy with high-flux membranes: here the steep pressure drop along the length of the dialyser results in an inversion of the pressure profiles such that, at the end of the dialyser proximal to the blood outlet, dialysis fluid enters the blood. This so-called backfiltration (described in the scientific literature since 1985 [41]) somewhat reduced the enthusiasm for high-flux membranes, and led to the development of low-flux counterparts of well-established, high-flux membrane polymers. Examples are Fresenius Polysulfone®, PMMA and, more recently, Polyamide S™ (now Polyamix™) – all membranes which were primarily developed solely as high-flux membranes. However, even a membrane with small pores is not capable of retaining all microbial products: microbial fragments of molecular weight under 5,000 can pass through low-flux membranes and can also be biologically active [42]. Cytokine generation (measured as interleukin-6 generation) was found to be higher during dialysis with low-flux regenerated cellulose than with high-flux polyacrylonitrile (PAN) when contaminated dialysis fluid was used [43]. The good adsorption capacity of the PAN membrane for microbial fragments (which is also a feature of many other synthetic membranes, e.g. polysulfone and polyamide) explains this observation [44]. This newly-discovered characteristic of some synthetic membranes opened up a novel application for highly permeable filters: the filtration of dialysis fluid to remove microbial substances that are potentially harmful for the patient. In the beginning, filters normally used for haemofiltration were used as endotoxin filters, but later special filters were developed specifically for filtering the inflowing dialysis fluid prior to its contact with the dialysis membrane (e.g. Diasafe® from Fresenius Medical Care).

Another aspect of biocompatibility is the sterilisation of the dialyser or filter. The first disposable dialysers employed in the nineteen seventies were sterilised using ethylene oxide (EtO). Due to the high content of polyurethane (PUR – the potting compound used in hollow fibre dialysers) which acts as a reservoir for the gas, EtO-sterilised dialysers induced the so-called "first use syndrome" in many patients, i.e. allergic reactions against EtO [45]. The PUR content has since been decreased to a minimum, and times for degassing have been increased to guarantee a safe level of residual EtO. Therefore, EtO-sterilisation has been improved so that dialysers sterilised in this way are still used. γ-irradiation is another cost-effective form of sterilisation; this requires a stabile membrane polymer in order to avoid membrane degradation, as was sometimes reported [46], as well as a particular potting material that does not release carcinogenic methylene dianiline (MDA) [47]. It appears that heat sterilisation is the most "biocompatible" method, but only cellulosic and polysulfone membranes are thermo stable polymers. Thus, this feature added to the excellent performance and biocompatibility characteristics of polysulfone membranes is making them immensely successful; this success is reflected by the fact that most membrane producers have started to develop their own particular polysulfone membrane.

From 1990 on, the quality aspect of dialysis therapy gained more and more importance. There was a rapid increase in the number of publications dealing with quality of life, hospitalisation of dialysis patients, morbidity and mortality (e.g. [48-51]). Initially, the difference in treatment modalities between countries was the main focus of attention [48]; later, interest turned to the influence of reuse on mortality [49]. Since 1994, the dialysis membrane and its impact on morbidity and mortality have been studied intensively, especially with respect to membrane biocompatibility (complement and cell activation, in particular) and permeability (high-flux or low-flux) (e.g. [50, 51]). Hakim and Schiffl reported that acute renal failure patients treated with membranes made from regenerated cellulose had a higher mortality rate than patients treated with synthetic membranes [52, 53]. Although these results were not confirmed in a later controlled, prospective, multicentre study of Jörres et al. [54], such studies inflamed a controversy in which various study designs were heavily criticised (e.g. [55]). Whereas the special group of acute renal failure patients is the focus of the above-cited studies, other investigations reported increased mortality for chronic haemodialysis patients when treated with low-flux rather than high-flux membranes (both polysulfone dialysers [56, 57]). However, the conditions under which such results were generated must be carefully analysed: patient collectives and treatment conditions (especially dialysis adequacy) must be comparable, and, ideally, membranes of the same polymer family should be used. Further insight into the possible benefits of using biocompatible, high-flux membranes regarding patient morbidity and mortality was expected, to be supplied by clinical trials, such as the HEMO study in the US (e.g. [58]) and the still ongoing MPO study in Europe [59]. The HEMO study failed to show any difference between low-flux and high-flux membranes (both biocompatible) with respect to mortality, but there are many points of criticism regarding study design etc. [60, 61]. Fact is, however, high-flux, synthetic membranes are now the most commonly used membranes, having long displaced the once predominant low-flux membranes made of regenerated cellulose (mainly Cuprophan®). In 2001, 55% of all membranes used in the USA, Japan and Europe were synthetic membranes and 50% of *all* membranes used were high-flux membranes [62]. These numbers increased again in 2002, i.e. worldwide numbers of high-flux and synthetic dialysers sold increased by 19% and 20%, respectively [63].

References

1. Graham T: Liquid diffusion applied to analysis. Phil Trans R Soc London 151: 183, 1861

2. Abel JJ, Rowntree LC, Turner BB: On the removal of diffusible substances from the circulating blood of living animals by dialysis. J Pharmacol Exp Ther 5: 275-316, 1914

3. Haas G: Versuche der Blutauswaschung am Lebenden mit Hilfe der Dialyse. Klin Wochenschrift 4: 13, 1925

4. Weingand R: Apparatus for manufacturing seamless flexible tubes from cellulose solutions. US Patent Nr. 1864006, 1932

5. Thalheimer W: Experimental exchange transfusion for reducing azotemia. Use of the artificial kidney for this purpose. Proc Soc Exp Biol Med 37: 641-643, 1937

6. Kolff WJ, Berk HTJ: De kunstmatige nier: een dialysator met groot oppervlak. Ned Tijdschr Geneeskd 87: 1684, 1943

7. Alwall N: On the artificial kidney I: apparatus for dialysis of blood in vivo. Acta Med Scand 128: 317-325, 1947

8. Alwall N, Norviit L: On the artificial kidney II: the effectivity of the apparatus. Acta Med Scand 196: 250, 1947

9. Kolff WJ, Watschinger B: Further development of the coil kidney. J Lab Clin Med 47: 969-977, 1956

10. Kiil F: Development of a parallel flow artificial kidney in plastics. Acta Chir Scand Suppl 253: 140-142, 1960

11. Stewart RD, Cerny JC, Mahon HI: An artificial kidney made from capillary fibres. Invest Urol 5: 614-624, 1966. Preliminary report. Univ Michigan Med Center J30: 116-118, 1964

12. Henderson LW, Besarab A, Michaels A, Bluemle LW: Blood purification by ultrafiltration and fluid replacement (diafiltration). Trans Amer Soc Artif Int Organs 13: 216-226, 1967

13. Man NK, Granger A, Rondon-Nucete M, Zingraff J, Jungers P, Sausse A, Funck-Brentano JL: One year follow-up of short dialysis with a membrane highly permeable to middle molecules. Proc Eur Dial Transplant Assoc 10: 236-245, 1973

14. Alwall N: A new disposable artificial kidney: experimental and clinical experience. Proc Eur Transplant Assoc 5:18-23, 1968

15. Clark WR, Hamburger RJ, Lysaght MJ: Effect of membrane composition and structure on solute removal and biocompatibility in hemodialysis. Kidney Int 56: 2005-2015, 1999

16. Babb AL, Farrell PC, Uvelli DA, Scribner BH: Haemodialyzer evaluation by examination of solute molecular spectra. Trans Am Soc Artif Organs 18: 98-105, 1972

17. Henderson LW, Colton CK, Ford CA: Kinetics of hemofiltration. II. Clinical characterization of a new blood cleansing modality. J Lab Clin Med 85 (3): 372-391, 1975

18. Leber HW, Wizemann V, Goubeaud G, Rawer P, Schütterle G: Simultanous hemofiltration/hemodialysis: an effective alternative to hemofiltration and conventional hemodialysis in the treatment of uremic patients. Clin Nephrol 9 (3): 115-121, 1978

19. Kaplow L, Goffinet J: Profound neutropenia during the early phase of hemodialysis. JAMA 203: 133-135, 1968

20. Craddock P, Fehr J, Dalmasso A, Brigham KL, Jacob H: Hemodialysis leukopenia: pulmonary vascular leucostasis resulting from complement activation of dialyser cellophane membranes. J Clin Invest 59: 879-888, 1977

21. Craddock P, Fehr J, Brigham KL, Kronenberg RS, Jacobs HS: Complement and leucocyte-mediated pulmonary dysfunction in hemodialysis. N Engl J Med 296: 769-774, 1977

22. Gurland HJ, Davison AM, Bonomini V, Falkenhagen D, Hansen S, Kishimoto T, Lysaght MJ, Moran J, Valek A: Definitions and terminology in biocompatibility. Nephrol Dial Transplant 9(Suppl 2): 4-10, 1994

23. Akzo Faser AG: Hemophan, a DEAE modified cellulose for dialysis. US-Patent No.4,668,396, European Patent No. 172,497

24. Lyman DJ, Metcalf LC, Albo D, Richards KF, Lamb J: The effect of chemical structure and surface properties of synthetic polymers on the coagulation of blood III. In vivo adsorption of proteins on polymer surfaces. Trans Am Soc Artif Organs 20: 474-478, 1974

25. Okano T, Kataoka K, Sakurai Y, Shimada M, Miyahara M, Akaike T, Shinohara I: Molecular design of block and graft co-polymers having the ability to suppress platelet adhesion. Artif Organs (Suppl 5): 468-470, 1981

26. Yui N, Tanaka J, Sanui K, Ogata N, Kataoka K, Okano T, Sakurai Y: Characterisation of the microstructure of poly(propylene oxide)-segmented polyamide and its suppression of platelet adhesion. Polym J 16: 119-128, 1984

27. Matsuda T: Biological responses at non-physiological interfaces and molecular design of biocompatible surfaces. Nephrol Dial Transplant 4: 60-66, 1989

28. Diamantoglou M, Platz J, Vienken J: Cellulose carbamates and derivatives as hemocompatible membrane materials for hemodialysis. Artif Organs 23(1): 15-22, 1999

29. Diamantoglou M, Lemke HD, Vienken J: Cellulose-ester as membrane materials for hemodialysis. Int J Artif Organs 17(7): 385-391, 1994

30. Vienken J, Diamantoglou M, Hahn C, Kamusewitz H, Paul D: Considerations on developmental aspects of biocompatible dialysis membranes. Artif Organs 19(5): 398-406, 1995

31. Deppisch R, Göhl H, Smeby L: Microdomain structures of polymeric surfaces – potential for improving blood treatment procedures. Nephrol Dial Transplant 13: 1354-1359, 1998

32. Geyjo F, Odani S, Yamada T, Homma N, Daito H, Suzuki Y, Nakagawa Y, Kobayashi H, Maruyama Y, Hirasawa Y, Suzuki M, Arakawa M: ß2-microglobulin:

a new form of amyloid protein associated with chronic hemodialysis. Kidney Int 30: 385-390, 1986

33. Jahn B, Betz M, Deppisch R, Janssen O, Hänsch GM, Ritz E: Stimulation of $beta_2$ -microglobulin synthesis in lymphocytes after exposure to Cuprophan dialyzer membranes. Kidney Int 40: 285-290, 1991

34. Wizemann V, Lotz C, Techert F, Uthoff S: On-line haemodiafiltration versus low-flux haemodialysis. A prospective randomized study. Nephrol Dial Transplant 15(Suppl 1): 43-48, 2000

35. Locatelli F, Marcelli D, Conte F, Limido A, Malberti F, Spotti D: Comparison of mortality in ESRD patients on convective and diffusive extracorporeal treatments. The Registro Lombardo Dialisi E Trapianto. Kidney Int 55(1): 286-293, 1999

36. Baz M, Durand C, Ragon A, Jaber K, Andrieu D, Merzouk T, Purgus R, Olmer M, Reynier JP, Berland Y: Using ultrapure water in hemodialysis delays carpal tunnel syndrome. Artif Organs 14(11): 681-685, 1991

37. Henderson LW, Koch KM, Dinarello CA, Shaldon S: Haemodialysis hypotension: the interleukin hypothesis. Blood Purification 1: 3-8, 1983

38. Shaldon S, Deschodt G, Branger B, Ouls R, Granolleras C, Baldamus CA, Koch KM, Lysaght M, Dinarello C: Haemodialysis hypotension: the interleukin hypothesis restated. Proc EDTA-ERA 22: 229-243, 1985

39. Laude-Sharp M, Caroff M, Simard L, Pusineri C, Kazatchkine MD, Haeffner-Cavaillon N: Induction of IL-1 during hemodialysis: transmembrane passage of intact endotoxins (LPS). Kidney Int 38: 1089-1094, 1990

40. Ureña P, Herbelin A, Zingraff J, Lair M, Man NK, Descamps-Latscha B, Drüeke T: Permeability of cellulosic and non-cellulosic membranes to endotoxins subunits and cytokine production during *in-vitro* hemodialysis. Nephrol Dial Transplant 7: 16-28, 1992

41. Stiller S, Mann H, Brunner H: Backfiltration in hemodialysis with highly permeable membranes. Contr Nephrol 46: 23-32, 1985

42. Lonnemann G, Koch KM: Pyrogenic reactions in *Replacement of renal function by dialysis*, 3rd ed., edited by Jacobs C, Kjellstrand CM, Koch KM, Winchester JF, Dordrecht, Kluwer Academic Publishers: 726-733, 1996

43. Pertosa G, Gesualdo L, Bottalico D, Schena FP: Endotoxins modulate chronically tumor necrosis factor α and interleukin 6 release by uraemic monocytes. Nephrol Dial Transplant 10: 328-333, 1995

44. Weber C, Linsberger I, Rafiee-Tehrani M, Falkenhagen D: Permeability and adsorption capacity of dialysis membranes to lipid A. Int J Artif Organs 20: 144-152, 1997

45. Dolovich J, Bell B: Allergy to a product(s) of ethylene oxide gas. Demonstration of IgE and IgG antibodies and hapten specificity. J Allergy Clin Immunol 62(1): 30-32, 1978

46. Takesawa S, Satoh S, Hidai H, Sekiguchi M, Sakai K: Degradation by gamma irradiation of regenerated cellulose membranes for clinical dialysis. Trans Am Soc Artif Intern Organs 33: 584-587, 1987

47. Shintani H, Nakamura A: Analysis of a carcinogen, 4,4′-methylenedianiline, from thermosetting polyurethane during sterilization. J Anal Toxicol 13: 354-357, 1989

48. Held PJ, Brunner F, Odaka M, Garcia JR, Port FK, Gaylin DS: Five-year survival for end-stage renal disease patients in the United States, Europe, and Japan, 1982 to 1987. Am J Kidney Dis 15(5): 451-457, 1990

49. Held PJ, Wolfe RA, Gaylin DS, Port FK, Levin NW, Turenne MN: Analysis of the association of dialyzer reuse practices and patient outcomes. Am J Kidney Dis 23(5): 692-708, 1994

50. Hakim RM, Held PJ, Stannard DC, Wolfe RA, Port FK, Daugirdas JT, Agodoa L: Effect of the dialysis membrane on mortality of chronic hemodialysis patients. Kidney Int 50: 566-570, 1996

51. Bloembergen WE, Hakim RM, Stannard DC, Held PJ, Wolfe RA, Agodoa LYC, Port FK: Relationship of dialysis membrane and cause-specific mortality. Am J Kidney Dis 33(1): 1-10, 1999

52. Hakim RM, Wingard RL, Parker RA: Effect of the dialysis membrane in the treatment of patients with acute renal failure. N Engl J Med 331: 1338-1342, 1994

53. Schiffl H, Lang SM, König A, Strasser T, Haider MC, Held E: Biocompatible membranes in acute renal failure: prospective case-controlled study. Lancet 344: 570-572, 1994

54. Jörres A, Gahl GM, Dobis C, Polenakovic MH, Cakalaroski K, Rutkowski B, Kisielnicka E, Krieter DH, Rumpf WK, Günther C, Gaus W, Hoegel J: Haemodialysis-membrane biocompatibility and mortality of patients with dialysis-dependent acute renal failure: a prospective randomised multicentre trial. Lancet 354: 1137-1341, 1999

55. Vanholder R, De Vriese A, Lameire N: The role of dialyzer biocompatibility in acute renal failure. Blood Purif 18: 1-12, 2000

56. Woods HF, Nandakumar M: Improved outcome for haemodialysis patients treated with high-flux membranes. Nephrol Dial Transplant 15(Suppl 1): 36-42, 2000

57. Port F: Mortality risk and dialysis membranes. USRDS report presented at the ISN-Meeting, Buenos Aires, 1999

58. Eknoyan G, Beck GJ, Cheung AK, Daugirdas JT, Greene T, Kusek JW, Allon M, Bailey J, Delmez JA, Depner TA, Dwyer JT, Levey AS, Levin NW, Milford E, Ornt DB, Rocco MV, Schulman G, Schwab SJ, Teehan BP, Toto R for the Hemodialysis (HEMO) Study Group: Effect of dialysis dose and membrane flux in maintenance hemodialysis. N Engl J Med 347(25): 2010-2019, 2002

59. Locatelli F, Hannedouche T, Jacobson S, La Greca G, Loureiro A, Martin-Malo A, Papadimitriou M, Vanholder R: The effect of membrane permeability on ESRD: design of a prospective randomised trial. J Nephrol 12: 85-88, 1999

60. Levin N, Greenwood R: Reflections on the HEMO study: the American viewpoint. Nephrol Dial Transplant 18(6): 1059-1060

61. Locatelli F: Dose of dialysis, convection and haemodialysis patients outcome–what the HEMO study doesn't tell us: the European viewpoint. Nephrol Dial Transplant 18(6): 1061-1065, 2003

62. Moeller S, Gioberge S, Brown G: ESRD patients in 2001: global overview of patients, treatment modalities and development trends. Nephrol Dial Transplant 17(12): 2071-2076, 2002

63. Moeller S, Grassmann A, Brown G: Patienten mit terminaler Niereninsuffizienz im Jahr 2002 - eine globale Betrachtung in: *Aktuelle Nephrologie*, edited by J. Passlick-Deetjen, Lengerich, Pabst Science Publishers, 2: 19-27, 2003

2. Membrane family overview and nomenclature

A wide spectrum of haemodialysers and filters together with a multitude of different membranes are currently available commercially. In the year 2002, more than 1000 different dialyser types with membranes made from at least 10 different polymer materials were on the market (see appendix: list of haemodialysers and **table 2.1**). Few would have the time to survey all the different types in order to evaluate the actual situation regarding membrane nomenclature. This chapter is intended to provide insight into the frequently inconsistent and confusing nomenclature of different membrane polymers and the various descriptions given.

The polymer essentially determines the chemical and physical behaviour of a dialysis membrane: the final dialyser sterilisation mode, resistance against chemical agents used during possible dialyser reprocessing, and device biocompatibility are all influenced by the type of polymer used to produce the membrane. The earliest dialysis membranes were manufactured from regenerated cellulose or cellulose acetate, originating from the spinning expertise of the textile industry. The ideal polymer for dialysis should enable the production of a biocompatible membrane family whose members are of considerable physical strength, have excellent diffusive and, where appropriate, convective properties, and have performance and biocompatibility profiles which are resistant to all chemicals and sterilising agents used in haemodialysis procedures, including heat sterilisation (121°C). In addition, recent literature demonstrates the importance of ultrapure dialysis fluid for the attenuation of long-term clinical consequences [1, 2]. Therefore, whenever ultrapure dialysis fluid cannot be guaranteed, as is still the case in many clinics, it is vital that modern haemodialysis membranes should adsorb endotoxins at the outer surface, as this provides added protection against transfer of bacterial derivates from the dialysis fluid to the patient in case of microbial contamination of the dialysis fluid.

Cellulosic		Synthetic		
Regenerated cellulose	**Modified cellulose**	**Polysulfones**	**Poly(aryl)ether-sulfones**	**Others**
Cuprophan® (Membrana)	CDA, Dicea (Teijin, Toyobo)	Fresenius Polysulfone® (FMC)	PEPA® (Nikkiso)	AN69®, AN69ST (Hospal)
Cuprammonium rayon (Asahi, Terumo, Teijin)	CTA, Tricea (Toyobo)	Helixone® (FMC)	Polyamix™ (PolyamideS™) (Gambro)	PAN (Asahi)
SCE (Teijin)	Hemophan® (Membrana)	α Polysulfone (Saxonia, B.Braun)	DIAPES® (Membrana)	PMMA (Toray)
G-O-P DIAFIL® (Renaselect*)	SMC® (Membrana)	Toraysulfone® (Toray)	Arylane (Hospal)	EVAL® (Kawasumi)
	PEG-RC (Asahi)	APS® (Asahi)		Polyamide (Gambro)
	Excebrane (Terumo)			

Table 2.1: Main dialysis membranes currently on the market. *SCE = saponified cellulose ester; CDA = cellulose diacetate; CTA = cellulose triacetate; Hemophan® = diethylamminoethyl cellulose; SMC® = benzyl cellulose = Polysynthane; PEG-RC = polyethyleneglycol grafted regenerated cellulose; EVAL® = ethylvinylalcohol copolymer; Excebrane = vitamin E coated regenerated cellulose; PAN = polyacrylonitrile; PEPA® = polyethersulfone / polyarylate; DIAPES®, Arylane = polyarylethersulfone syn. polyethersulfone, FMC = Fresenius Medical Care, *Renaselect former Gross-O-Pharm.*

As described in the previous chapter, which covered the history of almost 90 years haemodialyser and membrane development, modern haemodialysis membranes are highly-technical products which are tailored to the scientific demands of haemodialysis therapy. Even "early" materials, such as regenerated cellulose, are subject to permanent improvement by their manufacturers, and present types vary from their counterparts of some years ago in several aspects - although they may not achieve the demands of modern therapeutic modalities. Two classes of polymers are currently used for the production of dialysis membranes: cellulosic and synthetic as shown in **table 2.1**.

In addition to having different bulk polymers, physical differences also exist between cellulosic and synthetic membranes. Cellulosic membranes must be made relatively thin (wall thicknesses of the dry fibre in the range of 6.5 to

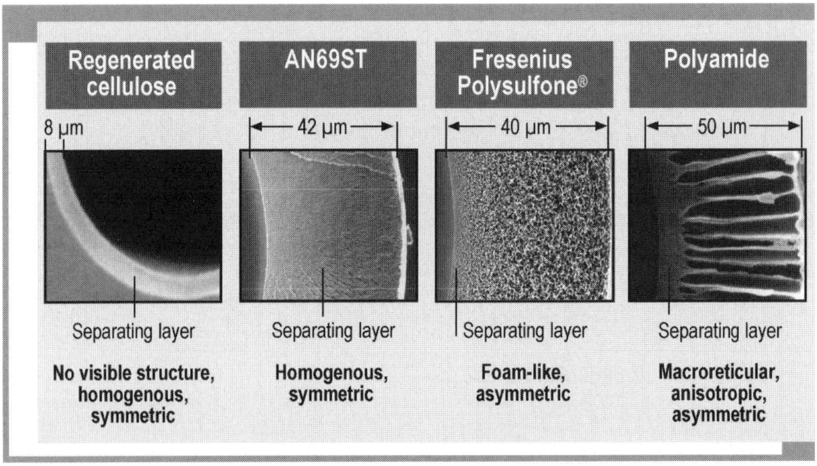

Figure 2.1: Dialysis membrane structures. *Dialysis membranes may be symmetric (e.g. nearly all cellulosic membranes, PMMA, AN69® and AN69ST) or asymmetric (e.g. Fresenius Polysulfone® or polyamide). Asymmetric structures have a thin inner separation layer on the blood side that essentially determines the sieving properties of the membrane, and at least one support layer (stroma), which provides mechanical strength. The size and morphology of this support layer can vary considerably from membrane to membrane. For high-flux membranes such as polyamide, Polyamix™, and Arylane the support layer is characteristically either a finger type or macrovoid structure. Membranes like the Fresenius Polysulfone® have a sponge-like (sometimes also termed "foam-like") structure, gradually increasing in porosity.*

15 μm) in order to achieve high diffusive solute transport and have a uniform (symmetric) structure of the fibre wall (from blood to dialysate side). Such membrane structure cannot generally accommodate the high ultrafiltration rates necessary in convective therapies. Therefore, most cellulosic membranes are not suitable for convective dialysis treatments, such as haemodiafiltration or haemofiltration. The only exception is the membrane made of cellulose triacetate (CTA). In contrast, synthetic membranes have a membrane thickness of 20 μm and more, and a structure which may be symmetric (e.g. AN69®, AN69ST, PMMA) or asymmetric (e.g. Fresenius Polysulfone®, Polyamide) (**figure 2.1**).

How are dialysis membranes produced?

Hollow fibre membranes can be manufactured in wet, dry-wet or dry (melt) spinning processes (**figure 2.2**). The dry-wet spinning process is used for most haemodialysis membranes, e.g. Cuprophan®, PAN and PMMA membranes. Here coagulation of the dissolved polymer is achieved by passing the solution through an air gap followed by immersion into the final coagulation bath. A core liquid (e.g. isopropylmeristate in cellulosic membranes, or dimethylsulfoxide in PMMA membranes, and water in AN69® membranes) is needed to support formation of the membrane dimensions. Chemical residues are removed in a series of post-treatment washing baths. In the production process of cellulosic membranes, glycerol is added as a plasticiser to maintain the structure of the membrane and the membrane is then dried [3]. Alternatively, cellulosic membranes (e.g. Xanthogenat, from Renaselect former Gross-O-Pharm) can be produced in a dry process by melt spinning: here cellulose is melted in sodium hydroxide and carbon sulphide (C_2S), coagulated in air after extrusion through the spinneret, and a co-extruded gas (nitrogen) forms the inner lumen of the fibre.

2.1 Cellulose-based membranes

2.1.1 Regenerated cellulose

For the production of cellulosic membranes, purified cellulose (e.g. from cotton linters) is dissolved in an ammoniac solution of cupric oxide (origin of the brand name Cuprophan®), and the cellulosic polymer chains are newly arranged during the subsequent spinning process - this explain the term "regenerated" cellulose. The result of both the dry-wet and dry spinning process

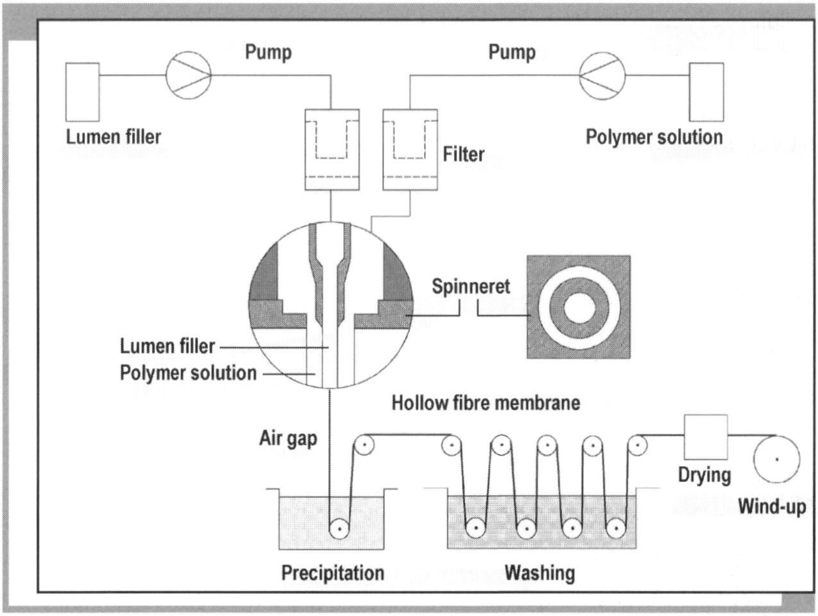

Figure 2.2: Dry-wet spinning process for hollow fibre membranes. *In the dry-wet process, the air gap induces a precoagulation that is terminated in a wet bath. In contrast, coagulation of the polymer occurs in a temperature-controlled air gap in the melt spinning process, and the developing hollow fibre is then only washed in a wet washing bath (not shown). In the wet spinning process, the spinneret touches the precipitation bath (not shown) (from [3] with permission).*

is a macroscopically homogenous membrane that is extremely hydrophilic, absorbs water and forms a hydrogel; diffusion of solutes actually takes place through water-swollen regions rather than pores as observed for synthetic membranes (**figure 2.3**; SEM picture of a Cuprophan® hollow fibre in **figure 2.1**, chemical structure in **figure 2.4**).

The Japanese manufacturers (Asahi, Teijin and Terumo) term their cellulosic membrane cuprammonium rayon, while the German manufacturer (Membrana) sells its product under the brand name Cuprophan®. Teijin produces a regenerated cellulose membrane with fin structures on the outer wall (in order to enhance uniform dialysis fluid flow, see chapter 6), as well as a saponified cellulose ester (SCE) that is, chemically, identical to regenerated cellulose. G-O-P DIAFIL® (Xanthogenat, Plasmaselect Germany) is also a regenerated cellulose membrane but is produced by melt spinning.

Originally, all cellulosic membranes had a low hydraulic permeability [4]. Due to their small membrane wall thickness, membranes made from regenerated cellulose have good diffusive low molecular weight clearance properties. In a well- designed dialyser, these clearances may be comparable, or even superior, to those of some low-flux synthetic membranes. Another advantage of membranes made from regenerated cellulose is that they can be sterilised by all common sterilisation procedures (EtO, γ-irradiation, steam). Disadvantages are their poor biocompatibility profiles and their inability to adsorb small bacterial products [5, 6].

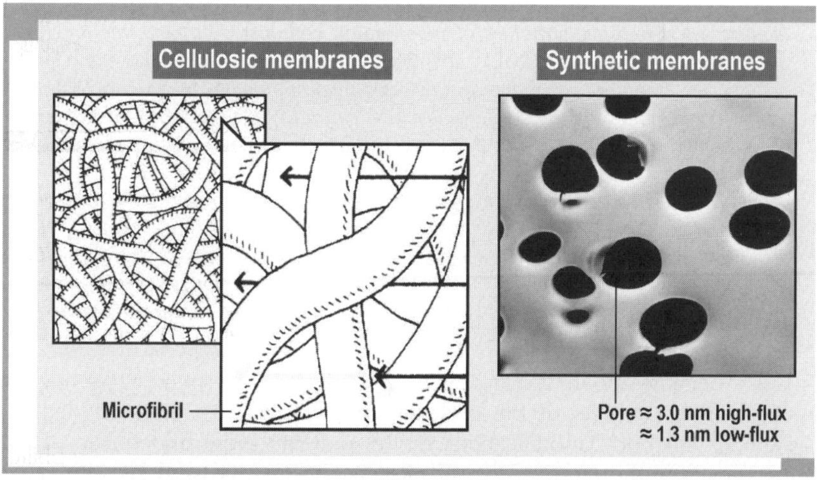

Figure 2.3: Differences in pore structure of cellulosic and synthetic membranes. *In cellulosic membranes, transport of solutes takes place through "spaces" formed by microfibrils. In contrast, synthetic membranes contain distinct pores that are formed during the spinning process. As a consequence, "pore sizes" in cellulosic membranes may vary widely, whereas those of synthetic membranes have a more narrow distribution.*

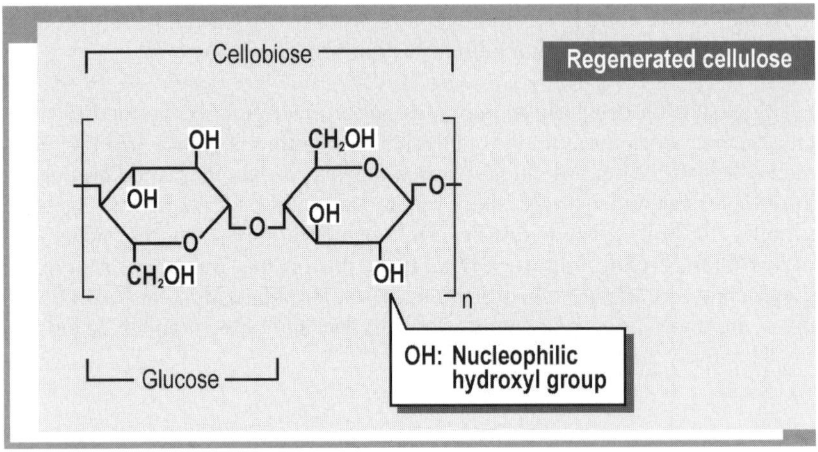

Figure 2.4: Chemical structure of regenerated cellulose. *The basic monomer of regenerated cellulose (RC) is cellobiose, a disaccharide naturally found in plants. RC (Membrana) or the synonymous cuprammonium rayon (Asahi, Terumo, Teijin) or G-O-P DIAFIL® (Renaselect) can also be termed 'unsubstituted cellulose', because they exhibit three free hydroxyl groups per glucose molecule (marked in the above figure) on the membrane surface. These are held responsible for the strong complement and cell activation observed with these kind of membranes.*

2.1.2 Modified regenerated cellulose (Hemophan®, SMC®)

As it became apparent that cellulosic materials, and especially the nucleophilic hydroxyl groups of the polymer, interact with e.g. the complement system of the body, modifications of the polymer were undertaken; these were mostly in the direction of substituting the hydroxyl groups with other less-reactive chemical groups.

Substitution of some hydroxyl groups by N,N,-diethylaminoethyl (DEAE) was the first modification of cellulosic membranes which was introduced specifically to increase its biocompatibility. The membrane is sold under the brand name Hemophan® from Membrana, and is available in dialysers from Baxter, Bellco/Sorin, Braun/Schiwa, Gambro, Haidylena, Cobe, IDEMSA, JMS, Kawasumi, Nephro System/Meditech, Nikkiso and Saxonia. In the bulk polymer, tertiary amino groups replace only 1.5% of all hydroxyl groups through ether bonds (**figure 2.5**) [7]. These positively charged groups constitute hydrophobic regions on a hydrophilic surface and sterically hinder the interac-

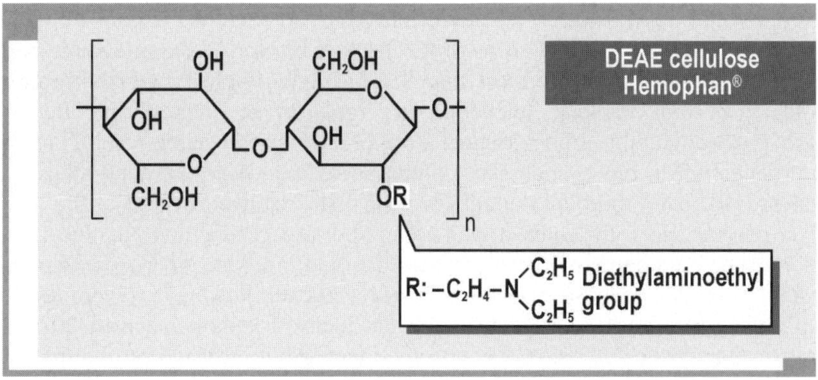

Figure 2.5: Chemical structure of diethylaminoethyl (DEAE) cellulose, Hemophan®. *In Hemophan® (Membrana), 1.5% of the hydrogen atoms of the hydroxyl groups of the glucose monomer are replaced by diethylaminoethyl groups. These are positively charged at physiological pH levels.*

tion of complement factors with the membrane: the result is a marked improvement in the membrane's biocompatibility profile compared to that of unsubstituted, regenerated cellulose membranes with comparable performance characteristics (e.g. [8]). However, the positive DEAE groups are suspected of causing increased heparin consumption during treatment; the reason is that heparin adsorbs from blood onto the DEAE cellulose surface [9,10]. This aspect will be discussed in more detail in chapter 8.

DEAE cellulose exhibits the good hydraulic properties of regenerated cellulose (Cuprophan®) and was once available in both low-flux and high-flux types (an example of the latter is the Hemophan HP membrane from Membrana which was available in two γ-wet Nikkiso housings with UF_{coeff}s of 24 and 32 ml/h•mmHg) [11]. Up until last year, two different membrane formats existed: hollow fibres and flat sheets; the latter were incorporated into Gambro plate dialysers but production of these has now ceased. The DEAE cellulose membrane can be sterilised by all the common sterilisation methods.

What is the chemical modification in SMC®?

SMC® (synthetically modified cellulose) is another example for the creation of hydrophobic domains onto a hydrophilic membrane surface. This membrane is produced by Membrana (Wuppertal, Germany) and is available in different housings from a variety of dialyser manufacturers (e.g. as Polysynthane™, PSN, by Baxter and as SMC® by Bellco/Sorin, B.Braun/Schiwa and Kawasumi). In this polymer, less than 1% of the hydrophilic hydroxyl groups ($-OH^-$) of the cellulosic backbone are replaced by hydrophobic benzyl groups through ether bonds (**figure 2.6**) [12]. This modification resulted in an improvement in biocompatibility compared to unmodified, regenerated cellulose. However, the biocompatibility profile still fell short of that of the low-flux polysulfone with which it was compared in a clinical investigation [13]. Surprisingly, the intra-treatment kinetics of some biocompatibility parameters (such as elastase release, complement activation and leukopenia) were found to differ from those usually observed: the nadir of leukopenia is at 30 min rather than around 15 min (as is observed with other modified or unmodified cellulosic membranes), and maximum complement activation and elastase release are also observed after 30 minutes [14]; this aspect ought to be taken into consideration when planning clinical studies.

This membrane type features all the favourable properties of cellulosic membranes (i.e. sterilisable with all current methods, good mechanical strength, good small solute clearances); it is only available in a low-flux version [15].

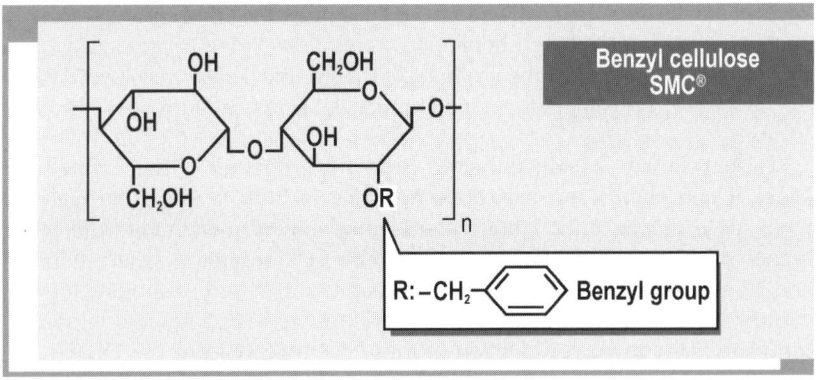

Figure 2.6: Chemical structure of benzyl cellulose – SMC® (Membrana) and Polysynthane™ (in Baxter dialysers). *In SMC® and Polysynthane™ (PSN), less than 1% of the hydrogen atoms of the hydroxyl groups of the glucose monomer are replaced by benzyl groups.*

2.1.3 Regenerated cellulose grafts (AM-BIO, Excebrane)

An improvement of cellulosic membrane biocompatibility was also achieved by grafting the cellulosic backbone of cuprammonium rayon with a polyethyleneglycol (PEG) layer (AM-BIO membrane, Asahi). Alkylether carboxylic acid (PEG acid) is esterified with its terminal carboxyl group to the

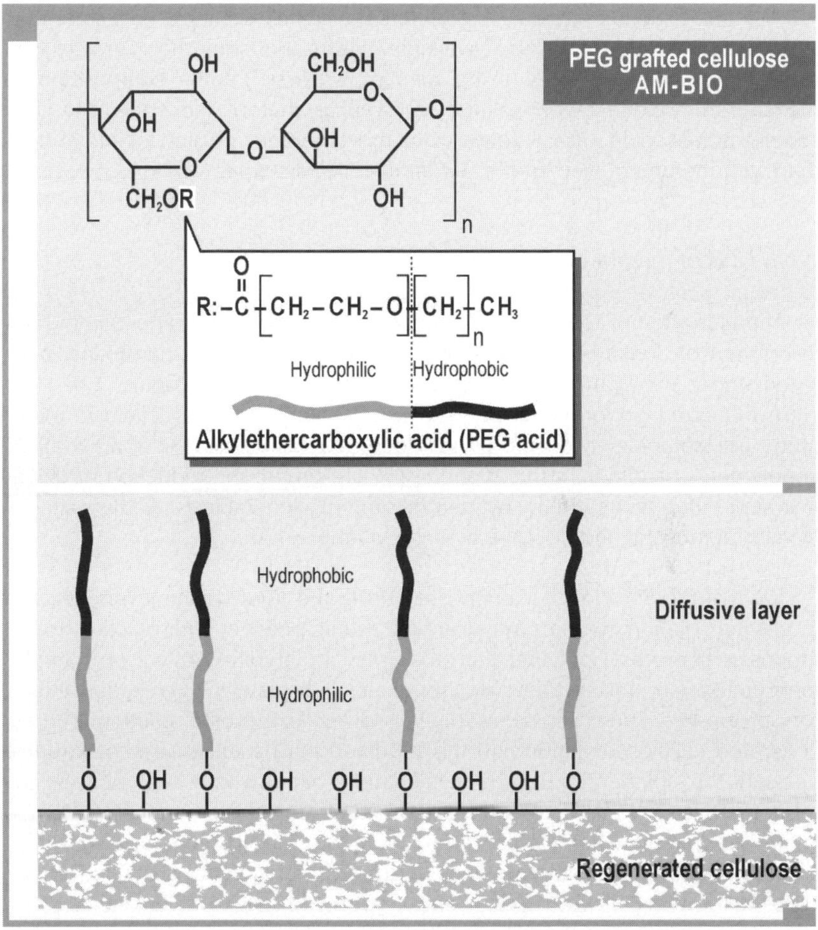

Figure 2.7: Chemical structure of PEG-grafted cellulose – AM-BIO (Asahi). *The backbone of regenerated cellulose is grafted with a polyethleneglycol (PEG) layer.*

hydroxyl group of the cellulose polymer (**figure 2.7**) [16]. These PEG chains form a so-called hydrogel layer on the cellulosic surface (thickness 2.4 nm); this may act as a buffer zone between the cellulosic backbone and blood, hindering the direct contact of plasma proteins with the membrane surface and leading to a reduction in platelet adhesion and complement activation [17].

The membrane is available with different pore size distributions, i.e. as low-flux and high-flux versions. In addition, a high-flux version with a smoother surface (AM-BIO HX) is also available. Here the smoother surface was achieved by altering stages of the spinning process, i.e. the composition of the cuprammonium rayon solution as well as that of the coagulant [18]. Platelet adhesion *in vitro* is lower with this smoother version of membrane than with the unmodified and PEG-grafted cellulosic types [18].

What kind of membrane is Excebrane?

The first attempt to create a "bioreactive" dialysis membrane was the development of a vitamin E (d-α-tocopherol)-coated cellulosic membrane, marketed under the brand name Excebrane (Terumo, Japan) (**figure 2.8**) [19]. Here the good performance properties of a highly porous cellulosic membrane are combined with the good biocompatibility features of a synthetic copolymer. In addition, a therapeutic goal is claimed: the reduction of oxidative stress during treatment by neutralising oxygen radicals at their site of development using the radical scavenger vitamin E [20].

Surface modification is carried out during the fibre spinning process: the modifying solution contains a hydrophilic acrylic polymer with reactive epoxy groups, a fluororesin polymer that possesses an inhibitory effect on complement activation, and an oleyl alcohol chain with platelet aggregation inhibitory properties. These substances are dissolved in the core solution. The regenerated cellulose solution and this modified core solution are co-extruded through the spinneret into the coagulation bath, where two phases are formed. The outer circumference of the hollow fibre is composed of the cellulosic membrane, while the primarily hydrophilic inside surface is covered by a hydrophobic layer of the modifier (**figure 2.8**). This coating is achieved by covalent bonding of the reactive epoxy group of the modifier with the hydroxyl groups of the cellulosic membrane. Around 150 mg/m^2 of vitamin E is immobilised to oleyl alcohol via hydrophobic bonding [21].

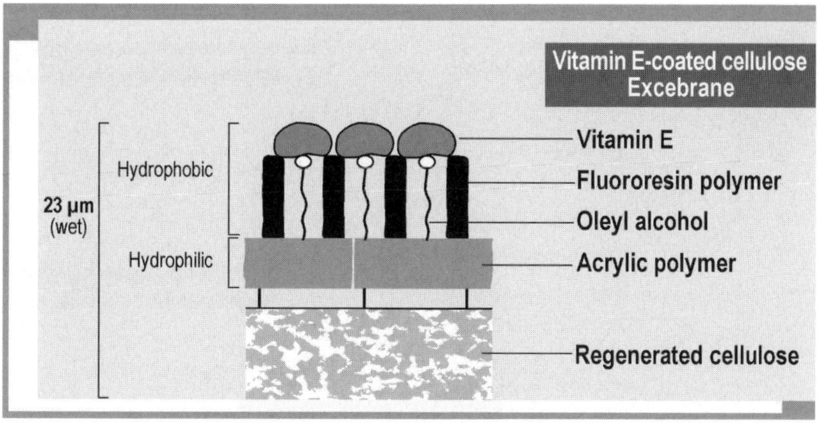

Figure 2.8: Chemical structure of the vitamin E-coated membrane – Excebrane (Terumo). *A hydrophilic acrylic polymer is brought onto the backbone of regenerated cellulose. The inner surface consists of a hydrophobic fluororesin polymer to which vitamin E is immobilised via an oleyl alcohol chain.*

The results of some clinical investigations involving this kind of membrane are already available: these show an improved biocompatibility compared to regenerated cellulose. However, the advantages and exact therapeutic effect of this kind of vitamin E supplementation need to be investigated further (discussed in more detail in chapter 10).

This membrane is available as a high-performance membrane with *in vitro* UF_{coeff}s ranging from 9.9 up to 14.5 ml/h • mmHg, depending on the size of dialyser. In the manufacturer's brochures, an *in vitro* sieving coefficient of 0.4 is cited for cytochrome C (a surrogate for ß2-m), measured with a filtrate flow of 10 ml/min. The mean pore size is 3.7 nm (according to manufacturer data).

2.1.4 Cellulose acetate

In cellulose acetate (CA) membranes, at least two (substitution grade 2) of the three hydroxyl groups of the cellulosic glucose monomer are replaced by acetyl groups (**figure 2.9**). In the presence of sulphuric acid, cellulose is treated with pure acetic acid and acetic anhydride to form a cellulose acetate ester. This ester bond is responsible for the thermolability and chemolability of the CA polymer: CA cannot be sterilised by steam and acetylation occurs

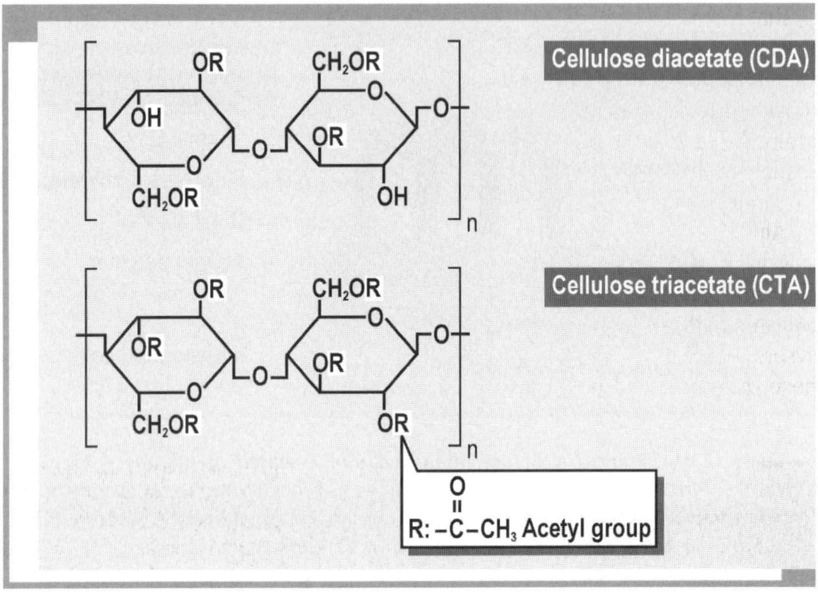

Figure 2.9: Chemical structure of cellulose diacetate (CDA) and cellulose triacetate (CTA). *In CDA, 2 to 2.4 hydrogen atoms of the 3 hydroxyl groups of the glucose monomer are replaced by acetyl groups (Toyobo, Teijin); all 3 are replaced in CTA (Toyobo).*

at strong basic pH-values, whereas hydrolysation of the polymer starts at acidic pH-values. Polymer degradation has been reported under special conditions: for example, failure to adhere to recommended storage times resulted in fragmentation of the polymer into acetylated carbohydrate derivatives which caused adverse reactions in patients within 24 hours after treatment (anaphylactic reactions, scleritis, iritis, tinnitus, conjunctivitis, red eye syndrome, visual loss and hearing loss; see chapter 10 for more details) [22]. Substitution of some hydroxyl groups with acetate makes the hydrophilic cellulosic backbone more hydrophobic, and allows some protein adsorption by the inner surface.

Several types of CA membranes are currently available commercially; these differ in their degree of hydroxyl substitution (i.e. their substitution grade), their hydraulic permeability and their manufacturing process (melt spun or dry-wet) (**table 2.2**). Measures to increase performance, such as the so-called fins on the outer surface of the fibres from Teijin, are other distinguishable parameters. All these differences may lead to some small advantage of one CA membrane over another (e.g. [23]). Altogether, most CA membranes exhibit the good performance characteristics of their unmodified cellulosic counterparts, but are more biocompatible. Nevertheless, they do not attain the excellent biocompatibility profile of some synthetic membranes (explained in chapter 8 in more detail).

Althin Medical AB (now Baxter) took over the Cordis Dow melt-spun process from 1963 and produced a symmetric *cellulose diacetate* membrane (substitution grade 2) under the brand name Althane®. The membrane was available in both high-flux and low-flux versions and was incorporated in dialysers with UF_{coeff}s ranging from 6.2 up to 40 ml/h•mmHg [24]. Recently, these dialysers were held responsible for a number of deaths among dialysis

Brand name	Substitution grade	Both low-flux and high-flux versions available?	Membrane manufacturer[1]/Dialyser manufacturer[2] /Distributer[3]
Cellulose diacetate	2.4	Low-flux	Toyobo[1] / Nipro / Nissho[2,3]
Dicea (Cellulose diacetate)	2.0	Low-flux	Toyobo[1] / Nipro / Nissho[2] Baxter[3]
Tricea (Cellulose triacetate)	3.0	Yes	Toyobo[1] / Nipro / Nissho[2] Baxter[3]
Cellulose acetate	2.4	Low-flux	Helbio
Cellulose diacetate	2.0	Yes	Helbio
Cellulose triacetate	3.0	High-performance/ high-flux	Helbio
Cellulose diacetate (Fibres with fin structure)	2.4	Low-flux / high-performance	Teijin[1] / Hospal[2,3] / Cobe[3]

***Table 2.2:* Different cellulose acetate membranes currently on the market.**

patients in Spain, Croatia, USA, Italy, Germany, Taiwan, and Colombia. Intensive investigations revealed that a processing fluid, perfluorohydrocarbon, was the reason for these fatal reactions [25-27]. The production of these dialysers and membranes was ceased as a result.

A melt spun *cellulose diacetate* is available from Teijin, now Gambro, (here with a substitution factor 2.4) and is incorporated into the Hospal Acepal dialysers. A clinical comparison of this membrane with a CA membrane with substitution factor of 2 (i.e. the Dicea membrane from Toyobo) did not reveal any statistically relevant differences with regard to complement activation [23]. Both low-flux membranes were able to remove small amounts of ß2-microglobulin (ß2-m sieving coefficients of around 0.02) [23], values which are too low to be of therapeutic relevance.

Cellulose triacetate (CTA) (substitution grade 3) membranes have a thin uniform skin structure and were first used exclusively for high-flux dialysis or haemodiafiltration (e.g. the Toyobo membrane in Nipro/Nissho housings). These were the first and only cellulosic membranes suitable for convective therapies. Today, low-flux versions of this membrane are also available (e.g. the Toyobo membrane in Nipro/Nissho housings, which is distributed in Europe and USA by Baxter). The highly permeable CTA version is also suitable for continuous renal replacement therapy [28].

2.2 Synthetic membranes

With the exception of ethylenevinylalcohol copolymer (EVAL®), all synthetic polymers currently on the market are hydrophobic in nature and have to be made more hydrophilic during their production by using additives or copolymers. The structural differences compared to cellulosic membranes have already been explained in **figure 2.1**. These structural differences and the membrane crystallinity are the result of phase separation during production, where phase inversion and immersion follows extrusion of the polymer mixture through a spinneret. Partial evaporation of the solvent is responsible for skin formation.

The main purpose of developing synthetic membranes was to create more porous membranes which could better simulate the filtration process of the natural kidney, thereby removing middle molecules and higher molecular weight uraemic toxins, such as ß2-m. The molecule radius (Stokes radius) of ß2-m is variously described as being 1.6 nm [23], 2.2 nm [29] or as being not round but rather elliptic (4.5 x 2.5 x 2.0 nm in size) [30]. Modern high-flux membrane development aims at providing pores that allow the passage of ß2-m while restricting the passage of albumin.

2.2.1 Polyacrylonitrile (PAN, AN69®, AN69 ST)

Rhône Poulenc was the first to manufacture a highly permeable, symmetric, synthetic membrane - a co-polymer of the hydrophobic polyacrylonitrile and the hydrophilic sodium metallylsulfonate (**figure 2.10**). A high density of medium-sized pores is distributed throughout the homogenous polymer, and glycerol is used as pore filler. This membrane, produced and marketed by Hospal under the brand name AN69®, has been a success since its introduction. Today, severe clinical limitations of the membrane are apparent (discussed below), and these have led to the development of the altered type AN69ST.

Asahi is the other producer of polyacrylonitrile (PAN) membranes. Their PAN membrane consists of hydrophobic acrylonitrile and methylacrylate monomers, and is rendered hydrophilic by the addition of acrylic acid (**figure 2.10**). Due to the special production process, the membrane is asymmetric in

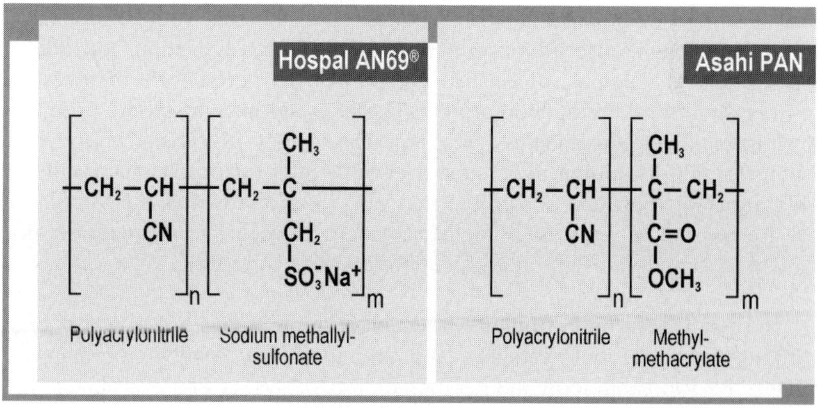

Figure 2.10: Chemical structure of polyacrylonitrile (PAN) – AN69® (Hospal) and Asahi PAN. *Polyacrylonitrile is made hydrophilic by co-polymerisation with sodium (Na)- methallylsulfonate in the case of AN69®, and with methyl-methacrylate and addition of acrylic acid in the case of Asahi PAN.*

structure and possesses a skin layer with a wide range of pore sizes. These determine the sieving properties of the membrane.

Up to the early nineteen-nineties, AN69® was believed to be one of the most biocompatible dialysis membranes available, despite it having the drawback that it, like all PAN membranes, is not sterilisable by heat. However, reports of anaphylactoid reactions with AN69® in combination with the consumption of ACE inhibitors have appeared since 1990 [31-35]. Bradykinin generation, resulting from contact phase activation of the kallikrein-kinin system by the negatively charged surface of the AN69 membrane, was identified as the underlying mechanism (explained in chapters 7 and 10 in more detail) [36]. Some of the effects of bradykinin are mediated by nitric oxide [37, 38]. Other factors, which influence the extent of reaction, are surface electronegativity (zeta potential) of the membrane, the pH of the rinsing solution, and the plasma dilution factor [35, 39]. It was then not surprising that the polyacrylonitrile membrane PAN DX from Asahi also led to bradykinin generation, but to a lower extent because of its lower zeta potential (-60 mV in comparison to –70 mV of AN69®) [36, 39].

AN69® exhibits a high adsorption capacity for proteins (especially positively charged) due to its microstructure and its surface electronegativity (electric negative charges of the sulfonate groups) [40, 41]. This has been shown specifically for complement factor D [42], ß2-m [41, 43] and low molecular weight proteins [40]. This is advantageous regarding complement activation and ß2-m elimination, but undesired in the case of high molecular weight kininogen adsorption, as it results in contact activation and higher residual blood volumes, at least in comparison to polysulfone membranes [44]. Furthermore, therapeutic proteins like EPO are also adsorbed, probably diminishing their effectiveness [45, 46]. This is not of clinical importance whenever EPO is administered subcutaneously after haemodialysis treatment [47]. Substantial protein adsorption may also be a disadvantage if the dialysers are reused, as aggressive chemicals, such as hypochlorite, must be employed to remove these proteins and fibre damage can result.

The Asahi and the Hospal polyacrylonitrile membranes are available only with highhydraulic permeabilities and are, therefore, suitable for high-flux dialysis, haemodiafiltration and haemofiltration. AN69® is also available as flat sheets in plate dialysers for acute haemofiltration.

In order to overcome problems with anaphylactic reactions, Hospal developed a new AN69® type by coating the polyacrylonitrile flat sheet membrane with poly(ethyleneimine) (PEI), a polycationic polymer (**figure 2.11**). PEI is sprayed onto the flat sheet membrane surface during the manufacturing process until a targeted concentration of 9 mg/m^2 is reached [49]. The zeta potential of the resultant AN69ST (ST stands for surface treated) is reduced to around −29 mV (48) or −15 ± 5 mV [50], depending on the source of information. In hollow fibre-membranes, the polycationic polymer is introduced by using a washing method [50]. Negatively charged sulfone groups of the AN69® polymer are masked by the polycationic polymer; the thickness of this layer also constitutes an additional steric barrier (**figure 2.11**) [48]. No hypersensitivity reactions were observed with such modified plate dialysers (Crystal ST) in the first clinical study, which also included patients on ACE-inhibitor therapy [49]. However, certain adverse reactions were also recently reported with the clinical use of AN69ST dialysers: according to the authors, these side effects resulted from insufficient treatment of the PEI modification [51].

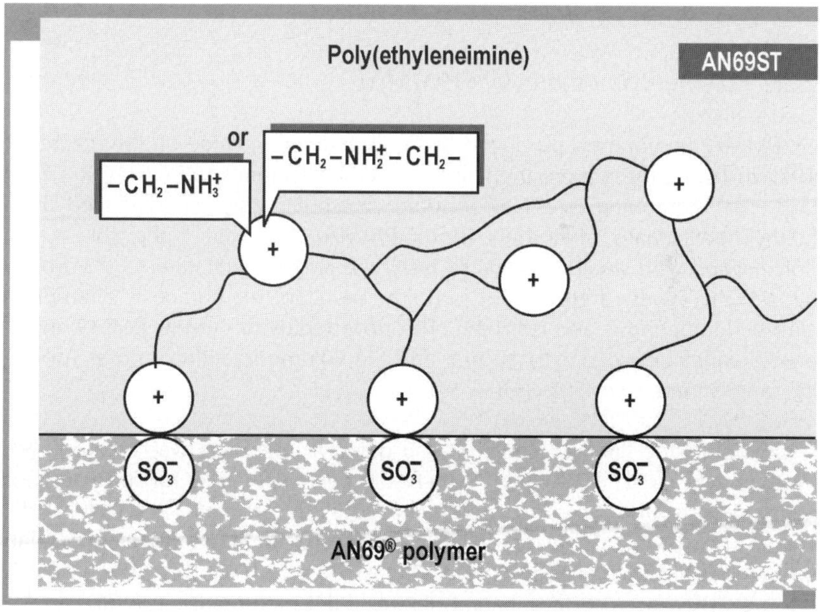

Figure 2.11: Surface coating of PAN (AN69®) to produce AN69ST (Hospal). *The cationic polymer polyethyleneimine is adsorbed onto the membrane through strong ionic interactions with the sulfonate groups of the AN69 polymer in order to reduce the negative surface charge (adapted from [48]).*

Coating of the membrane with a positively charged polymer had an additional effect: negatively charged heparin was bound to the membrane. First clinical trials show that no further systemic heparinisation was needed during treatment if heparin was bound onto the membrane during the priming procedure [52, 53]. A low heparin desorption from the membrane during dialysis treatment was detected in *vitro* and *in vivo* [54]. In human citrated plasma, 15% of unfractionated heparin and 50 - 100% of low molecular heparin desorbed from the membrane [50]. However, a 50% reduction of the reference heparin dose was reported for unfractionated as well as for low molecular weight heparin if the AN69ST dialysers were coated with this types of heparin during the priming procedure [53]. These reports must be confirmed in routine clinical practice.

The effect of introducing positive surface charges on the membrane biocompatibility compared to the "standard" AN69® type is of particular interest. A change in membrane biocompatibility will certainly result, as alterations in surface electronegativity have a marked impact on protein adsorption.

2.2.2 Polymethylmethacrylate (PMMA)

PMMA membranes, produced by Toray Industries, came on the market in 1977 in Japan; these were the first synthetic membranes to be γ-ray sterilised [55]. The membrane is a hydrophobic, non-polar polymer produced from methylmethacrylate monomers (homo-PMMA). In some types, this is co-polymerised with small amounts of p-styrene sodium sulfonate (co-PMMA in B2, B3, BG Types) (**figure 2.12**) [55]. The resultant membrane is symmetric, almost homogenous and isotropic. The pore radius of current PMMA membranes varies between 2 to 10 nm, and the volume fraction of pores (porosity) ranges from 50 to 70% [55].

A membrane family consisting of 9 different members was created with low-flux types (B2, B3 series), high-flux types (B1 series, mostly used for haemodialysis) and a version with increased ß2-m removal (BK series U/P/F). The last was produced by increasing the pore size so that adsorption of ß2-m throughout the entire membrane wall was possible [56]. This BK-F model is the highest ß2-m adsorbing haemodialysis (HD) membrane currently on the market; convective ß2-m removal is negligible [41, 43, 57]. The larger pores (10 nm) allow also the removal of larger uraemic toxins, as well as useful proteins (Stokes radius of albumin 3.6 nm). An erythropoiesis-inhibiting fraction, KR4-0, and its subfraction, YS-1 (MW 40,000), have been isolated from the dialysate after a PMMA BK-F haemodialysis treatment [58]. Whether this is a unique property of the BK-F membrane or is also a feature of other highly permeable membranes remains to be further seen. A multicentre, randomised, controlled trial with 84 patients for 12 weeks found no difference between this highly porous membrane and low-flux cellulose membranes regarding their effects on anaemia [59]. However, considerable amounts of albumin are also lost even during haemodialysis with this highly porous membrane (albumin loss is higher in highly convective treatment modes, i.e. haemofiltration or haemodiafiltration): an albumin loss of 5.9 g/session was reported for the Filtryzer BK-P dialyser, and the loss was even as high as 7.4 g/session with the BK-F type [60].

The strong adsorbing property of PMMA may not always be of advantage: it may result in an undesired adsorption of platelets, with all the subsequent effects on fibrin formation [61]. A higher residual blood volume was reported for PMMA membranes [59]. Furthermore, one case of anaphylactoid reactions was reported under ACE inhibitor therapy, probably due to the negative surface charge [63].

All PMMA dialysers are sterilised by γ-irradiation. The material is not steam or EtO sterilisable.

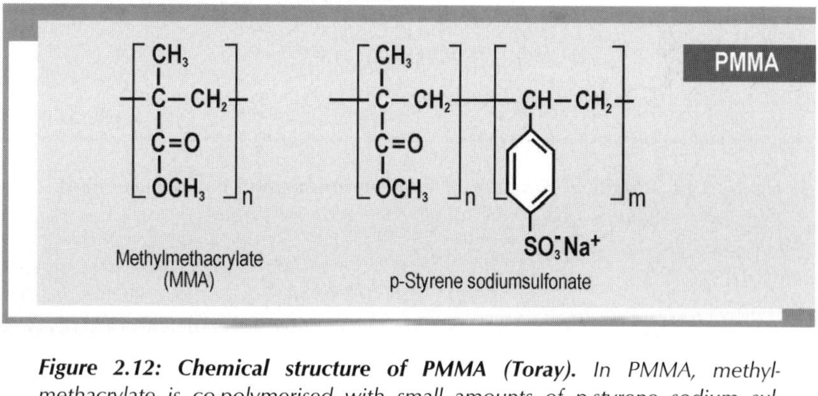

Figure 2.12: Chemical structure of PMMA (Toray). *In PMMA, methylmethacrylate is co-polymerised with small amounts of p-styrene sodium sulfonate (adapted from [55]).*

2.2.3 *Ethylenevinylalcohol copolymer (EVAL®)*

Membranes made from ethylenevinylalcohol copolymer (EVAL® from Kawasumi Laboratories, Kuraray Co, LTD) are naturally hydrophilic due to their hydroxyl groups (**figure 2.13**), but exhibit a much better biocompatibility than membranes made from regenerated cellulose [64]. One reason for this may be that the surface oxygen content, which is believed by some to be responsible for lower protein adsorption and lower activation of humoral systems, is lower (25.5%) than in regenerated cellulose (37.4%) [64].

The symmetric membrane EVAL® is available in three different types (D, C, m-type), differing in pore size. Most are low-flux membranes but some high performance varieties are available with UF_{coeff}s up to 15.3 ml/min•mmHg at surface areas of 1.8 m^2. Although some ß2-m removal was reported, no considerable change in plasma ß2-m concentration was observed with EVAL® dialysers in a clinical study [11].

EVAL® dialysers are sterilised by EtO or by γ irradiation.

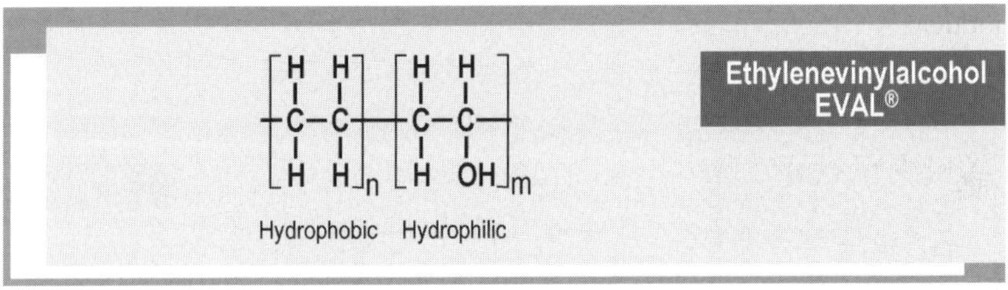

Figure 2.13: Chemical structure of ethylenevinylalcohol copolymer– EVAL®.
EVAL® (Kawasumi) is a copolymer of ethylene and vinylalcohol.

2.2.4 Polycarbonate polyether (Gambrane®)

The polycarbonate polyether membrane was marketed under the brand name Gambrane® by Gambro and was a copolymer of polycarbonate and polyethylene glycol (**figure 2.14**). Its production was recently ceased but it is mentioned here because several publications about these dialysers exist. The symmetric membrane was available only in flat sheet form in plate dialysers sterilised by EtO (Lundia Pro 100 - Pro 800). Although the membrane was a low-flux type (having ultrafiltration coefficients generally below 10 ml/mmHg), it was capable of removing small amounts of ß2-m [65]. A reduction in blood levels of ß2-m of 24% was reported after Gambrane® dialysis, corresponding to a total amount of 169 mg removed per session [66]. The mechanism of ß2-m removal was explained by the microdomain structure of the material: the hydrophobic polycarbonate adsorbed ß2-m, whereas ß2-m diffusion took place through hydrophilic polyether regions [66]. Some authors speculate that some large pores may be present through which ß2-m removal took place [66, 67].

Regarding biocompatibility, polycarbonate polyether holded an intermediate position: it was more biocompatible than regenerated cellulosic with respect to complement activation and leukopenia, but was more leukopenia-inducing than low-flux polysulfone membranes [66].

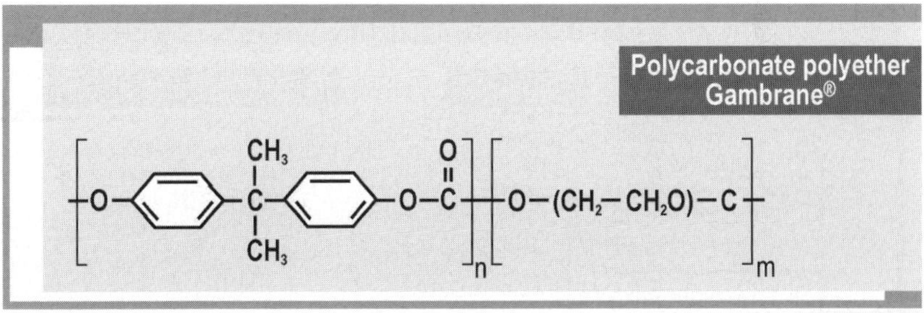

Figure 2.14: Chemical structure of polycarbonate polyether – Gambrane® (Gambro). *Gambrane is a co-polymer of polycarbonate and polyethyleneglycol.*

2.2.5 Polyamide

Polyamide membranes (in Polyflux dialysers, Hemoflux haemofilters and FH haemofilters from Gambro) consist of a hydrophobic, aromatic-aliphatic co-polyamide that is blended with hydrophilic polyvinylpyrrolidone (PVP) (**figure 2.15**) [68]. The membrane is asymmetric with 3 distinguishable regions: a thin skin of 0.1-0.5 µm on the blood side, followed by a sponge structure of 5 µm, which is supported by a finger structure of about 45 µm. Pore size increases dramatically from the blood side to the dialysate side, being smallest at the skin layer with around 5 nm [68].

First polyamide membranes were manufactured as flat sheets but today only hollow-fibre, high-flux membranes are available. Polyamide dialysers and filters exhibit good ß2-m removal with a S.C. of 0.6 [69]; this is due to their diffusive and convective performance characteristics, and not the result of adsorption as the membrane absorbs very little protein [70]. However, bacterial products are successfully rejected at the dialysate side [71].

The available polyamide dialysers and filters are all EtO sterilised only. In order to overcome this disadvantage, a polyarylethersulfone membrane with minute amount of polyamide was developed, that is sterilisable also by heat. The new membrane, firstly named Polyamide S™, now Polyamix™ , is, due to the significant portion of polyarylethersulfone, described in the previous section on polyarylethersulfone membranes.

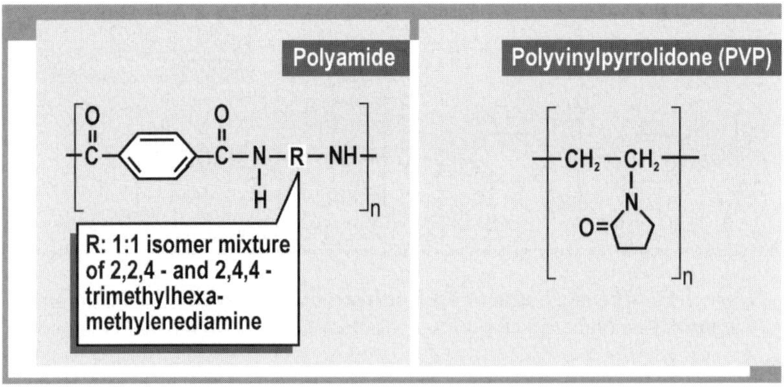

Figure 2.15: Chemical structure of polyamide (Gambro) and polyvinylpyrrolidone (PVP). *Polyamide is blended with PVP in order to make the polymer more hydrophilic (adapted from [68]).*

2.2.6 Polysulfones (Fresenius Polysulfone®, Helixone®, α polysulfone, Asahi polysulfone®, Toraysulfone®)

World-wide, there are more than 15 suppliers of polysulfone and poly(aryl)ethersulfone dialysers, underlining the great success and versatility of these membrane polymers (**table 2.3**). Polysulfone and poly(aryl)ethersulfone membranes meet most of the demands made on a modern membrane: they can be sterilised with all common methods (γ irradiation, β irradiation, EtO, steam), are biocompatible, and are of high physical strength and chemical resistance. Both the low-flux and the high-flux versions exhibit good performance characteristics, and the high-flux type removes considerable amounts of ß2-m by filtration. Moreover, polysulfones but not polyarylethersulfones are suitable for use as endotoxin adsorbers (eg. [72]). The great similarity between the polymers means that the terms polysulfone and polyethersulfone or polyarylethersulfone are often used synonymously, although this is not strictly correct.

In chemistry, the terminus polysulfone (PSu) comprises simply a group of polymers containing sulfone groups and alkyl or aryl (e.g. arylether) groups (see **figure 2.16** for the chemical structure). However, according to chemical convention, only all such polymers, which additionally contain isopropylidene groups, are termed polysulfones (Fresenius Polysulfone®, Helixone®, Asahi Polysulfone®, Toraysulfone®, α Polysulfone). Those dialysis membrane polysulfones which do not contain isopropylidene groups are termed polyarylethersulfones or, in short, polyethersulfones (DIAPES®, Arylane, Polyamix™ the former Polyamide S™) (**figure 2.16**). This is somewhat confusing because, as mentioned above, all dialysis membrane polysulfones include an arylether. **Table 2.3** provides an overview of the main manufacturers of polysulfones and poly(aryl)ethersulfones and some special features of the particular polymers.

Fresenius introduced the first high-flux polysulfone in 1983 [73], followed by the low-flux version in 1987 [74]. The latest improvement, Helixone®, was introduced into the market in 2000 [75, 76]. Due to patent protection, all polysulfones developed up to now had to differ from the original Fresenius Polysulfone®. Consequently, they differ in their basic co-polymer/polymer alloy, in the possible addition of polyvinylpyrrolidone (PVP) (polysulfone alone is hydrophobic and has to be made more hydrophilic, usually by blending the polymer with the hydrophilic PVP), and in their entire production processes that yield different membrane morphologies. Pore sizes are also different. Only the Fresenius (Fresenius Polysulfone®) and B. Braun (α Polysulfone) polysulfone membranes are currently available as low-flux types.

Manufacturer (Distributer)	Brand name (Polymer)	Sterilisation (Flux)	SEM picture
Fresenius Medical Care	Fresenius Polysulfone® (Polysulfone) Helixone® (Polysulfone)	Inline steam, EtO (High-flux Low-flux) In-line steam (High-flux Low-flux)	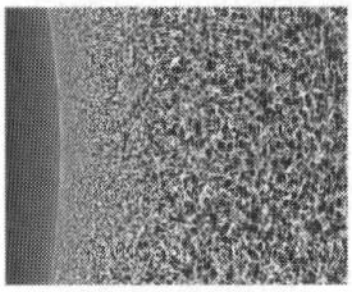
Asahi Medical (e.g. Diamed)	APS® (Polysulfone)	γ-wet (High-flux)	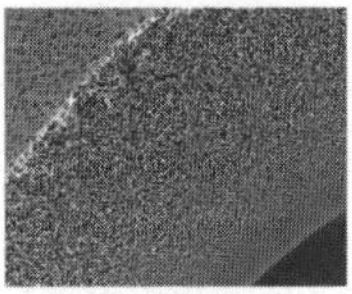
Toray Industries	Toraysulfone® (Polysulfone)	γ-wet (High-flux)	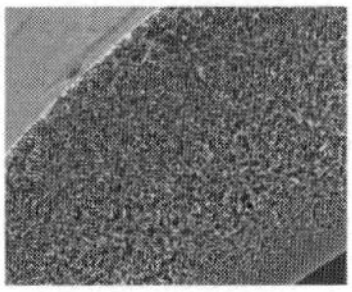
Saxonia (B. Braun)	α Polysulfone	γ-dry (High-flux)	
Membrana (Allmed, Baxter, Bellco, Helbio, Haidylena, Idemsa, Kawasumi Saxonia)	DIAPES® (Polyethersulfone)	ß-dry, γ-dry, heat, EtO (High-flux Low-flux)	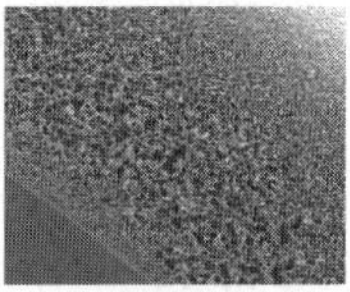
Hospal/Cobe	Arylane (Polyethersulfone)	γ-dry (High-flux)	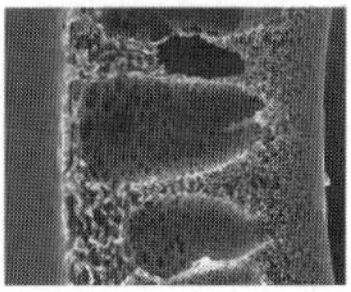
Kimal	Polyethersulfone	γ-dry (High-flux)	
Minntech	Minntech PS Polyphen® (Polyethers.)	EtO (High-flux) EtO (High-flux)	
Gambro	Polyamix™ * (Polyethersulfone)	Heat (High-flux Low-flux)	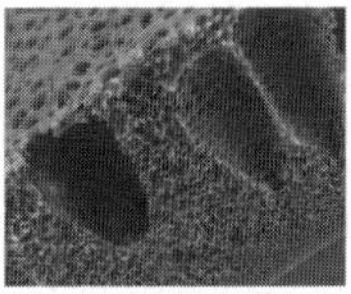
Nikkiso	PEPA® (Polyethersulfone)	γ-wet (High-flux)	

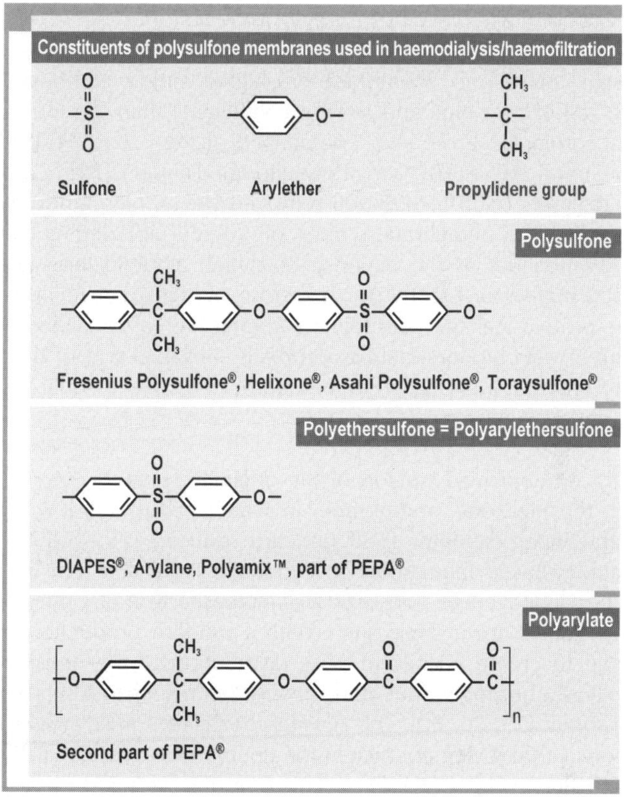

Figure 2.16: Chemical structure of different polysulfones. *Most of the various polysulfones currently available on the market differ only slightly in their basic polymer. According to the manufacturer's brochures, small amounts of polyamide are present in Polyamix™. With the exception of PEPA® which contains polyarylether all polysulfone or poly(aryl)ethersulfone membranes are blended with polyvinylpyrrolidone (chemical structure in* ***figure 2.15****).*

Table 2.3: *Membranes* ***of the polysulfone/poly(aryl)ethersulfone family currently on the market and their characteristics.*** **According to the manufacturer, Polyamide S™ is a co-polymer of polyarylethersulfone and only a small amount of polyamide; therefore, it is mentioned here under polysulfones [89]. With the exception of PEPA -a copolymer of polyethersulfone and arylate- all membranes contain polyvinylpyrrolidone (PVP) (data from [89]).*

How does polysulfone differ from polyarylethersulfone?

The Asahi Polysulfone® membrane has higher middle and large molecule clearances, reduction ratios and sieving coefficients than the Fresenius Polysulfone®, according to an *in vivo* comparison of the 1.3 m^2 F60S (Fresenius Polysulfone®) and APS-650 (Asahi Polysulfone) dialysers [77]. Compared to Helixone® dialysers (FX60), APS650S removed similar high amounts of ß2-m (more than 70% at ultrafiltration rates of 90 ml/min) during post-dilution haemodiafiltration but at the expense of a high albumin loss (about 3800 mg/4h; 2000 mg/4h for FX60) [78]. Therefore, in highly convective treatment modes, the protein leakage with this membrane has to be taken into consideration. The *in vitro* biocompatibility profile is similar to that of the Fresenius Polysulfone® membrane [79]. The membrane is available only as high-flux type in γ-sterilised housings.

Recently, an improved version of the original Fresenius Polysulfone® was developed, the Helixone® membrane, in which hollow fibre wall thickness (35 µm) and inner diameter (185 µm) are reduced [75, 76]. By applying nanotechnology-based fabrication procedures for the first time in haemodialysis, the nominal average pore size was increased from 3.1 nm in Fresenius Polysulfone® to 3.3 nm in Helixone®. With a modern production process, it was possible to create a uniform pore distribution at the dense innermost layer as well as a homogeneous pore size, which results in a sharper molecular weight cut-off [75, 76, 80]. The sieving coefficient for ß2-m was extended to 0.8, whereas the sieving coefficient for albumin was preserved in the range between 0.001 and 0.01 [81]. First clinical studies revealed the same excellent biocompatibility profile as Fresenius Polysulfone® [82, 83].

Toraysulfone® is a membrane which is available only as high-flux type in γ-sterilised dialysers. In a recent clinical study comparing Arylane, PEPA®, Fresenius Polysulfone®, Helixone®, DIAPES®, CTA, Asahi Polysulfone® and Polyamix™ dialysers, it was the membrane with the highest ß2-m removal rate (about 75% at an ultrafiltration rate of 90 ml/min in post-dilution haemodiafiltration) but also with the highest protein leakage (about 7000 mg/4h) [78].

The latest polysulfone on the market, α Polysulfone, is manufactured by Saxonia and sold in the γ-irradiated dialyser Diacap® by B.Braun [84, 85]. The membrane consists of a polysulfone-PVP-blend and is available in low-flux and high-flux versions.

2.2.7 Poly(aryl)ethersulfones (PEPA®, Arylane, DIAPES®, Polyamix™)

PEPA® (polyester-polymer alloy) produced by the Japanese company Nikkiso is a blend of polyethersulfone and polyarylate and is the only polyarylethersulfone membrane which does not contain PVP. Consequently, it exhibits some special characteristics: for example, it adsorbs ß2-m although this is uncommon for all other poly(aryl)ethersulfone or polysulfone membranes. However, despite this adsorption, removal rates for ß2-m are lower with this membrane than with the other polysulfone membranes [78, 86, 87]. The membrane is available as y-wet sterilised in the FLX-GWS and the recently developed FLY-GWS filter series.

Arylane® (polyarylethersulfone/PVP), which is available in the y-dry sterilised H and M filter series from Hospal/Cobe, removed less ß2-m than DIAPES®, Asahi Polysulfone®, Helixone® and Toraysulfone, but more than PEPA®, CTA or Polyamix™ in a recent investigation comparing dialysers with similar surface areas [78]. With regard to albumin loss, the membrane holds the same intermediate position as it does for ß2-m removal [78]. An older investigation reported a similar neutropenia and complement-activating potential for Arylane® and for Fresenius Polysulfone® and an equal ß2-m removal and protein loss (Hospal H4 vs. F60S) [88].

Polyamide S™, now Polyamix™, is a blend of poly(aryl)ethersulfone, PVP and low amounts of polyamide [89]. It has a moderate ß2-m removal ability and a very low protein loss [78]. Low- and high-flux versions are available in the heat-sterilised Polyflux S, H and L filter series from Gambro.

The DIAPES® membrane - a blend of poly(aryl)ethersulfone and PVP - is produced by the German manufacturer Membrana (Wuppertal) and available in dialyser housings from Allmed, Baxter, Bellco, Haidylena, Kawasumi, Nephros, Nikkiso and Saxonia. Low-flux, middle-flux (high-performance) and high-flux versions exist, sterilised by all common methods, depending on the provider. In order to further increase performances, spacer yarns are included in the fibre bundle. ß2-m removal was comparable to Fresenius Polysulfone® (about 77% during HDF with a 1.8 m^2 dialyser) and higher than with polyamide (ß2-m removal 71%), but the albumin loss with DIAPES® was higher (DIAPES® HF800: 5.7 ± 1.4 g/session) than with the other membranes in this investigation (Fresenius Polysulfone®: 3.5 ± 1.4 g/session; polyamide: 1.0 ± 0.7 g/session; blood flow: 250 ml/min, filtration/substitution volume: 60 ml/min) [90]. Another investigation comparing the ability of 8 different high-flux membranes to remove ß2-m reported a 65% removal rate for DIAPES® and 70%

for Helixone® (postdilution HDF; data for 60 ml/min ultrafiltration/substitution flow; blood flow of 292 ± 21 ml/min). Under these conditions, the albumin loss with DIAPES® amounted to 4000 mg/session, while it was only 300 mg/session with the Helixone® dialyser. At an ultrafiltration/substitution flow of 90 ml/min, DIAPES® exhibited - together with Toraysulfone® - the highest albumin loss of all membranes: almost 7000 mg in 4 hours (the loss with Helixone® was around 2000 mg in 4 hours) [78]. Even in the case of haemodialysis (blood flow 200 ml/min; dialysis fluid flow 500 ml/min), an albumin loss with DIAPES® HF 800 of 3100 mg in 4 h was reported (for the sake of comparison, this was only 200 mg with Fresenius Polysulfone® and Helixone®) [91].

Low-flux and high-flux DIAPES® membranes are not impermeable for bacterial products. Pyrogen transfer from saline in the dialysis fluid compartment into saline in the blood compartment (simulating the situation during predialysis rinsing procedures) was detected during *in vitro* dialysis in two different independent investigations using different sources of pyrogens. Under identical conditions, no transfer of endotoxins was detectable with Helixone® and Fresenius Polysulfone® [72, 92].

References

1. Lonnemann G: The quality of dialysate: an integrated approach. Kidney Int (Suppl 58): S112-119, 2000

2. Lonnemann G: Chronic inflammation in hemodialysis: the role of contaminated dialysate. Blood Purif 18: 214-223, 2000

3. Paul D, Vienken J: Capillary membranes for medical application in *Recent research developments in biomaterials,* edited by Ikada Y, Trivandrum: 179-220, 2002

4. Hoenich NA, Stamp S: Clinical investigation of the role of membrane structure on blood contact and solute transport characteristics of a cellulose membrane. Biomaterials 21: 317-324, 2000

5. Ureña P, Herbelin A, Zingraff J, Lair M, Man NK, Descamps-Latscha B, Drüeke T: Permeability of cellulosic and non-cellulosic membranes to endotoxin subunits and cytokine production during *in-vitro* haemodialysis. Nephrol Dial Transplant 7: 16-28, 1992

6. Weber C, Linsberger I, Rafiee-Tehrani M, Falkenhagen D: Permeability and adsorption capacity of dialysis membranes to lipid A. Int J Artif Organs 20: 144-152, 1997

7. Akzo Faser AG: Hemophan, a DEAE modified cellulose for dialysis. US-Patent No.4,668,396, European Patent No. 172,497

8. Oosterhuis WP, de Metz M, Wadham A, Daha MR, Go RH: In vivo evaluation of four hemodialysis membranes: biocompatibility and clearances. Dialysis & Transplantation 24(8): 450-458, 1995

9. Holland FF, Gidden HE, Mason RG, Klein E: Thrombogenicity of heparin-bound DEAE cellulose hemodialysis membranes. ASAIO J 1: 24-36, 1978

10. Nakagawa K, Inagaki O, Saian Y, Fujita Y: A study on heparin adsorption in Hemophan membrane dialyzer. Kidney 15: 71, 1992

11. Ward RA, Schaefer RM, Falkenhagen D, Joshua MS, Heidland A, Klinkmann H, Gurland HJ: Biocompatibility of a new high-permeability modified cellulose membrane for haemodialysis. Nephrol Dial Transplant 8(1): 47-53, 1993

12. Bowry SK, Rintelen TH: Synthetically modified cellulose (SMC): a cellulosic hemodialysis membrane with minimized complement activation. ASAIO J 44(5): M579-M583, 1998

13. Hoenich N, Woffindin C, Stamp S, Roberts SJ, Turnbull J: Synthetically modified cellulose: an alternative to synthetic membranes for use in haemodialysis? Biomaterials 18: 1299-1303, 1997

14. Mandolfo S, Tetta C, David S, Gervasio R, Ognibene D, Wratten ML, Tessore E, Imbasciati E: *In vitro* and *in vivo* biocompatibility of substituted cellulose and synthetic membranes. Artif Organs 20(11): 603-609, 1997

15. Clark WR, Shinaberger JH: Clinical evaluation of a new high efficiency hemodialyzer: Polysynthane™. ASAIO J: 288-292, 2000

16. Kishida A, Mishima K, Corretge E, Konishi H, Ikada Y: Interactions of poly(ethylen glycol)-grafted cellulose membranes with proteins and platelets. Biomaterials 13(2): 113-118, 1992

17. Fushimi F, Nakayama M, Nishimura K, Hiyoshi T: Platelet adhesion, contact phase coagulation activation, and C5a generation of polyethylene glycol acid-grafted high flux cellulosic membranes with varieties of grafting amounts. Artif Organs 22(10): 821-826, 1998

18. Fukuda M, Miyazaki M, Hiyoshi T, Iwata M, Hongou T. Newly developed biocompatible membrane and effects of its smoother surface on antithrombogenicity. J Appl Polym Sci 72: 1249-1256, 1999

19. Sasaki M, Hosoya N, Saruhashi M: Vitamin E modified cellulose membrane. Artif Organs 24(10): 779-789, 2000

20. Saruhashi M, Sasaki M: Antioxidant function of Viatmin E-modified dialyzer CL-EE. Jpn J Artif Organs 29(1): 161-165, 2000

21. Sasaki M, Hosoya N, Saruhashi M: Development of vitamin E-modified membrane in *Vitamin E-bonded membrane. A further step in dialysis optimization* edited by Ronco C, La Greca G, Contr Nephrol, Basel, Karger 127: 49-70, 1999

22. Averbukh Z, Modai D, Sandbank J, Berman S, Cohn M, Galperin E, Cohen N, Dishi V, Weissgarten J: Red eye syndrome: clinical and experimental experience in a new aspect of diffusive eosinophilic infiltration? Artif Organs 25(6): 437-440, 2001

23. Hoenich NA, Woffindin C, Cox PJ, Goldfinch ME, Roberts SJ. Clinical characterization of Dicea a new cellulose membrane for haemodialysis. Clin Nephrol 48(4): 253-259, 1997

24. Dameche L, Brunet P, George F, André-Pinon S, Bernard D, Sampol J, Berland Y: Meltspun cellulose diacetate and polysulfone membranes have the same effect on complement activation and expression of leukocyte adhesion molecules and complement receptors. Nephrol Dial Transplant 10(Suppl 10): 33-38, 1995

25. Canaud B: Performance liquid test as a cause for sudden deaths of dialysis patients: perfluorohydrocarbon, a previously unrecognized hazard for dialysis patients. Nephrol Dial Transplant 17: 545-548, 2002

26. Shaldon S, Koch KM: Understanding the epidemic of deaths associated with the use of the Althane dialyzer. Artif Organs 26(10): 894-895, 2002

27. Shaldon S, Koch KM: Dialyzer repair: A disastrous exercise in cost effectiveness. ASAIO J 48(5): 453-454, 2002

28. Ronco C, Brendolan A, Everard P, Irone M, Ballestri M, Cappelli G, Inguaggiato P, Bellomo R: Cellulose triacetate: another membrane for continuous renal replacement therapy J Nephrol 12: 241-247, 1999

29. Takeyama T, Sakai Y: Polymethylmethacrylate: One biomaterial for a series of membrane in: *Polymethylmethacrylate. A flexible membrane for a tailored dialysis,* edited by Ronco C, Contrib Nephrol, Basel, Karger 125: 9-24, 1998.

30. Becker J, Reeke N: Three-dimensional structure of ß2-microglobulin. Proc Natl Acad Sci 82: 4225-4229, 1985

31. Verresen L, Waer M; Vanrenterghem Y, Michielsen P: Angiotensin-converting-enzyme-inhibitors and anaphylactic reactions to high-flux membrane dialysis. Lancet 336: 1360-1362, 1990

32. Tielemans C, Madhoun P, Lenaers M, Schandene L, Goldman M, Vanherweghem JL: Anaphylactoid reactions during hemodialysis on AN69 membranes in patients receiving ACE inhibitors. Kidney Int 38: 982-984, 1990

33. Parnes EL, Shapiro WB: Anaphylactoid reactions in hemodialysis patients treated with the AN69 dialyzer. Kidney Int 40(6): 1148-1152, 1991

34. Brunet P, Jaber K, Berland Y, Baz M: Anaphylactoid reactions during hemodialysis and hemofiltration: role of associating AN69 membrane and angiotensin I converting enzyme inhibitors. Am J Kidney Dis 9: 444-447, 1992

35. Brophy PD, Mottes TA, Kudelka TL, McBryde KD, Gradner JJ, Maxvold NJ, Bunchman TE: AN-69 membrane reactions are pH-dependent and preventable. Am J Kidney Dis 1: 173-178, 2001

36. Krieter DH, Grude M, Lemke HD, Fink E, Bönner G, Schölkens BA, Schulz E, Müller GA: Anaphylactoid reactions during hemodialysis in sheep are ACE inhibitor dose-dependent and mediated by bradykinin. Kidney Int 53: 1026-1035, 1998

37. Coppo R, Amore A: Importance of the bradykinin-nitric oxide synthase system in the hypersensitivity reactions of chronic hemodialysis patients. Nephrol Dial Transplant 15: 1288-1290, 2000

38. Coppo R, Amore A, Cirina P, Scelfo B, Giacchino F, Comune L, Atti M, Renaux JL: Bradykinin and nitric oxide generation by dialysis membranes can be blunted by alkaline rinsing solutions. Kidney Int 58: 881-888, 2000

39. Renaux JL, Thomas M, Crost T, Loughraieb N, Vantard G: Activation of the kallikrein-kinin system in hemodialysis: role of membrane electronegativity, blood dilution, and pH. Kidney Int 55 (3): 1097-1103, 1999

40. Valette P, Thomas M, Déjardin P: Adsorption of low molecular weight proteins to hemodialysis membranes: experimental results and simulations. Biomaterials 20: 1621-1634, 1999

41. Moachon N, Boullanger C, Fraud S, Vial E, Thomas M, Quash G: Influence of the charge of low molecular weight proteins on their efficacy of filtratrion and/or adsorption on dialysis membranes with different intrinsic properties. Biomaterials 23: 651-658, 2002

42. Pascual M, Schifferli JA: Adsorption of complement factor D by polyacrylonitrile membranes. Kidney Int 43: 903-911, 1993

43. Klinke B, Röckel A, Abdelhamid S, Fiegel P, Walb D: Transmembranous transport and adsorption of beta-2-microglobulin during hemodialysis using polysulfone, polyacrylonitrile, polymethylmethacrylate and cuprammonium rayon membranes. Int J Artif Organs 12(11): 697-702, 1989

44. Leitienne P, Trzeciak MC, Adeleine P, Ville D, Dechavanne M, Traeger J, Zech P: Comparison of hemostasis with two high-flux hemocompatible dialysis membranes. Int J Artif Organs 14(4): 227-233, 1991

45. Mori H, Hiraoka K, Yorifuji R, Iwasaki T, Gomikawa S, Inagaki O, Inoue S, Takamitsu Y, Fujita Y: Adsorption of human recombinant erythropoietin on dialysis membranes *in vitro*. Artif Organs 18(10): 725-728, 1994

46. Cheung AK, Hohnholt M, Leypoldt JK, DeSpain M: Hemodialysis membrane biocompatibility: the case of erythropoietin. Blood Purif 9(3): 153-163, 1991

47. Opatrny K Jr, Krouzecky A, Wirth J, Vit L, Eiselt J: The effects of a polyacrylonitrile membrane and a membrane made of regenerated cellulose on the plasma concentrations of erythropoietin during hemodialysis. Artif Organs 22(10): 816-820, 1998

48. Thomas M, Valette P, Mausset A-L, Déjardin P: High molecular weight kininogen adsorption on hemodialysis membranes: influence of pH and relationship with contact phase activation of blood plasma. Influence of pre-treatment with poly(ethyleneimine). Int J Artif Organs: 29(1): 20-26, 2000

49. Maheut H, Lacour F: Using AN69 ST membrane: a dialysis center experience. Nephrol Dial Transplant 16(7): 1519-1520, 2001

50. Renaux JL, Atti M: The AN69ST dialysis membrane: a new approach for reducing systemic heparinization. In: Contrib Nephrol, edited by Ronco C, La Greca G, Basel Karger 137: 111-119, 2002

51. Des Grottes J-M, Molinaro G, Adam A, Muniz M-C, Nortier J, Thomas M, Tielemans C: A new type of adverse reactions (AR) during hemodialysis (HD) on AN69 hollow fiber dialysers. Solving the problem by a different membrane treatment procedure with polyethylene imine (PEI) (Abstract). J Am Soc Nephrol 13: 579A, 2002

52. Renaux JL, Thomas M, Crost T, Paris JM: Heparin adsorption on Nephral ST: in vivo/ex vivo results. Abstract book 38th EDTA, Vienna: 253, 2001 (abstract)

53. Lavaud S, Canivet E, Wuillai A, Maheut H, Randoux C, Bonnet J-M, Renaux J-L, Chanard J: Optimal anticoagulation strategy in haemodialysis with heparin-coated polyacrylonitrile membrane. Nephrol Dial Transplant 18: 2097–2104, 2003

54. Lavaud S, Canivet E, Mohajer M, Crost T, Wuillai A, Renaux J-L, Chanard J: Change in membrane electronegativity induces heparin sparing for hemodialysis. J Am Soc Nephrol 11: 281 A, 2000

55. Sugaya H, Sakai Y: Polymethylmethacrylate: from polymer to dialyzer in: *Polymethylmethacrylate. A flexible membrane for a tailored dialysis,* edited by Ronco C, Contrib Nephrol, Basel, Karger 125: 1-8, 1998

56. Ono T, Iwamoto N, Kataoka H, Yamada S, Sakai Y, Kunitomo T: Clinical significance of a dialysis membrane that can remove ß2-microglobulin (ß2m). Trans Am Soc Artif Intern Organs 34: 342-345, 1988

57. Campistol JM, Torregrosa JV, Ponz E, Fenollosa B: $ß_2$-microglobulin removal by hemodialysis with polymethylmethacrylate membranes. In: *Polymethylmethacrylate. A flexible membrane for a tailored dialysis,* edited by Ronco C, Contrib Nephrol, Basel, Karger 125: 76-85, 1998

58. Yamada S, Kataoka H, Kobayashi H, Ono T, Minakuchi J, Kawano Y: Identification of an erythropoietic inhibitor from the dialysate collected in the hemodialysis with PMMA membrane (BK-F) and its clinical effects. In: *Polymethylmethacrylate. A flexible membrane for a tailored dialysis,* edited by Ronco C, Contrib Nephrol, Basel, Karger 125: 159-172, 1998

59. Locatelli F, Andrulli S, Pecchini F, Pedrini L, Agliata S, Lucchi L, Farina M, La Milia V, Grassi C, Borghi M et al: Effect of high-flux dialysis on the anemia of haemodialysis patients. Nephrol Dial Transplant 15: 1399-1409, 2000

60. Bonomini M, Fiederling B, Bucciarelli T, Manfrini V, Di Ilio C, Albertazzi A: A new polymethacrylate membrane for hemodialysis. Int J Artif Organs 19: 232-239, 1996

61. Hoenich NA: Platelet and leukocyte behaviour during haemodialysis in: *Polymethylmethacrylate. A flexible membrane for a tailored dialysis,* edited by Ronco C, Contrib Nephrol, Basel, Karger 125: 76-85, 1998

62. Debrand-Passard A, Lajous-Petter A, Schmidt R, Herbst R, von Baeyer H, Krause AA, Schiffl H: Thrombogenicity of dialyzer membranes as assessed by residual blood volume and surface morphology at different heparin dosages in: *Improvements in dialysis therapy,* edited by Baldamus CA, Mion C, Shaldon S, Contrib Nephrol, Basel, Karger, 74: 2-9, 1989

63. Schwarzbeck A, Wittenmeier K-W, Hällfritzsch U, Frank J: Anaphylactoid reactions ACE inhibitors and extracorporeal hemotherapy. Nephron 65: 499-500, 1993

64. Sawada K, Malchesky PS, Guidubaldi JM, Sueoka A, Shimoyama T. *In vitro* evaluation of a relationship between human serum- or plasma-material interaction and polymer bulk hydroxyl and surface oxygen content. ASAIO J 39(4): 910-917, 1993

65. Zingraff J, Man NK, Jehenne G, Urena P, Drüeke T: $ß_2$-microglobulin: interaction of blood with different hemodialysis membranes. J Nephrol 2: 101-105, 1989

66. Klinkmann H, Buscaroli A, Stefoni S: $ß_2$microglonbulin and low-flux synthetic dialyzers. Artif Organs 22(7): 585-590, 1998

67. Ward RA, Buscaroli A, Schmidt B, Stefoni S, Gurland HJ, Klinkmann H: A comparison of dialysers with low-flux membranes: significant differences in spite of many similarities. Nephrol Dial Transplant 12: 965-972, 1997

68. Göhl H, Buck R, Strathmann H. Basic features of the polyamide membranes in: *Polyamide - The evolution of a synthetic membrane for renal therapy,* edited by Berlyne GM, Giovannetti S, Contrib Nephrol, Basel, Karger 96: 1-25, 1992

69. Floege J, Granolleras C, Deschodt G, Heck M, Baudin G, Branger B, Tournier O, Reinhard B, Eisenbach GM, Smeby LC, Koch KM, Shaldon S: High-flux synthetic versus cellulosic membranes for $ß_2$-microglobulin removal during hemodialysis, hemodiafiltration and hemofiltration. Nephrol Dial Transplant 4: 653-657, 1989

70. Deppisch R, Betz M, Hänsch GM, Rauterberg EW, Ritz E: Biocompatibility of the polyamide membrane in: *Polyamide - The evolution of a synthetic membrane for renal therapy,* edited by Berlyne GM, Giovannetti S, Contrib Nephrol, Basel, Karger 96: 26-46, 1992

71. Lonnemann G, Mahiout A, Schindler R, Colton CK: Pyrogen retention by the polyamide membranes in: *Polyamide - The evolution of a synthetic membrane for renal therapy,* edited by Berlyne GM, Giovannetti S, Contrib Nephrol, Basel, Karger 96: 47-63, 1992

72. Weber V, Linsberger I, Rossmanith E, Weber C, Falkenhagen D: Pyrogen transfer across high-and low flux hemodialysis membranes. Artif Organs to be published in February 2004

73. Streicher E, Schneider H: Polysulphone membrane mimicking human glomerular basement membrane. Lancet 11: 1136, 1983

74. Schaefer RM, Hörl WH, Gilge U, Konrad G, Heidland A: Biocompatibility profile of the polysulfone 400 membrane in: *Improvement in Dialysis Therapy,* edited by: Baldamus CA, Mion C, Shaldon S. Contrib Nephrol 74, Basel, Karger: 43-51, 1989

75. Ronco C, Bowry S: Nanoscale modulation of the pore dimensions, size distribution and structure of a new polysulfone-based high-flux dialysis membrane. Int J Artif Organs 24(10): 726-735, 2001

76. Bowry SK, Ronco C: Surface topography and surface elemental composition analysis of Helixone®, a new high-flux polysulfone dialysis membrane. Int J Artif Organs 24(11): 757-764, 2001

77. Klingel R, Ahrenholz P, Schwarting A, Röckel A: Enhanced functional performance characteristics of a new polysulfone membrane for high-flux hemodialysis. Blood Purif 20: 325-333, 2002

78. Ahrenholz PG, Winkler RE, Michelsen A, Lang DA, Bowry SK: Dialysis membrane-dependent removal of middle molecules during haemodiafiltration: the ß2-microglobulin/albumin relationship. Clin Nephrol accepted

79. Linnenweber S, Lonnemann G: Pyrogen retention by the Asahi APS-650 polysulfone dialyzer during in vitro dialysis with whole human donor blood. ASAIO J 46: 444-447, 2000

80. Ronco C, Nissenson AR: Does nanotechnology apply to dialysis? Blood Purif 19: 347-352, 2001

81. Ronco C, Bowry SK, Brendolan A, Crepaldi C, Soffiati G, Fortunato A, Bordoni V, Granziero A, Torsello G, La Greca G: Hemodialyzer: from macro-design to membrane nanostructure: the case of the FX-class of hemodialyzers. Kidney Inter 61(Suppl 80): S126-S142, 2002

82. Coli L, Donati G, Zambianchi L, Isola E, Manna C, Sestigiani E, Grammatico F, Marseglia CD, Iannelli S, Ramazotti E, Lang D, Pohlmeier R, Stefoni S: Assessment of the inflammatory response of FX60 versus F60S dialysers. Inter J Artif Organs 23 (8): 531, 2000 (Abstract)

83. Stefoni S, Coli L, Cianciolo G, Donati G, Ruggeri G, Ramazzotti E, Pohlmeier R, Lang D: Inflammatory response of a new synthetic dialyzer membrane. A randomised cross-overcomparison between polysulfone and helixone. Int J Artif Organs 26(1): 26-32, 2003

84. Mann H, Al-Bashir, Melzer H, Stiller S: Diacap® α-polysulfone HI PS: A new dialysis membrane with optimum ß2-microglobulin elimination. Int J Artif Organs 26(6): 461-466, 2003

85. Gastaldon F, Brendolan A, Crepaldi C, Frisone P, Zamboni S, Díntini V, Poulin S, Hector R, Granziero A, Martins K, Gellert R, Inguaggiato P, Ronco C : Effects of manufacturing technology on blood and dialysate flow distribution in a new low flux «α Polysulfone" hemodialyzer. Int J Artif Organs 26(2): 105-112, 2003

86. Sombolas K, Tsitsamidou Z, Kyriazis G, Karagianni A, Kantaropoulou M, Progia E: Clinical evaluation of four different high-flux hemodialyzers under conventional conditions in vivo. Am J Nephrol 17: 406-412, 1997

87. Stein G, Günther K, Sperschneider H, Carlsohn H, Hüller M, Schubert K, Schaller R: Clinical evaluation of a new dialyzer FLX-12 GW, with a polyester-polymer alloy membrane. Artif Organs 17(5): 339-345, 1993

88. Hoenich NA, Stamp S: Clinical performance of a new high-flux synthetic membrane. Am J Kidney Dis 35(2): 345-352, 2000

89. Gores F, Montag P, Schall C, Vienken J, Bowry SK: Verification of the chemical composition and specifications of haemodialysis membranes by NMR and GPC-FTIR-coupled spectroscopy. Biomaterials 23: 3131-3140, 2002

90. Samtleben W, Dengler C, Reinhardt B, Nothdurft A, Lemke HD : Comparison of the new polyethersulfone high-flux membrane DIAPES® HF800 with conventional high-flux membranes during on-line haemodiafiltration. Nephrol Dial Transplant 18: 2382-2386, 2003

91. Jaekel D, Kliem V, Reinhardt B, Sauer N, Lemke HD, Krieter DH: *In vivo* comparison of two new high-flux membranes in haemodialysis (HD). Nephrol Dial Transplant 18 (Suppl4): M618, 2003

92. Schindler R, Christ-Kohlrausch F, Frei U, Shaldon S: Differences in the permeability of high-flux dialyzer membranes for bacterial pyrogens. Clin Nephrol 59(6): 447-454, 2003

3. Dialyser constructions

The ideal dialyser should be highly effective regarding solute removal, exhibit constant performance over the whole treatment time, have a small blood priming volume and contain a biocompatible membrane [1]. Furthermore, it must be absolutely safe to use, be sterilised by steam in order to avoid hazards by possible sterilisation products (e.g. extracts after γ-irradiation, residual ethylene oxide (EtO) after EtO sterilisation) and should be made from materials which can be disposed of in an environmentally friendly manner. Current dialysers are available either as parallel-plate or, more commonly, as hollow-fibre devices (**figures 3.1** and **3.2**).

3.1. Parallel-plate dialysers

Parallel-plate dialysers are currently produced and sold only by the Gambro group (Hospal Crystal with AN69ST and the Hemospal series with AN69®). Production of the Lundia series with Cuprophan® (Alpha), Hemophan® (Aria), and Gambrane® (Pro) has been stopped. In parallel-plate dialysers, several layers of flat sheet membranes are stacked, supported by thin plates (**figure 3.1**). Plate dialysers do not contain polyurethane (PUR) and can, therefore, be more easily sterilised by EtO than hollow-fibre dialysers. This is because PUR acts as a reservoir for EtO, causing allergic reactions in some patients [2]. Therefore, the absence of PUR was considered a great advantage in the past, and plate dialysers were used for EtO sensitive patients. The incidence of anaphylactic reactions (type A first-use syndrome, allergic reactions to EtO) decreased significantly when plate dialysers were used instead of EtO-sterilised hollow-fibre devices [3]. Today, degassing techniques after EtO sterilisation have progressed and residual EtO is a rare problem, affecting only a few sensibilised patients. Furthermore, nearly all dialysers are available in alternative sterilisation modes.

A second theoretical advantage of plate dialysers is their reduced thrombogenicity compared to their hollow-fibre counterparts: this is expected as the shear stress experienced by the blood is lower in plate dialysers. How

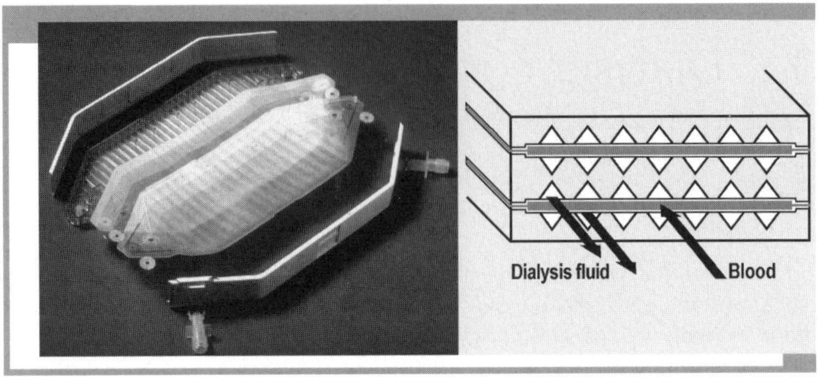

Figure 3.1: Components of a parallel-plate haemodialyser and flow conditions.

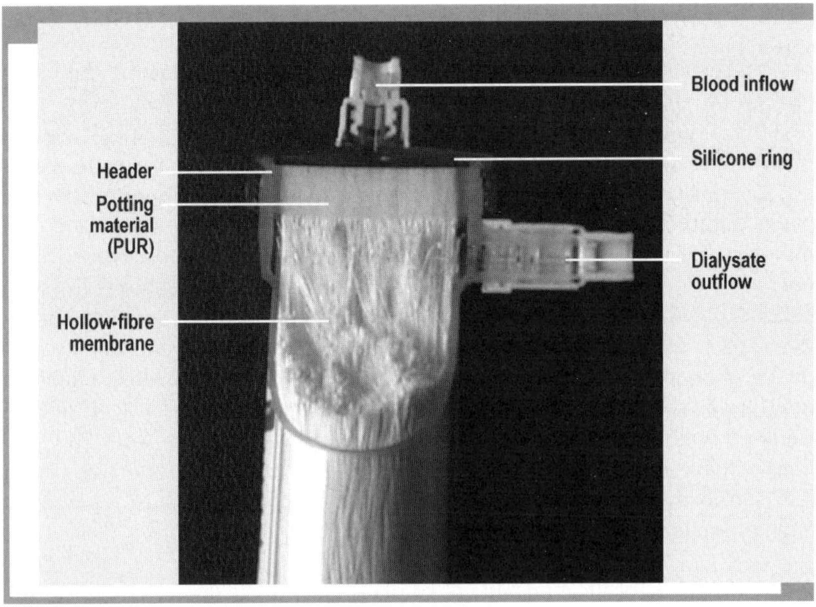

Figure 3.2: Components of a hollow-fibre dialyser. *PUR: polyurethan.*

ever, while this advantage was observed in comparisons with early hollow-fibre devices, it could not be confirmed in clinical practice with modern devices [4]. Regarding biocompatibility parameters (such as complement activation or platelet count), a comparison of Cuprophan® hollow-fibre and plate dialysers of the same surface area and sterilisation mode did not reveal any differences between the two geometries [4-6]. In summary, plate dialysers have no real advantage over hollow-fibre devices. Consequently, their usage declined year by year.

3.2 Hollow-fibre dialysers

A contemporary hollow-fibre dialyser consists of a housing containing a single membrane fibre bundle (**figure 3.2**). The bundle is embedded at both ends in polyurethane (PUR), which also fixes the bundle within the casing. A sophisticated cutting process is necessary to form a smooth end-surface - this ensures minimal activation of humoral or cellular systems in the blood. The end surfaces are covered by end caps, which contain the blood inlet and outlet ports and, in recent developments, also the dialysis fluid ports. In many dialysers, the two dialysis fluid ports are positioned directly on the housing, rather than on the end caps (**figure 3.2**). This relatively simple construction is the result of 60 years of dialysis experience and device development. The trend to miniaturise devices becomes evident when Kolff's artificial kidney from 1943 (**figure 1.4,** chapter 1) is compared with the latest dialyser of today. Nearly all components of current dialysers have been improved upon over the years.

Housing

The performance characteristics of each dialyser are primarily determined by the size and design of the fibre bundle included. The blood compartment volume has to be as low as possible, and each fibre should be surrounded by a uniform stream of dialysis fluid during dialysis. This is achieved in some newer housings by a so-called pinnacle design of the housing in the area of the end-caps. This special design facilitates a radial dialysis fluid stream around the whole fibre bundle (see chapter 6). The number of fibres and, consequently, the fibre bundle density increase with surface area until performance has reached a maximum. Then a longer and/or wider housing has to be used. In practice, fibre length or diameter are rarely increased in order to obtain a greater surface area. A comparison of dialysers from various manufacturers which contain the same membrane (e.g. Cuprophan®) and have the same clearance properties clearly demonstrates the differences in packing design which exist, and the advanced technology behind good housing designs.

A current trend in device technology is the use of materials which can be disposed of in an environmentally friendly manner. Polypropylene is such a material; this is used in the newest housings instead of polycarbonate (in FX-class housings, Fresenius Medical Care). Furthermore, comparing dialyser performances, housings have become smaller and smaller since the development of the first disposable hollow-fibre dialyser. This development rests on the availability of membranes with high performance characteristics – a consequence of reduced fibre wall thickness, smaller fibre diameter and special bundle designs. Smaller dialysers reduce waste, have a sparing effect on transport costs, and are beneficial for the patient because of reductions in the blood contact surface area and blood volume in the extracorporeal circuit. An additional advantage for the clinic is the saving of storage space.

Potting material

The composition of the potting compound has changed over the years. The main motivation behind this development was to minimise risks associated with toxic substances which may evolve after sterilisation of the PUR. In particular, irradiation with ß- or γ-beams may lead to the fission product 4,4'-methylene dianiline, a proven carcinogenic substance [7]. The amount of PUR used to embed the fibre bundle in the dialyser has been reduced considerably over time. Furthermore, the effective surface area is increased when less potting compound is used. Some manufacturers have developed advanced cutting techniques to ensure a smooth and effective cutting surface which minimises blood activation (e.g. Fresenius Medical Care FX class series). Also, polycarbonate and/or silicon rings were introduced to reduce the PUR content of hollow-fibre dialysers.

Fibre bundle

The quality of the fibre bundle construction is of considerable importance for the performance of a dialyser. Fibre bundle quality has improved dramatically in recent years. In early dialysers, kinked fibres, which were the result of poor potting techniques and bundle handling, were a major problem as these caused considerable thrombus formation. In modern, high quality dialysers, this problem has been overcome using sophisticated embedding and cutting procedures (**figure 3.3**). In addition, the fibre distribution is nearly uniform in such high quality products. In order to improve dialysis fluid flow around the fibres, several bundle configurations have been developed, tested and rejected: rectangular block arrangements, cross-flow configurations in which the dialysis fluid flowed across the fibres rather than along them, multiple bundles, use of a solid central core with fibres wounded in a spiral manner, or warp knitted hollow-fibre mats [8]. Today, newest fibre developments use an undulation of the fibre itself (also called „ moiré structure") in order to provide space for a continuous uniform flow of the dialysis fluid (e.g. [9]). Alternatively, fibres with fins and bundles with spacer yarns are also on the market (described in chapter 6 in more detail).

Fibre bundle size and swelling of the membrane determine the priming blood volume. This is an important parameter in the choice of dialyser for patients with low blood volume, especially children. Today, the blood volume of most dialysers is smaller than that of the blood tubing sets (blood volumes are given in the list of membranes and dialysers currently on the market in the appendix).

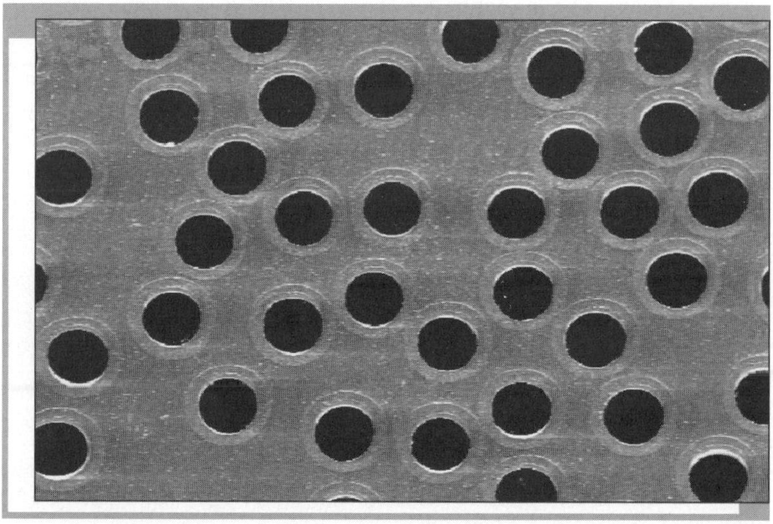

Figure 3.3: Cross-sectional view of the cutting area of a Fresenius Polysulfone® dialyser (F60).

Headers, connecting ports

Geometry and shape of the header determine the blood distribution within the housing and so influence the priming procedure. Therefore, headers were and still are a target for improvement. The newest headers have a lateral blood entry port rather than one on the top, allowing a radial inflow of blood (Hospal Arylane H/M series, Fresenius Medical Care FX class series).

Removable headers are appreciated in clinics that practice dialyser reuse because they allow a visible inspection of possibly clotted header regions and fibre ends. Manufacturers prefer sealed caps because sterility can be guaranteed better with this design. In some dialysers, O-rings are absent in order to minimise contact with foreign surfaces (e.g. Hospal Arylane H/M series).

References

1. Kessler M, Canaud B, Pedrini LA, Tattersall J, ter Wee PM, Vanholder R Wanner C: European best practice guidelines for haemodialysis (Part 1). Biocompatibility. Nephrol Dial Transplant 17(Suppl 7): 32-44, 2002

2. Ansorge W, Pelger M, Dietrich W, Baurmeister U: Ethylene oxide in dialyser rinsing fluid: effect of rinsing technique, dialyser storage time, and potting compound. Artif Organs 11(2): 118-122, 1987

3. Daugirdas JT, Potempa LD, Dinh N, Gandhi VC, Ivanovich PT, Ing TS: Plate, coil, and hollow-fiber cuprammonium cellulose dialyzers: discrepancy between incidence of anaphylactic reactions and degree of complement activation. Artif Organs 11(2): 140-143, 1987

4. Lins LE, Boberg U, Jacobson SH, Kjellstrand C, Ljungberg B, Skroder R: The influence of dialyzer geometry on blood coagulation and biocompatibility. Clin Nephrol 40(5): 281-285, 1993

5. Miranda VM, Miranda RM, Guerra L, Magro C: The influence of the geometry of the dialyzer and the composition of the dialysate in activating the complement system. Nephron 54(1): 26-31, 1990

6. Schaefer RM, Heidland A, Hörl WH: Effect of dialyzer geometry on granulocyte and complement activation. Am J Nephrol 7(2): 121-126, 1987

7. Wilski H: The radiation induced degradation of polymers. Int J Radiat Appl Instrum, Part C, Radiat Phys Chem 29(1): 1-14, 1987

8. Ronco, Ghezzi, Hoenich NA, Delfino: Membranes and filters for hemodialysis: Database 2001, Karger. 2001

9. Leypoldt JK, Cheung AK, Chiranathavat T, Gilson JF, Kamerath CD, Deeter RB : Hollow fibre shape alters solute clearances in high flux dialyzers. ASAIO Journal 81-87, 2003

4. Dialyser sterilisation

Dialysers must be sterilised before clinical use (i.e. microbial life, including highly resistant bacterial spores, must be totally destroyed). In practice, sterility is expressed as a statistic: a device is termed sterile when the chance of survival of a viable micro-organism is less than one in a million or, in other words, at most one device per million may theoretically contain one viable germ after sterilisation [1-3]. Manufacturers must supply dialysers in a sterilised form and thereby comply with strict criteria as stipulated by national and international regulatory commissions (e.g. DIN in Germany, EN in Europe and ISO internationally). Resterilisation of used dialysers in clinical environments (i.e. in dialyser reprocessing for multiple use) is another matter and is addressed in chapter 12 of this book.

Common sterilisation methods, as employed by dialyser manufacturers, are generally based on the use of ethylene oxide gas (EtO), irradiation (γ or ß) or heat (steam or dry heat). **Figure 4.1** provides an overview of the sterilisation methods employed in Europe between 1986 and 2002. Many dialysers are suitable for sterilisation by 2 or even all 3 of these methods, as indicated in **table 4.1**. Only the effect of the sterilisation procedure on the dialyser membrane is truly limiting, as other filter components can generally be exchanged to accommodate a particulate sterilisation method.

The performance data supplied by dialyser manufacturers refer to the sterilised device, i.e. the reported clearances, coefficients of ultrafiltration etc. are determined after sterilisation is completed. Consequently, the effect of the different sterilisation modes on dialyser performance is but of academic interest in clinical practice and will not be addressed here. Suffice it to say that values can be enhanced or reduced depending on the mode of sterilisation, whether wet or dry conditions are employed, the water content of the individual membranes, and which performance parameter is under investigation (e.g. [5-7]). However, the method by which a dialyser is sterilised is indeed of clinical interest and relevance when patient-specific sensitivities come to light; this explains why the same dialysers are sometimes supplied in more than one sterilisation form.

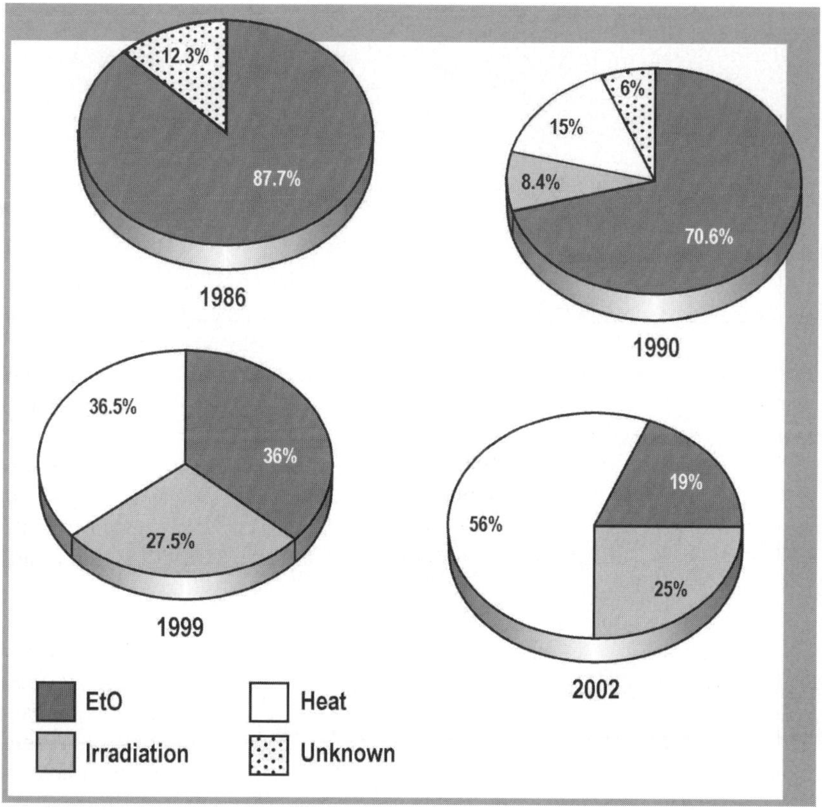

Figure 4.1: Sterilisation methods commonly employed in the European Union. *Sterilisation of new dialysers, as conducted between 1986 and 2002 in the European Community, shows a shift towards more heat (usually steam) and irradiation (usually γ) sterilisation at the expense of EtO sterilisation. EtO is the predominant sterilisation mode in North America, while all dialysers used in Japan are either irradiation or steam sterilised (from Fresenius Medical Care, with permission).*

Membrane polymer		Gamma irradiation	EtO	Heat
Cellulose-based polymers	Cellulose and modified cellulose (all except cellulose acetate)	+	+	+
	Cellulose acetate	+	+	-
Polysulfone-based polymers	Polysulfone	+	+	+
	Polyarylethersulfone (Arylane)	+	+	+
	PES (DIAPES®)	+	+	+
	Polyamide S™/Polyamix™*	+	+	+
	PEPA	+	+	+
Other synthetic polymers	PAN	+	+	-
	PMMA	+	-	-
	EVAL®	+	+	-
	Polycarbonate	+	+	-
	Polyamide	+	+	-

*PAN: polyacrylonitrile; PMMA: polymethylmethacrylate; EVAL®: ethylvinylalcohol copolymer; PES: polyethersulfone; PEPA®: polyethersulfone/polyarylate; *Polyamide S™: an alloy of the heat resistant polymer polyarylethersulfone with small amounts of polyamide, now called Polyamix™(see [36]).*

Table 4.1: Sterilisation methods possible for various common dialysis membranes *(adapted from [4]).*

4.1 Sterilisation with ethylene oxide gas

Exposure to ethylene oxide gas (EtO) was the most common method of sterilisation of new dialysers in Europe and America in the eighties, but alternative methods have gained significantly in popularity since then (**figure 4.1**). The highly diffusive nature of this gas makes sterilisation of devices in their packaging possible. Furthermore, dialysis membrane performance characteristics appeared to be unaffected by exposure to this sterilant, probably due to the low physical and thermal stress, making EtO a comfortable, inexpensive and relatively safe sterilisation method.

During EtO sterilisation, bacteria are killed by alkylation of sulphur-containing proteins [8] and the success of the method depends on five factors: concentration, time, temperature, humidity and pressure. Regarding concentration, EtO is usually (but not always) mixed with an inert gas in device sterilisation to reduce its toxicity and flammability. Typical commercial systems use either mixtures of 20% EtO with 80% carbon dioxide (CO_2), 12% EtO with 88% freon or pure EtO [9], whereby use of large quantities of CO_2 is generally favoured in the sterilisation of artificial kidneys, e.g. 10% EtO with 90% CO_2 [8]. Effective concentrations range between 400 and 1,600 mg/l (whereby many European manufacturers employ the maximum of 1,600 mg/l [9]) and are a function of the process temperature. Exposure time varies with the size of the steriliser, the load and the nature of the materials being sterilised. Exposure time is also a function of temperature, as the higher the temperature the faster the diffusion of EtO into the dialyser. Common operating temperatures range from 21.1°C to 65.5°C [9]. **Figure 4.2** shows how the temperature influences the exposure time and the gas concentration required. For example, increasing the temperature from 30°C to 50°C (which is only possible if the materials are thermostable at such temperatures) means that the gas concentration can be reduced by almost a third and the gasification time by almost 40% [2, 3]. An effective sterilisation of dialysers can be achieved, for example, with 10% EtO and 90% CO_2 applied for 4 hours at 40°C at 40% humidity [8].

The whole course of a low-pressure sterilisation procedure is summarised in **figure 4.3**. Particular attention should be paid to the humidity, as high levels of toxic ethylene glycol (which can be difficult to remove) may be produced at excessive levels [9]. The amount of residual gas is influenced by process parameters, such as frequency, degree of vacuum or time. Different postconditioning approaches to remove residual gas are adopted by manufacturers, but usually commercial aerators (or degassing units) are employed.

Alternatively, or additionally, the dialyser storage time can be increased and the amount of polyurethane used can be minimised, e.g. by replacing part of the potting compound in hollow fibre devices with a polycarbonate or silicon ring, or by exclusive use of the alternative support structures for all plate dialysers [10]. Some companies have developed their own specific procedures for postconditioning, such as that of Fresenius Medical Care, which involves increased temperatures and several air changes (see **figure 4.3**). Dialysers that are appropriately designed and correctly postconditioned contain very low amounts of residual ethylene oxide as early as 2 weeks after sterilisation [2].

Thorough rinsing of the whole extracorporeal circuit is still highly recommended before clinical application of products sterilised by EtO in order to further reduce residual levels of the gas itself and of possible EtO sterilisation by-products, such as ethylene glycol, ethylene chlorohydrin or diethylene glycol [9]. In the past, residues of EtO were identified as a common cause of allergic reactions in a number of dialysis patients: in roughly 70% of severe allergic reactions, elevated levels of EtO-specific IgE antibodies were meas-

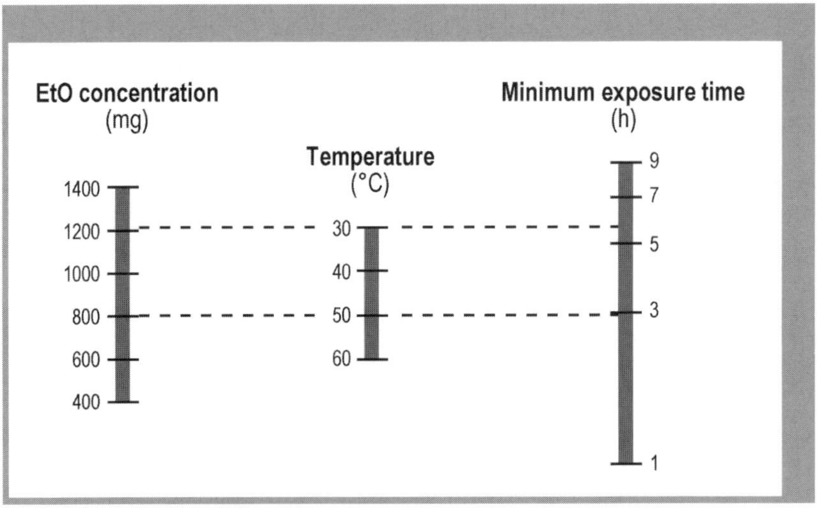

Figure 4.2: Nomogram of relationship between temperature, concentration and exposure time in ethylene oxide sterilisation procedures. *Increasing the temperature from 30°C to 50°C means that the gas concentration can be reduced by almost a third and the gasification time by almost 40% (adapted from [3]).*

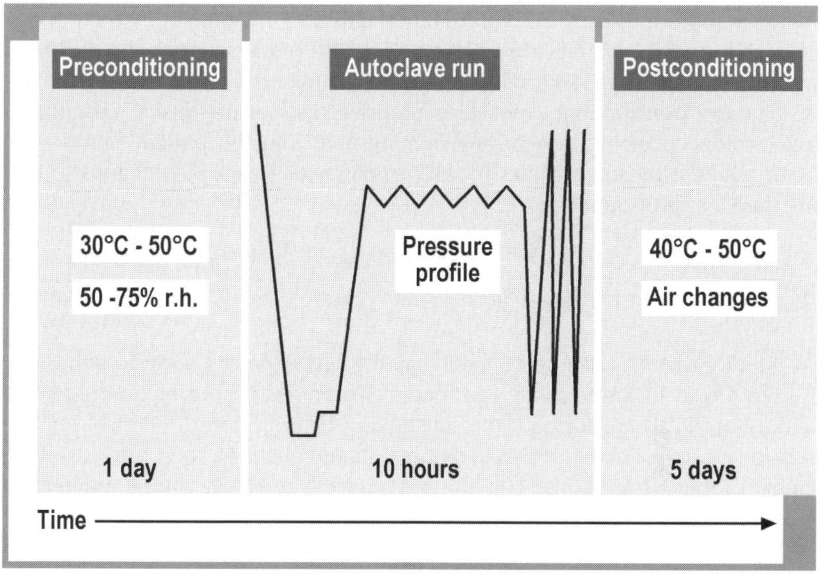

Figure 4.3: The ethylene oxide sterilisation process. *In the preconditioning phase, the dialysers are brought up to specified temperature and moisture values to ensure complete penetration of the gas. In the autoclave phase, a vacuum is generated (indicated by the fall in the pressure curve) and steam is added to increase humidity, when necessary. The actual sterilisation time starts after the introduction of the gas (indicated by the recovery of pressure) and, after a defined contact time, the gas is removed from the autoclave in several evacuation and aeration steps (indicated by the quick variations in pressure). Postconditioning to reduce residual levels of the gas according to manufacturer-specific procedures follows (here the conditions typical of Fresenius Medical Care are indicated). r.h.: relative humidity (from [2]).*

ured in patient blood ([11-17], see also chapters 7.3.5 and 9.2). The problem was mainly based on the adsorption and inadequate or slow release of EtO by some specific membrane polymers and by the potting material used in many dialysers [8, 18, 19]. For example, EtO levels in polypropylene (used in some casings), polyurethane (used as a potting compound in hollow fibre devices) and PMMA membranes were found to take up to 24 hours, 60 days and 3.5 years, respectively, to decrease to one tenth of their initial value [20, 21]. The risk for patient health led to a partial renunciation of devices sterilised by this method, especially for certain patients. However, these observations also resulted in the definition of maximal permissible residue levels by national authorities (e.g. 2 ppm in France and Italy, 10 ppm by the European pharmacopoeia) and the introduction of costly organisational and technical measures at the manufacturing sites to assure minimal residue levels [2, 10]. As an extra precautionary measure, intensive dialyser pre-rinsing procedures and avoidance of infusion of any priming fluid into the patient blood have been adopted by some clinics for EtO sterilised dialysers, as reactions to EtO are then less pronounced [19].

4.2 Radiation sterilisation

Medical devices can be radiation sterilised by exposing them to either γ or ß rays: atoms in the irradiated products are ionised by the high energy rays and free radicals are formed; the subsequent dimerisation of DNA bases and scission or cross-linking of the sugar-phosphate backbone then prevents replication of micro-organisms [10]. The procedure is relatively simple, offers high microbiological safety and can be conducted on already packed devices. Use of γ irradiation to sterilise medical devices has long been common practice in Japan (where the first γ-sterilised dialyser (PMMA) appeared on the market in 1988) and has now also become popular in the western world. ß irradiation is not so common, being only employed by a few companies, such as Fresenius Medical Care North America (for some polysulfone dialysers), Helbio (for polysulfone and cellulose acetate based membranes) and Meditech (for polyethersulfone and Cuprophan® dialysers). Historically, this was due to the limited depth of penetration and uneven absorption, but recent advances in accelerator design have overcome these shortcomings so that the electrons from newer devices have a penetrating power similar to that of the γ radiation produced from cobalt 60. The main advantage of ß radiation over γ radiation is the possibility to more precisely dose and target the required sterilisation [22]. While γ radiation is still recommended for heat sensitive and higher density materials, exposure times are shorter with ß irradiation, implying that less material damage is likely [9].

The degree of sterilisation is always directly related to the amount of radiation adsorbed. This was traditionally measured in rads and the equivalent SI unit is the gray (Gy). One gray is defined as the absorbed dose when the energy per gram imparted to matter by ionising radiation is one joule per kilogram. ß irradiation is a stream of high energy electrons accelerated by means of a linear accelerator and produced using normal electrical energy (also called e-beam sterilisation). In γ radiation, the radiation source is a radioactive isotope - either cesium 137 or cobalt 60; the latter is more popular as a greater quantity of cesium 137 is required to obtain the same radiation level, and because cobalt 60 is produced in abundance in nuclear reactors and has a relatively slow decay rate of 12.5% per annum [9]. The devices to be sterilised are placed close to the radiation source for a time appropriate to attain the required irradiation dosage – this is a few seconds for ß radiation and minutes to hours for γ radiation. The γ radiation dose targeted is generally 25 KGy (or 2.5 Mrads) [2, 3, 5, 23]. Membrane degradation was found to increase with increasing dosage [6, 23, 24], and this has motivated some manufacturers to reduce dosages down to 20 - 15 KGy or less [5, 9] or to consider using ß irradiation with its significantly shorter exposure times. Field data published in 1983 showed that bacteria could be controlled using 3 KGy, spores using 15 KGy, and most resistant spores with 21 KGy [9]. It should be remembered, however, that the radiation intensity falls with distance from the source due to dispersion and adsorption so, in order to guarantee minimal radiation levels throughout the device, points nearer the source are often subjected to significantly higher doses [10, 25].

How are the membrane polymers affected by irradiation?

Currently little has been published on the effects of ß radiation on membrane polymers used in dialysis, while this has been examined extensively in the case of γ radiation. The stabilities of some commonly used membrane polymers that are sensitive to γ irradiation are summarised in **table 4.2**. The numerous types and purities of polymers presently employed to produce dialysis membranes, as well as the variety of additive systems and formulations developed for stability during sterilisation and end use, makes the formulation of general statements about the radiation resistance of polymers used for dialysis membranes extremely difficult. Damage caused by ionising radiation is often based on one of the two basic mechanisms, cross-linking and chain scission (**figure 4.4**). To minimise damage, stabilisers must be added; these chemicals react with the first radicals formed, thereby blocking follow-up reactions [2]. Sensory perceptible radiation effects, such as discoloration or odour, can usually be effectively suppressed, but the formation of toxicologically questionable molecules has been reported In *In vitro* studies of γ ray sterilised regenerated cellulose dialysers [6, 26]. This aspect deserves further investigation. It is less of a problem in wet-sterilised devices (where leachables present can be more readily removed) than in dry-sterilised ones (see section 4.4 for details). It should be noted that the added stabilisers themselves might constitute a toxicological risk factor [2, 3].

Monomer / Polymer	Effect of gamma irradiation
Acrylic monomers (e.g. PAN membranes)	Increase in permeability to higher molecular weight molecules
Cellulose	Chain scission
Polyamide	Transient bluish discoloration; cross-linking
Polymethyl-methacrylate (PMMA)	Chain scission; reduction in permeability to higher molecular weight molecules (10^6 to 10^5 by 35 kGy)
Polyethylene (e.g. EVAL® and housing)	Cross-linking; oxidated hydrocarbons cause the formation of aldehydes and organic acids.
Polycarbonate (housing)	Darkening
Polyvinylchloride (PVC; e.g. housing)	Chain scission; darkening; release of hydrochloric acid; leaching of partially decomposed additives may occur, leading to unpleasant odour and accelerated ageing.
Polyurethane (PUR; potting material)	Release of mutagenic compounds, especially from aromatic PURs

Table 4.2: Effects of gamma irradiation on the stability of some sensitive materials used in renal replacement therapy. *As γ sterilisation is conducted on the whole packaged dialyser, the effect of irradiation on all components is of interest (adapted from [2, 3, 8]).*

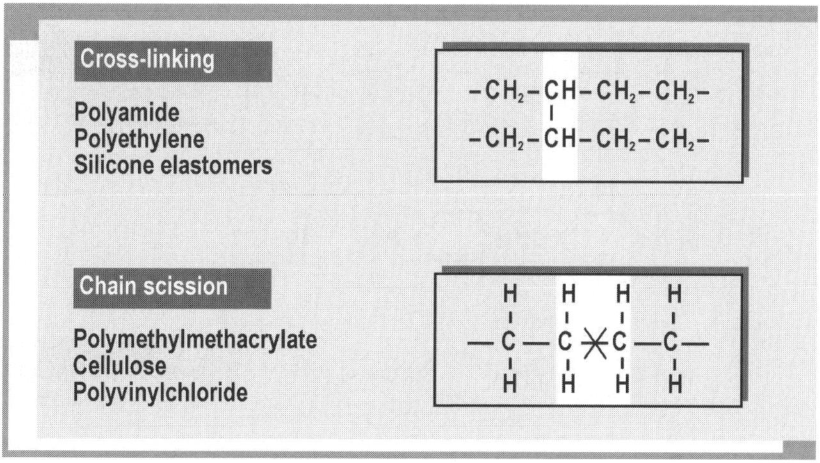

Figure 4.4:** γ **irradiation-induced changes in polymers. *Some polymers, e.g. polyamides, have a preferential tendency towards cross-linking upon γ radiation; here radicals of various different chains recombine, resulting in an increase in average mole mass. Other polymers are more susceptible to chain scission in γ radiation, e.g. polymethylmethacrylate and cellulose: here radicals formed by the breakage of bonds in the main chain become stable without forming new bonds, resulting in a reduction of the average mole mass [2, 3]. Stabilisers must be added to prevent cross-linking and chain scission during radiation sterilisation of polymers used in extracorporeal blood treatment (from Fresenius Medical Care, with permission).*

Why is the nature of the potting compound of particular interest?

As in the case of EtO sterilisation, the effect of irradiation on the potting compound used in hollow fibre devices is a cause for concern: carcinogenic 4,4'-methylene dianiline (MDA) was found to be released following irradiation with γ rays from the aromatic polyurethane used in some hollow fibre dialysers [27]. The polyurethane in question is that composed of 4,4'-diphenylmethane diisocyanate (MDI), and MDA formation is attributed to the fact that radiation cleaves urethane linkage proximal to terminal free amino groups (**figure 4.5**) (although the probability of cleaving two successive urethane linkages to form MDA is small) [28]. The amount of MDA formed is related to the irradiation dose by a second order equation [28, 29]. It also stands in inverse relationship to the rigidity of the potting material, i.e. the more pliant the material, the greater the amount of MDA extracted [28], possibly because of easier access to the inner areas of the potting material.

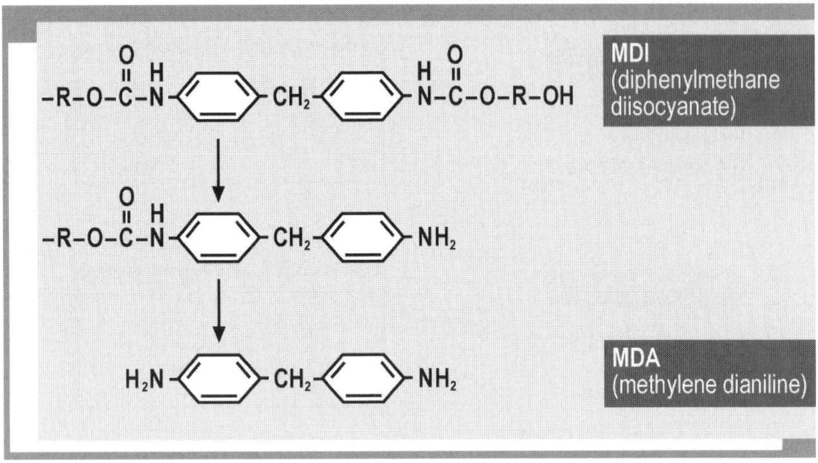

Figure 4.5: Proposed mechanism for the formation of methylene dianiline (MDA) by gamma rays. *The mechanism for the formation of MDA in polyurethane potting compound made from 4,4'-diphenylmethane diisocyanate (MDI) is probably based on cleavage of the urethane linkage proximal to terminal free amino groups by the γ rays [28].*

Migration of the released MDA, with all its documented carcinogenic, mutagenic and toxic properties, into patient blood during dialysis is highly likely [28, 29]. Therefore, steps should be taken to avoid this, such as using the least possible yet effective radiation dose and the least possible amount of polyurethane. MDA release can be totally avoided by choosing a polyurethane mix composed of isocyanates other than MDI. However, of the two alternative isocyanates, toluene diisocyanate (TDI) and aliphatic isocyanate, the former is also a toxic and mutagenic compound, and there are some reports (albeit conflicting and not of recent origin) regarding the possible contribution of antibodies against TDI to allergic reactions in patients who tested negative for EtO antibodies [13, 28, 30-34]. Thus use of aliphatic isocyanate to produce polyurethane potting compound appears the most promising at the moment. Indeed, one study reported that carcinogenic responses in rats to implanted polyurethanes were much less pronounced for aliphatic polyurethanes than for aromatic ones [35]. In addition, intensive prerinsing of the dialysers (particularly the γ-dry sterilised devices) immediately prior to use is essential, not only to reduce levels of any sterilisation by-products but also to remove all micro-organisms destroyed by the irradiation.

Contrary to very early reports, no MDA is formed in thermosetting polyurethane after autoclave sterilisation, even if the sterilisation time is increased from 30 mins to 1 hour (temperature of t = 121°C unchanged [29]).

4.3 Thermal sterilisation

In thermal sterilisation, micro-organisms are destroyed by heat denaturation of their cell walls and proteins. Heat sterilisation of thermally stable devices is free from all risks of chemical residuals, is highly effective, and avoids any changes to the dialyser materials possibly caused by gamma rays (e.g. [28, 29]). It is therefore considered by many to be the best sterilisation method.

For sterilisation by steam (as opposed to dry heat), the dialysers are placed in a pressurised autoclave (normally 1-2 bar) at a temperature and for a time sufficient to assure inactivation of any micro-organisms which could be present. In general, the higher the temperature, the less time is required to assure effective sterilisation. Normally temperatures of up to around 121°C and times of 20-90 minutes are used to ensure steam penetration of the whole device plus packaging [5, 7, 29]. The autoclave/steam process itself is summarised schematically in **figure 4.6**. This is technically the simplest method of heat sterilisation; in dry heat sterilisation, higher temperatures (e.g. 180°C) and/or times are necessary to achieve sterilisation – this method is not commonly employed in the medical device industry [3, 22]. When such standard steam or dry heat sterilisation processes are employed, dialysers must be thoroughly rinsed with saline before use. This is to ensure removal of destroyed micro-organisms, extracts dislodged during sterilisation, pore-fillers (e.g. glycerol) and softeners (used to protect the membrane from degradation during the application of such high temperatures) [5].

As an alternative to standard steam or dry heat sterilisation, dialysers containing thermostable membranes can be heat sterilised by the so-called "INLINE steam sterilisation" process (**figure 4.7**, Fresenius Medical Care). In this approach, every point of each dialyser is subjected to 121°C hot steam for at least 15 minutes during production, and the devices are then vented, cooled and dried before the specially constructed and sterile closure caps are closed, thereby making the dialysers impervious to micro-organisms [10]. This method is superior to other steam sterilisation processes in that the extensive rinsing of the blood and dialysis fluid compartments with steam assures that heat-resistant endotoxins and other pyrogens are flushed out of the device

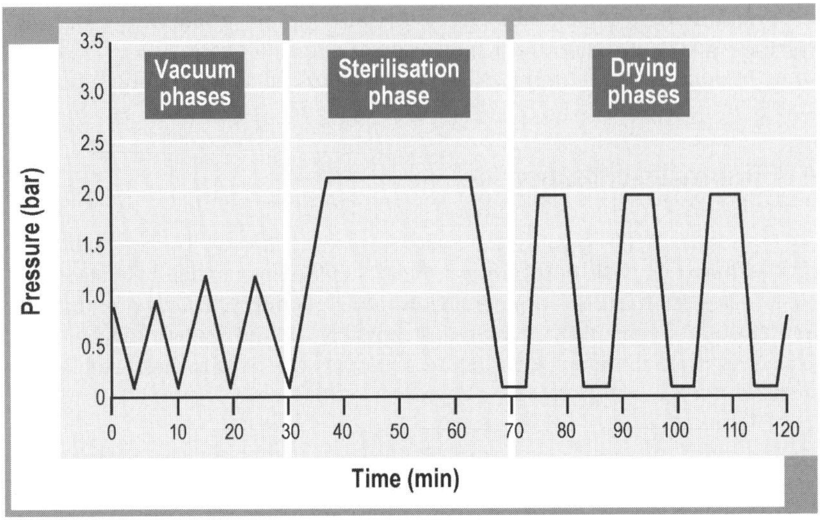

Figure 4.6: The standard steam (autoclaving) sterilisation process. *The dialysers are first subjected to several vacuuming phases in the autoclave (indicated by the abrupt changes in pressure) to remove air and thereby facilitate the exposure of all items in the chamber to steam. Sterilisation follows under high pressure after the chamber is filled with saturated steam. Several venting, cooling and drying with hot air phases follow this (from [2]).*

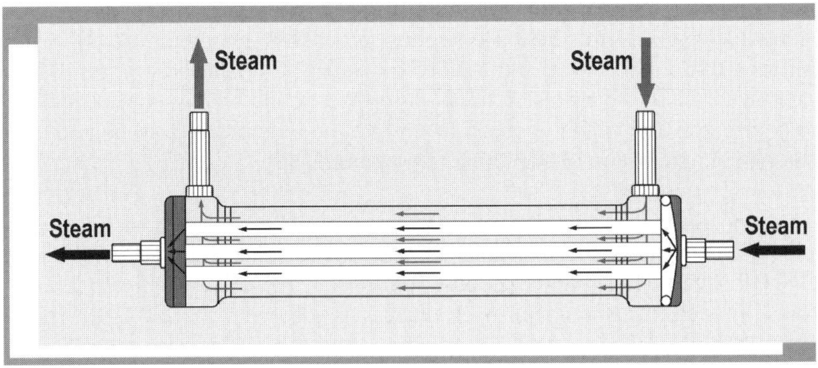

Figure 4.7: The INLINE steam sterilisation process. *121°C hot steam streams through the blood and dialysis fluid compartments of the dialyser for at least 15 minutes during production. The devices are then vented, cooled, dried and the specially constructed closure caps are closed (with permission from Fresenius Medical Care).*

[10]. Moreover, the intactness of all capillaries can be tested during sterilisation, the use of glycerol as a pore-filler becomes obsolete, and the time-consuming prerinsing of the dialyser is significantly reduced, saving also saline [2, 10].

4.4 Comparison of sterilisation procedures

As depicted in **table 4.1**, not all dialyser membranes can be sterilised by each of the procedures discussed. Reasons for the inapplicability of a particular method vary from dialyser to dialyser and are determined primarily by the choice of dialyser membrane and secondarily by the nature of the potting compound. Typical grounds are chemical residues, discoloration, membrane degradation and formation and release of sterilisation by-products. Widely accepted strengths and weaknesses of the three commonly employed methods are summarised in **table 4.3**.

From a clinical point of view, heat or steam sterilisation of dialysers appears to be superior to EtO or γ irradiation sterilisation. The lack of sterilisation by-products is the winning factor, and the intensive rinsing with steam in the described INLINE steam sterilisation procedure has added advantages regarding assured freedom from any pyrogenic substances. The ease of quality management inspires further confidence in this procedure. Unfortunately, not all dialyser membranes and casings are sufficiently thermostable to withstand the high temperatures involved. Furthermore, the method is costly from the production point of view, and this may be reflected in higher product prices. Sterilisation with ethylene oxide gas or γ irradiation are safe, well tested and easily conducted alternatives, and the documented release of sterilisation by-products or residues can be reduced to negligible levels in modern, quality-conscious production facilities and by adherence to stipulated predialysis rinsing procedures.

What is meant by "wet" and "dry" sterilisation?

In addition to choosing between different sterilisation modes, the manufacture can also opt for "wet" or "dry" sterilisation insofar as heat or radiation sterilisation is performed (EtO sterilised products are always "dry"). Sterilisation methods termed "heat (wet)" generally refer to wet steam sterilisation whereby the dialysers are generally filled with an aqueous solution after sterilisation, while dry steam sterilised devices do not contain any fluid. In the

	Gamma irradiation	EtO	Heat
Microbiological efficacy	High	High	High
Effect on dialyser materials	Intermediate material stress	Very low mechanical and no thermal stress	High thermal stress (not suitable for heat susceptible and highly porous materials; possible thermal degradation of pore-fillers or softens)
Release of sterilisation by-products	Cytotoxic compounds from some dialysers; MDA from aromatic polyurethane in some potting compounds	Residual EtO if degassing not adequate and/or materials adsorb much gas (e.g. potting compound, PMMA)	None
Ease of quality management	Good (few process parameters) -: official "Environmental safety" and "Safety at work" regulations	Poor due the need for comprehensive validation of a high number of process parameters	Good (few process parameters)
Environmental risks	High	High	None
Pharmacopoeia recommendation	–	Only when no alternative is available	Recommended whenever possible

	Gamma irradiation	EtO	Heat
Postconditioning	Not necessary	Degassing	Not necessary
Ease of conduction	Good +: possible in final packaging -: need protective measures	Very good +: possible in final packaging	Fair -: need protective measures* -: not suitable for closed systems
Cost of equipment	High	Low	High

**Except for the special INLINE steam procedure employed by Fresenius Medical Care, Germany. MDA: 4,4'-methylene dianiline.*

Table 4.3: Strengths and weaknesses of the 3 common sterilisation methods for blood purification devices. *The documented release of sterilisation by-products in the cases of γ irradiation and EtO sterilisation makes intensive pre-rinsing of these dialysers necessary. In this respect, γ-wet sterilised devices have an advantage over their γ-dry sterilised counterparts. +: positive aspect; -: negative aspect (adapted from [2] and [8]).*

case of γ-wet sterilisation, the membranes are wetted by introducing an aqueous solution into the blood and dialysis fluid compartments of the device prior to sterilisation. Both wet types have the advantage that sterilisation by-products or impurities can diffuse into the solution during transport and storage, and are removed with the fluid at the start of dialysis. Furthermore, pre-rinsing procedures need not be as intensive as in the case of dry dialysers, and recently a reduction in circulating microemboli (possibly air bubbles) in the subclavian vein of patients undergoing dialysis was reported with wet dialysers compared to dry dialysers [37]. On the negative side, the weight of the wet dialysers and the sensitivity of the aqueous solution to high and low temperatures often make transport and, sometimes, storage of such dialysers more expensive (i.e. frequent need for air-conditioned containers). In addition, the aqueous filling solution can constitute an additional source of contamination if not of high microbiological purity, and wet cellulose membranes sterilised by γ rays can be more susceptible to damage due to a reported significant reduction in tensile strength [6]. Although dry sterilisation is by far more common than wet sterilisation in western countries, γ wet sterilisation is the norm in Japan.

References

1. Bland LA, Favero MS: Microbiologic and endotoxin considerations in hemodialyzer reprocessing in *AAMI standards and Recommended Practices,* vol. 3 Dialysis, 2nd ed., Arlington, VA, AAMI: 293-300, 1993

2. Kümmerle W, Heilmann K, Nederlof B: Importance of sterilisation procedures for extracorporeal devices in *Blood-material interaction: A basic guide from polymer science to clinical application* edited by Falkenhagen D, Klinkmann H, Piskin E, Opatrny Jr. K, Glasgow, International Faculty for Artificial Organs (INFA): 100-105, 1998

3. Dawids S, Handlos VN: Practical aspects of sterility and medical device sterilization in *Polymers - their properties and blood compatibility,* Kluwer Academic Publishers: 347-368, 1989

4. Klinkmann H, Vienken J: Membranes for dialysis. Nephrol Dial Transplant 10 (Suppl 3): 39-45, 1995

5. Hoenich NA, Woffindin C, Ronco C: Haemodialysers and associated devices in *Replacement of renal function by dialysis,* 4th ed., edited by Jacobs C, Kjellstrand CM, Koch KM, Winchester JF, Dordrecht, Kluwer Academic Publishers: 188-230, 1996

6. Takesawa S, Satoh S, Hidai H, Sekiguchi M, Sakai K: Degradation by gamma irradiation of regenerated cellulose membranes for clinical dialysis. Trans Am Soc Artif Intern Organs 33(3): 584-587, 1987

7. Takesawa S, Ohmi S, Konno Y, Sekiguchi M, Shitaokoshi S, Takahashi T, Hidai H, Sakai K: Varying methods of sterilisation, and their effects on the structure and permeability of dialysis membranes. Nephrol Dial Transplant 1(4): 254-257, 1987

8. Vienken J: Survey on sterilization methods and associated adverse reactions. (Presentation) Dialysis Academy, Germany, April 1999

9. Landfield H: Sterilization of medical devices based on polymer selection and stabilization techniques in *Biocompatible Polymers, Metals and Composites,* edited by Szycher M, PA, Technomic Publ Inc: 975-999, 1983

10. Information brochure from Fresenius Medical Care, Germany: Sterilisation methods and selected criteria

11. Grammer LC, Patterson R: IgE against ethylene oxide-altered human serum albumin (ETO-HSA) as an etiologic agent in allergic reactions of hemodialysis patients. Artif Organs 11(2): 97-99, 1987

12. Dolovich J, Marshall CP, Smith EKM, Shimizu A, Pearson FC, Sugona MA, Lee W: Allergy to ethylene oxide in chronic hemodialysis patients. Artif Organs 8: 334-337, 1984

13. Mujais SK, Ing T, Kjellstrand C: Acute complications of hemodialysis and their prevention and treatment in *Replacement of renal function by dialysis,* 4th ed., edited by Jacobs C, Kjellstrand CM, Koch KM, Winchester JF, Dordrecht, Kluwer Academic Publishers: 688-725, 1996

14. Lemke H-D, Grassmann A, Vienken J, Shaldon S: Biocompatibility - clinical aspects in *Replacement of renal function by dialysis,* 4th ed., edited by Jacobs C, Kjellstrand CM, Koch KM, Winchester JF, Dordrecht, Kluwer Academic Publishers: 734-749, 1996

15. Lemke H-D: Mediation of hypersensitivity reactions during hemodialysis by IgE antibodies against ethylene oxide. Artif Organs 11(2): 104-110, 1987

16. Grammer LC: Hypersensitivity. Nephrol Dial Transplant 9 (Suppl 2): 29-35, 1994

17. Bommer J, Ritz E: Ethylene oxide (ETO) as a major cause of anaphylactoid reactions in dialysis (A review). Artif Organs 11(2): 111-117, 1987

18. Ing TS, Daugirdas JT: Extractable ethylene oxide from cuprammonium cellulose plate dialyzers: importance of potting compound. Trans Am Soc Artif Intern Organs 32(1): 108-110, 1986

19. Ansorge W, Pelger M, Dietrich W, Baurmeister U: Ethylene oxide in dialyzer rinsing fluid: effect of rinsing technique, dialyzer storage time, and potting compound. Artif Organs 11(2):118-122, 1987

20. Vienken J: Polymers in nephrology. Characteristics and needs. Int J Artif Organs 25(5): 470-479, 2002

21. Handlos H: Hazards of ethylene oxide sterilisation. Proceedings Concept Symposium on sterilisation procedures, Heidelberg: 90-92, 1981

22. Gavioli G, Gennari M, Bruns S: Methods of sterilization and their effects on membrane performance and safety in *Contributions to Nephrology – Hemodialysis Technology,* edited by Ronco C, La Greca G, Basel, Karger: 137: 78-84, 2002

23. Bommer J, Miltanburger HG, Hourner V, Kilian S: Cytotoxicity of γ-ray sterilised dialysis devices. (Abstract) J Am Soc Nephrol 5: 408, 1994

24. Klimentov AS, Martynenko AI, Fiodorov AL, Ershov BG: Influence of γ-radiation on the molecular-mass distribution of cellulose. Radiochem Radioanal Let 48(3-4): 137-142, 1981

25. Woolston J: Sterilisation technology choices during product design and development. Med Device Technol 12(2): 18-21, 2001

26. DeSoi CA, Umans JG: Does the dialysis prescription influence phosphate removal? Seminars in Dialysis 8(4): 201-203, 1995

27. Daka JN, Chawla AS, Hinberg I: Release of methylene dianiline from hemodialyzers under static conditions. ASAIO Abstracts 22: 91, 1993

28. Shintani H, Nakamura A: Formation of 4,4'-methylenedianiline in polyurethane potting materials by either γ-ray or autoclave sterilization. J Biomed Mater Res 25(10): 1275-1286, 1991

29. Shintani H, Nakamura A: Analysis of a carcinogen, 4,4'-methylenedianiline, from thermosetting polyurethane during sterilization. J Anal Toxicol 13(6): 354-357, 1989

30. Piento RJ., Shah MJ., Lebherz WB., Andrews AW: Correlation of bacterial mutagenicity and hamster cell formation with tumorigenicity induced by 2,4-toluenediamine. Cancer Lett 3: 45-52, 1977

31. Shanmugam K, Subrahmanyam S, Tarakad SV, Kodandapani N, Stanly DF: 2,4-Toluene diamines - their carcinogenicity, biodegradation, analytic techniques and an approach towards development of biosensors. Anal Sci 17(12): 1369-1374, 2001

32. Grammer LC, Harris KE, Shaughnessy MA, Dolovich J, Patterson R, Evans S: Antibodies to toluene diioscyanate in patients with and without dialysis anaphylaxis. Artif Organs 15(1): 2-4, 1991

33. Chanard J, Lavaud S, Lavaud F, Toupance O, Kochman S: IgE antibodies to isocyanates in hemodialyzed patients. Trans Am Soc Artif Intern Organs 33: 551-553, 1987

34. Butcher BT, Reed MA, O'Neill CE, Leech S, Pearson FC: Immunologic studies of hollow-fiber dialyzer extracts. Artif Organs 8: 318-324, 1984

35. Gogolewski S: Selected topics in biomedical polyurethanes. Colloid Polym Sci 267: 757-785, 1989

36. Gores F, Montag P, Schall C, Vienken J, Bowry SK: Verification of the chemical composition and specifications of haemodialysis membranes by NMR and GPC-FTIR-coupled spectrscopy. Biomaterials 23: 3131-3140, 2002

37. Droste DW, Beyna T, Frye B, Schulte V, Ringelstein EB, Schaefer RM: Reduction of circulating microemboli in the subclavian vein of patients undergoing haemodialysis using pre-filled instead of dry dialysers. Nephrol Dial Transplant 18: 2377-2381, 2003

Section B.
Dialyser Performance

5. Performance parameters

In clinical practice, dialysis efficiency is usually assessed by the attending physician on the basis of either Kt/V or urea reduction ratio values (URR) (see appendix for details). These measurements were traditionally conducted at regular intervals (e.g. weekly or every 1 to 4 months, whereby at least monthly assessments are generally recommended [1, 2]), but the development of sophisticated on-line clearance tools has made continuous supervision of Kt/V during each dialysis now possible [3, 4]. At the other end of the scale, predialysis blood urea nitrogen (BUN) levels are sometimes still used instead of Kt/V or URR, but with documented disadvantages [5]. Irrespective of the method employed, should an increase in dialysis efficiency be deemed judicious, then the shunt situation is critically assessed, dialysis time is extended (if practical) or blood flow is increased (if possible). If the desired increase in dialysis efficiency is still not attained, the next step is generally to exchange the dialyser for another of larger surface area, thereby increasing the urea clearance (K).

Although dialyser performance is traditionally focused on urea clearance (whereby urea is simply used as a generic low molecular weight solute for the quantification of dialysis dose), the removal of larger molecules from the blood has gained more and more attention over the past years. Generally, molecules of molecular weight below 300-500 are termed "small solutes", while there is more ambiguity concerning the classification of larger molecules into "middle molecules" and "large solutes" (e.g. [6-10]). **Table 5.1** summarises the categorisation of small, middle and large molecules used throughout this book; the range of molecular weights taken to define "middle molecules" is such that the much-discussed solute ß2-microglobulin (MW 11,818) falls into the "middle molecule" class. Recently, the European Uremic Toxin Work Group (EUTox) published a comprehensive list of all uraemic toxins known to date [10]. Of the 92 compounds identified, 68 fall into the low molecular weight range, whereby as many as 23 of these are protein-bound. Twelve toxins were of middle molecular weight, and the remaining 12 had molecular weights in excess of 15,000.

Classification	Molecular weight range
Small molecules e.g. urea (60), creatinine (113), phosphate (134)	**< 500**
Middle molecules e.g. vitamin B_{12} (1355), vancomycin (1448), inulin (5200), endotoxin fragments (1000-15,000), parathormone (9425), ß2-m (11,818)	**500 - 15,000**
Large molecules e.g. myoglobin (17,000), RBP (21,000), α1-m (26,700), EPO (30,000), albumin (66,000), transferrin (90,000)	**> 15,000**

Table 5.1: Classification of small, middle and large solutes as employed in this work. *Varying definitions are employed throughout the scientific literature, e.g. upper limits of 300 for small solutes and 12,000 for middle molecules. ß2-m: beta$_2$-microglobulin; RBP: retinol binding protein; α1-m: alpha$_1$-microglobulin; EPO: erythropoietin [6-10].*

As the dialyser coefficient of ultrafiltration (UF_{coeff}), frequently just termed "flux", characterises the "openness" of a membrane, this term is commonly used as an indication of the ability of a dialyser to remove middle molecules and large solutes, in addition to it being a measure of the dialyser hydraulic permeability. The limitations of this association will be discussed - a more reliable measure than UF_{coeff} for middle and large solute removal by a dialyser is necessary; more refined alternatives which are commonly used are sieving coefficients, percentage reductions and clearances of middle molecular marker molecules, such as vitamin B_{12}, inulin and ß2-microglobulin. An indication of dialyser impermeability for proteins which should be *retained* in the blood would also be of practical interest, i.e. for molecules of molecular weight greater or equal to that of albumin (66,000), as solutes of such sizes are effectively held back by the healthy glomerular membrane.

Surface area class	Increases in ultrafiltration coefficient	Increases in small solute clearance (urea)	Increases in middle molecule clearance (vitamin B_{12})
< 1.2 m^2	154%	47%	74%
> 1.2 m^2	133%	12%	63%

Table 5.2: Improvements in dialyser performance between 1973 and 1994. *Values result from the comparison of 23 haemodialysers with surface areas between 0.6 and 2.5 m^2 evaluated in the early 1970s and 18 dialysers with surface areas between 0.6 and 1.8 m^2 evaluated during 1993-1994. Ultrafiltration coefficients and middle molecule clearances were measured* in vitro; *small solute clearances were determined* in vivo. *Increases in creatinine clearances were similar to those shown for urea (from [11]).*

The dialyser performance data of paramount interest to the physician in everyday clinical practice are then (a) its coefficient of ultrafiltration (flux), (b) its ability to remove urea and other low molecular weight molecules normally eliminated in the urine (small solute clearance), (c) its proficiency in expelling middle molecules, and (d) its ability to retain albumin and larger substances. These performance characteristics of dialysers have changed significantly over the past 30 years. Woffindin and Hoenich summarised improvements reported in ultrafiltration coefficients, small solute clearances and middle molecule clearance between 1973 and 1994 (**table 5.2**); these developments, which have continued to today, exemplify the changing face of "standard" dialysers and the consequent varying definitions of dialyser categories regarding flux and middle molecules.

5.1 Ultrafiltration coefficients

One aim of dialysis therapy is the removal of excess water from the overhydrated dialysis patient. To achieve this, the dialysis membrane should be highly permeable for water, i.e. be of good hydraulic permeability. This is defined as the volumetric flow rate of water per unit area of membrane per unit pressure gradient (ml/min/cm^2/mmHg). Understandably, its magnitude is particularly sensitive to the "openness" of the membrane (i.e. its porosity).

In practice, however, the membrane ultrafiltration coefficient (UF_{coeff}) is used to characterise the water permeability of a dialyser: this is simply the product of the hydraulic permeability (L_h) and the surface area (A) of the membrane embedded in the particular dialyser casing, i.e.

UF_{coeff} ultrafiltration coefficient	=	L_h hydraulic permeability	·	A surface area	**[5.1]**

The ultrafiltration coefficient is so termed as it is the number which was originally used with the transmembrane pressure gradient (TMP) to yield the ultrafiltration rate (Q_F) (also called filtrate flow) during dialysis:

Q_F ultrafiltration rate	=	UF_{coeff} ultrafiltration coefficient	·	TMP transmembrane pressure gradient	**[5.2]**

Thus, a specified transmembrane pressure gradient (whether applied directly or resulting from automatic ultrafiltration control units) will trigger a filtrate flow through the membrane, and the size of this filtrate flow is dependent on the ultrafiltration coefficient of the particular membrane. The ultrafiltration rate per unit membrane area is approximately proportional to the fourth power of the mean membrane pore radius [12]. Thus small changes in pore size have large effects on the membrane UF_{coeff}.

As is clear from eqn. 5.1, the UF_{coeff} is a direct function of the membrane surface area. Consequently, the UF_{coeffs} of membranes of varying surface area can be easily compared by simply dividing the values by the effective surface area (i.e. the total membrane surface area minus the loss of area due to the presence of potting compound). As the surface area is an integral part of the definition of membrane ultrafiltration coefficient, knowledge of the ultrafiltration coefficient makes information on the surface area redundant for the attending physician, at least for fluid removal considerations (not true for solute removal and biocompatibility, see section 5.2 and chapter 8).

5.1.1 Standard values

The conditions under which ultrafiltration coefficients of dialysis membranes are measured by device manufacturers are summarised in **table 5.3**. The relationship between TMP and ultrafiltration rate is linear at relatively low TMPs for all membranes, but membrane deterioration due to blood protein and cell deposition places an upper limit on the achievable filtrate flow, as demonstrated in **figure 5.1** [18-20]. Normally, the ultrafiltration rate is measured at various different TMPs, and the dialyser UF_{coeff} is defined as the slope of the linear portion of the Q_F versus TMP curve [17]. Alternatively, some device manufacturers calculate the UF_{coeff} from the ultrafiltration rate measured at a specific TMP, i.e. according to equation 5.2. Values may vary by as much as ± 20% of that stated by the manufacturer [15]. One cause for concern in using the UF_{coeff} determined under these standardised conditions for comparison of devices is that the corresponding blood flow is not strictly specified nor, indeed, always reported in the dialyser data sheets. Traditionally, most manufacturers provide the UF_{coeff} measured at Q_B = 200 ml/min, in analogy with the stipulations for clearance measurements (section 5.2). However, dialyser characterisation using an UF_{coeff} corresponding to blood flows of 300 ml/min has become quite popular; the result is an augmented UF_{coeff} value (due to the steeper UFR vs. TMP curve as shown in **figure 5.1**), which makes the filter appear more suitable for convective therapies than competitor devices and which complicates comparison.

What are "low-flux", "high-flux" and "high-performance" dialysers?

Nowadays, classification of low-flux, high-flux and high-performance dialysers on the basis of their UF_{coeff} is less than strict. However, by convention, low-flux dialysers have low ultrafiltration coefficients, e.g. under 10 ml/h/mmHg in Europe [16, 23] and under 8 ml/h/mmHg in the United States [17]. The ultrafiltration coefficients of high-flux dialysers lie in the 8 (or 10) to > 50 ml/h/mmHg range, although higher values are stipulated by some countries or organisations (e.g. > 14 ml/h/mmHg by the American National Institute of Health hemodialysis (HEMO) study group [21], > 20 ml/h/mmHg in Germany since 2000 [22], and even > 40 ml/h/mmHg by some authors (e.g. [23])). Frequently, some specifications are imposed on high-flux devices regarding their abilities to remove ß2-microglobulin, but the commonly used definition is UF_{coeff}-based only (see section 5.3 for ß2-microglobulin removal stipulations for some high-flux dialysers).

UF_{coeff} test parameter	Standard	Exceptions observed in data sheets
Test type	*In vitro*	*In vivo*
Test medium	Blood (bovine or human)	Saline***
Concentration of test medium	Haemocrit 32 ± 2%* Protein content > 60 g/l*	Haemocrit 25%
Temperature of test medium	37 ± 1.5°C (USA) 37 ± 1°C (Europe)	
Blood flow (Q_B)#	Range given by manufacturer*	*Rarely mentioned in data sheet but information is desirable*
Dialysis fluid flow (Q_D)	0 ml/min	
Filtrate flow (Q_F)	That resulting from the set TMP	
Basis of measurement	Measurements of Q_F at various TMPs; UF_{coeff} is the slope of the linear portion of the Q_F vs. TMP curve**	Measurements of Q_F at different or at only one TMP (e.g. 50, 100 or 150 mmHg); UF_{coeff} is QF/TMP.

**European standards [13]; not specified in the USA. **German standards specify TMPs of 100, 200 and 300 mmHg [14]; this approach is only recommended where a linear relationship is found. ***Dialysis fluid was also mentioned as test medium in the literature, but was not found in data sheets. #The published UF_{coeff} is usually the value corresponding to Q_B = 200 ml/min, but this is not stipulated so that some device manufacturers report the higher values measured at Q_Bs of 300 ml/min or higher (see figure 5.1 for comparison).*

Table 5.3: Standard test conditions for the determination of dialyser ultrafiltration coefficients. *Standard conditions for the measurement of dialyser ultrafiltration coefficients (UF_{coeff}) by manufacturers as stipulated by regulatory authorities (AAMI, DIN 58352, EN 1283, ISO 8637) and exceptions as reported in individual data sheets [13-15, 17]. Measurements should be made after the dialyser membranes have been wetted (usually with dialysis fluid) for at least 10 minutes [15].*

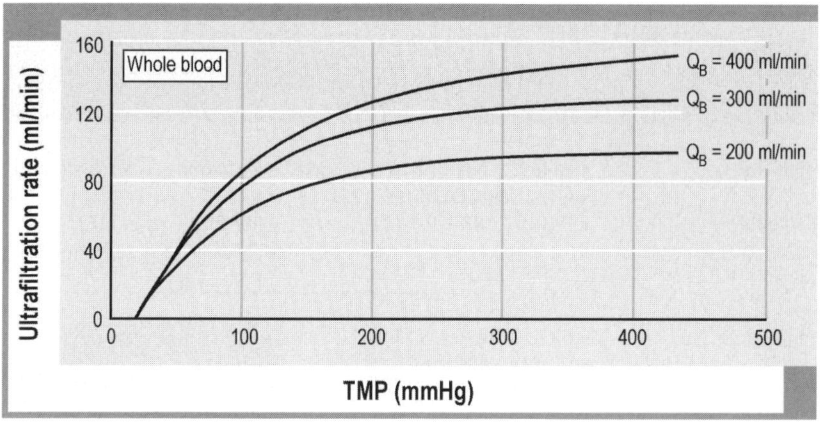

Figure 5.1: Relationship between ultrafiltration rate and transmembrane pressure at different blood flows. *The relationship between ultrafiltration rate and transmembrane pressure (TMP) is linear at relatively low TMPs for all membranes, but membrane deterioration due to protein and cell deposition places an upper limit on the achievable filtrate flow in the presence of blood or plasma [18]. Higher filtrate flows can be obtained by increasing the blood flow.*

Some dialysers are referred to as "high-performance" or "high-efficiency" – these terms are somewhat ambiguous as two to three different definitions exist: (1) for dialysers with ultrafiltration coefficients higher than those of low-flux dialysers and in the lower range of those of high-flux dialysers, i.e. generally between 10 and 20 ml/h/mmHg (Europe) or between 8 and 15 ml/h/mmHg (USA [17]); (2) for large surface area dialysers, e.g. with membrane surface areas ≥ 2 m^2 (>1.5 m^2 is also accepted in some countries, e.g. Germany [24]), as the ultrafiltration coefficient is directly related to the membrane surface area (eqn. 5.1); and (3) sometimes to characterise dialysers suitable for short-time dialysis, i.e. dialysis with high blood flows, typically around 400 ml/min [25, 26] – these can be dialysers with high ultrafiltration coefficients and/or large surface areas. **Table 5.4** shows examples of dialysers in the different UF_{coeff} categories, taking the surface areas of the dialysers into consideration.

High-flux dialysers can have ultrafiltration coefficients even greater than 50 ml/h/mmHg (e.g. the HF, HdF and some FX dialysers from Fresenius Medical Care, the APS, BLS, SYNTRA™and Polyflux series from Asahi, Bellco, Baxter and Gambro, respectively). Such devices are particularly suited for

Classification	Examples of membranes / dialysers (UF_{coeff} in ml/h/mmHg)	
High-flux 10-50 ml/h/mmHg***	• AN69® / Nephral ST 200 (33) • CTA / TRICEA 110 G (25) • PMMA / BK-1.0 P (21)	• Polyamide S™/ Polyflux 11 S (53) • PES / Bio 1000 (36) • Fresenius Polysulfone® / F 50 (30)
High-performance 10-20 ml/h/mmHg**	• CTA / FB- 90 U (17.9) • PMMA / BK-1.0 F (13) • PES / P 100 (12)	Large surface area devices ($\geq 2m^2$): • Fresenius Polysulfone® / F 10 HPS (18) • Hemophan® / HG 700 (11) • SMC® / PSN 210 (10.7)
Low-flux < 10 ml/h/mmHg*	• PES / Quartz 100 S (8.4) • PMMA / B3-1.0 A (7) • Cuprammonium rayon with PEG / AM-BIO- 500 (5.7) • EVAL® / KF 101 1.0 D5 (5.5) • Cellulose acetate / CA 110 (5.3) • Cuprophan® / NT 1175 (4.5)	• Fresenius Polysulfone® / F 5 (4.0) • Hemophan® / HAT 100 (4.0) • SMC® / NC 0985 G (2.9)

**USA: < 8 ml/h/mmHg. **USA: 8 - 15 ml/h/mmHg. ***USA: 8 - 50 ml/h/mmHg; more strict definitions are commonly used: >20 ml/h/mmHg in Germany and >14 ml/h/mmHg in the USA.*

Table 5.4: Classification of membranes / dialysers according to their ultrafiltration coefficients alone. *Examples of membranes / dialysers of comparable surface area (between 0.9 and 1.1 m^2) with ultrafiltration coefficients (shown in brackets) in the European low-flux, high-flux and high-performance ranges [17, 21, 22]. Some commonly used high-performance membranes / dialysers are only classified as such in practice as their surface areas are sufficiently high to raise the UF_{coeff} to within the defined range; examples of these are given in the dark grey box. PEG: polyethylenglycol layer; CTA: cellulose triacetate; PAN: polyacrylonitrile; EVAL®: ethylenevinylalcohol copolymer; PES: polyethersulfone; SMC®: synthetically modified cellulose; PMMA: polymethylmethacrylate. Data taken from manufacturers' data sheets.*

predominantly convective modes of blood purification, and the extreme ultrafiltration rates involved necessitate the infusion of a substitution solution ([27] for example). Nowadays, dialysers with high ultrafiltration coefficients are often also called "haemofilters" or "haemodiafilters" (rather than high-flux haemodialysers) whenever substitution fluid is required during their use.

Are the terms "high-flux" and "low-flux" interchangeable with the terms "synthetic" and "cellulosic", respectively?

Historically, the first membranes commonly used for dialysis were cellulose-based and low-flux in nature (i.e. Cuprophan®); high-flux membranes were developed later and were made from the then available synthetic materials. This sequence of development led to a perception which still lingers in part of the dialysis community, i.e. that "cellulose" and "low-flux" are interchangeable descriptions of a membrane, as are the terms "synthetic" and "high-flux". The present state of affairs is clear from **table 5.4**. The fact that cellulose-based membranes dominate in the low-flux segment for membranes of surface area between 0.9 and 1.1 m^2, and that almost all very high-flux membranes in the same surface area range are synthetic, is somewhat in keeping with this perception. However, the table also clearly shows that there is now a variety of synthetic membranes with very low ultrafiltration coefficients (e.g. EVAL®, PMMA and some low-flux polyethersulfone and polysulfone membranes), and that some cellulose-based membranes have ultrafiltration coefficients in the high-performance range and even in the pure high-flux range (e.g. cellulose triacetate membranes and higher surface area SMC® and Hemophan®).

5.1.2 *Ultrafiltration coefficients* in vivo

In vivo ultrafiltration coefficients of dialysers can differ from the published *in vitro* values for a number of reasons. One is the inexactness of the *in vitro* values stated by the manufacturer: variations between produced batches exist (e.g. deviations of ± 8-10% have been reported [28]) and values are influenced by storage conditions (e.g. temperature and humidity [29]). Consequently, variations of up to ± 20% are officially permitted [15]. Such deviations from the stated *in vitro* values will be reflected in different *in vivo* values.

Different *in vivo* ultrafiltration coefficients can also result from deviations of the patient's blood composition from that of the test medium (i.e. haematocrits and protein contents different from 32% and 60 g/l, respectively) and from factors that affect membrane hydraulic permeability and surface area.

As the blood moves through the dialyser, water is continually removed by filtration; the resultant increases in blood haematocrit and percentage plasma protein content along the length of the dialyser and as dialysis progresses are such that the plasma oncotic pressure can be augmented to an extent which reduces the membrane ultrafiltration coefficient. Furthermore, the membrane's hydraulic permeability depends on the membrane porosity (ρ); this is a function of pore number and size, but is particularly sensitive to the latter, being defined [17] as

$$\underbrace{\rho}_{\text{membrane porosity}} = \underbrace{N}_{\text{number of pores}} \cdot \pi \cdot \underbrace{r_p^2}_{\text{pore radius}} \qquad \textbf{[5.3]}$$

Therefore, treatment parameters which enhance or diminish any pore blockage will be responsible for variations in a dialyser's coefficient of ultrafiltration [12, 30]. The most notable of these are the actual filtrate flow and the blood flow. During dialysis, cell components and proteins in the patient blood assemble at the membrane surface, thereby blocking pores otherwise open to water transport (this is often referred to as membrane "deterioration" or "fouling" (e.g. [31])). When filtrate flow is high, e.g. especially during haemofiltration and haemodiafiltration, plasma protein concentrations and pore blockage can increase significantly; the oncotic pressure thus generated is opposed to the much greater forced removal of water from the patient during treatment. These effects can be minimised by increasing the blood flow: the higher blood flow increases membrane shear stress, displaces this cell component protein-cake and partly reverts the system to a hydrostatic pressure controlled regime [32]. *In vivo* coefficients of ultrafiltration may be 20-25% lower than *in vitro* values due to such variations in the oncotic pressure and in the amount of protein that is adsorbed onto the membrane [28].

While dialyser manufactures usually publish the effective membrane surface areas as measured in the dry state, surface areas change *in vivo* due to wetting of the membrane with saline, blood or dialysis fluid (e.g. swelling of hollow-fibre cellulose by 13.5% in internal diameter and 100% in wall thickness [33]). However, such changes in surface area can be ignored with respect to their effect on the membrane ultrafiltration coefficient, as standard UF_{coeff} determinations are conducted on wet membranes after allowing at least 10 minutes for swelling [15]. *In vivo* factors which affect the surface area accessible by the blood and dialysis fluid (but which are difficult to take into consideration) are the presence of clots on the blood side, air bubbles on the dialysis fluid side and channelling of blood and dialysis fluid flow: these reduce the membrane surface area available for water and solute removal and, consequently, negatively affect the membrane ultrafiltration coefficient in clinical practice. However, such losses in membrane UF_{coeff} can be minimised by appropriate anticoagulation, conscientious filling of the dialysis fluid compartment and choosing filters with good designs (i.e. designs that ensure optimal blood and dialysis fluid flow (see chapter 6)).

5.1.3 Association between ultrafiltration coefficient and solute removal

Some confusion exists concerning the relevance of the membrane's ultrafiltration coefficient in describing its solute removal capacity. By definition, the dominant solute removal mechanism in haemodialysis is diffusion – a mechanism which is driven solely by a concentration gradient across the membrane and which occurs in the absence of any transmembrane fluid motion. In contrast, solutes are removed by convection during haemofiltration, i.e. together with fluid moving along a transmembrane pressure gradient (solvent drag principle). This fluid will contain solutes in the same concentration as the plasma water - with the exception of those solutes too large to pass unhindered through the membrane. Practical haemodialysis is a mixture of diffusion and convection as the need to restore fluid homeostasis means that a TMP gradient is added on the concentration gradient (either directly, as in older machines, or indirectly via volume control units in machine with volumetric control of ultrafiltration).

In general, the degree to which convection augments total solute removal is proportional to solute molecular weight, and solute diffusivity decreases with increasing solute size [34, 35]. Therefore, the higher the ultrafiltration rate, the greater the contribution of convection to solute removal, and the more the movement of large solutes is supported. This association led to the common assumption that high ultrafiltration coefficients automatically mean good removal of middle molecules. However, this can be misleading: while the dialyser's ultrafiltration coefficient is a reliable measure of its ability to remove water, it is only an *indirect* measure of its solute removal capability. Indirect, and indeed unreliable, because it refers only to convective removal and because of ambiguity concerning the size of the solutes that can be removed. Regarding the latter, equations 5.1 and 5.3, and **figure 5.2** show us that an increase in UF_{coeff} does not necessarily reflect an increase in pore size

– it can also result from an increase in membrane surface area or pore number or a combination of all these parameters. Indeed, high UF_{coeffs} were found to be largely unrelated to high middle molecule permeability in a clinical study involving 8 common high-flux membranes [35]. Similarly, membranes with rather low ultrafiltration coefficients could possibly remove also large solutes, such as ß2-microglobulin, if the ultrafiltration coefficient is the result of few, large pores: this was thought to be the case for a particular low-flux membrane with an ultrafiltration coefficient of only 6.1 ml/h/mmHg (flat sheet Gambrane®, LunDia Pro 600 – no longer produced) which also achieved a 20-30% reduction in plasma ß2-m [17, 36, 37].

These observed dissociations between hydraulic permeability and solute permeability demonstrate the necessity for independent measures for middle and large solute removal properties of membranes, particularly high-flux membranes.

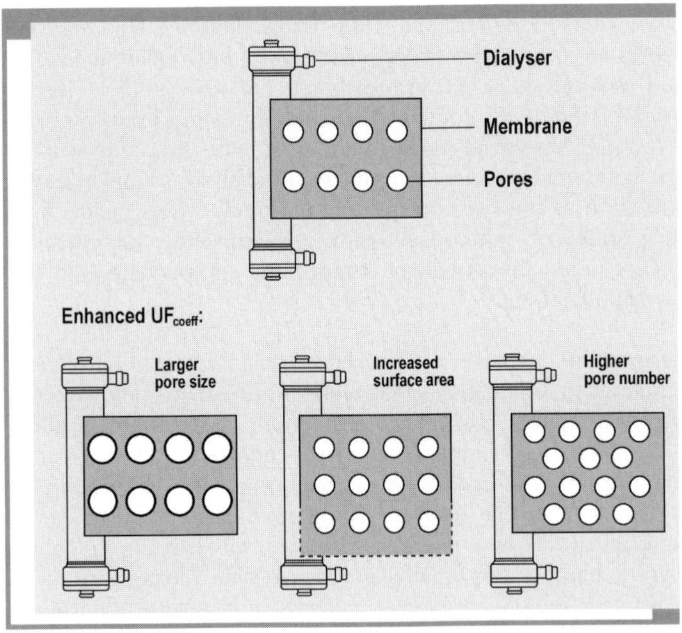

Figure 5.2: Pore size, surface area and pore number define the ultrafiltration coefficient of a dialyser. *Increasing the pore size, the membrane surface area and/or the number of pores in the dialysis membrane can enhance the ultrafiltration coefficient (UF_{coeff}).*

5.1.4 The role of the ultrafiltration coefficient in backfiltration

The phenomenon of backfiltration appeared with the advent of high-flux dialysers and gained significance due to the dangers attributed to the flux of potential contaminants from dialysis fluid to blood during treatment with this type of filter. "High ultrafiltration coefficients" and "backfiltration" have since then gone hand in hand.

The term backfiltration describes the movement of fluid from the dialysis fluid compartment into the blood compartment of the dialyser in that section of the dialyser distant from the blood inlet port. The driving force is a trans-

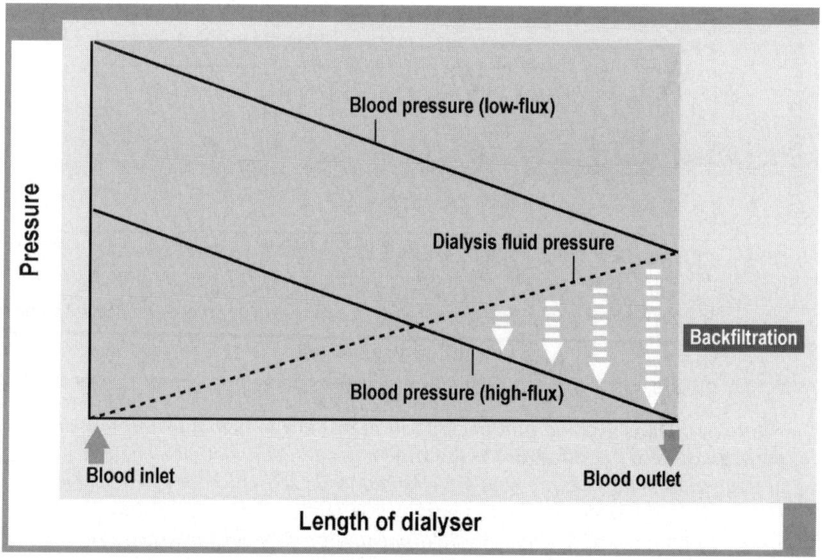

Figure 5.3: The principle of backfiltration: crossed blood and dialysis fluid pressure profiles trigger backfiltration of dialysis fluid into the blood compartment. *Due to the low hydraulic permeability of low-flux dialysers, pressure in the blood compartment is generally higher than pressure in the dialysis fluid compartment along the complete length of the dialyser, ensuring filtration of fluid from the blood. The high water permeability of high-flux dialysers means that less blood pressure is necessary to achieve fluid removal. The drop in pressure along the length of the high-flux dialyser is such that the dialysis fluid pressure exceeds the blood pressure at some point along the dialyser length. Backfiltration of dialysis fluid into the blood follows [40]. In practice, the pressure profiles are actually non-linear (see next figure).*

membrane pressure gradient, which is such that the dialysis fluid pressure is higher than the blood pressure – this is in the reverse direction of the TMP set (either manually or automatically by ultrafiltration control units) for the removal of fluid from the patient's blood. At the blood inlet port, the blood pressure will always exceed the dialysis fluid pressure, so filtration from blood to dialysis fluid occurs. However, pressures drop along the length of the dialyser (from inlet to outlet) and the blood pressure may become lower than the dialysis fluid pressure at some point in the dialyser [38, 39]. Backfiltration of dialysis fluid into blood results (**figure 5.3**).

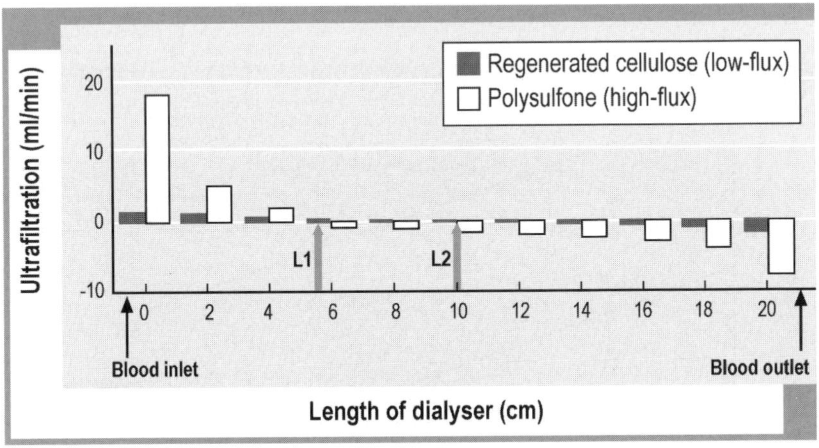

Figure 5.4: Ultrafiltration and backfiltration profiles in high-flux and low-flux dialysers at zero net filtration. *In this experimental set-up, net ultrafiltration and average transmembrane pressure were forced to be zero in order to identify positions along the dialysers where backfiltration begins. The result of this forced crossing of the blood and dialysis fluid pressure profiles (which would not normally occur during low-flux dialysis in clinical practice, as the TMPs are always positive along the length of the low-flux dialyser) is equal filtration near the blood inlet and backfiltration near the blood outlet. Total filtration and total backfiltration were 6.79 and 6.61 ml/min, respectively, for low-flux regenerated cellulose (RC), and were 30.6 and 30.9 ml/min, respectively, for high-flux polysulfone (PSu). Maximum filtration occurs near the blood inlet (0 cm) and decreases to zero at different positions along the length of the dialyser for the different membranes (L1 for PSu, L2 for RC). Backfiltration begins at these points and increases to a maximum at the blood outlet (20 cm) (adapted from [41]).*

The role played by the membrane ultrafiltration coefficient in this scenario is fairly straightforward: the higher the ultrafiltration coefficient (i.e. the more "open" a membrane is), the less TMP is necessary to instigate fluid movement across the membrane; and the lower the TMP, the more difficult it becomes to avoid crossing of the blood and dialysis fluid compartment hydrostatic pressure profiles. Such a crossing of the pressure profiles does not normally occur during low-flux dialysis, but is unavoidable during high-flux dialysis, and irrevocably results in backfiltration of dialysis fluid into patient blood during treatment.

The volume of backfiltered fluid was originally estimated from measurements of the pressure ratios at the blood and dialysis fluid ports. Now we know that these calculations overestimated the amount of backfiltration as the blood and dialysis fluid pressures do not, as was assumed, fall linearly along the length of the dialyser (**figure 5.4**). This non-linear shape of the profiles results from changes in blood viscosity, variations in fibre diameter along the length of the dialyser and the progressively greater impact of oncotic pressure as water is removed by ultrafiltration; the profiles are therefore particularly non-linear for high-flux membranes [39, 41-44].

5.2 Clearance, dialysance and K_oA

The clearance of a dialyser is defined as its volumetric rate of removal of a particular blood solute, i.e. the amount of solute removed from the blood per unit time, divided by the incoming blood concentration [45]. It can be calculated by [13, 15, 28, 46]:

$$K = Q_{Bi}((C_{Bi}-C_{Bo})/C_{Bi}) + Q_F(C_{Bo}/C_{Bi}) \quad \text{ml/min} \qquad [5.4]$$

or

$$K = Q_{Di}((C_{DFi}-C_{DFo})/C_{Bi}) + Q_F(C_{DFo}/C_{Bi}) \quad \text{ml/min} \qquad [5.5]$$

clearance = diffusive term + convective term

In the absence of adsorption, the ultrafiltration rate (Q_F) in eqn. 5.4 is given by

$$Q_F = Q_{Bi} - Q_{Bo} \qquad [5.6]$$

Q_F: ultrafiltration rate; Q_{Bi}: blood inlet flow; Q_{Bo}: blood outlet flow

The nomenclature is: K for clearance; Q for flow; C for concentration; subscripts B, DF and F for blood, dialysis fluid and filtrate, respectively; and subscripts i and o for fluids flowing into and out of the dialyser, respectively. The first parts of both equations reflect solute clearance by diffusion, while the last parts represent the convective components of solute transport - the equations are reduced to their first parts in the absence of filtrate flow. Clearance of a dialyser is mostly characterised by its diffusive clearance values alone (i.e. is measured in the absence of filtration).

Which solute clearances are generally measured?

There is widespread agreement about which solutes must be employed by manufacturers for clearance measurements on haemodialysers: regulatory authorities world-wide require data sheets to provide clearance values for urea, creatinine, phosphate and vitamin B_{12} (cyanocobalamin) - data for inulin and ß2-microglobulin is also supplied by some manufacturers for haemofilters and haemodiafilters (i.e. very high-flux dialysers used in haemofiltration and haemodiafiltration). Of all these solutes, only urea - the main nitrogenous end-product of protein metabolism - is considered in measurements of dialysis efficiency (Kt/V and Urea Reduction Ratio).

The choice of mainly low molecular weight marker solutes in haemodialysis (**table 5.5**) reflects the focus on diffusive removal in this therapy mode. However, the larger the solute, the more convection contributes to its removal. The consequence of this and, possibly, solute removal via adsorption onto the membrane, is that measurements of the diffusive clearance of larger molecules do not provide reliable information on their actual removal from the blood. Alternative measures are necessary for such molecules, such as percentage reduction or sieving coefficients (see section 5.3), but total clearances (convective plus diffusive) are also informative and are sometimes provided by dialyser manufactures for high-flux dialysers, as these target enhanced removal of such larger molecules.

Marker molecule	Molecular weight	
Urea	60	For all haemodialysers
Creatinine	113	
Phosphate	134	
Vitamin B_{12}	1355	
Inulin	5200	Only for haemofilters and haemodiafilters
ß2-microglobulin*	11,818	
Myoglobin	17,000	
Albumin	66,000	

Table 5.5: Marker molecules for dialyser and haemofilter clearance characterisation. **Generally not required by authorities.*

When is "dialysance" used instead of "clearance"?

Instead of clearance, the term dialysance (D) is sometimes employed by device manufactures; its definition is the same as that of clearance, but it applies to the special case when the concentration of a solute in the dialysis fluid entering the dialyser is greater than zero [15]. The formulae are identical to those of clearance, except that the denominators are reduced by concentrations in the incoming dialysis fluid:

$$D = Q_{Bi}((C_{Bi}-C_{Bo})/(C_{Bi}-C_{DFi})) + Q_F(C_{Bo}/(C_{Bi}-C_{DFi}))\ \text{ml/min} \quad [5.7]$$

or

$$= Q_{DFi}((C_{DFi}-C_{DFo})/(C_{Bi}-C_{DFi})) + Q_F(C_{DFo}/(C_{Bi}-C_{DFi}))\ \text{ml/min} \quad [5.8]$$

dialysance — diffusive term — convective term

Dialysance is, therefore, more appropriate than clearance in studies of the transmembrane transport of solutes which are present in *both* blood and the dialysis fluid, e.g. sodium, potassium, calcium, magnesium, chloride, buffer or glucose. It is also commonly used to compare solute removal under varying blood and dialysis fluid flow configurations (e.g. single-pass versus recirculation set-ups). However, regarding the removal of uraemic toxins from patient blood, the clinical relevance of dialysance is much reduced due to the almost exclusive use of single-pass systems in haemodialysis treatment: in such systems C_{DFi} = 0, so that clearance and dialysance are identical [28]. In dialysis fluid recirculation systems, clearance and dialysance are only identical at the very start of treatment.

Dialysance has gained in popularity in recent years as it can be easily and reliably measured using conductivity probes [1, 47-51] and this allows it to be incorporated into new technologies for on-line dialysis control. An example of such is the on-line clearance monitor (OCM) from Fresenius Medical Care: here the direct correlation between urea and sodium dialysances is utilised to determine the effective urea clearance, the dialysis dose (Kt/V) and the plasma sodium concentration on-line during dialysis [3]. Dialysance exceeds clearance: for blood values [28],

$$\underset{\text{clearance}}{K} = \underset{\text{concentration factor}}{((C_{Bi}-C_{DFi})/\,C_{Bi})} \cdot \underset{\text{dialysance}}{D} \quad \text{ml/min} \qquad \textbf{[5.9]}$$

5.2.1 Typical dialyser clearance values

From equations 5.4 and 5.5 it is obvious that solute clearance is particularly sensitive to the flows Q_B, Q_{DF} and Q_F. Thus, in order to compare the clearances of different dialysers, these must be measured under comparable, repeatable conditions. Such conditions are stipulated by national authorities, such as the AAMI in the U.S.A. and the EN 1283 in Europe. A summary of common measurement conditions for device manufacturers is given in **table 5.6**.

The fact that positive filtrate flow is a precondition for standard clearance measurements in America but not in Europe, and the fact that various filtrate flows are actually published in dialyser data sheets (see **table 5.6**), complicates a comparison of dialyser clearances for the clinic staff. **Figure 5.5** shows the ranges of diffusive clearances (Q_F = 0 ml/min) of the marker solutes for 13 low- and 7 high-flux dialysers of comparable surface area from different manufacturers, as published in official dialyser data sheets [28]. This will hopefully provide the reader with some conception of typical low and high clearance values for the individual substances. The clearance ranges shown in **figure 5.5** are mostly narrow, indicating that the different dialysers with their different membranes have relatively similar small molecule clearances. This has also been confirmed in clinical studies (e.g. [35, 52]). It is of particular interest that

Clearance test parameter	Standard	Exceptions observed in data sheets
Test type	*In vitro*	
Test medium	Dialysis fluid enriched with urea, creatinine, phosphate and vitamin B_{12}	
Concentrations of test substances#	Urea: 100 mg/dl Creatinine: 10 mg/dl Phosphate: 5 mg/dl Vitamin B_{12}: 5 mg/dl	
Temperature of test medium	37 ± 1.5°C (USA) 37 ± 1°C (Europe)	
pH of test medium	7.4 ± 0.1***	
Blood flow (Q_B)	200 ± 4* ml/min	300 ml/min
Dialysis fluid flow (Q_D)	500 ± 10* ml/min	
Filtrate flow (Q_F)	0 ml/min** (Europe)	7, 10 and 60 ml/min
	Q_Fs corresponding to a TMP of 100 mmHg (USA)	

Range from [14]. **Zero ultrafiltration is stipulated by the European norm (EN 1283) but is ignored by many dialyser producers; should measurements with zero ultrafiltration not be possible, then good standardised solutions are generally available, e.g. an ultrafiltration-corrected clearance value calculated from two different clearances (K_1 and K_2) measured at different ultrafiltration rates (Q_{F1} and Q_{F2}) according to the following: $K = K_1 - Q_{F1} \cdot ((K_2-K_1)/(Q_{F2}-Q_{F1}))$ (Germany [14]). * From [15], important for phosphate measurements. #From [14] and [15].*

Table 5.6: Test conditions for the determination of dialyser clearance values. *Standard conditions for the measurement of dialyser clearances by manufacturers, as stipulated by regulatory authorities (AAMI, DIN 58352, EN 1283, ISO 8637), together with exceptions reported in individual data sheets. Equation 5.4 is generally used to calculate clearances, whereby C_{Bi} and C_{Bo} are measured after the system has been stabilised for 10 minutes [13, 15].*

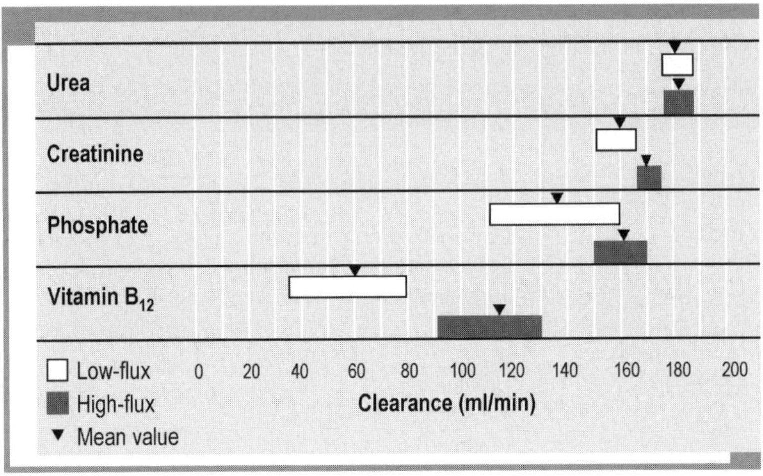

Figure 5.5: Typical* in vitro *clearance ranges of low- and high-flux dialysers. *Clearance ranges of 13 different low-flux and 7 different high-flux dialysers with surface areas between 1.3 m² and 1.35 m² are shown for standard haemodialyser marker solutes. All measurements were made under the conditions of Q_B = 200 ml/min, Q_D = 500 ml/min and Q_F = 0 ml/min. Average values are indicated by arrows (data from dialyser data sheets, see appendix).*

the range of values for phosphate in low-flux dialysers is wider than those of other solutes; indeed the long-ongoing discussion about whether particular dialysers are better phosphate removers than others has more or less closed with the consensus that the dialysis membrane alone cannot remove clinically relevant quantities of phosphate (see section 5.2.2).

How does membrane surface area affect solute clearance?

Surface areas of dialysers vary between as little as 0.3 m^2 and as much as 2.6 m^2, but most are in the 0.8 - 1.4 m^2 range [53]. As small solute clearance is achieved by diffusion, it is governed by Fick's Law (see appendix) and is, consequently, a direct function of solute diffusivity and membrane surface area. Assuming equal blood, dialysis fluid and filtrate flows, small solute clearance has been shown to increase linearly with surface area up to about 1.2 - 1.4 m^2 and to then flatten off [46]. Thus only dialysers of comparable surface areas should be used when comparing filter clearances. Alternatively, comparison of dialysers of different surface area can be conducted using formulae involving mass transfer area coefficients (KoA) (see section 5.2.3 for details of this parameter).

Augmented diffusive clearances can also be achieved nowadays with the use of thinner membranes or with dialysers of more efficient design, such that dialysis fluid flow around the individual fibres is optimised (see chapter 6 for details). Therefore, focus on surface area is considered by some to be of less significance for small solutes, which are predominately removed from patient blood by diffusion, than for larger solutes [54]. As solute size increases, solute diffusivity decreases and convection contributes more and more to total clearance. Here filtrate flow (Q_F) is all-important, and membrane surface area is an integral part thereof (eqns 5.1 and 5.2). Consequently, total clearance (i.e. diffusive plus convective clearance) of middle or large solutes is more sensitive to membrane surface area than small solute clearance at a given blood and dialysis fluid flow [55-57].

What do the dialyser data sheets reveal about in vitro phosphate clearances?

A closer look at the data sheets available reveal a wide range of phosphate clearance values for dialysers of comparable ultrafiltration coefficient and surface area *in vitro*: 101 to 160 ml/min for low-flux dialysers and 140 to 180 ml/min for high-flux dialysers of surfaces areas between 1.3 to 1.35 m^2, for example (**table 5.7**).

Membranes with a negative surface charge, such as PMMA and PAN (AN69®), tend to be at the lower end of the range of phosphate clearances. It has been postulated that this is the result of clearance-inhibiting charge interactions between the negatively charged phosphate ion and the negatively charged PMMA and polyacrylonitrile membranes (e.g. [58]). The phosphate clearance range for low-flux dialysers is topped by SMC® (partly due to the presence of fibre bundle spacer yarns which enhance phosphate clearance by about 5% [59]) and Hemophan® (which is positively charged, possibly assisting phosphate removal), while various polysulfones and cellulose triacetate are at the upper end of the high-flux range.

The kinetics of phosphate removal during clinical dialysis are more complicated than in these *in vitro* measurements: phosphate transport out of cells places a limit on the amount of phosphate accessible for removal by the dialyser during treatment (details in section 5.2.2).

Low-flux Dialysers (UF_{coeff} < 10 ml/h·mmHg)		**High-flux Dialysers** (UF_{coeff} > 20 ml/h·mmHg)	
Membrane material (manufacturer)	***In vitro* phosphate clearances (mean) (ml/min)**	**Membrane material (manufacturer)**	***In vitro* phosphate clearance (mean) (ml/min)**
Cellulose acetate (Nipro)	101*, 111 (mean **106**)	PMMA (Toray)	140*, 140* (mean **140**)
PMMA (Toray)	**121***	PAN - AN69® (Hospal/Cobe)	139*, 146* (mean **143**)
Cellulose diacetate (Nipro)	120, 138 (mean **129**)	Cellulose with PEG (Asahi)	**150**
EVAL® (Kawasumi)	125*, 134* (mean **130**)	Cellulose - Bioflux® (Membrana)	148#, 158#* (mean **153**)
Polysulfone (Fresenius Medical Care)	123, 140 (mean **132**)	Polysulfone (Minntech)	**154**
Cellulose - Cuprophan® (Membrana)	135, 139*, 139, 140, 140, 144 (mean **140**)	PAN (Asahi)	156, 174# (mean **165**)
Cellulose with PEG (Asahi)	**142**	Polyarylethersulfone - ARYLANE* (Hospal/Cobe)	**167**
Cellulose - SMC® (Membrana)	**150#**	Polysulfone (Asahi)	**170**
Cellulose - Hemophan® (Membrana)	141*, 148*, 159*, 160*, 160 (mean **154**)	Polysulfone (Fresenius)	**170**
		Cellulose triacetate (Nipro)	**175**
		Polysulfone (Toray)	179* 180* (mean **180**)

*PEG = polyethylenglycol. PAN = polyacrylonitrile. EVAL® = ethylenevinylalcohol copolymer. #Dialysers with fibre bundle spacer yarns (enhance clearance). *Measurements made at positive filtration rates.*

How relevant are diffusive clearance values?

For low-flux dialysers, diffusive clearances are reliable measures of solute clearance by diffusion. However, this is not the case for high-flux dialysers: in these, blood and dialysis fluid pressure profiles cross within the dialyser and, even when $Q_F = 0$ ml/min, both filtration of fluid from blood to dialysis fluid (so-called "internal filtration") and backfiltration of dialysis fluid into the blood compartment (so-called "internal backfiltration") always occurs; the consequence is that diffusive clearance measurements (i.e. clearances at $Q_F = 0$ ml/min) are influenced by this internal filtration and backfiltration and the effect thereof on solute concentration profiles within and along the membrane [60]. Measurement of the magnitude of this effect is complicated, so this aspect is generally neglected altogether. However, the ambiguity it introduces into diffusive clearance measurements of high-flux dialysers makes the measurement of total clearances ($Q_F > 0$ ml/min) appear more attractive.

As the diffusion rate of solutes is inversely proportional to the square root of the solute molecular weight, there is also some concern that measurements of the pure diffusive clearances of solutes the size of vitamin B_{12} and inulin are of limited practical value [34, 35]. However, in contemporary dialysis with high flows and thinner membranes, there is sufficient data available which proves that diffusion is still by far the dominant mode of removal for these solutes and also for the potential vitamin B_{12} substitute for *in vitro* investigations, vancomycin (see next paragraph) [17, 60-62]. On the other hand, the contribution of convection to total solute removal increases with increasing molecular size and, although it is not dominant for these solutes, it is indeed significant [60]. In clinical practice, filtration is an integral part of both low-and high-flux dialysis, so that some dialyser manufactures, and indeed regulatory authorities (e.g. the AAMI in the USA [15]), prefer to supply

Table 5.7:* In vitro *phosphate clearances of various low- and high-flux membranes according to data sheets. In vitro *phosphate clearance values from the data sheets of 9 low-flux (UF_{coeff} < 10 ml/h/mmHg) and 11 high-flux (UF_{coeff} > 20 ml/h/mmHg) hollow-fibre dialysers of 1.3 or 1.35 m^2 surface area. Only values measured at blood flows of 200 ml/min and dialysis fluid flows of 500 ml/min were considered. As phosphate is predominately removed from blood by diffusion, measurements at a variety of filtrate flows were included in the analysis (i.e. Q_Fs of 0 or 10 ml/min, or those corresponding to a TMP of 100 mmHg). However, an asterisk indicates measurements made at positive filtration rates as phosphate removal is known to be enhanced by this factor.* In vivo *clearances differ (also section 5.2.2).*

total clearance measurements conducted under defined filtration conditions rather than diffusive clearances alone.

Although the diffusive clearance of vitamin B_{12} is frequently used as a marker for middle molecule removal, its relevance for the *clinical* assessment of dialyser performance is further reduced by the fact that it cannot be measured with whole blood or *in vivo* due to its extensive binding to plasma proteins [17]. The search for alternative middle molecule surrogates is ongoing, as there is some evidence that the loss of appetite common in uraemic patients is mediated by retention of molecules of similar molecular weight [63]. Vancomycin, an antibiotic commonly used in acute and chronic renal failure, has been employed with success as such a middle molecule surrogate [17, 62]. This has a molecular weight of 1449, low protein binding and a small distribution volume [64, 65]. Therefore, diffusive clearance of vancomycin could be employed as an alternative to vitamin B_{12} diffusive clearance in dialyser tests.

In summary, diffusive clearances are more clinically relevant and informative for small solutes and low-flux membranes than for middle molecules or large solutes and high-flux membranes. Consideration of the contribution of convection to net removal by high-flux membranes would be preferable for membrane data sheets in the future.

What about total clearance measurements for middle molecules and high-flux membranes?

The discussed short-comings of pure diffusive clearance for high-flux membranes and for solutes larger than approximately 500 makes the use of *total* clearance measurements (i.e. diffusive plus convective clearances, $Q_F \neq 0$ in eqn 5.4) for middle molecules (500 - 15,000) meaningful. American authorities presently recommend that *all* clearance measurements be conducted at a TMP of 100 mmHg – the Q_F in eqn. 5.4 is then given by the product of this TMP and the dialyser's ultrafiltration coefficient. Some companies provide such clearance values for a selection of their dialysers, e.g. Asahi, Baxter, Gambro, Hospal (just for vitamin B_{12}), Idemsa, Kawasumi, Nikkiso, Teijin, Terumo and Toray. Some of these and other companies supply total clearance information from measurements made at defined ultrafiltration rates (Q_F) - usually 10 ml/min (e.g. Baxter, Bellco, Hospal, Kawasumi, Nikkiso, Terumo and Toray). Other Q_Fs reported in dialyser data sheets for total clearance measurements are 7 ml/min (Baxter) or 60 ml/min (Fresenius Medical

Care for the very high-flux haemofilters HF80 (S) and HDF 100S). These values are of limited clinical significance as actual ultrafiltration rates and TMPs vary widely from patient to patient and indeed from dialysis to dialysis, but they support device comparison to a certain extent.

A common definition of low- and high-flux membranes in the USA specifies a limit for ß2-m clearance as well as ultrafiltration coefficient: high-flux dialysis membranes and haemofilters should have total ß2-m clearances of > 20 ml/min during first use together with high UF_{coeffs} (i.e. > 14 ml/h/mmHg), as measured under the standard conditions employed in the USA (**tables 5.3** and **5.6** [21]). However, *in vitro* values of ß2-m clearance are very rarely supplied in dialyser data sheets - membrane ultrafiltration coefficients and vitamin B_{12} clearances, although insubstantial measures for middle molecule removal, are the parameters commonly employed in practice. Recently, a more reliable alternative to these - the membrane sieving coefficient for ß2-m - has gained acceptance by both dialyser producers and the medical community. This will be discussed in section 5.3.

5.2.2 Dialyser clearance in vivo

Standard dialyser clearances measured *in vitro* using aqueous solutions are generally higher than those measured using blood under otherwise identical conditions. This is because only a fraction of the blood is available for solute removal during its passage through the dialyser, as cells and plasma proteins occupy space, and because, depending on the cell permeability for individual solutes, the distribution space of some solutes is compartmentalised.

Predicted and measured changes in urea clearance *in vitro* as a function of blood haematocrit are shown in **figure 5.6** [66]. In the range of clinically relevant haematocrit values (approx. 20 to 40%), the decrease in urea clearance is only 5%. Similar insignificant reductions over this range were measured in other studies (e.g. [67, 68]). This slight loss of urea clearance can be compensated by increasing the blood flow by 5 - 10% or by increasing the membrane area [66].

However, urea is highly diffusible across red blood cell membranes so that a uniform distribution in a single compartment can be assumed [69]. This is not so for all solutes. There is a concentration gradient between red cells and

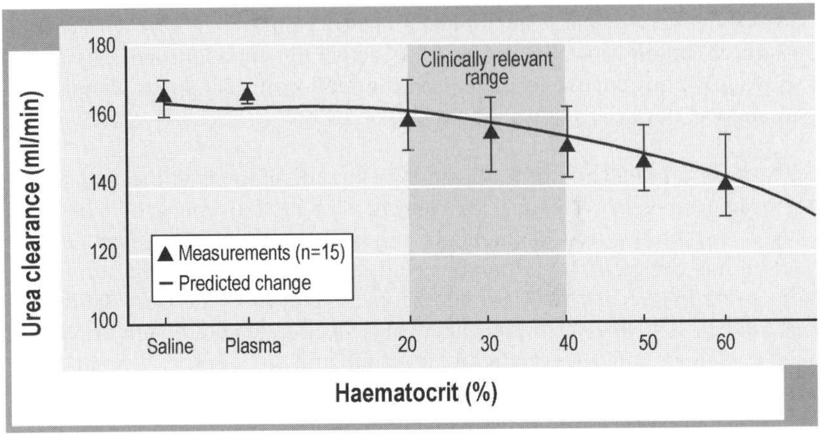

Figure 5.6: Predicted and measured changes (*in vitro*) in urea clearances with increasing haematocrit. *The continuous line depicts changes in urea clearance predicted by a model which incorporates blood, membrane and dialysis fluid side resistances. Experimentally obtained values (plus standard deviations) are plotted for measurements performed in saline, plasma and whole fresh human blood at serial haematocrits of 20%, 30%, 40%, 50% and 60% on 5 low-flux Cuprophan® dialysers in each series. The decrease in clearance in the clinically relevant range of 20% to 40% haematocrit is only 5%. This range is even narrower for dialysis patients (30 - 35%) (adapted from [66]).*

plasma for solutes which diffuse more slowly across the erythrocyte membrane, and clearance of these solutes will be more negatively affected by haematocrit increases than the clearance of urea [67]. This has been demonstrated *in vivo* for creatinine [67]. Morcos and Nissenson derived a correction factor for Q_B which considers the impact of haematocrit on the clearance of such solutes, and of solutes for which the red blood cell membrane is impermeable and which are distributed exclusively in plasma water (e.g. inulin, ß2-microglobulin) [70]. For the latter, precise calculations of clearance should use plasma flow (Q_P) instead of blood flow (Q_B). The situation for creatinine and, especially, phosphate is more complicated: the red cell membrane resistance is such that some creatinine and phosphate will diffuse from the cells into the plasma during blood passage through the dialyser - the effective flow for clearance calculations is then between Q_P and Q_B [71]. However, corrections to Q_B are not routinely applied in practice, even when indicated. In fact, it is common clinical practice to mix solute plasma concentrations with blood flows in clearance calculations [72].

In vivo, low- and high-flux membranes have comparable small solute clearances (i.e. urea and creatinine) under conditions of similar haematocrit, predialysis plasma solute levels, dialyser surface area and blood, dialysis fluid and filtrate flows (e.g. [35-37, 52, 56, 73, 74]). Creatinine clearances are typically around 80-90% of urea clearances. Although the *in vivo* clearances of dialysers are lower than the equivalent *in vitro* values (e.g. by 7% for urea [28, 75]), use of blood flows higher than 200 ml/min can easily mask such differences.

What about phosphate clearance in vivo?

Phosphate partitioning in the body is complex (e.g. [69, 76-78]), and *in vivo* dialyser phosphate clearances appear to vary more than those of other uraemic toxins (both between dialysers and intradialytically), despite the clearances being proportional to the very low plasma phosphate level [69, 79-81]. As already mentioned in section 5.2.1, *in vitro* data suggest some membrane-specific trends regarding phosphate clearance, i.e. (1) negatively charged membranes (PMMA, AN69®/PAN) have low clearances, (2) for the low-flux membranes, SMC® and Hemophan® have the best phosphate clearance and cellulose acetate the worst, and (3) various polysulfones and cellulose triacetate appear to be superior high-flux membranes in this respect. These *in vitro* trends in the low-flux dialyser case were only partially seen *in vivo*. For example, the low-flux PMMA (Toray) membrane was found to be less effective in removing phosphate than a regenerated cellulose (Cuprophan®, Membrana/Gambro) membrane in two *in vivo* studies, under conditions of comparable predialysis plasma levels, dialysis times and dialyser surface areas [36, 37]. Two other *in vivo* studies, comparing 6 and 4 low-flux membranes, reported a high phosphate removal with Hemophan® and lower values for cellulose acetate, but these differences failed to reach statistical significance [73, 82]. Regarding the high-flux membranes, clinical investigations found no statistically significant differences in phosphate removal [69, 77].

Whether particular membranes are really more efficient phosphate removers than others in their clinical application is actually of more academic than practical interest: only a daily average of 250 - 325 mg of phosphate can be removed from a mild to moderately hyperphosphataemic patient by standard 3-5 hour, thrice-weekly haemodialysis or haemodiafiltration, while an adequate diet already provides about 500 - 900 mg of phosphate daily [83]. Control of plasma phosphate levels is more efficiently achieved by dietary compliance and the use of oral phosphate binders [76]. Standard dialysis prescriptions can at best only constitute an additional small removal as dialytic removal is known to be effective only in the initial phase of the dialysis session; after that, the slow transfer rate for phosphate from the intracellular space to the plasma becomes the rate-limiting factor, and there is a rebound phenomenon 1 - 2 hours after the end of dialysis [77, 78, 84]. It is, therefore, not surprising that more frequent treatments, or possibly long slow treatments that give phosphate time to move from the intracellular to the extracellular compartment, will go further towards enhancing phosphate removal than standard 4-hour dialyses [69, 78, 85-88].

In addition, phosphate clearance has been shown to be more sensitive to the ultrafiltration rate and the dialyser surface area than creatinine or urea clearances, as indicated in **figure 5.7** for surface area changes [35, 57, 81, 89]. In fact, one group reported that the use of aluminium-based phosphate binders could be totally avoided by switching to dialysers with larger surface

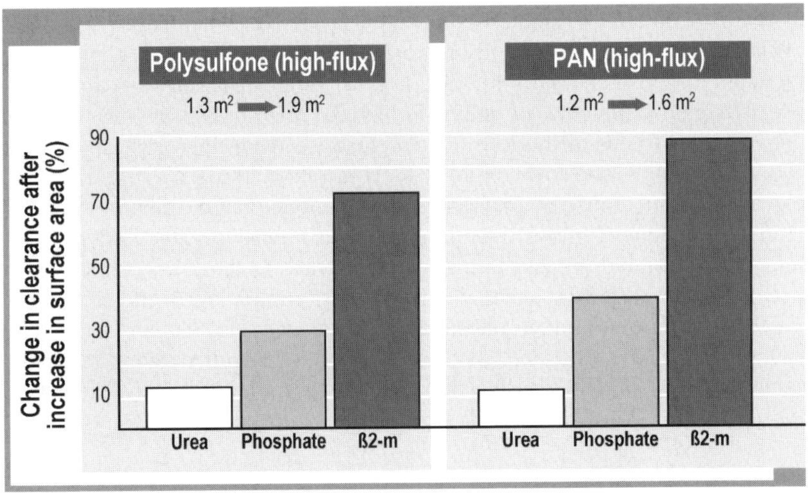

Figure 5.7: Effect of surface area on phosphate, urea and ß2-m clearances. *Clearance measurements were conducted at zero ultrafiltration on two high-flux dialysers (Fresenius Polysulfone® and AN69®) of two different surface areas each in vivo. Comparison with measurements of urea clearances reveal that phosphate clearance is more sensitive to increases in membrane surface area than is clearance of the smaller molecule urea. The surface area effect is even more pronounced for the larger molecule ß2-m (adapted from [35]).*

areas (1.7 m^2 vs. 1.4 m^2) and increasing the blood flow by 13%, but keeping the dose of calcium-based phosphate binders constant [89]. The results depicted in **figure 5.7** for the larger molecule, ß2-m, indicate that this is probably due to the enhanced contribution of convection (filtration or "internal filtration" in high-flux membranes) with increasing molecular weight. Therefore, in addition to more frequent and/or longer dialysis treatments, dialytic removal of phosphate can be improved by the use of larger surface area dialysers. The sensitivity of phosphate to convective transport casts doubt on the reliability of diffusive clearance measurements even for this small solute. Indeed, it is debatable whether the distribution space of phosphate and its intra- to extracellular transfer rate makes even total clearance an acceptable measure for the removal of this solute - other parameters (e.g. total solute extraction or mass transfer) may be more appropriate, although these too have their limitations [56, 77, 84, 85].

What about middle molecule clearance in vivo?

Vitamin B_{12} clearance, although commonly used as a marker for middle molecule removal, cannot be measured reliably *in vivo* due to its extensive binding to plasma proteins [17]. Alternatives, such as vancomycin, are currently under investigation.

In vivo clearances of ß2-m for dialysers defined as low-flux on the basis of their ultrafiltration coefficients alone are, as a rule, generally negligible, being below 10 ml/min (e.g. 3.1 ± 11 and 1.7 ± 11.3 ml/min for low-flux cellulose acetate (CA 210) and low-flux polysulfone (F8), respectively [21]). Clearances by high-flux dialysers vary considerably, being highly sensitive to the membrane pore size, the degree to which ß2-m is adsorbed by the membrane, the membrane surface area and the treatment mode chosen (i.e. haemodialysis, haemodiafiltration or haemofiltration). Whether or not the contribution of convection to clearance is taken into consideration greatly affects values for middle and large molecules [35, 90]. Values for membranes made from very similar materials (e.g. polyacrylonitrile) even differ significantly [35], and clearances also tend to change during the course of treatment.

Figure 5.8 shows ß2-m total clearances measured during the course of dialysis using two high-flux membranes: PMMA, which has a high adsorptive capacity for ß2-m, and polysulfone. The 65% decline in clearance for PMMA and 19% decline for polysulfone from 30 to 180 minutes of treatment result from membrane deterioration due to adsorption of blood proteins onto the

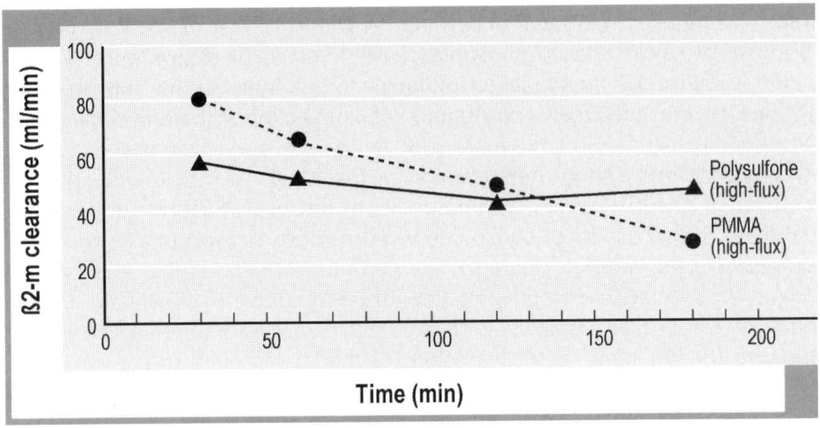

Figure 5.8: Changes in the ß2-m clearances of two high-flux membranes during the course of dialysis. In vivo *ß2-m clearances with high-flux Fresenius Polysulfone® (Hemoflow F80, 1.8 m²) decreased by 19% between 30 and 180 minutes of treatment, while those with high-flux PMMA (BK-2.1P, 2.1 m²) fell by 65%. Loss of clearance is due to the adsorption of blood proteins by the membranes. Dialysis conditions: Q_B = 300 ml/min, Q_D = 500 ml/min and Q_F varied according to clinical indications (adapted from [91]).*

surface and into the pore structure of the high-flux membranes [91]. These *in vivo* results reveal that, although total clearance is an advance over pure diffusive clearance for middle molecules and high-flux membranes, *in vitro* total clearance measurements using aqueous solutions will but poorly reflect the true middle molecule removal ability of such membranes. Alternative approaches to measuring the ability of a dialyser to remove middle molecules are available; these will be addressed in section 5.3. At present, it appears that knowledge of the specific characteristics of each membrane (such as its ultrafiltration coefficient and the extent to which it can adsorb ß2-m) is necessary to choose the appropriate method for determining its middle molecule performance *in vivo*.

How does recirculation affect in vivo clearances?

Even solute clearances that are determined using blood can differ from those measured in the actual clinical situation, due to the effects of cardiopulmonary and access recirculation. Recirculation reduces the solute concentration of the blood entering the dialyser, and thus diminishes solute elimination. The reducing effect of access recirculation on clearance is more pronounced for small molecules, as shown schematically in **figure 5.9** ([71], also [28, 92]). Gotch derived a correction factor for *in vivo* clearance which allows consideration of blood recirculation in fistula, needles and blood tubing [92]. Recirculation is often considered a deterrent to using high blood flows, but even in stenotic accesses the urea clearance is enhanced significantly by increasing the blood flow [93]. Nonetheless, careful testing must be done to ensure that the level of recirculation does not unacceptably compromise dialysis efficiency.

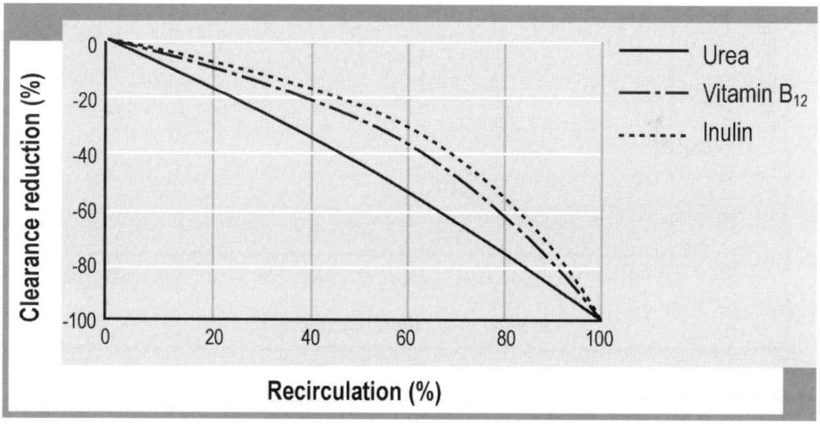

Figure 5.9: Effect of recirculation on solute clearance during dialysis. *Blood recirculation in the dialyser due to access problems will result in a decrease in solute clearance, particularly small molecule clearance (with permission from [71]).*

5.2.3 Effect of flow conditions on dialyser clearance – the K_oA concept

As is obvious from the equations for clearance shown at the start of this chapter, solute clearance is a direct function of blood flow and dialysis fluid flow and, in the case of simultaneous ultrafiltration, also filtrate flow. These are fixed at predefined values in *in vitro* measurements for the characterisation of dialyser performance, but vary *in vivo* according to the particular clinical situation. The manner in which these influence dialyser clearance is described in the following.

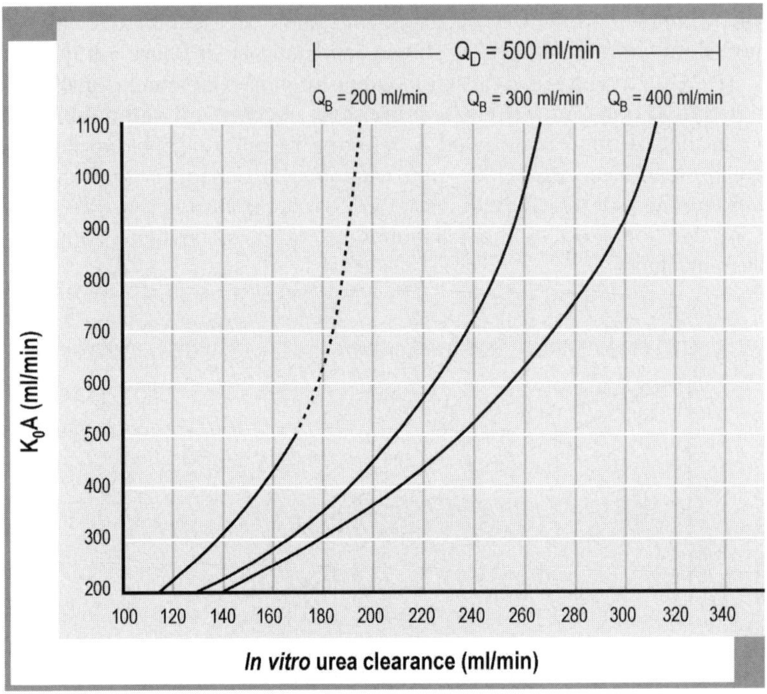

Figure 5.10: Nomogram of relationship between mass transfer area coefficient (K_OA) and* in vitro *urea clearance. *K_OA was calculated from clearances reported in manufacturer's data sheets using eqn. 5.10 under varying blood flows and, in this case, a fixed dialysis fluid flow (Q_D) of 500 ml/min. To use, find the urea clearance on the x-axis, rise vertically to the appropriate blood flow curve (Q_B), and read the corresponding K_OA off the y-axis. The 200 ml/min blood flow curve should not be used for clearances above 170 ml/min (adapted from [95]).*

K_OA stands for "mass transfer area coefficient"; it is a measure of dialyser performance which enables one to estimate clearances of a dialyser under various flow conditions. The standard formula for this extension of the pure diffusive clearance concept for urea (Q_F = 0 ml/min) is that published by Sargent and Gotch [94]:

K_OA	=	$[Q_B/(1-Q_B/Q_D)]$	·	$\ln[(1-K/Q_D)/(1-K/Q_B)]$	**[5.10]**
mass transfer area coefficient		blood and dialysis fluid factor		flow-adapted *in vitro* urea clearance factor	

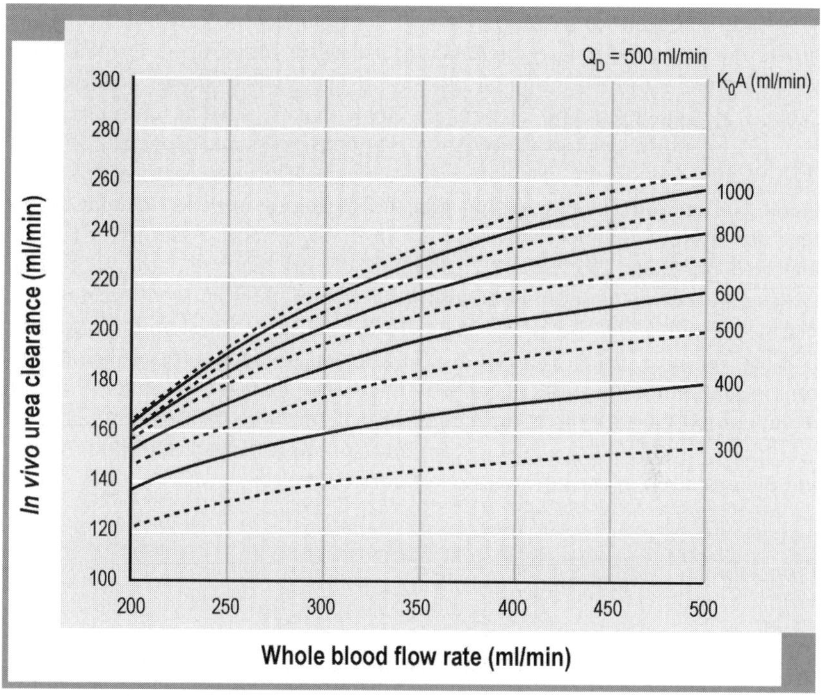

Figure 5.11: Nomogram for estimation of the* in vivo *urea clearance from the dialyser mass transfer area coefficient (K_0A). *In this nomogram, estimation of* in vivo *urea clearances is based on a dialysis fluid flow (Q_D) of 500 ml/min, the nominal blood flow, and the K_0A calculated from eqn. 5.10 or read from the nomogram in figure 5.10. To use, find the relevant blood flow on the x-axis, rise vertically to the appropriate K_0A curve, and read the corresponding estimate of the* in vivo *clearance off the y-axis. The* in vivo *estimations are based on a wide range of assumptions and corrections (see text for details) (adapted from [95]).*

Alternatively, K_0A can be read from a clearance versus K_0A nomogram computed from the *in vitro* clearances published by the dialyser manufacturer (e.g. **figure 5.10** for urea, a Q_D of 500 ml/min, and specified Q_B values). In addition to taking the blood and dialysis fluid flows into account, K_0A has another advantage over clearance measurements: it allows easy comparison of the solute removal characteristics of dialysers of different sizes. To do this, the K_0A values must simply be divided by the individual dialyser surface areas (A).

Using a number of assumptions and corrections, one can use K_0A to estimate the expected *in vivo* clearance of a dialyser based upon the known *in vitro* clearance and the nominal blood and dialysis fluid flows. This was described by Daugirdas and Depner in 1994, making specific corrections to, first, Q_B for errors related to negative prepump pressure, especially at Q_B > 200 ml/min, then to the calculated clearances to allow for the effect of blood water content and, finally, to this adjusted clearance in order to take the effect of cardiopulmonary recirculation into consideration. Assumptions made included particular blood pump calibration errors, an haematocrit of 30%, effective urea distribution volumes of 0.80 and 0.93 in erythrocytes and plasma, respectively, use of an arteriovenous access, a systemic blood flow (cardiac output - fistula blood flow) of 4 l/min, no access recirculation, and no loss of membrane surface area due to protein coating or clotting [95]. The *in vivo* urea clearances thus estimated for dialysers with various K_0A values at blood flows ranging from 200 to 600 ml/min and a dialysis fluid flow of 500 ml/min are given in the nomogram in **figure 5.11**.

Blood flow

The relationship between blood flow and clearance is curvilinear, i.e. the increase in clearance levels off at high blood flows. With modern dialysers, significant clearance increases have been shown with Q_B values of up to 600 ml/min [93]. **Figure 5.12** demonstrates the effect of increasing the blood flow on the total clearances of urea and the much larger middle molecule inulin (MW 5200) at 2 different ultrafiltration rates. The enhancing effect of blood flow on clearance appears to level off at lower blood flows for solutes the size of inulin; this is because the contribution of convection to total clearance increases as molecular size increases, and convective clearance is less sensitive to changes in blood flow (see eqns. 5.5 and 5.6) than to changes in other parameters, e.g. filtrate flow and surface area [55, 97].

K_0A was long considered to be constant, i.e. independent of blood and dialysis fluid flow and, indeed, no significant changes in urea K_0A during clinical use were observed by Ouseph and Ward upon increasing Q_B from 300 to 400 ml/min [98]. However, significant increases in dialyser K_0A for urea, creatinine and phosphate were reported when the blood flow was increased from 200 to 300 ml/min during clinical dialysis [45]. These results possibly indicate that blood flows of 300 ml/min or higher are necessary to ensure homogeneity of blood flow in the capillaries and/or an effective reduction of the blood-membrane stagnant layer.

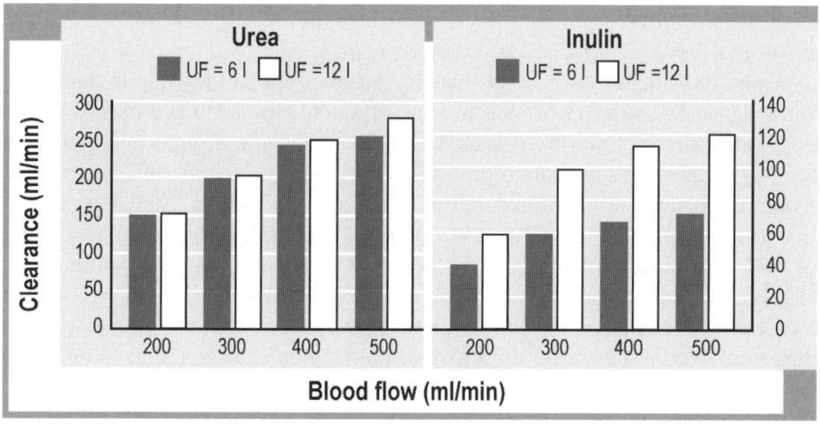

Figure 5.12: Influence of blood flow and ultrafiltration on small and large molecule clearances. *The effects of 4 different blood flows and of 2 different ultrafiltration volumes on the* in vitro *urea and inulin clearances of a high-flux polysulfone dialyser (F60 from Fresenius Medical Care) are depicted (adapted from [96]).*

Nowadays blood flows higher than the 200 ml/min stipulated by regulatory authorities to characterise dialyser clearance can be readily attained due to developments in access surgery and equipment, e.g. the Cimino Brescia shunt, implantation of prosthetic grafts, individual needle size and type, and larger temporary or permanent implantable, double lumen central venous catheters. Consequently, a Q_B of 300 - 450 ml/min is not uncommon and values even up to 600 ml/min are sometimes (albeit rarely) used, especially in modern high-flux and high-efficiency dialysis and in ultra-high-efficiency dialysis aiming to shorten treatment time [28, 93, 99, 100]. However, use of high blood flows can increase the risk of recirculation if the vascular access is problematic, and is not recommended for some patient groups due to the danger of inducing a disequilibrium syndrome, e.g. children, elderly and diabetic patients, and patients with severe acidosis and/or high urea levels [93]. The decision on which blood flow to use will then depend on the type of dialysis being performed (e.g. high-efficiency), on the quality of the vascular access, and on the ability/inability of the patient to tolerate higher blood flows.

Dialysis fluid flow

Early investigations showed that the optimal choice of dialysis fluid flow with regard to solute clearance is approximately twice the blood flow – values higher than $2{\cdot}Q_B$ were long believed to have only a slight enhancing effect on small solute clearance [55, 76, 101]. More recent *in vitro* and *in vivo* work has proven the positive effect of increasing dialysis fluid flow to between $2{\cdot}Q_B$ and $3{\cdot}Q_B$ on solute clearance [98, 102-104]. For example, at a Q_B of 300 ml/min, increasing Q_D from 500 to 800 ml/min results in an increase in K_oA (originally believed to be fixed for each dialyser) and, consequently, an increase in small solute clearance. It was postulated that the higher dialysis fluid flow (a) decreases the thickness of the stagnant dialysis fluid layer at the outer membrane surface, thus reducing the total membrane-associated resistance to solute movement and (b) acts to more equally distribute flow around the hollow fibres in bundles which do not already have spacer yarn or wave structure, thus yielding a larger effective membrane surface area [98]. The consequence is that use of dialysis fluid flows higher than the traditional 500 ml/min have been recommended to optimise dialyser performance [104]. Many modern dialysis machines offer a choice of Q_D of 300, 500 or 800 ml/min.

Increasing dialysis fluid flow to over 2 times the blood flow means more dialysis fluid concentrate is required per dialysis, and thus increases the cost of treatment. Recent developments in dialyser design improve the distribution of dialysis fluid around the individual fibres and hinder the formation of stagnant fluid layers; use of such designs could well have the same beneficial effect on solute clearance as increasing the dialysis fluid flow above twice the blood flow. These developments are discussed in chapter 6.

Filtrate flow

When $Q_F \neq 0$, as is the case for clearances published by many manufacturers, a mixture of diffusive and convective transport across the dialysis membrane occurs. These two mechanisms of solute removal interfere with each other continually; for example, convection causes an accumulation of membrane-impermeable solutes at the membrane surface, thus affecting concentration gradients for diffusion and diffusion lengths, and diffusion changes local solute concentrations, consequently affecting their net convective transport. It is therefore difficult to specify the exact contribution of convection (filtrate flow) to net dialyser solute clearance. However, filtrate flow will certainly have a greater effect on large solutes, which do not diffuse easily, than on smaller solutes. A number of groups have published theoretical calculations of the contribution of filtrate flow to total solute clearance (e.g. [60, 105]). Actual *in vitro* measurements are shown in **figure 5.12**; this also shows that the higher the blood flow, the greater the influence of Q_F on the clearance of middle molecules. Filtrate flow is limited by the blood flow (eqn. 5.6) and the degree of membrane fouling (i.e. loss of membrane permeability due to pore blockage).

Comparison of strict haemodialysis (with Q_F = 0 ml/min for clearance measurements), haemofiltration (where Q_D = 0 ml/min) and haemodiafiltration (with both Q_D and Q_F > 0 ml/min) also provides insight into the roles of flows in clearance measurements. **Figure 5.13** is a schematic diagram of the corresponding clearances as a function of solute molecular weight [106]. Haemofiltration is a pure convection based technique, as is reflected in the poor clearance of small solutes compared to haemodialysis. As haemodiafiltration combines the good diffusive removal of low molecular weight solutes with the good convective removal of larger solutes, clearance values for all solutes are generally higher than in haemodialysis. Comparing HDF and HD, the improvement in clearance of very low molecular weight solutes due to

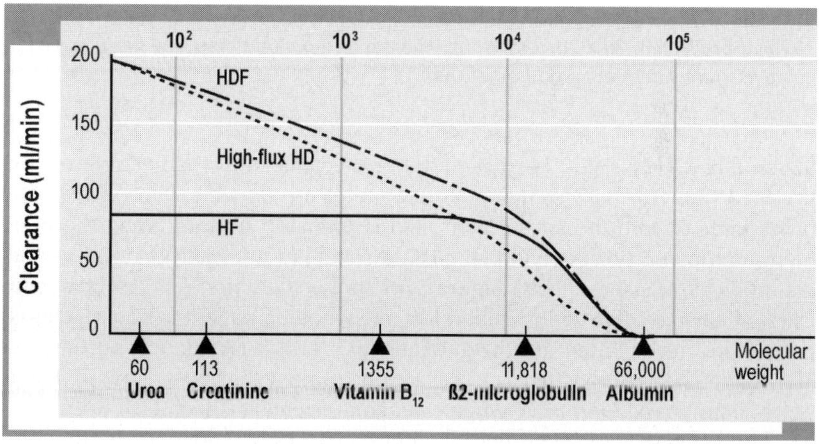

Figure 5.13: Schematic diagram of the clearances achieved with different dialysis therapies. *Clearance is presented as a function of molecular weight for haemodialysis (HD), conventional haemofiltration (HF) and haemodiafiltration (HDF) therapies using high-flux membranes (F60 - Fresenius Polysulfone®) (adapted from [106]).*

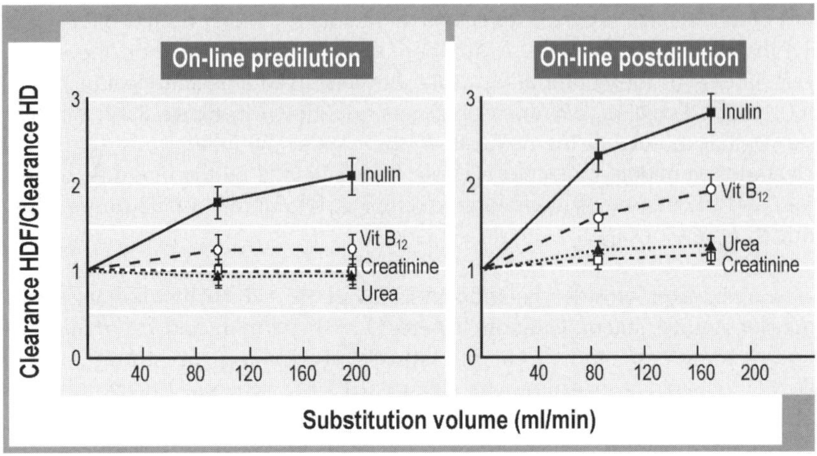

Figure 5.14: Differences in clearances between haemodialysis and on-line haemodiafiltration treatment modes. *In vitro clearances of small, middle and large solutes measured during haemodiafiltration (HDF) using a high-flux polysulfone membrane (F60) are divided by the corresponding measurements made during haemodialysis (HD). Blood and dialysis fluid flows were 200 and 800 ml/min, respectively. The resultant HDF/HD clearance ratios only exceed 1 when clearance by HDF is higher than that by HD. Both pre- and postdilution HDF approaches are shown; postdilution HDF yields higher clearance values than predilution HDF (provided that haemoconcentration does not cause problems in the filter) (adapted from [109]).*

filtrate flux is only slight, as expected, but is significant for larger solutes (**figure 5.13** [20, 106, 107]). Higher filtration rates are possible with *on-line* HDF procedures (where the substitution fluid is prepared on-line during the treatment) compared to conventional HDF, resulting in a further increase in middle molecule transport [109]. **Figure 5.14** shows that the clearance characteristics of on-line HDF differ depending on whether patient blood is diluted before or after it enters the haemofilter (pre- and postdilution approaches). These and other studies (e.g. [109, 110]) document that post-dilution HDF is better than pre-dilution HDF when targeting maximal clearance of both small and large solutes. However, the inherent danger of haemoconcentration and subsequent membrane clogging with proteins in postdilution procedures can cause a reduction in clearances, so that this advantage may be lost.

5.3 Specific measures for the removal of middle molecules

The shortcomings of using *in vitro* ultrafiltration coefficients and standardised clearance measurements (i.e. at zero or small filtrate rates) to describe the ability of a modern membrane/dialyser to remove middle molecules from patient blood led to the search for other measures. The most commonly used alternatives are the membrane sieving coefficient (SC) and the percentage reduction over a complete dialysis session (PR) in plasma levels of marker molecules. The absolute amount of solute removed by the dialyser *in vivo* is sometimes (but rarely) measured in this context. These specific approaches to characterise middle molecule removal by filters will be discussed and critically compared.

Although vitamin B_{12} and inulin are middle molecules according to the definition used in this work and many others, attention over the past 2 decades have been focused on the particular middle molecule ß2-m (11,818), which has a molecular weight at the upper end of the middle molecule range (see **table 5.1**). The reason for this is its probable involvement in the devel-

Dialyser type	UF_{coeff} (ml/h/mmHg)	ß2-m sieving coefficient	Surface area (m^2)
Low-flux	< 10		
High-performance	> 10		> 1.5
High-flux	> 20*	> 0.6**	
Haemofilter	> 20	> 0.6	

**Changed from 10 ml/h/mmHg to 20 ml/h/mmHg in 2000. **Up to 2000, had only be specified for those high-flux membranes used in haemofilters, haemodiafilters and haemoconcentrators.*

Table 5.8: German classification of dialysers and haemofilters according to their ultrafiltration coefficients and ß2-m sieving coefficients. *Specifications for low-flux, high-performance and high-flux dialysers and haemofilters according to the German standards authorities [13, 22, 24].*

opment of dialysis-related amyloidosis (e.g. [111]). As a consequence of it being targeted for removal, various commissions have extended their definitions of high-flux membranes/dialysers to include specifications regarding ß2-m removal. For example, the American HEMO study group and the German dialysis standard specify that particular high-flux membranes must have a ß2-m clearance of > 20 ml/min or a sieving coefficient for ß2-m of at least 0.6, respectively ([21] and [24], respectively; see also **table 5.8**).

5.3.1 Membrane sieving coefficient

The sieving coefficient (SC) of a membrane is derived from the convective term of the clearance equation (eqn. 5.4). As middle molecule removal is chiefly achieved via ultrafiltration (solvent drag), the sieving coefficient is generally defined to be the ratio of the solute concentration in the *ultrafiltrate* (C_F) to that in incoming blood (C_{Bi}) [72], i.e.

SC	=	C_F/C_{Bi}	**[5.11]**
sieving coefficient		concentration ratio	

A SC of 1 for a given substance represents unhindered transport through the membrane, while a value of zero means that the membrane is impermeable for this substance. Values are dimensionless and are generally only officially required for middle molecules and for those high-flux membranes used in convection-based therapies, i.e. haemofiltration, haemodiafiltration and haemoconcentration [13, 15].

Dialyser producers must use a more accurate formula incorporating the average plasma solute concentration to calculate the sieving coefficients for membranes [13, 112]:

SC	=	$2C_F$	/	$(C_{Pi}$	+	$C_{Po})$	**[5.12]**
sieving coefficient		concentration in filtrate plasma		concentration in incoming plasma		concentration in outgoing	

The plasma concentrations of $ß_2$-m measured at any time "t" after start of treatment should be corrected for haemoconcentration due to ultrafiltration. Assuming that all plasma proteins are confined to the vascular space, a suitable correction is [113]:

$$\text{Corrected } C_P(t) = C_P(t) \cdot (TP(t_0) / TP(t)) \qquad [5.13]$$

Corrected $C_P(t)$	=	$C_P(t)$ measured plasma concentration at time "t"	·	$(TP(t_0) / TP(t))$ ratio of total plasma protein at start of dialysis (t_0) to that at time "t"

Unfortunately, SC measurements have the disadvantage that solute removal by membrane *adsorption* is very difficult to detect – only that portion of the adsorbed quantity that is swept into the filtrate will be recognised (see section 5.3.4 for more details on the limitation of this measure). The *in vitro*

Sieving coefficient test parameter	German standard
Test type	*In vitro*
Test medium	Blood (bovine or human)
Contents of test medium	Protein content > 60 g/l
	Fixed amounts of the test substances albumin, inulin, myoglobin and vitamin B_{12}
Temperature of test medium	37 ± 1°C
Blood flow (Q_B)	Maximum specified by manufacturer (e.g. 300 ml/min)
Dialysis fluid flow (Q_D)	0 ml/min
Filtrate flow (Q_F)	20% of Q_B

Table 5.9: Test conditions for the determination of dialyser/haemofilter sieving coefficients. *Standard conditions for the measurement of sieving coefficients (SC) by manufacturers as stipulated by the German regulatory authority (EN 1283). Other countries prefer the use of measures other than SCs (e.g. clearances in the USA).*

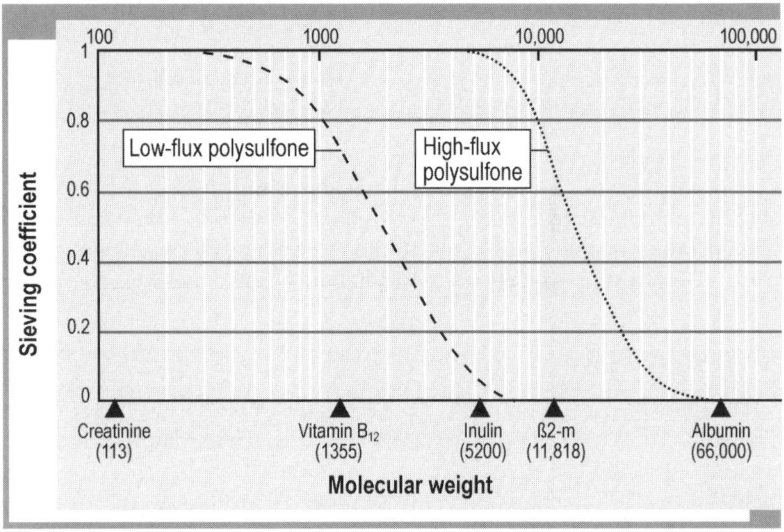

Figure 5.15: Schematic diagram of sieving coefficient profiles of low- and high-flux polysulfone membranes. *(Fresenius Polysulfone®, adapted from [115]).*

test conditions for the measurement of sieving coefficients as employed in Germany are summarised in **table 5.9**. The exact blood flow used in the determination of this parameter is not strictly specified; values of 300 ml/min appear to be common [114]. SC measurements are not requested in many countries (e.g. total clearance values are used exclusively in the USA).

Figure 5.15 shows the sieving coefficient profiles of low-flux and high-flux polysulfone dialysis membranes as a function of solute molecular weight. Obviously, the small pores in the low-flux membrane effectively inhibit the passage of middle molecules. As opposed to this, the high-flux membrane allows almost free passage of some middle molecules (e.g. inulin) and good removal of other solutes (e.g. ß2-microglobulin).

How do SCs change in vivo?

As in the case of ultrafiltration coefficients, *in vivo* measurements of SC will vary from their *in vitro* counterparts due to the different composition of the patient blood, the different flow conditions and secondary membrane formation. Mean *in vivo* haemofiltration and high-flux haemodialysis values for ß2-m are generally between 0.3 and 0.8 for different high-flux membranes of varying surface areas [114, 116-121]. As shown in **figure 5.16**, haemofiltration as conducted in this study tends to yield higher values than haemodialysis, with haemodiafiltration taking an intermediate position (except for cellulose triacetate). This reflects the fact that ß2-m removal is achieved predominantly by convection/filtration in these dialysers but that diffusion plays the domi-

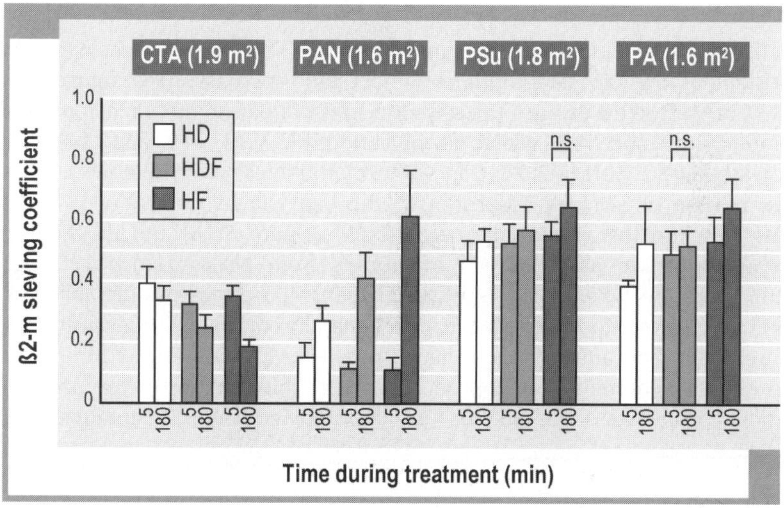

Figure 5.16: Change in ß2-microglobulin sieving coefficients during haemodialysis, haemodiafiltration and haemofiltration with 4 different high-flux membranes. *Except for cellulose triacetate (CTA, FB 190 U from Nipro), haemofiltration tends to yield higher sieving coefficients than haemodialysis, with haemodiafiltration taking an intermediate position (whereby the higher ultrafiltration rate of ~ 170 ml/min used in HF compared to that of ~ 116 ml/min in HDF favour HF for ß2-m removal in this study). The other membranes/dialysers tested were polyacrylonitrile (PAN, here AN69®, Filtral 1.6 from Hospal-Cobe), polysulfone (PSu, HF 80 from Fresenius Medical Care), and polyamide (PA, Polyflux 160 from Gambro). N = 6 for PAN, PSu and PA, N = 5 for CTA. Postdialysis levels were corrected for the change in total plasma protein during treatment using eqn. 5.13. All changes with increasing treatment time were statistically significant (p < 0.05), except for those marked n.s. (not significant) (adapted from [113]).*

Note: *absolute values serve the comparison of the effects of dialysis time and ß2-m removal procedure; they are not necessarily typical of present-day membranes.*

nant role for cellulose triacetate under the high blood flow conditions tested (450 ±35 ml/min) [113]. Low SCs may indicate that a membrane has a high adsorptive capacity for ß2-m, or that the membrane has become plugged with proteins during the course of treatment, making it less penetrable. The latter was postulated as the reason for the reduction in values observed with cellulose triacetate when filtrate flow was added in **figure 5.16** (i.e. lower values with HDF or HF than with HD). Thus haemofiltration and haemodiafiltration techniques will only significantly enhance ß2-m removal if the appropriate membrane is used.

Sieving coefficients for ß2-m may decrease, increase or remain roughly constant as the blood-membrane contact time increases (see **figure 5.16**) [113, 116]. Decreases are probably due to secondary membrane formation, osmotic stress and transcellular disequilibrium [52, 113, 119, 122-124]. Large increases in SC were observed in some membranes which remove a significant portion of ß2-m by adsorption in the early stages of treatment and release this into the filtrate later, e.g. AN69® (**figure 5.16**) and the high-flux polyester-polymer alloy (PEPA®) membrane from Nikkiso [113, 120, 125, 126]. Therefore, when using sieving coefficients to characterise the ability of a particular dialyser to remove ß2-m, one generally compares values at the start of treatment and after a defined time span, e.g. 30 minutes, 1-3 hours or at the end of treatment. This approach provides information on the particular removal properties of the dialyser throughout the course of the treatment.

5.3.2 Percentage reduction during dialysis

As effective removal of large molecules across dialysis membranes will be reflected in altered plasma levels of the molecule in question, pre- to post-dialysis percentage reduction (PR) in these levels is sometimes used as an measure of membrane middle molecule removal ability (analogous to the urea reduction ratio usually measured in the clinic). This is not recommended as an *in vitro* measurement by regulatory agencies, but is commonly used *in vivo* to gauge the effectiveness of dialyser middle molecule removal and in comparing different devices. As only plasma levels are measured, removal by diffusion, convection and adsorption are all taken into account. An appropriate formula is

$$PR = [(C_{pre} - C_{post})/ C_{pre})] \cdot 100 \qquad \textbf{[5.14]}$$

percentage reduction	predialysis and postdialysis plasma concentrations

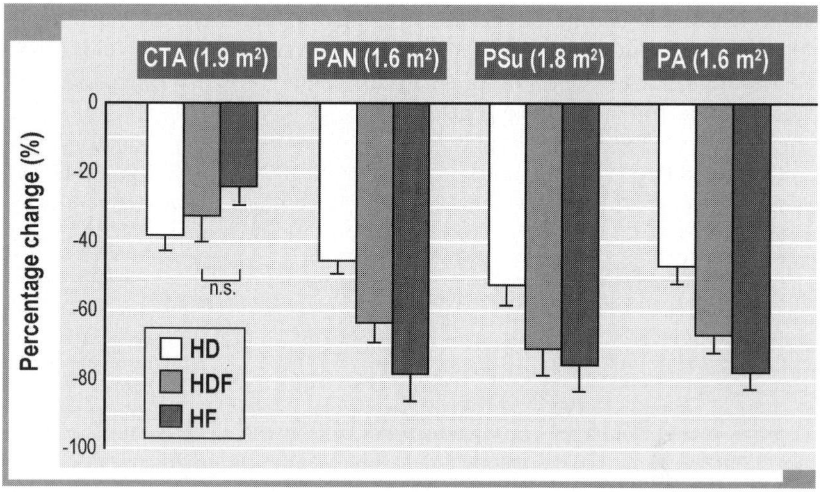

Figure 5.17: Comparison of percentage reductions in ß2-microglobulin levels during haemodialysis, haemodiafiltration and haemofiltration with 4 different high-flux membranes. *Plasma levels of ß2-m were measured at the entrance to the dialyser/haemofilter. Except for cellulose triacetate (CTA, FB 190 U from Nipro), haemofiltration tends to yield greater reductions than haemodialysis, with haemodiafiltration taking an intermediate position (whereby the higher ultrafiltration rate of ~ 170 ml/min used in HF compared to that of ~ 116 ml/min in HDF favour HF for ß2-m removal in this study). Postulated reasons are given in the text. N = 6 for polyacrylonitrile (PAN, here AN69®, Filtral 1.6 from Hospal/Cobe), polysulfone (PSu, HF 80 from Fresenius Medical Care), and polyamide (PA, Polyflux 160 from Gambro); N = 5 for CTA. Postdialysis levels were corrected for the change in total plasma protein during treatment using eqn. 5.13. The differences between the three treatment modes were statistically significant ($p < 0.05$ or $p < 0.01$) for each membrane group, except where indicated (n.s.) (adapted from [113]).*

Note: *values serve the comparison of different ß2-m removal procedures; they are not necessarily typical of present-day membranes.*

Here postdialysis plasma concentrations must be corrected for haemoconcentration resulting from ultrafiltration. Different correction factors appear in the literature, for example the popular correction for ß2-microglobulin supplied by Bergström and Wehle [127]:

$$\text{Corrected } C_{post} = \text{Measured } C_{post} / [1 + (BW_{pre} - BW_{post})/(0.2 \cdot BW_{post})] \quad \textbf{[5.15]}$$

postdialysis plasma conc. corrected for haemoconcentration	measured postdialysis plasma ß2-m concentration	change in body weight during dialysis	postdialysis body weight

or that given in eqn. 5.13 and used by Lesaffer et al. [52], Floege et al. [113] and others.

Such *in vivo* values are sensitive to predialysis levels, dialysis time and flow conditions, so that "typical values" of particular membranes/dialysers cannot be supplied (e.g. [123]). Plasma levels of ß2-microglobulin are determined using enzyme immunoassays, and reductions of 13-48% were often reported for high -flux membranes in the past (e.g. see [57, 121, 128-130, 132]). A PR of around 70% for ß2-m with high-flux membranes is considered very high, but values close to this (after correction for haemoconcentration) have been measured after haemodialysis with the high-flux membranes polysulfone (F60, Fresenius Medical Care), polyamide (Polyflux HDF 139, Gambro), and following on-line haemodiafiltration [57, 90, 117, 131, 133]. Once again, haemofiltration and haemodiafiltration generally reduce plasma levels of ß2-m more than haemodialysis (see **figure 5.17** and [134], for example), except in the case of cellulose triacetate (probably for the reasons given in the last section).

5.3.3 Total amount of solute removed

Studies reporting ß2-m removal generally employ measurements ranging from diffusive clearances, over total clearances and sieving coefficients to percentage reduction during dialysis – absolute values of ß2-m removed by transmembrane transfer into the dialysis fluid are rarely measured due to the practical difficulties involved. As in the case of sieving coefficients, such dialysis fluid-based measurements fail to take removal by membrane adsorption into account.

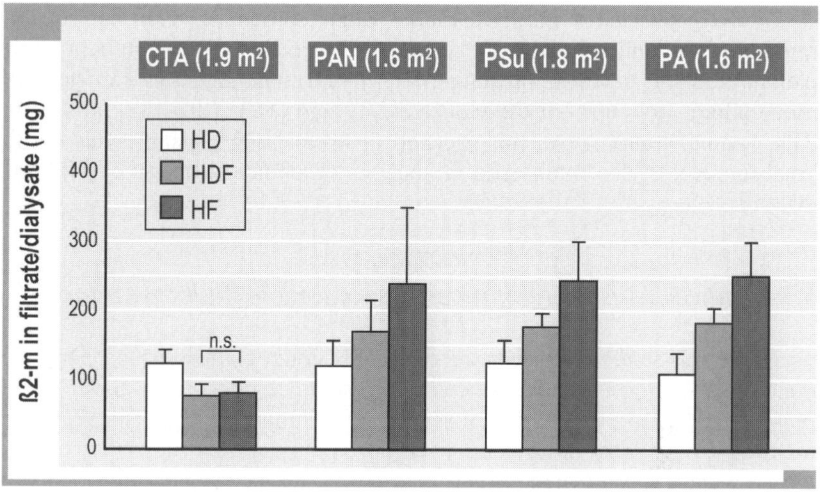

Figure 5.18: Comparison of ß2-microglobulin amounts collected in ultrafiltrate/dialysate after haemodialysis, haemodiafiltration and haemofiltration with 4 different high-flux membranes. *Except for cellulose triacetate (CTA, FB 190 U from Nipro), haemofiltration tends to remove higher quantities than haemodialysis, with haemodiafiltration taking an intermediate position (whereby the higher ultrafiltration rate of ~ 170 ml/min used in HF compared to that of ~ 116 ml/min in HDF favour HF for ß2-m removal in this study). Postulated reasons are given in the text. N = 6 for polyacrylonitrile (PAN, here AN69®, Filtral 1.6 from Hospal/Cobe), polysulfone (PSu, HF 80 from Fresenius Medical Care), and polyamide (PA, Polyflux 160 from Gambro); N = 5 for CTA. All differences between the three treatment modes for each dialyser were statistically significant ($p < 0.05$ or $p < 0.01$), the only exception being those between HDF and HF with CTA (adapted from [113]).*

Note: *values serve the comparison of different ß2-m removal procedures; they are not necessarily typical of present-day membranes.*

Absolute quantities of ß2-m reported to be removed per haemodialysis session with high-flux membranes lie between 42 and 350 mg (**figure 5.18**, also [56, 113, 117, 120, 121, 123, 126, 129, 135]). As in the case of PR, these values vary with dialysis time, predialysis levels and flow conditions (e.g. [123, 136]). Again, particularly high values are achieved by most high-flux membranes in haemodiafiltration and haemofiltration procedures ([90, 113, 137] - see also **figure 5.18**): for example, 259 and 350 mg per post-dilution haemofiltration session involving exchange volumes of 20 litres and blood flows of 300 ml/min with polysulfone and AN69® membranes, respectively [137].

Total removal is of particular value when comparing ß2-m production rates and its dialytic removal: the average daily production of ß2-m by a 60 kg patient is in the 180-360 mg range; intermittent haemodialysis can only remove about 50 - 60% of the weekly ß2-m load [123, 128, 132], and even daily haemofiltration does not succeed in normalising plasma levels [136]. Total removal is also often used in analyses of albumin leakage by high-flux dialysers.

5.3.4 Critical assessment of measures for middle molecule removal

Numerous studies of dialytic removal of ß2-microglobulin have been conducted, so that now certain general conclusions can be drawn about membrane transport properties for molecules of comparable size. First, low-flux membranes generally remove no or negligible amounts of molecules of molecular weight greater than 10,000 (e.g. [36, 37, 60]). Second, the dominant mechanism by which ß2-m is removed by high-flux membranes varies between diffusion (e.g. some cellulose triacetate membranes, particularly at high blood flows [17, 113, 138]), convection (e.g. high-flux polysulfone [35, 113, 117, 139, 140]) and adsorption (e.g. PMMA [17, 35, 138, 140]). Usually removal is achieved by a combination of two or all of these mechanisms (e.g. polyacrylonitrile (AN69®), where adsorption dominates in the early stages of treatment and convection overrules later [112, 113]). Third, when removal is achieved by adsorption or convection, use of high ultrafiltration rates in haemofiltration and haemodiafiltration enhances removal compared to standard haemodialysis [113, 141].

Clearly the measure used for quantifying ß2-m removal should take the various membrane-specific removal mechanisms into consideration. The matter of membrane adsorption appears to come up short in this light.

When does adsorption play a role in the removal of middle and large molecules?

Discrepancies between blood-side and dialysis fluid-side clearance measurements for some membranes indicated that adsorption can be a factor of considerable clinical relevance in solute removal. It is now known that the adsorptive surface of a membrane resides primarily in its pore structure rather than in its nominal surface area, and that adsorption of any middle or low molecular weight protein will depend on it having access to the membrane's internal pore structure [17, 60]. This is thought to explain why PMMA and PAN (AN69®) membranes can adsorb more ß2-m (MW 11,818) than EPO (MW approx. 30,000) [142]. Consequently, the tighter inner membrane surfaces of low-flux synthetic membranes do not allow these to adsorb large molecules. There is also some indication that hydrophobic synthetic membranes have particularly good adsorptive characteristics [17].

Adsorption is solely responsible for ß2-m removal by PMMA membranes [17, 35, 140]. It also plays a major role in ß2-m removal with some PAN membranes (e.g. AN69®, see also low initial SCs in **figure 5.16**, which indicate adsorption in the initial stages of treatment), but here filtration was found to contribute significantly to net removal later in the dialysis [17, 56, 112, 120, 125, 139, 140]. Another study showed significant adsorption of ß2-m also onto polyester-polymer alloy (PEPA®) membranes [56]. Adsorption plays only a minor role in ß2-m removal by the Fresenius Polysulfone® membrane: here the good removal values are achieved predominantly by filtration [35, 113, 117, 139, 140].

Adsorption of plasma proteins other than ß2-m can have a negative effect on the performances of the individual membranes or dialysers. Protein adsorption onto the membrane during treatment, as well as the eventual retention of such proteins even after reprocessing, leads to so-called "membrane fouling". This term is generally used to describe the deterioration of membrane performance by the presence of a secondary layer of plasma components. This layer increases the diffusive length for blood solutes (thus decreasing diffusion) and blocks pores - whereby membrane hydraulic permeability, adsorptive capacity for ß2-m and convective removal properties are negatively affected (e.g. [143]).

How do the measurements compare?

Examples of ß2-m SC, PR and total amount removed by each of 4 different high-flux dialysers are shown in **figure 5.16 - figure 5.18**. Clearance, SC and PR values for 8 high-flux membranes all investigated under identical conditions are shown in **table 5.10**. The results indicate that a high/low SC goes hand in hand with a high/low clearance and a high/low PR, at least for membranes which remove ß2-m predominantly by convection or diffusion.

These parameters are, however, equivocal when adsorption is the predominant removal mode. For example, as sieving coefficient measurements are dependent on transmembrane solute movement, dialysers which remove ß2-m almost entirely by adsorption (i.e. PMMA) will have lower sieving coefficients than membranes that remove less ß2-m in this manner (e.g. polysulfone) [112, 140]. Similarly, clearance values will be in more or less agreement with PR values for adsorbing membranes, depending on whether blood or dialysis fluid side formulae are used, respectively (i.e. eqn. 5.4 rather than eqn. 5.5). As the clearance values reported in **table 5.10** are diffusive clearances (i.e. Q_F = 0 ml/min) which were determined using dialysis fluid concentrations of ß2-m (eqn. 5.5), ß2-m removal by adsorption is not recognised. It is, therefore, understandable that zero clearance was measured for PMMA in this study despite a PR of 32%. **Figure 5.19** shows the results of a detailed analysis of the adsorption capacity of different dialysis membranes for ß2-microglobulin. The results shown prove that adsorption contributes significantly to the overall elimination of ß2-microglobulin by PMMA and PAN membranes, whereby differences between different PAN (i.e. Asahi PAN and AN69®) membranes exist [144].

Clearly, the various specific measures used for middle molecule removal by membranes/dialysers are not equally applicable or informative. While PR is appropriate for the characterisation of all membranes, including those that remove ß2-m mostly by adsorption, SC and diffusive clearance are suitable only for membranes that remove ß2-m primarily by convection and diffusion, respectively. Regarding diffusive removal, it should be pointed out that, nowadays, high flow conditions are common and that highly permeable dialysis membranes are thinner and/or more porous than their older counterparts (e.g. [145]); the consequence is a significant diffusive clearances of ß2-m, which can even exceed the respective convective clearance. This was demonstrated for the cellulose triacetate (in the Baxter CT-190GA), regenerated cellulose (in the Asahi Medical AMNeo-2001UP), polyacrylonitrile (in the Asahi Medical PAN-12CX1) and EVAL® (in the Kuraray KF-201-12C) membranes in an *in vitro* study using ^{3}H-labelled water and ^{125}I-labelled ß2-m [146].

There remains an outstanding need for a universally recognised and utilised measure of middle molecule removal that is generally applicable for all membrane types and facilitates comparison thereof. PR takes total removal irrespective of modus into account, and is especially attractive due to it being clinical in nature and easy to measure. However, errors due to inexact or no correction for haemoconcentration resulting from ultrafiltration must be ruled out. Measurement of total clearance using blood-side measurements (so that adsorption is recognised) and positive Q_Fs is a good alternative.

Dialyser membrane (manufacturer - surface area)	UF_{coeff} ml/mmHg·h	Sieving coefficient	Diffusive clearance ml/min	Percentage removal
PMMA (Toray - 2.1 m^2)	40	0	0	-32.0 ± 5
Cellulose acetate (Nipro - 2.1 m^2)	10	0	0	-
PAN (Asahi - 1.4 m^2)	45	0	4.3 ± 0.4	+9.2 ± 4
MCA (Cordis-Dow - 1.4 m^2)	15	0.27 ± 0.04	11.4 ± 1.6	-12.0 ± 4
PAN (AN69®) (Hospal - 1.2 m^2)	45	0.21 ± 0.01	17.3 ± 1.2	-5.4 ± 3
Polysulfone (Fresenius - 1.3 m^2)	40	0.47 ± 0.01	31.3 ± 0.6	-43.0 ± 4
PAN (AN69®) (Hospal - 1.6 m^2)	54	0.31 ± 0.04	36.1 ± 5.0	-32.5 ± 3
Polysulfone (Fresenius - 1.9 m^2)	60	0.43 ± 0.01	54 ± 3.6	-54.0 ± 4

PMMA: polymethylmethacrylate; PAN: polyacrylonitrile; MCA: modified cellulose acetate

Table 5.10. Comparison of measures for ß2-m removal in various high-flux dialysers of difference surface areas. *ß2-microglobulin diffusive clearances, percentage removals (PR) and sieving coefficients (SC) of for 8 different high-flux (UFcoeff ≥ 10 ml/mmHg·h) dialysers on the market in 1989 are shown. Diffusive clearances were measured at zero ultrafiltration using dialysis fluid measurements. The negative sign before the PR values indicates a reduction in serum levels by dialysis - values were not corrected for haemoconcentration and this may explain the increase measured after dialysis with Asahi PAN. SCs were measured after 40 to 45 minutes of dialysis and in the absence of dialysis fluid (adapted from [35]).*

Note: *values do not reflect actual removal characteristics of these dialysers today, but simply serve the purpose of comparing the different method of measurement.*

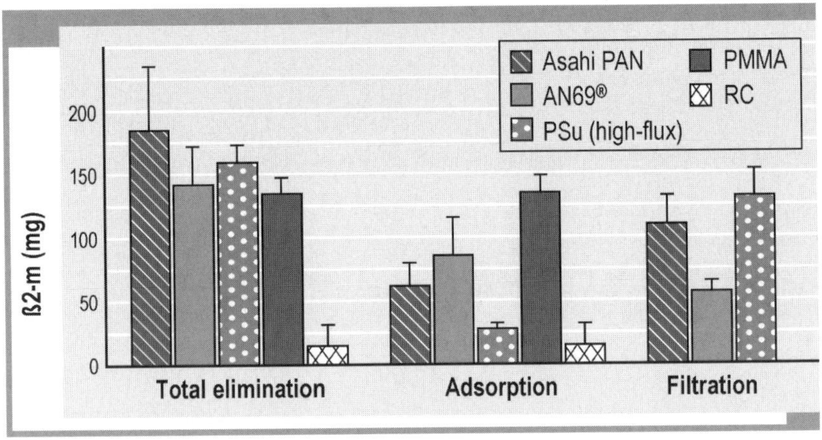

Figure 5.19: Contribution of adsorption and filtration to total ß2-microglobulin removal* in vivo *by one low-flux and four different high-flux membranes. *Adsorption contributes considerably to the overall elimination of ß2-microglobulin by PMMA and PAN (Hospal and Asahi) membranes.*
Note: *values serve the comparison of different ß2-m removal procedures; they are not necessarily typical of present-day membranes (adapted from [144]).*

5.4 Retention of large solutes

In analogy to the natural glomerular filter, artificial kidney membranes should be impenetrable for solutes of molecular weight as high or higher than that of albumin (66,000). However, in the natural kidney, most middle and large solutes are reabsorbed in the renal tubulus, so that early artificial kidneys aimed at the removal of small solutes only. Later recognition that certain middle molecules are uraemic retention solutes with detrimental effects on patient health led to an opening of the artificial kidney membrane to allow the removal of solutes in the middle molecular weight range. Although identification of those molecules which should be targeted for removal is a subject of ongoing investigations that reveal the complexity of the matter (e.g. [8, 10, 52, 147-150]), the present generally accepted picture of an optimal dialyser membrane is one which allows the removal of small and middle molecules while preventing the loss of those larger solutes of nutritional and energy donating value.

5.4.1 Albumin leakage and amino acid loss

Today, high-flux filters aim at achieving a high removal of ß2-m while retaining as much albumin as possible (see **figure 5.15** for typical sieving coefficient profiles of low- and high-flux dialysers). Albumin is an important carrier for essential nutrients, and low plasma levels indicate malnutrition and are taken as a prediction of mortality in haemodialysis patients. *In vivo* investigations have revealed that only small amounts of albumin are lost with most membranes during haemodialysis if they are not reused, i.e. albumin losses are generally < 1 g/ session in single use [56, 151]. Higher losses during single dialyser use have been reported with the membranes polyethersulfone (DIAPES®, 3.1 g/session), cellulose triacetate (1.5, 2.1 and 2.7 g/session), polysulfone (Minntech polysulfone, 1.7 g/session), and polyester-polymer alloy (PEPA®, 1.8 g/session) [56, 152].

Dialyser reuse, especially with bleach, has been reported to augment albumin loss with cellulose triacetate membranes and older versions of the Fresenius Polysulfone® membrane: here maximum losses reported were 4.25 g/session and 20 g/session, respectively [151, 154]. This aspect is discussed in detail in chapter 12.

The trend in some countries towards more convective modes of solute transport (i.e. haemofiltration and haemodiafiltration) means augmented removal of middle molecules (see **figure 5.17**, for example) but also bears the risk of excessive loss of albumin. Albumin concentrations in *in vitro* haemofiltration filtrates varying from 50 to 700 mg/l were reported for various high-flux polysulfones (Fresenius Medical Care, Minntech), Polyamide S™ (Gambro), PEPA® (Nikkiso) and Excebrane (Terumo) [155]. Total albumin losses in haemofiltration of 5.47 ± 0.69 g/session were measured *in vivo* [156]. In haemodiafiltration, total albumin losses per treatment of between 0.4 ± 0.2 g and as high as even 18.9 ± 3.5 g were reported using various high-flux membranes and operation modes [133, 153, 157-160]. High losses can be reduced by variations in the actual haemodiafiltration procedure, e.g. by changing to "programmed filtration" or pressure-controlled push/pull approaches; by changing from the postdilution to the predilution mode (see **figure 5.20**); and by reducing the rate of ultrafiltration (**see figure 5.21**) [131, 153, 160, 161]. However, ß2-m removal is then most probably also compromised. A recently conducted study of ß2-m removal rates and albumin losses with eight different high-flux dialysers of surface areas between 1.3 and 1.5 m^2 during haemodiafiltration treatments yielded some very interesting results: plots of the ß2-m removal rate against the albumin loss of each dialyser at various ultrafiltration rates allowed the identification of dialysers with a good or poor balances between ß2-m removal and albumin loss (**figure 5.21** [131]). In this study, both ß2-m removal and albumin loss values were shown to be sensitive to the ultrafiltration rate. The membranes with the best balance between ß2-m removal and albumin loss are those in the upper-left box of the figure. These were Asahi Polysulfone (APS®, at a filtration rate of 60 ml/min), Polyamide S™ from Gambro/Hospal (at a filtration rate of 100 ml/min), and Helixone® from Fresenius Medical Care (at ultrafiltration rates of 60 and 80 ml/min).

Regulatory authorities have not yet stipulated a recommendation for an upper limit of acceptable albumin loss. While some authors find losses of up to 8 - 10 g per treatment, irrespective of procedure, to be acceptable [162], others prefer to target losses lower than 5 g per treatment [157]. Definition of a maximum acceptable albumin loss is urgently required.

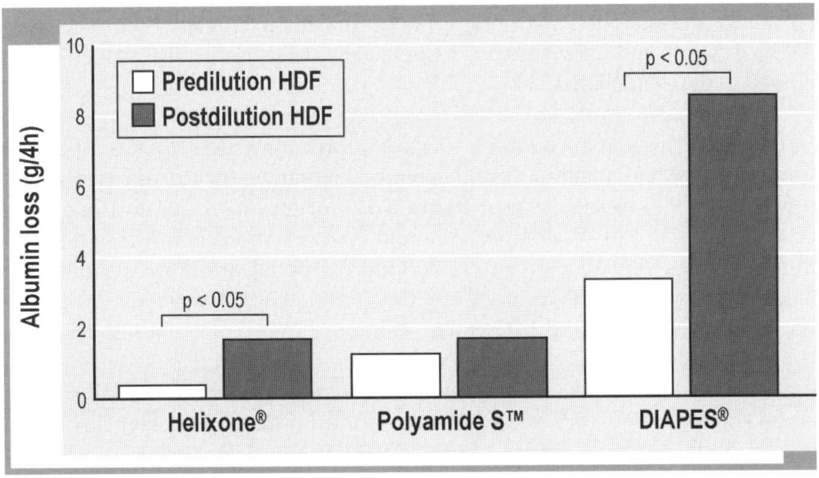

Figure 5.20:* In vivo *loss of albumin into the dialysis fluid during haemodiafiltration with 3 different membranes in pre- and post-dilution modes *The membranes tested were Fresenius Helixone® (FX80, 1.6 m²), polyamide S™ from Gambro (Polyflux 17S, 1.7 m²) and DIAPES® from Baxter/Membrana (Syntra 160, 1.6 m²). Differences between DIAPES® and the other two membranes were statistically significant (adapted from [153]).*

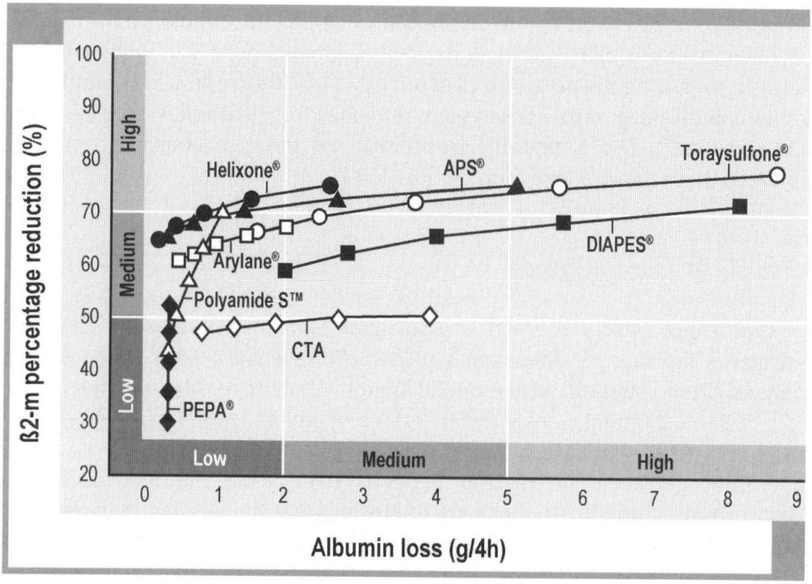

Figure 5.21: The relationship between ß2-microglobulin removal rate and albumin loss in post-dilution haemodiafiltration with 8 different dialysers. *Three dialysis patients were each treated in 32 haemodiafiltration sessions with the following 8 dialysers in total: Fresenius Helixone® (FX60, 1.4 m^2), Toraysulfone® (BS-1.3U, 1.3 m^2), DIAPES® from Bellco (BLS814 G, 1.4 m^2), PEPA® from Nikkiso (FLX-15 GWS, 1.5 m^2), polysulfone from Asahi (APS®-650, 1.3 m^2), Polyamide S™from Gambro/Hospal (Polyflux 14S, 1.4 m^2), Arylane® from Hospal (H4, 1.35 m^2), and cellulose triacetate (CTA) from Baxter/Nipro (CT 150G, 1.5 m^2). The curves describe the balance between ß2-m removal and albumin loss at increasing total ultrafiltration rates of (from left to right) 20, 40, 60, 80 and 100 ml/min. Values were calculated by regression analysis, whereby ß2-m removal followed a linear regression (removal rate = $38.39 + 0.318 \cdot Q_F$; $R^2 = 0.345$, $p = 0.005$) and albumin loss followed an exponential regression ($y = 175.32e^{0.027x}$; $R^2 = 0.7187$) (adapted from [131]).*

Care must be taken to ensure that new membranes and technologies do not aggravate the present situation. A clear advance towards increasing middle molecule removal while simultaneously restricting albumin loss is the application of nanotechnology-based principles in the production of dialysis membranes. Whereas attempts to increase the permeability of a membrane for ß2-microglobulin are normally based on increasing the mean pore size of the membrane, and thus also its permeability for albumin (as pores exist as a distribution of sizes and not as an absolute size), nanotechnology-based fabrication procedures allow an increase in the nominal pore size while simultaneously narrowing the pore size distribution [114]. This approach is employed in the newest generation of dialysis membranes from Fresenius Medical Care (i.e. Helixone®), and is possibly responsibe for the good balance reported between ß2-m removal and albumin loss [131].

What about amino acid loss?

One factor often discussed in association with malnutrition and albumin leakage is the loss of amino acids, especially essential amino acids, during dialysis, haemofiltration or haemodiafiltration. Dialysis results in a mean loss of 3 - 12% of the total weekly dietary intake of amino acids [163, 164], or in a loss of 6 - 13 g of amino acids per dialysis [165-167]. The quantity of amino acid removed from the plasma depends directly on the individual pre-treatment level, and it is particularly interesting that the amount recovered in the dialysis fluid or filtrate is generally higher than that expected from the observed decreases in plasma levels, i.e. protein catabolism appears to be stimulated during treatment ([163, 165-167], chapter 10). The question to be addressed regarding performance is whether amino acid loss is also sensitive to the physical characteristics of the various membranes.

Given that free amino acids are much smaller than proteins, one would expect them to be removed by low- and high-flux membranes to comparable extents. Two major studies investigated amino acid losses by a selection of membranes: one comparing two low-flux membranes (regenerated cellulose and PMMA) with one high-flux membrane (polysulfone) [165] and one comparing a low-flux membrane (regenerated cellulose) with two high-flux membranes (polysulfone and polyacrylonitrile) [163]. While the first study initially indicated a higher amino acid loss into the dialysis fluid with the high-flux membrane (8 ± 2 g (PSu) vs. 7.2 ± 2.6 g (RC) and 6.1 ± 1.5 g (PMMA)), this could be explained by its significantly larger surface area (1.8 m^2 (PSu) vs. 1.5 m^2 (RC and PMMA)) and the higher blood flow employed during treatment (400 ml/min (PSu) vs. 300 ml/min (RC and PMMA)). The second study reported relatively high losses into the dialysis fluid with one high-flux membrane (PAN, 6.1 ± 2.3 g), but amino acid losses with the other high-flux membrane (polysulfone) were comparable with those measured with the low-flux membrane (3.8 ± 1.3 g and 3.7 ± 1.3 g, respectively). Nonetheless, some evidence does exist that indicates that amino acid loss is enhanced in membranes of higher permeability: increases in membrane permeability due to dialyser reuse were accompanied with increases in amino acid loss [165], and one paper reported that losses were greater during acute high-flux dialysis than acute low-flux dialysis [168].

Analysis of changes in levels of specific amino acids during treatment indicates a contribution of membrane charge to amino acid loss: losses of the positively charged amino acid lysine were observed to be higher with the negatively charged PAN membrane than with the polysulfone and regenerated cellulose membranes of neutral charge. However, there were no differences regarding the losses of the negatively charged glutamate [163].

Further research is necessary to clarify the role of membrane physicochemical and permeability characteristics in amino acid loss. Factors which affect the measurements and complicate comparison of studies and dialysers are incomplete recovery of the amino acids, common failure to distinguish between free and peptide-bound amino acids, and differences in surface area of the dialysers, dialysis duration, flow conditions (especially blood flow), degree of correction of metabolic acidosis and food intake during treatment [163, 165]. The presence of glucose in the dialysis fluid has also been reported to affect the measurements of amino acid loss. The postulated association here is that the sparing effect of enhanced plasma glucose on protein catabolism results in reduced levels of amino acids, making them less available for removal by dialysis [166, 169].

References

1. Gotch F, Peter H, Panlilio F, Folden T, Keen M: On-line measurement of delivered Kt/V during dialysis. (Abstract) JASN 6(3): 600, 1995

2. National Kidney Dialysis Outcome Quality Initiative (DOQI): Clinical practice guidelines: hemodialysis adequacy and peritoneal dialysis adequacy. Am J Kid Dis 30(3, Suppl 2): S1-S64, 1997

3. Product brochure from Fresenius Medical Care Deutschland GmbH: On-line clearance monitor. Dialysis dose: here and now. January 2001.

4. Lipps B, Frydrych A, Gandhi V, Gotch FA, Ing TS, Levin NW: Comparison of urea clearance as determined by online conductivity monitoring to that predicted by urea kinetic modeling. (Abstract) J Am Soc Nephrol 13: 234A, 2002

5. Gotch FA, Sargent JA, Keen ML: Whither goest Kt/V? Kidney Int 58 (Suppl 76): S3-18, 2000

6. Vanholder R: Middle molecules as uremic toxins: still a viable hypothesis? Seminars in Dialysis 7(1): 65-68, 1994

7. Vanholder R, De Smet R, Hsu C, Vogeleere P, Ringoir S: Uremic toxicity: the middle molecule hypothesis revisited. Sem Nephrol 14(3): 205-218, 1994

8. Vanholder R, De Smet R, Lameire NH: Redesigning the map of uremic toxins in *Dialysis, dialyzers and sorbents. Where are we going?*, edited by Ronco C, Winchester JF, Basel, Karger, Contrib Nephrol 133: 28-41, 2001

9. Vanholder R, De Smet R, Vogeleere P, Hsu C, Ringoir S: The uraemic syndrome in *Replacement of renal function by dialysis*, 4th ed., edited by Jacobs C, Kjellstrand CM, Koch KM, Winchester JF, Dordrecht, Kluwer Academic Publishers: 1-33, 1996

10. Vanholder R, De Smet R, Glorieux G, Argilés A, Baurmeister U, Brunet P, Clark W, Cohen G, De Deyn PP, Deppisch R, Descamps-Latscha, Henle T, Jörres A, Lemke HD, Massy A, Passlick-Deetjen J, Rodriguez M, Stegmayr B, Stenvinkel P, Tetta C, Wanner C, Zidek W: Review on uremic toxins: classification, concentration, and interindividual variability. Kidney Int 63: 1934-1943, 2003

11. Wolffindin C, Hoenich NA: Hemodialyzer performance: a review of the trends over the past two decades. Artif Organs 19(11): 1113-1119, 1995

12. Lysaght MJ: Hemodialysis membranes in transition. Contrib Nephrol 61: 1-17, 1988

13. European standards for haemodialysers, haemodiafilters, haemofilters, haemoconcentrators and associated blood tubing systems, DIN, EN 1283:1996

14. German standards for haemodialysis: DIN 58352, Part 3, 1988

15. AAMI (Association for the Advancement of Medical Instrumentation) recommendations, vol. 3: dialysis, RD16 (First use hemodialyzers), 1996

16. Schönweiß G: High-Flux-Dialyse in *Dialyse Fibel*, 2nd ed., Bad Kissingen, Abakiss Verlag: 416, 1996

17. Clark WR, Hamburger RH, Lysaght MJ: Effect of membrane composition and structure on solute removal and biocompatibility in hemodialysis. Kidney Int 56: 2005-2015, 1999

18. Fresenius Medical Care Deutschland GmbH: Data sheet and Instructions for Use for the F-series high-flux capillary dialysers. May 1998.

19. Colton CK, Henderson LW, Ford CA, Lysaght MJ: Kinetics of hemodiafiltration. I. In vitro transport characteristics of a hollow-fiber blood ultrafilter. J Lab Clin Med 85(3): 355-371, 1975

20. Henderson LW, Colton CK, Ford CA: Kinetics of hemodiafiltration II. Clinical characterization of a new blood cleansing modality. J Lab Clin Med 85: 372, 1975

21. Cheung AK, Agodoa LY, Daugirdas JT, Depner TA, Gotch FA, Greene T, Levin NW, Leypoldt JK and the HEMO study group: Effects of hemodialyzer reuse on clearances of urea and β_2-microglobulin. J Am Soc Nephrol 10: 117-127, 1999

22. Dialysestandard der Arbeitsgemeinschaft Klinische Nephrologie e.V. and the Dialysegesellschaft Niedergelassener Ärzte e.V. (German dialysis standards), 2000

23. Ronco C, Ghezzi PM, Hoenich NA, Delfino P: Computerized selection of membranes and hemodialysers in *Dialysis, dialyzers and sorbents. Where are we going?*, edited by Ronco C, Winchester JF, Basel, Karger, Contrib Nephrol 133: 119-130, 2001

24. Dialysestandard der Arbeitsgemeinschaft Klinische Nephrologie (German dialysis standards), 1993

25. Mactier RA, Madi AM, Allam BF: Comparison of high-efficiency and standard haemodialysis providing equal urea clearances by partial and total dialysate quantification. Nephrol Dial Transplant 12: 1182-1186, 1997

26. Shinaberger H, Miller JH, von Albertini B, Gardner PW, Coburn JW: Phosphate (P) removal by conventional dialysis (CHD), high efficiency dialysis (HEHD) and high flux hemodiafiltration (HFHDF). (Abstract) ASN: 245, 1999

27. Ronco C: What clinically important advances in understanding and improving dialyzer function have occurred recently? Seminars in Dialysis 14(3): 164-169, 2001

28. Hoenich NA, Woffindin C, Ronco C: Haemodialysers and associated devices in *Replacement of renal function by dialysis,* 4th ed., edited by Jacobs C, Kjellstrand CM, Koch KM, Winchester JF, Dordrecht, Kluwer Academic Publishers: 188-230, 1996

29. Sato H, Kidaka T: Effect of moisture on and kinetic features of the ultrafiltration rate of dialysis membrane. Artif Organs 5(3): 286-289, 1981

30. Vaussenat F, Bosc JY, LeBlanc M, Canaud B: Data acquisition system for dialysis machines: a model for membrane hydraulic permeability. ASAIO J 43(6): 910-915, 1997

31. Osuga T, Zetta L, Gussoni M, Greco F, Obata T, Ikehira H, Homma K, Yamane S, Kinugasa E, Sakamoto H, Naito H: Precise analysis of dialysis membrane and dialysate flow in a hollow fiber dialyzer using ^{1}H magnetic resonance imaging. (Abstract) Artif Organs 23(7): 654, 1999

32. Vaussenat F, Canaud B, Bosc JY, LeBlanc M, Leray-Moragues H, Garred L: Intradialytic glucose infusion increases polysulphone membrane permeability and post-dilutional haemodiafiltration performances. Nephrol Dial Transplant 15: 511-516, 2000

33. Sigdell JE: Operating characteristics of hollow-fiber dialyzers in *Clinical Dialysis,* 2nd ed., edited by Nissenson AR, Fine RN, Gentile DE, Connecticut, Appleton Lange: 97-117, 1990

34. Colton CK, Lysaght MJ: Membranes for hemodialysis in *Replacement of renal function by dialysis,* 4th ed., edited by Jacobs C, Kjellstrand CM, Koch KM, Winchester JF, Dordrecht, Kluwer Academic Publishers: 101-113, 1996

35. Jindal KK, McDougall J, Woods B, Nowakowski L, Goldstein MB: A study of the basic principles determining the performance of several high-flux dialyzers. Am J Kidney Dis 14(6): 507-511, 1989

36. Ward RA, Buscaroli A, Schmidt B, Stefoni S, Gurland HJ, Klinkmann H: A comparison of dialysers with low-flux membranes: significant differences in spite of many similarities. Nephrol Dial Transplant 12: 965-972, 1997

37. Klinkmann H, Buscaroli A, Stefoni S: $ß_2$-microblobulin and low-flux synthetic dialyzers. Artif Organs 22(7): 585-590, 1998

38. Stiller S, Mann H, Brunner H: Backfiltration in hemodialysis with highly permeable membranes in *Proceeding of the Conference of Optimization of Blood Purification,* Rostock, Germany, 1987

39. Leypoldt JK, Schmidt B, Gurland HJ: Net ultrafiltration may not eliminate backfiltration during hemodialysis with highly permeable membranes. Artificial Organs 15(3): 164-170, 1991

40. Klinkmann H, Ebbighausen H, Uhlenbusch I, Vienken J: High-flux dialysis, dialysate quality and backtransport. Contrib Nephrol 103: 89-97, 1993

41. Ronco C, Brendolan A, Feriani M, Milan M, Conz P, Lupi A, Berto P, Bettini MC, La Greca G: A new scintigraphic method to characterize ultrafiltration in hollow fiber dialyzes. Kidney Int 41: 1383-1393, 1992

42. Bonnie-Schorn E, Grassmann A, Uhlenbusch-Körwer I, Weber C, Vienken J: Water quality in hemodialysis, 1st ed., edited by Vienken J, Lengerich, Pabst Science Publishers, 1998

43. Leypoldt JK, Schmidt B, Gurland HJ: Measurement of backfiltration rates during hemodialysis with highly permeable membranes. Blood Purif 9: 74-84, 1991

44. Ofsthun NJ, Leypoldt JK: Ultrafiltration and backfiltration during hemodialysis. Artif Organs 19(11): 1143-1161, 1995

45. Choong LHL, Leypoldt JK, Cheung AK: Dialyzer mass transfer-area coefficients (KoA) during clinical haemodialysis (HD) are dependent on both blood flow (Qb) and dialysate flow (Qd) rates. (Abstract) J Am Soc Nephrol 10: 189A, 1999

46. Ronco C, Ghezzi PM, Hoenich NA, Delfino P: Additional reading in *Membranes and filters for hemodialysis*, Basel, Karger, CD Database 2001

47. Di Filippo S, Manzoni C, Locatelli F: Kt/V or solute removal index: problems in measuring and interpreting the results. Nephrol Dial Transplant 13: 2199-2202, 1998

48. Manzoni C, Di Filippo S, Locatelli F: Ionic dialysance as a method for the on-line monitoring of delivered dialysis without blood sampling. Nephrol Dial Transplant 11: 2023-2030, 1996

49. Peticlerc T, Béné B, Jacobs C, Jaudon MC, Goux N: Non-invasive monitoring of effective dialysis dose delivered to the haemodialysis patient. Nephrol Dial Transplant 10: 212-216, 1995

50. Katopodis KP, Hoenich NA: Accuracy and clinical utility of dialysis dose measurement using online ionic dialysance. Clin Nephrol 57(3): 215-220, 2002

51. Wuepper A, Tattersall J, Kraemer M, Wilkie M, Edwards L: Determination of urea distribution volume for Kt/V assessed by conductivity monitoring. Kidney Int 64: 2262-2271, 2003

52. Lesaffer G, De Smet R, Lameire N, Dhondt A, Duym P, Vanholder R: Intradialytic removal of protein-bound uraemic toxins: role of solute characteristics and of dialyser membrane. Nephrol Dial Transplant 15: 50-57, 2000

53. Van Stone JC: Hemodialysis apparatus in *Handbook of dialysis*, 2nd ed., edited by Daugirdas JT, Ing TS, Boston, Little, Brown and Company: 30-52, 1994

54. Locatelli F, Valderrábano F, Hoenich N, Bommer J, Leunissen K, Cambi V: Progress in dialysis technology: membrane selection and patient outcome. Nephrol Dial Transplant 15: 1133-1139, 2000

55. Lysaght M: in Kirk Othmer Encyklopedia, 1993

56. Sombolos K, Tsitamidou Z, Kyriazis G, Karagianni A, Kantaropoulou M, Progia: Clinical evaluation of four different high-flux hemodialyzers under conventional conditions in vivo. Am J Nephrol 17: 406-412, 1997

57. Mandolfo S, Malberti F, Imbasciati E, Cogliati P, Gauly A: Impact of blood and dialysate flow and surface area on performance of new polysulfone hemodialysis dialyzers. Int J Artif Organs 26(2): 113-120, 2003

58. Okada M, Takesawa S, Watanabe T, Imamura K, Tsurumi T, Suma Y, Sakai K: Effects of zeta potential on the permeability of dialysis membranes to inorganic phosphate. Trans Am Soc Artif Intern Organs 35: 320-322, 1989

59. SMC product brochure: *Which dialysis membrane stands out from the rest?*, Membrana GmbH, Wuppertal, 1999

60. Ofsthun NJ, Zydney AL: Importance of convection in artificial kidney treatment in *Contributions to Nephrology - Effective hemodiafiltration: new methods*, edited by Maeda K, Shinzato T, Basel, Karger: 108: 53-70, 1994

61. Scott MK, Mueller BA, Sowinski KM, Clark WR: Dialyzer-dependent changes in solute and water permeability with bleach reprocessing. Am J. Kidney Dis 33(1): 87-96, 1999

62. Scott MK, Mueller BA, Clark WR: Vancomycin mass transfer characteristics of high-flux cellulosic dialysers. Nephrol Dial Transplant 12(12): 2647-2653, 1997

63. Anderstam B, Mamoun AH, Södersten P, Bergström J: Middle-sized molecule fractions isolated from uremic ultrafiltrate and normal urine inhibit ingestive behavior in the rat. J Am Soc Nephrol 7(11): 2453-2460, 1996

64. De Bock V, Verbeelen D, Maes V, Sennesael J: Pharmacokinetics of vancomycin in patients undergoing haemodialysis and haemofiltration. Nephrol Dial Transplant 4: 635-639, 1989

65. Lanese DM, Alfrey PS, Molitoris BA: Markedly increased clearance of vancomycin during hemodialysis using polysulfone dialyzers. Kidney Int 35: 1409-1412, 1989

66. Schmidt B, Ward RA: The impact of erythropoietin on hemodialyzer design and performance. Artif Organs 13(1): 35-42, 1989

67. Woffindin C, Hoenich NA, Kerr DNS: The effect of hematocrit on the clearance of small molecules during hemodialysis. Int J Artif Organs 6(3): 127-130, 1983

68. Delano BG, Lundin AP, Galonsky R, Quinn RM, Rao TKS, Friedman EA: Dialyzer urea and creatinine clearances not significantly changed in r-HuEPO treated maintenance hemodialysis (MD) patients. (Abstract ASN) Kidney Int 33: 219, 1988

69. Ritz E: Phosphate removal during dialysis - does the membrane matter? Clin Nephrol 42 (Suppl 1): 57-60, 1994

70. Marcos AWB, Nissenson AR: Erythropoietin and high-efficiency dialysis in *Contemporary Issues in Nephrology 27 - Hemodialysis High-efficiency Treatments,* edited by Bosch JP, New York, Churchill Livingstone: 151, 1993

71. Krämer M, Wüpper A: What is the meaning of clearance and Kt/V? EDTA symposium 'How to quantify dialysis dose and optimise outcome in haemodialysis', Nice, September 17-20, 2000

72. Henderson LW: Biophysics of ultrafiltration and hemofiltration in *Replacement of renal function by dialysis*, 4th ed., edited by Jacobs C, Kjellstrand CM, Koch KM, Winchester JF, Dordrecht, Kluwer Academic Publishers: 114-145, 1996

73. Kerr PG, Lo A, Chin MM, Atkins RC: Dialyzer performance in the clinic: comparison of six low-flux membranes. Artif Organs 23(9): 817-821, 1999

74. Hoenich NA, Woffindin C, Cox PJ, Goldfinch M, Roberts SJ: Clinical characterization of Dicea a new cellulose membrane for haemodialysis. Clinical Nephrology 48(4): 253-259, 1997

75. Hoenich NA, Stamp S: Clinical investigation of the role of membrane structure on blood contact and solute transport characteristics of a cellulose membrane. Biomaterials 21: 317-324, 2000

76. Grassmann A, Uhlenbusch-Körwer I, Bonnie-Schorn E, Vienken J: *Composition and management of hemodialysis fluids*, edited by Vienken J, Lengerich, Pabst Science Publishers, 2000

77. Chauveau P, Poignet JL, Kuno T, Bonete R, Kerembrun A, Naret C, Delons S, Man NK, Rist E: Phosphate removal rate: a comparative study of five high-flux dialysers. Nephrol Dial Transplant (Suppl 2): 114-115, 1991

78. Pohlmeier R, Vienken J: Phosphate removal and hemodialysis conditions. Kidney Int 59 (Suppl 78): S190-S194, 2001

79. Hou SH, Zhao J, Ellman CF, Hu J, Griffin Z, Spiegel DM, Bourdeau JE: Calcium and phosphorus fluxes during hemodialysis with low calcium dialysate. Am J Kidney Dis 18(2): 217-224, 1991

80. Pogglitsch H, Petek W, Ziak E, Sterz F, Holzer H: Phosphorus kinetics during haemodialysis and haemofiltration. Proc EDTA-ERA 21: 461-468, 1984

81. Zucchelli P, Santoro A: Inorganic phosphate removal during different dialytic procedures. Int J Artif Organs 10(3): 173-178, 1987

82. Oosterhuis WP, de Metz M, Wadham A, Daha MR, Go RH: In vivo evaluation of four hemodialysis membranes: biocompatibility and clearances. Dialysis and Transplantation 24(8): 450-458, 1995

83. DeSoi CA, Umans JG: Does the dialysis prescription influence phosphate removal? Seminars in Dialysis 8(4): 201-203, 1995

84. Man NK, Chauveau P, Kuno T, Poignet JL, Yanai M: Phosphate removal during hemodialysis, hemodiafiltration, and hemofiltration. ASAIO Transactions 37: M463-M465, 1991

85. Fabris A, La Greca G, Chiaramonte S, Feriani M, Brendolan A, Bragantini L, Milan M, Pellanda MV, Crepaldi C, Ronco C: Total solute extraction *versus* clearance in the evaluation of standard and short hemodialysis. Trans Am Soc Artif Intern Organs 34: 627-629, 1988

86. Mucsi I, Hercz G, Uldall R, Ouwendyk M, Francoeur R, Pierratos A: Control of serum phosphate without any phosphate binders in patients treated with nocturnal home dialysis. Kidney Int 53: 1399-1404, 1998

87. Galland R, Traeger J, Ferrier ML, Delawari E: Control of phosphatemia with short daily hemodialysis. (Abstract) World Congress of Nephrology, Berlin: W413, 2003

88. Fajardo L, Campistrús N, Ríos P, Gómez T: Evolution of serum phosphate in long intermittent hemodialysis. Kidney Int 63 (Suppl 85): S66-S68, 2003

89. Joeris B, Neman I, Renner D: Phosphate reduction and avoidance of aluminium containing phosphate binders by the use of large surface area dialyzers. Nieren- und Hochdruckkrankheiten 25(1): 21-26, 1996

90. Lornoy W, Becaus I, Billiouw JM, Sierens L, Van Malderen P, D'Haenens P: On-line haemodiafiltration. Remarkable removal of $ß_2$-microglobulin. Long-term clinical observations. Nephrol Dial Transplant 15: 49-54, 2000

91. Lian JD, Cheng CH, Chang YL, Hsiong CH, Lee CJ: Clinical experience and model analysis on beta-2-microglobulin kinetics in high-flux hemodialysis. Artif Organs 17(9): 758-763, 1993

92. Gotch FA: Models to predict recirculation and its effect on treatment time in single-needle dialysis in *First International Symposium on Single-Needle Dialysis,* edited by Ringoir S, Vanholder R, Ivanovich V, Cleveland, Int Soc Artif Organs Press: 47-62, 1984

93. Barth RH: Pros and cons of short, high efficiency, and high flux dialysis in*Replacement of renal function by dialysis,* 4th ed., edited by Jacobs C, Kjellstrand CM, Koch KM, Winchester JF, Dordrecht, Kluwer Academic Publishers: 418-453, 1996

94. Sargent JA, Gotch FA: Principles and biophysics of dialysis in *Replacement of renal function by dialysis,* 4th ed., edited by Jacobs C, Kjellstrand CM, Koch KM, Winchester JF, Dordrecht, Kluwer Academic Publishers: 188-230, 1996

95. Daugirdas JT, Depner TA: A nomogram approach to hemodialysis urea modeling. Am J Kid Dis 23: 33-40, 1994

96. Ronco et al : in *Contemp Issues in Nephrol* 27: 219-233, 1993

97. Von Albertini B, Miler JH, Gardner PW, Shinaberger JH: Performance characteristics of the Hemoflow F60 in high-flux hemodiafiltration. Contr Nephrol 46: 169-173, 1985

98. Ouseph R, Ward RA: Increasing dialysate flow rate increases dialyzer urea mass transfer-area coefficients during clinical use. Am J Kidney Dis 37(2): 316-320, 2001

99. Levin NW, Kupin WL, Zasuwa G, Venkat KK: Complications during hemodialysis in *Dialysis therapy*, edited by Nissenson AR, Fine RN, Gentile DE, Norwalk, Connecticut, Appleton & Lange: 172-210, 1990

100. Van Stone JC, Daugirdas JT: Physiologic principles in *Handbook of dialysis*, 1st ed., edited by Daugirday JT, Ing TS, Boston, Little Brown and Company: 11-20, 1988

101. Sigdell JE, Tersteegen B: Clearance of a dialyzer under varying operating conditions. Artif Organs 10(3): 219-225, 1986

102. Leypoldt JK, Cheung AK, Agodoa LY, Daugirdas JT, Greene T, Keshaviah PR: Hemodialyzer mass transfer-area coefficients for urea increase at high dialysate flow rates. Kidney Int 51(6): 2013-2017, 1997

103. Leypoldt JK, Cheung AK: Effect of low dialysate flow rate on hemodialyzer mass transfer area coefficient for urea and creatinine. Home Hemodial Int 3: 51-54, 1999

104. Hauk M, Kuhlmann MK, Riegel W, Köhler H: In vivo effects of dialysate flow rate on Kt/V in maintenance hemodialysis patients. Am J Kidney Dis 35(1): 105-111, 2000

105. Sargent JA, Gotch FA, Lipps BJ, et al.: Evaluation of experimental high flux artificial kidney in *Proceedings of the Fifth Annual Contractors Conference* edited by the Artificial Kidney Program, Washington, D.C., National Institute of Arthritis and Metabolic Diseases, p. 12, 1972

106. Sprenger KG, Stephan H, Kratz W, Huber K, Franz HE: Optimising of hemodiafiltration with modern membranes?. Contr. Nephrol 46: 43-60, 1985

107. Mishkin MA, Mishkin GJ, Lew SQ: Solute removal in hemodiafiltration compared to standard high flux dialysis: combined analysis of 2 cross over studies. (Abstract) J Am Soc Nephrol 13: 238A, 2002

108. Wizemann V: Hemodiafiltration - an avenue to shorter dialysis? Contrib Nephrol 44: 49-56, 1985

109. Ahrenholz P, Winkler RE, Ramlow W, Tiess M, Muller W: .On-line hemodiafiltration with pre- and postdilution: a comparison of efficacy. Int J Artif Organs 20(2): 81-90, 1997

110. Wizemann V, Külz M, Techert F, Nederlof B: .Efficacy of haemodiafiltration. Nephrol Dial Transplant 16 (Suppl 4): 27-30, 2001

111. Floege J, Koch KM: ß2-microglobulin associated amyloidosis and therapy with high flux hemodialysis membranes. Clin Nephrol 42 (Suppl 1): 52-56, 1994

112. Klinkmann H, Vienken J: Membranes for dialysis. Nephrol Dial Transplant 10 (Suppl 3): 39-45, 1995

113. Floege J, Granolleras C, Deschodt G, Heck M, Baudin G, Branger B, Tournier O, Reinhard B, Eisenbach GM, Smeby LC, Koch KM, Shaldon S: High-flux synthetic versus cellulosic membranes for $ß_2$-microglobulin removal during hemodialysis, hemodiafiltration and hemofiltration. Nephrol Dial Transplant 4: 653-657, 1989

114. Ronco C, Bowry S: Nanoscale modulation of the pore dimensions, size distribution and structure of a new polysulfone-based high-flux dialysis membrane. Int J Artif Organs 24(10): 726-735, 2001

115. High-flux dialysatoren - Fresenius Polysulfon®. Product brochure from Fresenius Medical Care, Bad Homburg, Germany.

116. Krämer BK, Pickert A, Hohmann C, Liebich HM, Müller GA, Hablitzel M, Risler T: *In vivo* clearance and elimination of nine marker substances during hemofiltration with different membranes. Int J Artif Organs 15(7): 408-412, 1992

117. Schaefer RM, Gilge U, Goehl H, Heidland A: Evaluation of a new polyamide membrane (Polyflux 130) in high-flux dialysis. Blood Purif 8: 23-31, 1990

118. Röckel A, Abdelhamid S, Fliegel P, Walb D: Elimination of low molecular weight proteins with high flux membranes in *Contributions to Nephrology - Highly permeable membranes* edited by Streicher E, Seyfart G, Basel, Karger, 46: 69-74, 1985

119. Röckel A, Hertel J, Fiegel P, Abdelhamid S, Panitz N, Walb D: Permeability and secondary membrane formation of a high flux polysulfone hemofilter. Kidney Int 30: 429-432, 1986

120. Kandus A, Ponikvar R, Drinovec J, Pavlin K, Ivanovich P: Beta 2-microglobulin elimination characteristics during hemofiltration with acrylonitrile and polysulfone membrane hemofilters. Int J Artif Organs 13(4): 200-204, 1990

121. Kes P, Zibcic A, Ratkovic-Gusic I, Prsa M, Sefer S: The effect of hollow-fiber dialyzer Plivadial Altra-Flux 140 on beta-2-microglobulin removal. Acta Med Croatica 51(2): 105-109, 1997

122. Mahiout A, Ludat K, Ghal GM, Schultze G: Effect of sodium dialysate concentration on beta$_2$ microglobulin during haemodialysis. (Abstract) Nephrol Dial Transplant 2: 448, 1987

123. Raj DS, Ouwendyk M, Francoeur R, Pierratos A: ß2-microglobulin kinetics in nocturnal haemodialysis. Nephrol Dial Transplant 15: 58-64, 2000

124. Kirkwood RG, Kunitomo T, Lowrie EG: High rates of controlled ultrafiltration combined with optimal diffusion: recent advances in hemodialysis technique. Nephron 22: 175-181, 1978

125. Kandus A, Malovrh M, Bren AF: Influence of blood flow on adsorption of ß$_2$-microglobulin onto AN69 dialyzer membrane. Artif Organs 21(8): 903-906, 1997

126. Stein G, Günther K, Sperschneider H, Carlsohn H, Hüller M, Schubert K, Schaller R: Clinical evaluation of a new dialyzer, FLX-12 GW, with a polyester-polymer alloy membrane. Artif Organs 17(5): 339-345, 1993

127. Bergström J, Wehle B: No change in corrected ß$_2$-microglobulin concentration after Cuprophane haemodialysis. Lancet March 1: 628-629, 1987

128. Odell RA, Slowiaczek P, Moran JE, Schindhelm K: Beta$_2$-microglobulin kinetics in end-stage renal failure. Kidney Int 39: 909-919, 1991

129. Schaefer RM, Huber L, Gilge U, Bausewein K, Vienken J, Heidland A: Clinical evaluation of a new high-flux cellulose acetate membrane. Int J Artif Organs 12(2): 85-90, 1989

130. Lornoy W, Becaus I, Billiouw JM, Sierens L, De Winter H, Van Malderen P: Beta$_2$ microglobulin kinetics with six different permeability membranes in six anuric haemodialysis patients. (Abstract) Nephrol Dial Transplant 2: 448, 1987

131. Ahrenholz PG, Winkler RE, Michelsen A, Lang DA, Bowry SK: Dialysis membrane-dependent removal of middle molecules during haemodiafiltration: the ß2-microglobulin / albumin relationship. Clinical Nephrology, submitted August 2003.

132. Mann H, Al-Bashir A, Melzer H, Stiller S: Diacap® -polysulfone Hl PS: A new dialysis membrane with optimum ß2-microglobulin elimination . Int J Artif Organs 26(6): 461-466, 2003.

133. Samtleben W, Dengler C, Reinhardt B, Nothdurft A, Lemke H.-D: Comparison of the new polyethersulfone high-flux membrane DIAPES® HF800 with conventional high-flux membranes during on-line haemodiafiltration . Nephrol Dial Transplant 18 : 2382-2386, 2003.

134. Schiffl H, D'Agostini B, Held E: Removal of beta 2-microglobulin by hemodialysis and hemofiltration: a four year follow up. Biomater Artif Cells Immobilization 20(5): 1223-1232, 1992

135. Bardin T, Zingraff J, Kuntz D, Drüeke T: Dialysis-related amyloidosis. Nephrol Dial Transplant 1: 151-154, 1986

136. Canaud B, Assounga A, Kerr P, Aznar R, Mion C: Failure of daily haemofiltration programme using a highly permeable membrane to return beta 2-microglobulin concentrations to normal in haemodialysis patients. Nephrol Dial Transplant 7(9): 924-930, 1992

137. Chanard J, Lavaud S, Toupance O, Melin JP, Gillery P, Revillard JP: $ß_2$-microglobulin-associated amyloidosis in chronic haemodialysis patients. Lancet 1: 1212, 1986

138. Mineshima M, Hoshino T, Era K, Kitano Y, Suzuki T, Sanaka T, Teraoka S, Agishi T, Ota K: Difference in $ß_2$-microglobulin removal between cellulosic and synthetic polymer membrane dialyzers. ASAIO Trans 36(3): M643-646, 1990

139. Ronco C, Heifetz A, Fox K, Curtin C, Brendolan A, Gastaldon F, Crepaldi C, Fortunato A, Pietribasi G, Caberlotto A, Brunello A, Milan Manani S, Zanella M, La Greca G: Beta 2-microglobulin removal by synthetic dialysis membranes. Mechanisms and kinetics of the molecule. Int J Artif Organs 20(3): 136-143, 1997

140. Chanard J, Caudwell V, Valeire J, Vincent C, Randoux C, Wuillai A, Wynckel A: Kinetics of ^{131}I-$ß_2$ microglobulin in hemodialysis patients: assessment using total body counting. Artif Organs 22(7): 574-580, 1998

141. David S, Canino F, Ferrari ME, Cambi V: The role of adsorption in beta 2-microglobulin removal. Nephrol Dial Transplant 6 (Suppl 2): 64-68, 1991

142. Mori H, Hiraoka K, Yorifuji R, Iwasaki T, Gomikawa S, Inagaki O, Inoue S, Takamitsu Y, Fujita Y: Adsorption of human recombinant erythropoietin on dialysis membranes in vitro. Artif Organs 18(10): 725-728, 1994

143. Clark WR, Gao D: Low-molecular weight proteins in end-stage renal disease: potential toxicity and dialytic removal mechanisms. J Am Soc Nephrol 13: S41-S47, 2002

144. Klinke B, Röckel A, Abdelhamid S, Fliegel P, Walb D: Transmembranous transport and adsorption of beta-2-microglobulin during hemodialysis using polysulfone, polyacrylonitrile, polymethylmethacrylate and cuprammonium rayon membranes. Int J Artif Organs 12(11): 697-702, 1989

145. Lee WCR, Uchino S, Fealy N, Baldwin I, Panagiotopoulos S, Goehl H, Morgera S, Neumayer H.-H, Bellomo R: ß2-microglobulin clearance with super high flux hemodialysis: an *ex vivo* study. Int J Artif Organs 26(8): 723-727, 2003

146. Naitoh A, Tatsuguchi T, Okada M, Ohmura T, Sakai K: Removal of beta-2-microglobulin by diffusion alone is feasible using highly permeable dialysis membranes. Trans Am Soc Artif Intern Organs 34: 630-634, 1988

147. Hörl WH: Are new toxins appearing on the horizon? in *Dialysis, dialyzers and sorbents. Where are we going?*, edited by Ronco C, Winchester JF, Basel, Karger, Contrib Nephrol 133: 42-70, 2001

148. Vanholder R, de Smet R, Jacobs V, van Landschoot N, Waterloos MA, Vogeleere P, Ringoir S: Uraemic toxic retention solutes depress polymorphonuclear response to phagocytosis. Nephrol Dial Transplant 9: 1271-1278, 1994

149. Blankestijn PJ, Vos PF, Rabelink TJ, van Rijn HJ, Jansen H, Koomans HA: High-flux dialysis membranes improve lipid profile in chronic hemodialysis patients. J Am Soc Nephrol 5(9): 1703-1708, 1995

150. Mujais SK: Protein permeability in dialysis. Nephrol Dial Transplant 15 (Suppl 1): 10-14, 2000

151. Kaysen GA, Dubin JA, Müller HG, Mitch WE, Rosales LM, Levin NW, and the HEMO group: Relationships among inflammation nutrition and physiologic mechanisms establishing albumin levels in hemodialysis patients. Kidney Int 61: 2240-2249, 2002

152. Jaekel D, Kliem V, Reinhardt B, Sauer N, Lemke H.-D, Krieter DH: In vivo comparison of two new high-flux membranes in haumodialysis (HD). Nephrol Dial Transplantthe new polyethersulfone high-flux membrane DIAPES® HF800 with conventional high-flux membranes during on-line haemodiafiltration . (Abstract) Nephrol Dial Transplant 18 (Suppl 4): 197, 2003

153. Ahrenholz P, Tiess M, Ramlow W, Winkler RE: Removal characteristics of synthetic high-flux dialysers in pre- and post-dilution hemodiafiltration (HDF). (Abstract) J Am Soc Nephrol 13: 239-240A, 2002

154. Kaplan AA, Halley SE, Larkin RA, Graeber CW: Dialysate protein losses with bleach processed polysulphone dialyzers. Kidney Int 47: 573-578, 1995

155. Beck W, Deppisch R, Göhl H: May albumin loss through dialyzer membranes contribute to low serum albumin levels in hemodialysis patients?. (Abstract) Blood Purif 16: 231, 1998

156. Nensel U, Roeckel A, Hillenbrand T, Bartel J: Dialyzer permeability for low-molecular weight proteins: comparison between polysulfone, polyamide and cuproammonium rayon dialyzers. Blood Purif 12(2):128-134,1994

157. Combarnous F, Tetta C, Chapuis Cellier C, Wratten ML, Custaud MA, De Catheu T, Fouque D, David S, Carraro G, Laville M: Albumin loss in on-line hemodiafiltrationInt J Artif Organs 25(3): 203-209, 2002

158. Shinzato T, Miwa M, Nakai S, Takai I, Matsumoto Y, Morita H, Miyata T, Maeda K: Alternate repetition of short fore- and backfiltrations reduces convective albumin loss. Kidney Int 50(2):432-435, 1996

159. Hillion D, Terki NH, Savoiu C et al: Albumin loss with high flux dialysers is under estimated. J Am Soc Nephrol 10: A283, 1999

160. Miwa M, Shinzato T: Push/pull hemodiafiltration: technical aspects and clinical effectiveness. Artif Organs 23(12): 1123-1126, 1999

161. Kim ST, Yamamoto C, Taoka M, Takasugi M: Programmed filtration, a new method for removing large molecules and regulating albumin during hemodiafiltration treatment. Am J Kidney Dis 38 (4 Suppl 1):S220-223, 2001

162. Lebedo I: Does convective dialysis therapy applied daily approach renal blood purification?. Kidney Int 59 (Suppl 78): S286-S291, 2001

163. Navarro JF, Marcén R, Teruel JL, del Río RM, Gámez C, Mora C, Ortuño J: Effect of different membranes on amino-acid losses during haemodialysis. Nephrol Dial Transplant 13: 113-117, 1998

164. Tepper T, Van der Hem GK, Tuma GJ, Arisz L, Donker AJ: Loss of amino acids during hemodialysis: quantitative and qualitative investigations. Clin Nephrol 10(1): 16-20, 1978

165. Ikizler TA, Flakoll PJ, Parker RA, Hakim RM: Amino acid and albumin losses during hemodialysis. Kidney Int 46(3): 830-837, 1994

166. Gutierrez A: Protein catabolism in maintenance haemodialysis: the influence of the dialysis membrane. Nephrol Dial Transplant 11 (Suppl 2): 108-111, 1996

167. Navarro JK, Mora C, León C, Del Río RM, Marcia ML, Gallego E, Chahin J, Méndez ML, Rivero A, Gracía J: Amino acid losses during hemodialysis with polyacrlyonitrile membranes: effect of intradialytic amino acid supplementation on plasma amino acid concentrations and nutritional variables in nondiabetic patients. Am J Clin Nutr 71: 765-773, 2000

168. Hynote ED, McCamish MA, Depner TA, Davis PA: Amino acid losses during hemodialysis: effects of high-solute flux and parenteral nutrition in acute renal failure. J Parent Ent Nutr 19: 15-21, 1995

169. Kopple JD, Swendseid ME, Shinaberger JH, Umezawa CY: The free and bound amino acids removed by hemodialysis. Trans Am Soc Artif Org 19: 309-313, 1973.

6. Performance-enhancing designs

Although most dialysers today have a close physical resemblance to those hollow-fibre devices used over 30 years ago, a number of new variations in design aimed at optimising filter performance have appeared in recent years. Most of these innovations are not obvious as they pertain to the interior of the filter casing, only those affecting the filter exterior being conspicuous. Unfortunately, ambiguity of the nomenclature used to describe dialyser features has led to some degree of confusion regarding actual developments: nowadays a variety of sometimes synonymous terms are used to describe constructions aimed at increasing filter performance (examples are given in **figure 6.1**). The practising clinician cannot be faulted for suspecting marketing gimmickry at times. This chapter aims at elucidating the scientific bases of new developments and the superfluity of terms used. Generally, improvements in either (1) the dialysis fluid flow around and throughout the fibre bundle, (2) blood access to and contact with the membrane, or (3) transmembrane transport as determined by fibre geometry and structure are targeted.

6.1 Constructions for optimising dialysis fluid flow within the dialyser

Optimally, each hollow fibre within a fibre bundle in a dialyser should be completely bathed in moving dialysis fluid for it to perform best. However, a number of observations made in recent years have shown that dialysis fluid flow is sub-optimal in practice. For example, increasing the dialysis fluid flow from 500 ml/min to 800 ml/min in a number of dialysers was found to result in significant increases in urea mass area transfer coefficient (K_oA) *in vitro* and *in vivo* (see chapter 5.2.3 for details) [1-5]. This increase could be due to a decrease in the stagnant dialysis fluid layer along the membrane (due to increased shear rates) and/or an increase in effective surface area (due to improved perfusion of the fibre bundle), whereby the former reason was indicated in a recent study [5, 6]. Increasing dialysis fluid flow is costly and alternative designs were sought which could ensure high dialysis fluid flow along the length of the fibres as well as good penetration of dialysis fluid through the fibre bundle, i.e. avoid channelling and non-uniform distribution of dialysis fluid flow. A number of different strategies are followed to achieve this; these focus on either the fibre bundle, the fibre itself or the dialyser casing, as summarised in **table 6.1**.

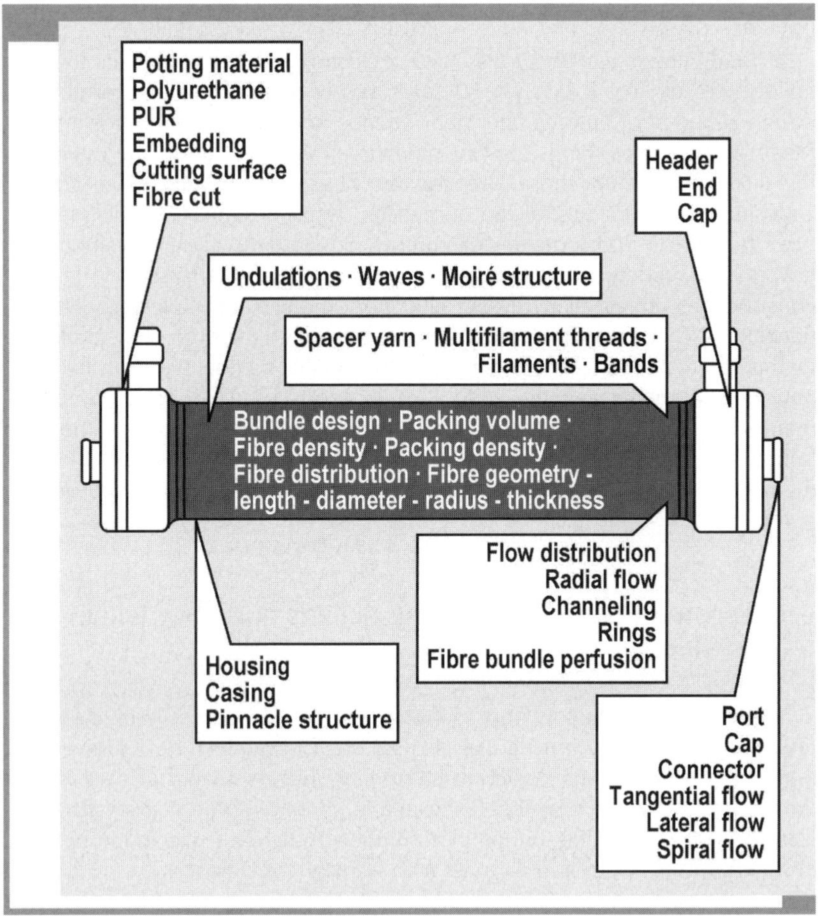

Figure 6.1: Variety of terms associated with performance-enhancing features of dialyser design. *The various nomenclatures used to describe changes in design that aim at improving dialyser performance can be confusing.*

Filter part affected	Feature names	Figure		Some companies supplying such dialysers and examples of the membranes involved
Fibre bundle	Spacer yarn Multifilament yarn Filaments	**Figure 6.2**	Asahi Baxter Bellco Cobe Haidylena Kawasumi Meditech Nipro/Nissho Saxonia Toray	PAN SMC®*, DIAPES®* SMC®*, DIAPES®* Some PES/Arylane® PES* SMC®*, DIAPES®* PES* PES DIAPES®* Some PMMA
Hollow fibre	Undulations Waves Moiré structure	**Figure 6.3**	Fresenius Medical Care Gambro B.Braun	Fresenius Polysulfone®, Helixone® Polyamix™ α Polysulfone
	FIN structure FINs	**Figure 6.6**	Teijin Hospal/Cobe	Cell. diacetate Cell. diacetate from Teijin
Casing	Pinnacle structures Radial flow Flow distributor	**Figure 6.7**	Fresenius Medical Care	Helixone®

**membranes produced by Membrana, Germany*

Table 6.1: Designs for improving dialysis fluid flow along and throughout the fibre bundle in dialysers. *PAN: polyacrylonitrile; PES: polyarylethersulfone, PMMA: polymethylmethacrylate.*

Spacer yarn versus waved fibres

A common approach to improving dialysis fluid flow throughout the dialyser interior appears to be the use of multifilament spacer yarns. These are placed within the fibre bundle to separate the fibres, thereby ensuring a more uniform dialysis fluid flow distribution around them. Two common but different forms of such spacer yarns are depicted in **figure 6.2**. A somewhat different configuration involving winding of the spacer yarn around the hollow fibres has been adopted by Toray for some PMMA dialysers. Dialyser performance was demonstrated to be much improved with the use of spacer yarn: for example, urea, creatinine, phosphate and inulin clearances increased by about 20%, 16%, 20% and 32%, respectively, in Asahi's PAN 650 SF dialyser when spacer yarn was employed [8]. The greater impact on inulin clearance than on urea clearance suggests that improved dialysis fluid penetration of the fibre bundle, rather than increased shear rates, is responsible for the enhancement in performance, as clearances of higher molecular weight solutes are more dependent on surface area than is the clearance of urea. Also, the undesired channelling of dialysis fluid, which was observed in the peripheral region of hollow fibre bundles, was significantly reduced when spacer yarn was included [8]. Significant increases in clearances were also reported in some Membrana products (e.g. DIAPES® and SMC® membranes) when spacer yarn was introduced into their fibre bundles [9-11].

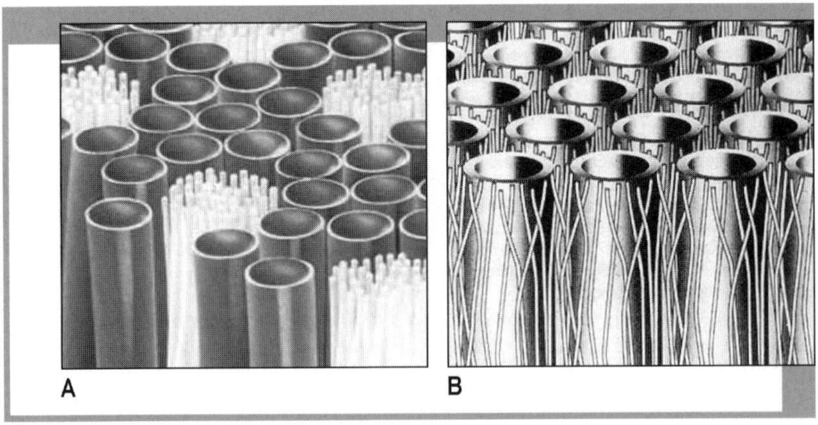

Figure 6.2: Two types of multifilament spacer yarn. *The multifilament yarn is positioned within the fibre bundle in order to separate the fibres and thus ensure a more homogeneous dialysis fluid flow distribution around them (A: with permission from Membrana GmbH, Germany; B: adapted from [7]).*

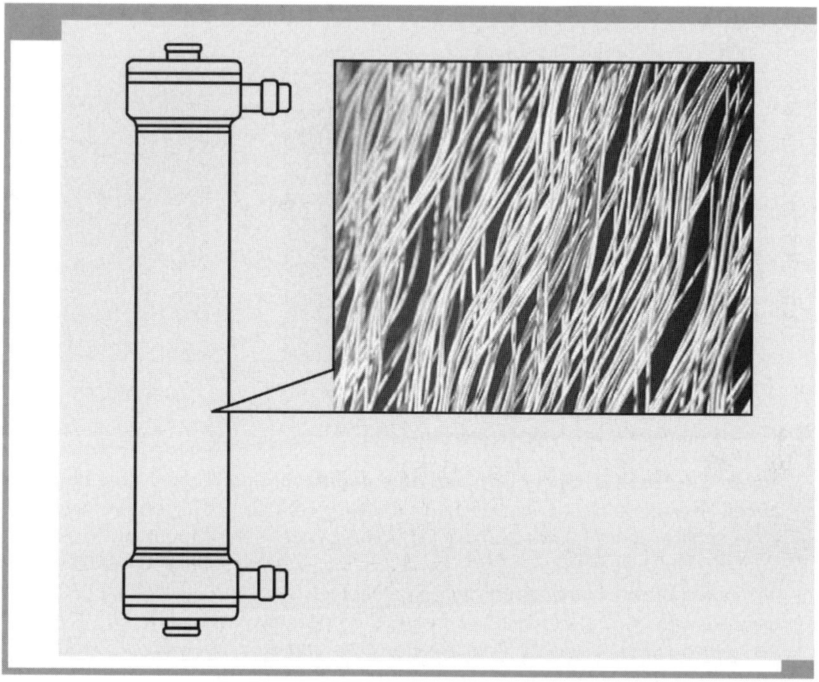

Figure 6.3: "Moiré structure" or "undulations" or "waves". *The fibres in the dialyser have a wavy or undulated form. This impedes the formation of a stagnant dialysis fluid layer at the membrane surface and ensures good spacing of the fibres (with permission from Fresenius Medical Care Deutschland GmbH).*

Another common approach to optimising dialysis fluid flow in the fibre bundle and reducing channelling is to give the fibres themselves a wavy or undulated or moiré structure (**figure 6.3**). The formation of a stagnant dialysis fluid layer (also called dialysis fluid boundary layer) at the outer membrane surface is then hampered, thus reducing mass transfer resistance on the dialysis fluid side of the membrane. Close aligning of the fibres is also avoided, which facilitates good inter-fibre dialysis fluid flow and increases the effective surface area. Fibre waving has also been reported to yield urea clearance increases of up to 20% (**figure 6.4**) [12]. A comparison using computerised tomography-based techniques of this type of dialyser with conventional dialysers and ones with spacer yarn revealed that flow distribution was most homogenous in dialysers with wavy fibres and least homogenous in conven-

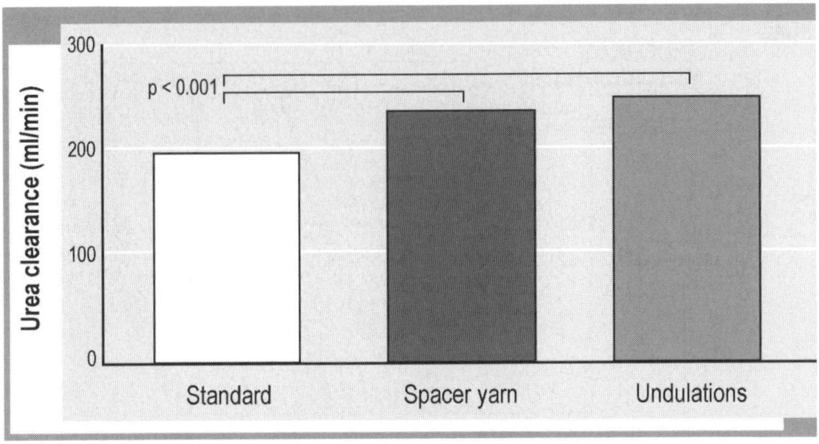

Figure 6.4: Effect of spacer yarn and fibre undulations on dialyser urea clearances. *Average values of urea clearance obtained with the 3 dialysers of comparable surface area (1.3 m^2) and packing density but with different or no performance-enhancing features are shown. The dialysers are Asahi PAN 65DX dialysers without performance-enhancing technology (standard), Asahi PAN 650SF dialysers with spacing yarn external to the fibres (spacer yarn) and FB 130 dialysers with cellulose diacetate from Nissho/Nipro and with wavy fibres (undulations). Measurements were made at Q_B = 300 ml/min and Q_D = 500 ml/min (adapted from [12]).*

tional dialysers, with dialysers containing spacer yarn holding an intermediate position (**figure 6.5**) [13]. A recent comparison of dialysers containing polysulfone membranes with a wave and the same polysulfone membranes with increased wave frequency but lower wave amplitude (the so-called microcrimping) showed that mass transfer characteristics of dialysers can be further enhanced by altering the actual shape of the undulations [5].

What about "fins" and other structures?

Another less common technique for improving bundle perfusion with dialysis fluid by securing space between fibres and keeping these separated is the construction of fin-like structures at the outer surfaces of the individual fibres (**figure 6.6**). The effect of this technology on filter performance has not been well documented, and did not appear to be significant in one study

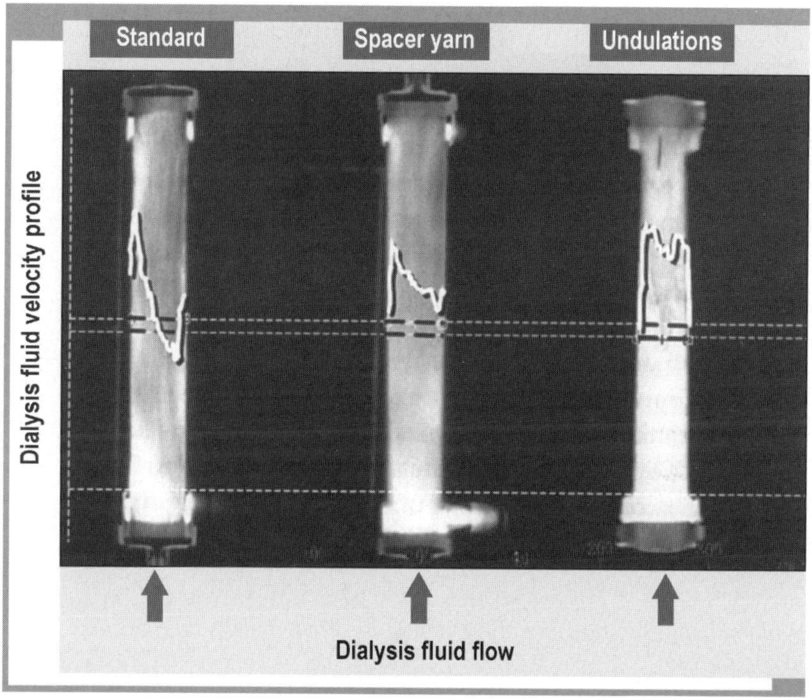

Figure 6.5: Effect of spacer yarn and fibre undulations on dialysis fluid flow. *Distributions of dialysis fluid flow in the dialysis fluid compartments of the three dialysers described in the previous figure were measured with computerised tomography-based techniques. The profiles show that, as the flow distribution pattern builds up, the standard dialyser displays an inhomogeneous distribution of the dye with higher velocity in the peripheral regions of the dialyser. The pattern is improved when spacer yarn is included in the bundle, and is improved even further when the fibres are undulated in the absence of spacer yarn (from [14] with permission).*

published [16]. Attempts to enhance performance by weaving a small number of fibres with a filament to form "bands" of fibres within the bundle have now been largely abandoned because of the technical complexity. However, crossing of fibres at a certain angle in combination with undulations has been adopted by Gambro for their Polyflux dialysers [17].

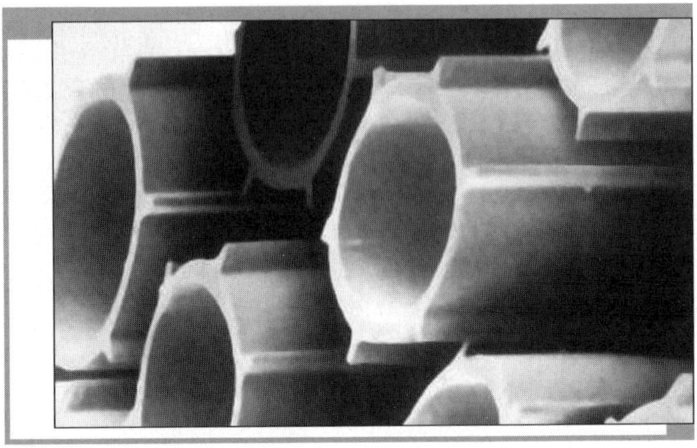

Figure 6.6: Fins at the ends of fibres. *The fin-like structure at the outer surfaces of the cellulose diacetate hollow fibres in dialysers from Teijin (Hospal/Cobe) aim at enhancing bundle perfusion and keeping the fibres straight (adapted from [15]).*

Which changes in housing construction improve dialysis fluid access to the fibres?

Observations of channelling of dialysis fluid in dialysers, e.g. higher flow in the region external to the fibre bundle and lower to even stagnant flow in the interior of the bundle (e.g. **figure 6.5**), led also to new fibre housing constructions. One attempt is the use of rings within the dialyser casing, which aim at evenly distributing the dialysis fluid. However, an even more innovative performance-enhancing construction to minimise dialysis fluid channelling is the "pinnacle structure" of the ends of the polypropylene casing of the Fresenius Helixone® dialysers (**figure 6.7**). This construction (together with the fibre undulations and improved fibre distribution) facilitates equal dialysis fluid flow distribution around the fibre bundle, thus improving conditions for good internal perfusion thereof with dialysis fluid [18].

Dialysers with 2 -3 different effective membrane surface areas from the same company are frequently supplied in housings of the same size. This means that variations in packing density are common, and this can be expected to affect the fibre bundle perfusion with dialysis fluid. Studies have shown that low packing densities result in shunting of dialysis fluid past the fibre bundle [6, 19], and excessively high packing densities may lead to

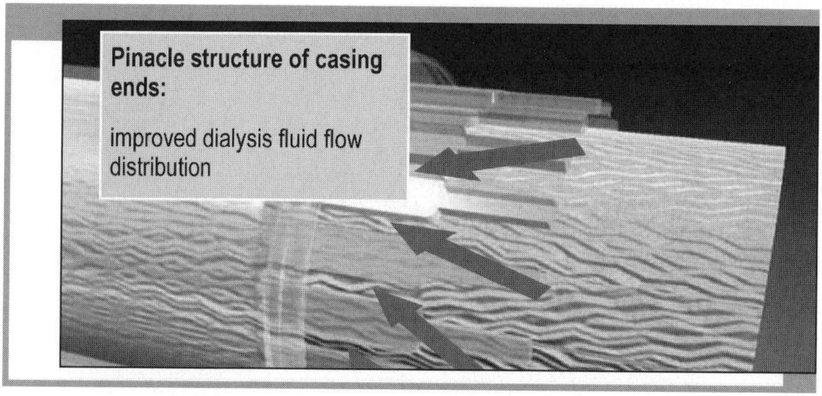

Figure 6.7: Pinnacle structure of dialyser housing ends. *The pinnacle structure of the ends of the polypropylene casing in the new FX class polysulfone dialysers from Fresenius Medical Care makes the dialysis fluid flow distribution more homogenous around the fibre bundle, thus improving conditions for good internal perfusion thereof (with permission from Fresenius Medical Care Deutschland GmbH, Germany).*

practically stagnant flow, thereby inducing channelling [6, 20]. Ideally, optimal dialyser dimensions and subsequent packing density should be determined for each dialyser individually, and theoretical calculations for such have long been available [21]. However, the practicalities of using standard casings for a narrow range of different "size" dialysers are convincing; disadvantages of doing so can be reduced by using modern, sophisticated potting techniques which ensure homogenous and optimal fibre distribution, such as are employed by some leading producers of dialysers (**figure 6.8**).

6.2 Approaches to optimise blood access to the membrane

Blood flow distribution in some hollow fibre dialysers was recently assessed using computerised tomography-based techniques: blood flow was found to be higher in the central regions of the dialysers than at the fibre bundle periphery, and this parabolic flow profile became more evident with increasing haematocrit ([13], **figure 6.9**). This flow pattern enhances the mismatch between blood and dialysis fluid flows which already exists due to maldistribution of dialysis fluid flow, e.g. in cases of excessive or packing density (**figure 6.10**). One feasible explanation for the observed parabolic

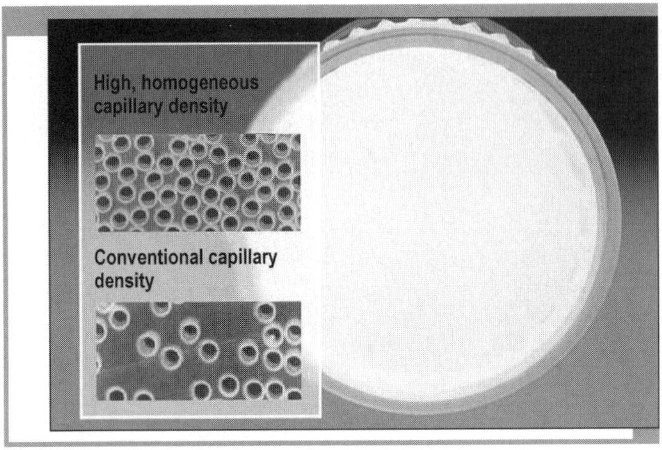

Figure 6.8: Optimal packing density of fibres within a given dialyser housing is homogenous. *The optimal packing density of hollow fibre dialysers is reflected in a tightly packed but homogenous potting (with permission from Fresenius Medical Care Deutschland GmbH, Germany).*

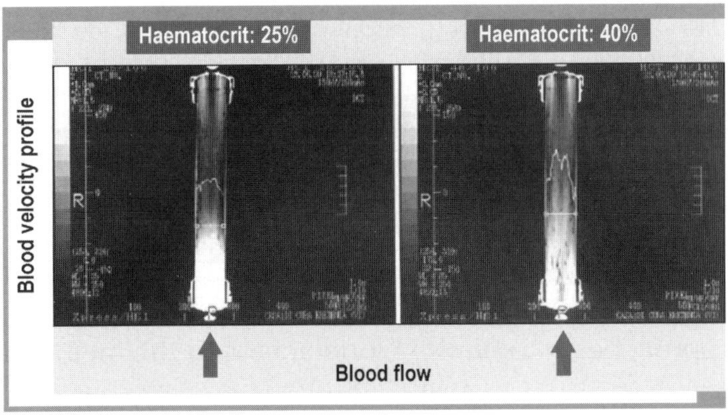

Figure 6.9: Blood flow is higher in the central fibres of a bundle than at the periphery. *Dye was injected into the blood compartment of a hollow fibre dialysers and circulated at 300 ml/min. The haematocrit was 25% in one experiment (left) and 40% in the other (right). Distributions of flow in the blood compartment were measured with computerised tomography-based techniques. The profiles show that the flow velocity distribution is parabolically shaped, and that this shape becomes more exaggerated in the case of higher haematocrit (from [14] with permission).*

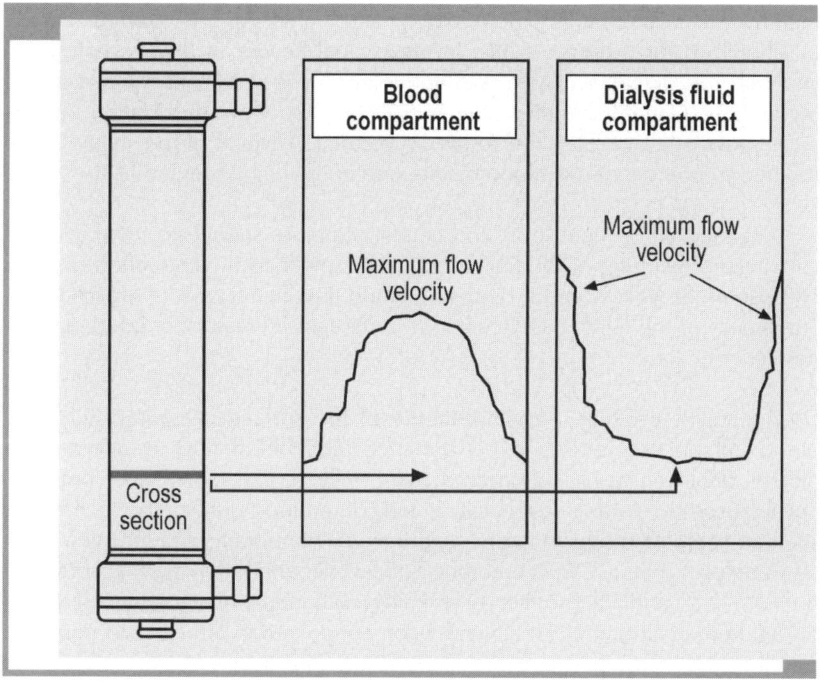

Figure 6.10: Mismatch between blood and dialysis fluid flow distributions. *Sub-optimal packing of hollow fibres can result in higher dialysis fluid flows at the periphery of the dialyser compared to the central regions. Coupled with the inverse blood flow profile found especially at high haematocrits, a mismatch of flows results which has detrimental effects on dialyser performance (from [14] with permission, velocity profiles here refer to blood and dialysis fluid flowing from the bottom to the top of the dialyser).*

blood flow profile is poor blood distribution at the arterial header region of the dialyser. This stimulated the development of new header designs, especially for the arterial ports, which aim at minimising dead spaces and totally avoiding irregularities in the internal structure. Recently, novel header designs that change the blood flow profile were introduced by the leading filter manufacturers Fresenius Medical Care and Hospal. In the new headers from both companies, the blood enters the dialyser through a laterally positioned-blood port of similar external appearance. In the case of the Fresenius Medical Care header on the FX-class dialysers, a helicoidal distributor built into the header region forces the inflowing blood to turn around a cylindrical helix, thereby maximising radial blood velocity and increasing homogenous access to all hollow fibres (**figure 6.11**). In the Hospal header on the Arylane H/M and cellulose diacetate dialysers, blood inlet flow is at a sharper angle to the bundle, i.e. tangential rather than radial [18, 22]. Flow distribution studies have shown that at least the former construction (spiral blood inflow) contributed to homogeneous blood distribution in the header region [18].

A refined blood entry port and header structure should go hand in hand with accurate cutting of the fibres: poor cutting results in obstruction or even collapse of the hollow fibres, hindering blood flow unnecessarily (**figure 6.12**). The quality of the cutting surface is now a recognised feature of good dialyser design.

Generally speaking, the smoothness of the surface in contact with the blood influences membrane performance (e.g. blood flow is affected by platelet adhesion at rough surfaces [23]), as does the loss of filter performance caused by clotting - especially in long-time blood purification techniques such as haemofiltration in acute renal failure. Membrane coating with polyethylenglycol (PEG) [23], membrane surface heparinisation during fibre production [24], and haemofilter prepriming with heparinised saline or heparinised human albumin [25] have all been conducted in attempts to minimise performance losses due to such effects, but no improvements were observed.

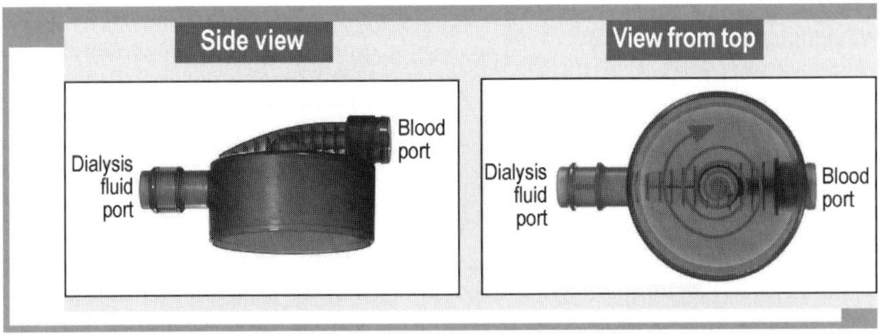

Figure 6.11: New header design with lateral blood inlet port and spiral blood flow. *The novel header employed by Fresenius Medical Care for their FX class dialysers has a laterally positioned blood port. A helicoidal distributor forces inflowing blood to more or less spirally access the complete face of the bundle. The blood flow distribution within the fibre bundle is thus improved compared to that in conventional headers (from Fresenius Medical Care with permission).*

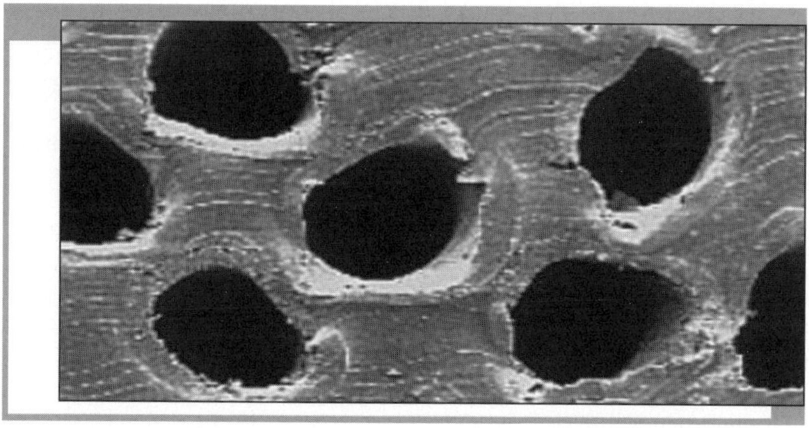

Figure 6.12: Poor cutting surface of a commercially available hollow fibre bundle in potting compound. *Poor cutting of the potting compound can result in partial or complete obstruction of blood flow into the hollow fibres, as well as in uneven and deformed fibre openings.*

6.3 Changes in fibre geometry and membrane structure aimed at improving transmembrane transport

Clearance values and ultrafiltration coefficients provide the clinician with clinically relevant performance data for a dialyser of a particular size - information on actual fibre wall thickness, diameter and length is only of academic interest in clinical practice, as this information is an integral part of the standard performance values. The same holds for the membrane structure itself. However, an understanding of new filter designs often necessitates an awareness of how these factors contribute to good removal performance.

Fibre thickness

As Fick's Law (see appendix) governs solute diffusion, the fibre wall thickness will affect diffusion insofar as it increases the diffusion length, thereby effectively reducing the concentration gradient driving diffusion. Essentially, the thicker the membrane, the lower the diffusive clearance. Differences in membrane thickness probably explain the higher urea mass transfer coefficient (K_oA) observed with a high-flux cellulose triacetate dialyser (15 µm) compared to the high-flux synthetic (40 μm) dialyser [1]. Reductions in fibre wall thickness have been shown to augment urea and creatinine clearance to such an extent that dialysers of smaller surface area could be used [26, 27].

Care must be exercised when referring to absolute values for membrane thickness. For example, the difference between the actual membrane thickness of cellulosic and synthetic membranes is complicated by the fact that synthetic membranes are composed of very thin skins (inner and/or outer) and a spongy outer matrix which lends them mechanical support, and which may or may not be counted as "membrane thickness" in solute removal mechanisms. Also, cellulose membranes swell when wet, increasing wall thickness by about 100% [28].

Highly permeable dialysis membranes tend to be now thinner and/or more porous than their older counterparts, allowing significant diffusive clearances of ß2-m, which can even exceed the respective convective clearances at times [29-33]. For membranes that remove solutes via adsorption (e.g. ß2-m removal by PMMA), an increase in porosity is targeted rather than a reduction in fibre thickness, as the adsorptive surface of a membrane lies primarily in its pore structure.

Fibre diameter

When an increase in fibre diameter means an increase in membrane surface area, diffusive and convective transmembrane solute transport will be enhanced correspondingly, as previously discussed. However, under conditions of constant surface area, increasing fibre diameter goes hand in hand with a reduction in the number of fibres or the fibre length, as hollow fibre surface area is defined as

$$\underset{\text{surface area}}{A} = 2 \cdot \pi \cdot \underset{\text{fibre radius}}{r} \cdot \underset{\text{fibre length}}{\Delta l} \cdot \underset{\text{fibre number}}{N} \qquad \textbf{[6.1]}$$

These variations should have no effect on diffusive solute transport in low-flux dialysers, as this is a simple function of membrane surface area (see Fick's Law in appendix). However, convection is the dominant mode of solute removal for middle and large solutes, especially in high-flux dialysers, and this is sensitive to the exact relationship between fibre diameter, number and length, being a function of the transmembrane pressure gradient. From analysis of the relevant equations (especially Hagen-Poiseuille's Law depicted in **figure**

6.13, eqn. 6.1 for surface area and eqn. 5.3 for membrane porosity), one can conclude that increases in fibre length, pore number and pore size will augment convective removal, as will decreases in fibre radius. (Note: the positive effect of fibre number on fibre surface area is negated by its presence in the denominator of the Hagen-Poiseuille equation, and the negative effect of fibre radius on convective transport is exaggerated due to its fourth power in the denominator of the Hagen-Poiseuille equation.) This, and the fact that reducing fibre diameter results in an increased average flow per fibre and consequent higher wall shear rates [14], explains recent developments by some manufacturers concerning reductions in fibre diameter with the aim of improving convective clearance. For example, a reduction in the inner diameter of polysulfone hollow fibres from 200 µm to 185 µm was shown to increase solute removal, especially that of ß2-m [34]. Reductions down to 175 µm resulted in significant increases of in vivo convective clearances of vitamin B_{12} and inulin of more than 30% (**figure 6.14**) [35]. Similar effects of reduced membrane diameter have been observed by others [36]; here measurements

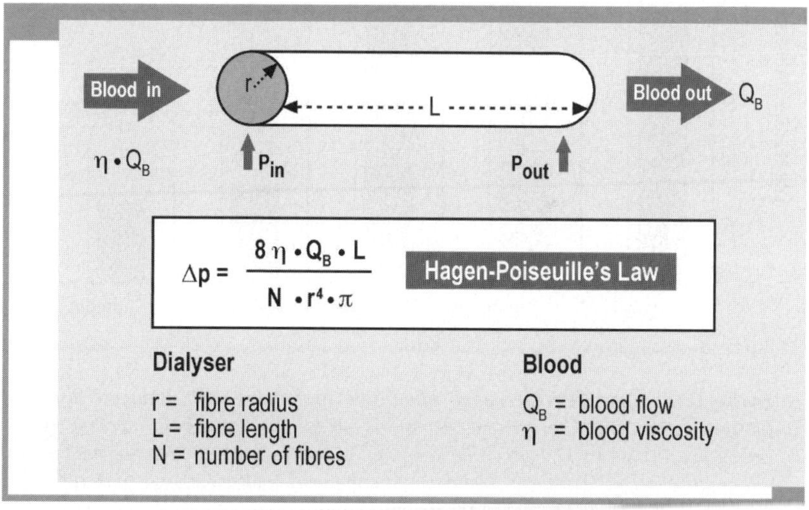

Figure 6.13: Increased pressure drop with reduced fibre diameter. *The pressure drop along the length of a hollow fibre can be estimated using Hagen-Poiseuille's Law. Decreasing fibre radius (r) results in an increased pressure drop. In general, the higher the pressure drop, the greater the convective transport of solutes from the blood into the dialysis fluid or filtrate.*

of hydrostatic pressures and longitudinal reductions therein proved that the pressure drop, and therefore convective removal, is significantly greater when the fibre diameter is narrowed.

Correspondingly, dialysers with fibres of larger inner diameter have smaller changes in pressure along their length, and therefore reduced filtration. These are mostly used in paediatric dialysis, in arteriovenous circuits and for patients treated with continuous replacement therapies because the filtration volume is reduced at a given blood flow and the degree of heparinisation necessary is reduced [14]. For example, fibres of even 1100 µm and 570 µm lumen are commercially available for acute dialysis of infants and children, respectively.

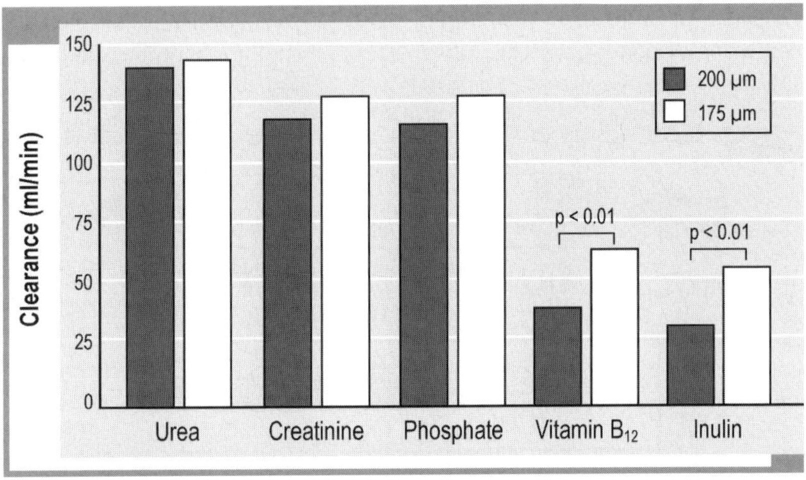

Figure 6.14: Increased clearance of middle molecules with reduced fibre diameter. *Reducing the internal diameter of Fresenius Polysulfone® hollow fibres from 200 µm to 175 µm while keeping the dialyser surface area constant at 0.5 m^2 resulted in statistically significantly enhanced total clearances (i.e. diffusive plus convective clearances) for the middle molecules vitamin B_{12} and inulin (adapted from [14]).*

Fibre length

Once again, diffusive transport is described by Fick' Law (see appendix) and as such is directly related to membrane surface area (eqn. 6.1). Consequently, dialysers of equal surface area with identical membranes should have equal diffusive clearances, irrespective of their specific fibre length. However, convective removal, as described above, is a direct function of fibre length and, as a result, convective transport can be expected to be higher in dialysers with long fibres than in dialysers with short fibres of the same surface area.

These theoretical considerations were supported in a recent *in vivo* study addressing the possible advantages of using *short* fibres for *acute* renal failure patients: the pressure drop along the length of the fibres was greater for long fibres (23 cm) than for short fibres (14 cm) in 2 polysulfone dialysers of equal surface area (0.7 m^2) [37]. The conditions in continuous therapies with low blood flow circuits are such that the use of filters with many short fibres would then appear to be preferable in order to avoid excess filtration and resultant clotting. However, an unexpected finding of this investigation of venovenous haemofiltration in acute renal failure patients was that the shorter dialysers had an *increased* transmembrane pressure (despite having a lower pressure drop along the dialyser) and *shorter* running time until clotting than the longer ones, i.e. they failed to show the expected lower transmembrane pressure gradient and consequent prolongation of running time. The authors offered a plausible explanation involving the influence of the blood pump in the CVVH treatment, but exact investigations into this unexpected result remain to be undertaken. In the meanwhile, there is no clear indication for the use of particularly short dialysers in intensive care units.

Membrane structure

The specific characteristics of the various membrane structures have been described already in this book (chapter 2). However, there is one development worth mentioning with regard to performance-enhancing advances, i.e. the application of modern nanotechnology in membrane production facilities. For example, nano-controlled spinning technology (NCS™) was employed by the producers of the new Helixone® membrane (Fresenius Medical Care) to modulate and control the number, size and size distribution of pores on the inner surface of the polysulfone hollow fibre [18, 32, 38-40]. The *in vitro* studies performed to date document that the result is a polysulfone membrane that is more permeable to ß2-microglobulin than high-flux polysulfone without compromising the albumin retention characteristics [18, 32]. First *in vivo* measurements of different sized Helixone® dialysers have confirmed the high ß2-m removal and good albumin retention of this new membrane [18, 41, 42]. The secret to this success is a marginal increase of the mean pore size (by 0.2 nm) coupled with a simultaneous narrowing of the pore size distribution (**figure 6.15**, [32]). The effect on the sieving coefficient of the membrane is illustrated in **figure 6.16**: this technology offers clear advantages for the production of highly-permeable, safe membranes for high-flux dialysis, haemofiltration and haemodiafiltration.

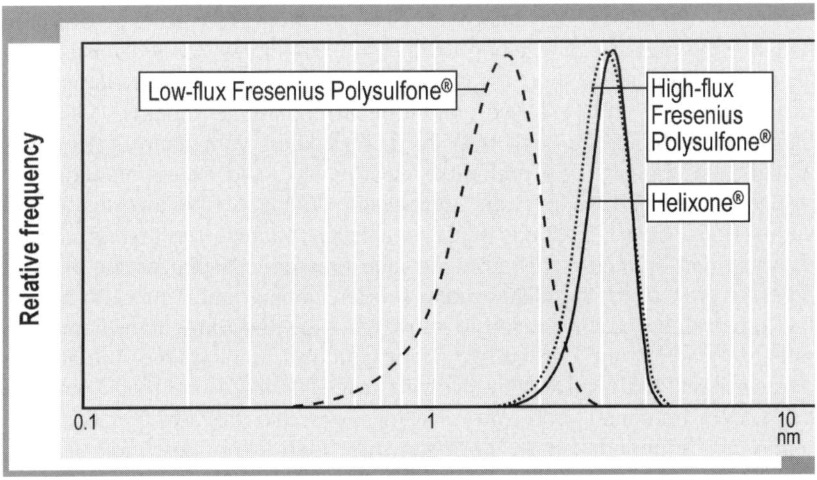

Figure 6.15: Improved pore structure of hollow fibre inner surface due to the application of nanotechnology. *The application of nanotechnology fabrication principles and procedures has enabled the development of a new polysulfone membrane (Helixone®) with a higher mean pore size (by 0.2 nm, as indicated by the peak at 3.3 nm rather than at 3.1 nm) and an overall narrower pore size range (as indicated by the reduced peak width) than the high-flux Fresenius Polysulfone® membrane. This enhances the passage of ß2-microglobulin and restricts the loss of proteins such as albumin (from Fresenius Medical Care with permission).*

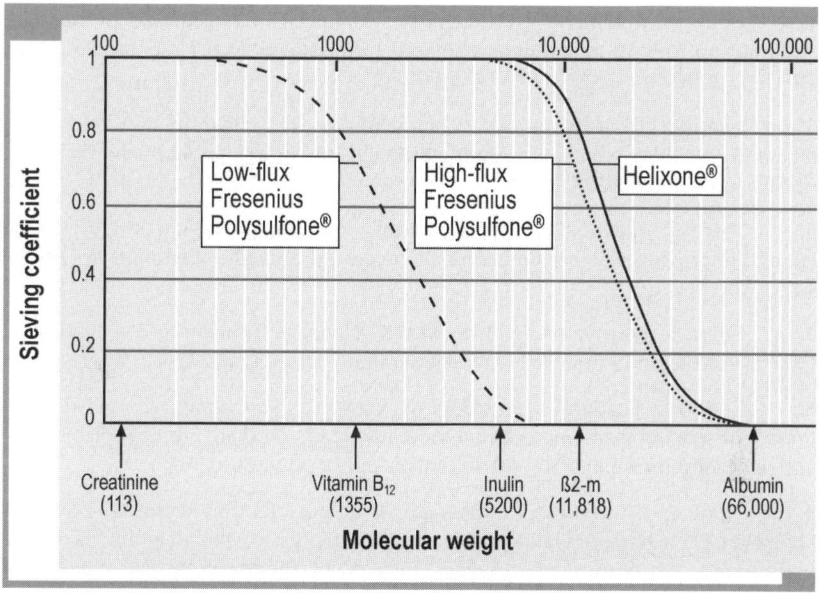

Figure 6.16: Effect of nanotechnology-based production on the sieving coefficients of the Helixone® membrane. *The changes in pore number, size and size distribution achieved by the application of nanotechnology in the production of the Helixone® membrane result in augmented sieving coefficients for middle molecules with simultaneous good retention of albumin (from Fresenius Medical Care with permission).*

References

1. Leypoldt JK, Cheung AK, Agodoa LY, Daugirdas JT, Greene T, Keshaviah PR: Hemodialyzer mass transfer-area coefficients for urea increase at high dialysate flow rates. Kidney Int 51(6): 2013-2017, 1997

2. Ouseph R, Ward RA: Increasing dialysate flow rate increases dialyzer urea mass transfer-area coefficients during clinical use. Am J Kidney Dis 37(2): 316-320, 2001

3. Choong LHL, Leypoldt JK, Cheung AK: Dialyzer mass transfer-area coefficients (KoA) during clinical haemodialysis (HD) are dependent on both blood flow (Qb) and dialysate flow (Qd) rates. (Abstract) J Am Soc Nephrol 10: 189A, 1999

4. Hauk M, Kuhlmann MK, Riegel W, Köhler H: In vivo effects of dialysate flow rate on Kt/V in maintenance hemodialysis patients. Am J Kidney Dis 35(1): 105-111, 2000

5. Leypoldt JK, Cheung AK, Chirananthavat T, Gilson JF, Kamerath CD, Deeter RB: Hollow fiber shape alters solute clearances in high flux hemodialyzers. ASAIO Journal 49: 81-87, 2003

6. Ward RA, Leypoldt JK: What clinically important advances in understanding and improving dialyzer function have occurred recently?. Seminars in Dialysis 14(3): 160-162, 2001

7. Ohira S, Nagayama M, Iwayama K, Hanai T, Enokimoto Y, Nitadori Y: Clinical evaluation of new PAN-DX dialyser. Jpn J Artif Organs 22(1): 3-7, 1993

8. Ronco C, Scabardi M, Goldoni M, Brendolan A, Crepaldi C, La Greca G: Impact of spacing filaments external to hollow fibers on dialysate flow distribution and dialyzer performance. Int J Artif Organs 20(5): 261-266, 1997

9. Günther C, Ansorge W, Blümich B, Blümler P, Chwatinski C, Bowry S, Lemke H.-D.: Characterization of a new technique to enhance the clearance performance of all modern dialyzers using NMR spectroscopy. (Abstract) Artif Organs 23(7): 650, 1999

10. Clark WR, Shinaberger JH: Clinical evaluation of a new high efficiency hemodialyzer: Polysynthane™. ASAIO J 46: 288-292, 2000

11. Günther C, Ansorge W, Blümich B, Blümler P, Chwatinski C, von Harten B, Lemke H-D: New highly effective technique to enhance the clearance performance in modern dialyzers. (Abstract) ERA-EDTA Congress: No. 270, 1999

12. Ronco C, Brendolan A, Crepaldi C, Rodighiero M, Everard P, Ballestri M, Cappelli G, Spittle M, la Greca G: Dialysate flow distribution in hollow fiber hemodialyzers with different dialysate pathway configurations. Int J Artif Organs 23(9): 601-609, 2000

13. Ronco C: What clinically important advances in understanding and improving dialyzer function have occurred recently? Seminars in Dialysis 14(3): 164-169, 2001

14. Vienken J, Ronco C: New developments in hemodialyzers in *Dialysis, dialyzers and sorbents. Where are we going?*, edited by Ronco C, Winchester JF, Basel, Karger, Contrib Nephrol 133: 105-118, 2001

15. Hosmed Medizintechnik GmbH product brochure for TFU-FIN dialysers. Distributed at the Dialysis Nurse Congress in Ulm, Germany, 1993

16. Hoenich NA, Woffindin C, Cox PJ, Goldfinch M, Roberts SJ: Clinical characterization of Dicea a new cellulose membrane for haemodialysis. Clinical Nephrology 48(4): 253-259, 1997

17. Ronco C, Crepaldi C, Brendolan A, Bragantini L, d'Intini V, Inguaggiato P, Bonello M, Krause B, Deppisch R, Goehl H, Scabardi A: Evolution of synthetic membranes for blood purification: the case of the Polyflux family. Nephrol Dial Transplant 18 (Suppl 7): vii10-vii20, 2003

18. Ronco C, Bowry SK, Brendolan A, Crepaldi C, Soffiati G, Fortunato A, Bordoni V, Granziero A, Torsello G, La Greca G: Hemodialyzer: From macro-design to membrane nanostructure; the case of the FX class of hemodialyzers. Kidney Int 61 (Suppl 80): S126-S142, 2002

19. Noda I, Brown-West DG, Gryte CC: Effect of flow maldistribution on hollow fiber dialysis - experimental studies. J Membr Sci 5: 209-225, 1979

20. Noda I, Gryte CC: Mass transfer in regular arrays of holow fibers in countercurrent dialysis. AIChE J 25(1): 113-122, 1979

21. L, Zaltzman S: Optimum geometry for artificial kidney dialyzers. Chem Eng Prog Symp Ser 64(84): 101-104, 1968

22. Hospal product brochure: Arylane H/M series - A design for unmatched performance. EDTA congress, Nice, 2000

23. Tsunoda N, Kokubo K-I, Sakai K, Fukuda M, Miyazaki M, Hiyoshi T: Surface roughness of cellulose hollow fiber dialysis membranes and platelet adhesion. ASAIO Journal: 418-423, 1999

24. Józwiak A, Ciechanowska A, Sabalinska S, Werynski A, Wójcicki J: Experimental heparinized hollow fiber membrane, evaluation of the filtration efficiency. (Abstract) Artif Organs 23(7): 651, 1999

25. Reeves JH, Seal PF, Voss AL, O'Connor C: Albumin priming does not prolong hemofilter life. ASAIO Journal: 193-196, 1997

26. *Contributions to biocompatibility 1: Membranes for dialysis*, edited by Vienken J, Baurmeister U, Akzo, Wuppertal, Germany, April 1989.

27. Baurmeister U, Vienken J, Ansorge W, Luttrell A: Cellulose versus synthetic membranes: a reasonable comparison? Artific Organs 13(1): 52-57, 1989

28. Sigdell JE: Operating characteristics of hollow-fiber dialyzers in *Clinical Dialysis*, 2nd ed., edited by Nissenson AR, Fine RN, Gentile DE, Connecticut, Appleton Lange: 97-117, 1990

29. Naitoh A, Tatsuguchi T, Okada M, Ohmura T, Sakai K: Removal of beta-2-microglobulin by diffusion alone is feasible using highly permeable dialysis membranes. Trans Am Soc Artif Intern Organs 34: 630-634, 1988

30. Akizawa T, Kinugasa E, Sato Y, Kohjiro S, Naitoh H, Azuma M, Mizutani S, Ideura T: Development of a new cellulose triacetate membrane with a microgradient porous structure for hemodialysis. ASAIO Journal: M584-586, 1998

31. Borst S, Breuer B: Effektivitätssteigerung in der Dialyse und Dialysatordesign. Dialysefachtagung Ulm, March 2001

32. Ronco C, Bowry S: Nanoscale modulation of the pore dimensions, size distribution and structure of a new polysulfone-based high-flux dialysis membrane. Int J Artif Organs 24(10): 726-735, 2001

33. Garcia H, Hernandez-Jaras J, Maduell F, Calvo C, Ferrero JA: Interaction of the mechanisms of beta 2-microglobulin convection, diffusion and adsorption in line hemodiafiltration. Nefrologia 20(1): 59-65, 2000

34. Vienken J, Pohlmeier R: How to improve convective removal of LMW proteins during hemodialysis. (Abstract) Artif Organs 23(7): 658, 1999

35. Ronco C, Brendolan A, Lupi A, Metry G, Levin NW: Effects of a reduced inner diameter of hollow fibers in hemodialyzers. Kidney Int 58(2): 809-817, 2000

36. Dellanna F, Wuepper A, Baldamus CA: Internal filtration - advantage in haemodialysis? Nephrol Dial Transplant 11(2): 83-86, 1996

37. Düngen HD, von Heymann C, Ronco C, Kox WJ, Spies CD: Renal replacement therapy: physical properties of hollow fibers influence efficiency. Int J Art Organs 24(6): 357-366, 2001

38. Bowry S, Ronco C: Surface topology and surface elemental composition analysis of Helixone®, a new high-flux polysulfone dialysis membrane. Int J Artif Organs 24(11): 757-764, 2001

39. Ronco C, Nissenson AR: Does nanotechnology apply to dialysis? Blood Purif 19: 347-352, 2001

40. Bowry SK: Nano-controlled membrane spinning technology: regulation of pore size, distribution and morphology of a new polysulfone dialysis membrane in *Contributions to Nephrology - Hemodialysis Technology*, edited by Ronco C, La Greca G, Basel, Karger: 137: 85-94, 2002

41. Meffert G, Huber A, Bock A: New polysulfone filter design (Fresenius FX) increases urea and ß2 microglobulin clearance: a prospective randomised cross-over study. (Abstract) J Am Soc Nephrol 13: 601A, 2002

42. Martin K, Bosc JY, Krieter DH, Leray H, Senecal L, Canaud B: Performance of a new high flux dialyzer "FX" in HD and HDF. (Abstract) J Am Soc Nephrol 13: 602A, 2002

Section C. Dialyser biocompatibility

7. Basic principles of biocompatibility assessment

The biocompatibility of a dialyser, particularly that of its membrane, is one of the main criteria for choosing a particular dialyser. During the Consensus Conference on Biocompatibility held in 1993, biocompatibility was defined as "the ability of a material, device or system to perform without a significant host response in a specific application" [1]. The addition of the term "significant" made the definition less strict than earlier ones, which demanded the absence of all host responses, and reflects the realisation that all foreign materials available at present induce some kind of reaction in the host. In renal replacement therapy, interactions between blood and the artificial surface (also termed blood compatibility or haemocompatibility, a sub-division of the more general term biocompatibility) are especially important due to the chronic character of the treatment.

Several well-accepted markers for the evaluation of biocompatibility are presently available, but new ones are being introduced from time to time. Furthermore, methods of assessment are becoming more and more sensitive. In the early years of chronic haemodialysis treatment, biocompatibility issues such as thrombogenicity and haemolysis were the main matters of concern for physicians [2]. Manufacturers focused on the development of surfaces that were less thrombogenic and on the toxicity of the materials used, which should not liberate plasticisers and chemical additives. In the late 1970s, hypersensitivity reactions were observed in response to EtO sterilisation of dialysers [3]. At the same time, activation of the complement system gained attention, and was linked to transient leukopenia and sequestration of neutrophils in the lungs during dialysis with cellulosic membranes [4, 5]. The influence of chronic haemodialysis treatment on the immune system received further recognition over the following years, with the formulation of the "Interleukin Hypothesis" in 1983 being a milestone in this kind of research [6]. Stimulation of immune cells during dialysis, the release of mediators (such as cytokines) and the pathological consequences thereof then became topics of intensive research. In the early 1990s, the significance of adverse interactions between the extracorporeal circuit and some pharmaceutical drugs began to become clinically evident: anaphylactoid reactions were observed in patients on ACE-inhibitor therapy in combination with the use of a certain negatively charged dialysis membrane which, until then, had been considered "biocompatible" [7]. Investigations revealed that the kallikrein-kinin-system was involved in this side effect, adding bradykinin to the list of biocompatibility parameters.

What, then, are the biocompatibility parameters of contemporary interest? Some parameters can be measured relatively easily in the clinical setting, such as the differential cell count – while factors of the complement and clotting cascades need specialist laboratories. On a more in-depth scientific level, investigations into gene expression of, for example, cytokines and ß2-microglobulin, and into the stimulation of immune cells and their reactions (i.e. receptor expression, generation of reactive oxygen species etc.) have become state-of-the-art.

Which pathways and cells are triggered by blood contact with foreign surfaces?

The contact of blood with artificial surfaces initiates the activation of several pathways, such as the clotting cascade or the complement system. Furthermore, immune cells, like neutrophils and monocytes, and platelets are activated either by products of the complement or clotting cascades, or by direct membrane contact (**figure 7.1**). These processes are explained in more detail in the following.

7.1 Membrane thrombogenicity

The haemostatic system in the body is well balanced between activation in times of injury on the one side (procoagulatory activity: platelet activation, platelet adhesion, aggregation and blood coagulation with thrombus formation), and mechanisms against these processes located in the endothelium and plasma on the other side (anticoagulatory activity: e.g. fibrinolytic activity). In extracorporeal treatment, triggering of the haemostatic systems starts with the insertion of a cannula as this cannot be performed without vascular injury. Once triggered, the haemostatic system activation continues with

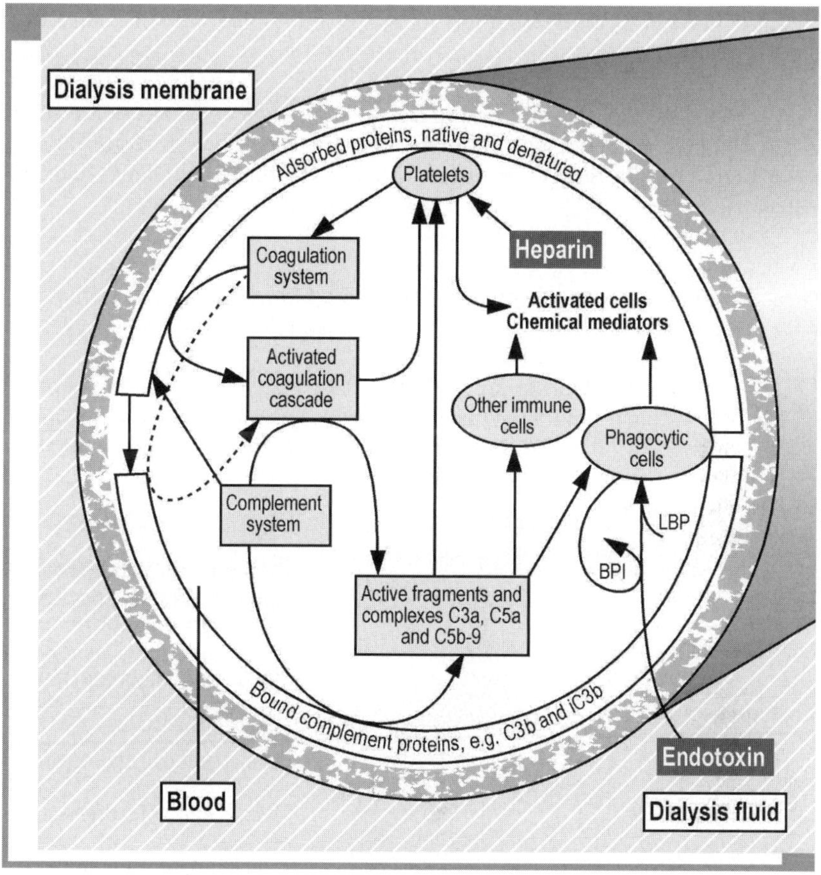

Figure 7.1: Interrelations of major biochemical pathways induced after contact of blood with dialyser and haemofilter membranes. *Several biochemical pathways (explained in more detail in the relevant sections of this chapter) are activated after blood-membrane interaction. Main inducers of this activation are adsorbed proteins and artifical membrane-bound complement factors, such as C3b and iC3b. The physicochemical characteristics of the membrane, e.g. surface charge, functional groups on its surface etc., determine which proteins are adsorbed and the extent of adsorption. Membrane porosity and the membrane's adsorptive capacity are important if the dialysis fluid is contaminated with bacterial products, such as endotoxins: these may cross the membrane and stimulate phagocytic cells of the immune system via lipopolysaccharide binding protein (LBP) and the bactericidal permeability increasing protein (BPI) (adapted from [8]).*

repeated contact of blood with the surface of the tubing and, of course, the dialysis membrane [9].

Whereas the clinical relevance of some parameters activated in the body is still a matter of discussion, thrombus formation, resulting in clotted fibres, has a direct negative impact on dialysis efficiency and can sometimes even be visually detected.

How does the haemostatic system react when blood comes into contact with foreign surfaces?

The exposure of blood to an artificial surface results in a rapid adsorption of proteins within seconds (**figure 7.2**) [10]. According to Vroman, initial protein deposition on artificial surfaces takes place in the sequence albumin,

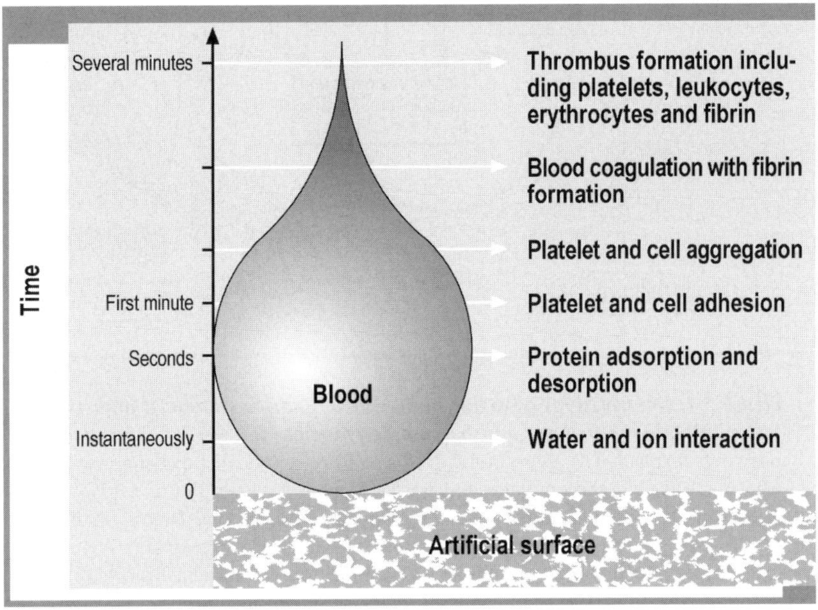

Figure 7.2: The sequence of thrombogenic events following blood-material interaction. *When blood comes into contact with foreign surfaces, a variety of systems are activated. These vary in their time course and with the protein layer that is built up on the surface. Cells that adhere and aggregate on the artificial surface are mainly white blood cells like monocytes (adapted from [11]).*

immune globulin G (IgG), fibrinogen, fibronectin, factor XII and high molecular weight kininogen (HMWK), whereby a process of adsorption is followed by desorption caused by the subsequent arrival of a higher affinity protein [12]. Furthermore, the adsorption of thrombin in its active form may activate the clotting cascade [13]. However, the exact composition of the protein layer is dependent on the surface hydrophobicity/hydrophilicity and the protein layer itself is considered to exert a controlling influence during further blood-material interactions, e.g. fibrinogen, at a critical adsorption thickness of approximately 200 nm, supports platelet adherence [14]. After adhesion to this layer of adsorbed proteins, platelets undergo a morphological change, release platelet factors and aggregate. Parallel to this, the coagulation cascade may be activated mainly via adsorbed proteins and, to a minor extent, by platelet release factors. This results in the formation of fibrin, which is stabilised to a fibrin clot within several minutes of blood-surface contact.

7.1.1 Platelet activation

Platelets are essentially bound to artificial surfaces via the von-Willebrandt-factor (vWF), an oligomeric plasma glycoprotein that adsorbs onto the surface. vWF, together with the specific glycoprotein GPIb/IX (or CD42 a-d in the CD antigen nomenclature) that is expressed by platelets, functions as a bridge between the surface and the activated platelet (**figure 7.3**) [15]. In cases of activation and adhesion, platelets change their morphology: they form pseudopodia to which other platelets attach via fibrinogen bridges, which is itself bound by the platelet receptors GPIIb (CD41) and GPIIIa (CD61). Often this reversible aggregation of platelets is mediated by adenosin diphosphate (ADP) and enhanced by collagen, adrenalin and platelet-activating factor (PAF), the last being secreted by activated leukocytes. At the same time, thromboxane synthesis and irreversible aggregation of platelets is initiated by thrombin. This further leads to degranulation and liberation of a number of biologically active substances that accelerate thrombin formation (**figure 7.4**). Platelet adhesion and aggregation is responsible for the measurable drop in the number of platelets during dialysis; this drop is often partially reversible due to disaggregation and detachment from the surface over treatment time [10].

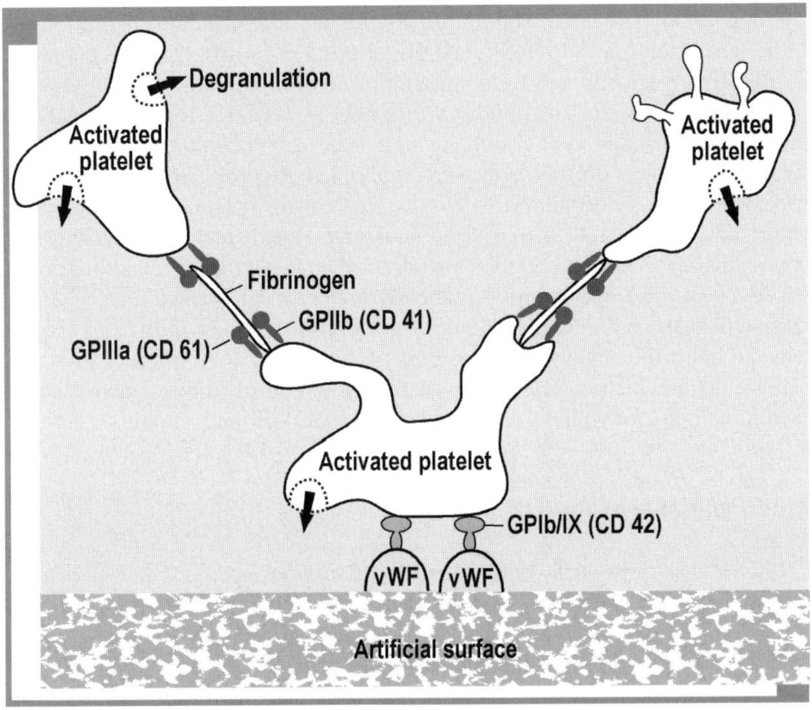

***Figure 7.3: Platelet adhesion and aggregation on artificial surfaces**. Platelet adhesion to artificial surfaces is mediated by the von-Willebrandt-factor (vWF) and the platelet receptor glycoprotein (GP) GPIb/IX (in the CD nomenclature CD42a-d). Adherent platelets then release preformed granule constituents and generate* de novo *mediators which regulate platelet activation, lead to a change in platelet shape and conform the GPIIb/IIIa complex (CD41/CD61) so that it binds fibrinogen, thus linking adjacent activated platelets (adapted from [15]).*

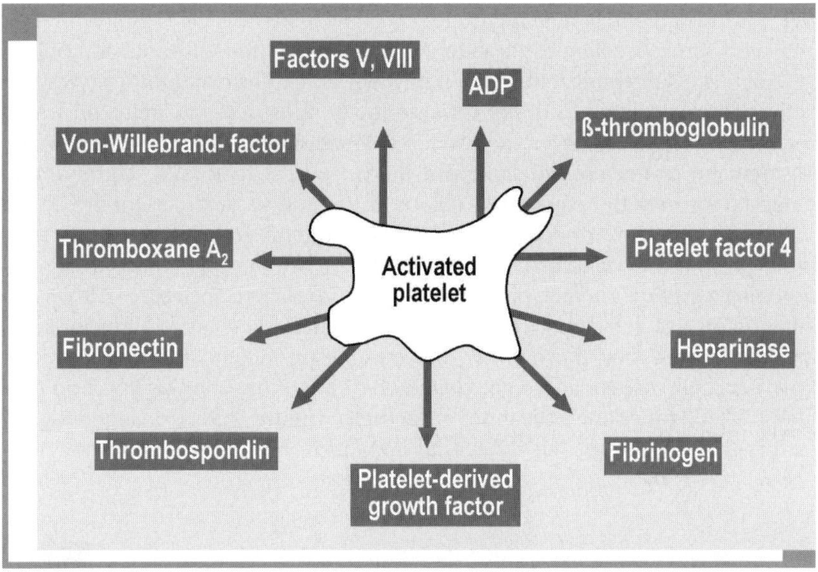

Figure 7.4: Platelet release reaction after activation. *After adhesion, platelets undergo a morphological change and release vasoactive substances (such as adenosine diphosphate (ADP) and thromboxane A_2), which are produced in cases of activation. Furthermore, the activated platelet surface is an essential catalytic surface for several coagulation reactions that generate thrombin. Thrombin, along with thromboxane A_2 and ADP, activates surrounding quiescent platelets, thereby amplifying platelet aggregation, fibrin formation and vasoconstriction. Furthermore, various inert platelet markers are released, such as ß-thromboglobulin and platelet factor 4; these are useful markers of platelet adhesion and activation (adapted from [14, 16]).*

7.1.2 Coagulation activation and thrombus formation

Parallel to the activation of platelets, plasma coagulation proteins are activated to initiate secondary haemostasis, i.e. the formation of a fibrin clot. The coagulation pathway consists of a series of reactions, each requiring the formation of a surface-bound enzyme complex. In these reactions, inactive precursor proteins (proenzymes, namely the clotting factors XII, XI, X, IX, VII and II (prothrombin)) are transformed into active proteases (so-called enzyme factors, namely XIIa, XIa, Xa, IXa, VIIa and IIa (thrombin)) by limited proteolysis. Factors VII, IX, X and prothrombin require vitamin K for their synthesis (i.e. for post-translational modification of the protein) and divalent cations (Ca^{2+},

Mg^{2+}) for their biologic activity. Factors V and VII are co-factors which, in their activated form, accelerate the catalytic reaction. Factor VIII (antihaemophilic globulin) is a substrate-factor. Two pathways, an extrinsic and intrinsic way, of activation exist (**figure 7.5**): *the extrinsic (exogenous) system* is initiated within seconds by the cell membrane-anchored tissue factor which is exposed during damage of the endothelium and then activates factor VII. Furthermore, tissue factor may be exposed in response to agonists such as endotoxin, interleukin-1 and tumor necrosis factor [17]. *The intrinsic (endogenous) system* is activated within minutes by artificial surfaces [18] through factor XII, a reaction also termed "contact phase activation" (explained in **figure 7.5** on the left). In cases of activation, platelets express negatively charged phospholipids on their surface, and these either enhance the proteolytic activity of prekallikrein and high-molecular weight kininogen or trigger the clotting cascade by a factor XII-independent activation of factor IX (**figure 7.5**). Consequently, all factors that activate platelets have an impact on coagulation activation. This

Figure 7.5: Simplified scheme of the blood coagulation cascade. *In cases of local injuries of the endothelium, the clotting cascade is triggered via both the extrinsic system and the intrinsic system. The extrinsic system is triggered by the expression of phospholipoproteins (tissue factor) from tissue cells and activation of factor VII, while the intrinsic system is initiated by the negative charges of phospholipids expressed at the surface of activated platelets or, as in extracorporeal treatment, by negatively charged artificial surfaces. Four factors are necessary for this so-called contact phase activation: (1) a negatively charged surface which induces a conformational change in (2) factor XII, rendering it highly susceptible to proteolytic cleavage of (3) prekallikrein and (4) high molecular weight kininogen (HMWK). Surface bound activated factor XII (i.e. XIIa) then activates factor XI. Factor XIa activates factor IX which, together with substrate factor VIII and calcium ions, forms an enzyme complex (intrinsic tenase). This complex is able to activate factor X. Factor X can also be activated by the tissue factor-VIIa-complex (extrinsic tenase). In the presence of calcium ions, membrane-bound factor Xa forms a complex with co-factor Va and prothrombin (prothrombinase, not shown) on the phospholipid membrane. The developing thrombin is a pluripotent substance with several functions. In the context of haemodialysis, we want to emphasise its thrombogenic potential as it is able to split fibrinogen into the fibrin monomers fibrinopeptide A and fibrinopeptide B. These molecules polymerise to a soluble form of fibrin that is cross-linked by the action of substrate factor XIIIa (which is itself activated by thrombin). A thrombus is formed after retraction of the fibrin mesh and trapping of erythrocytes and platelets (adapted from [17]).*

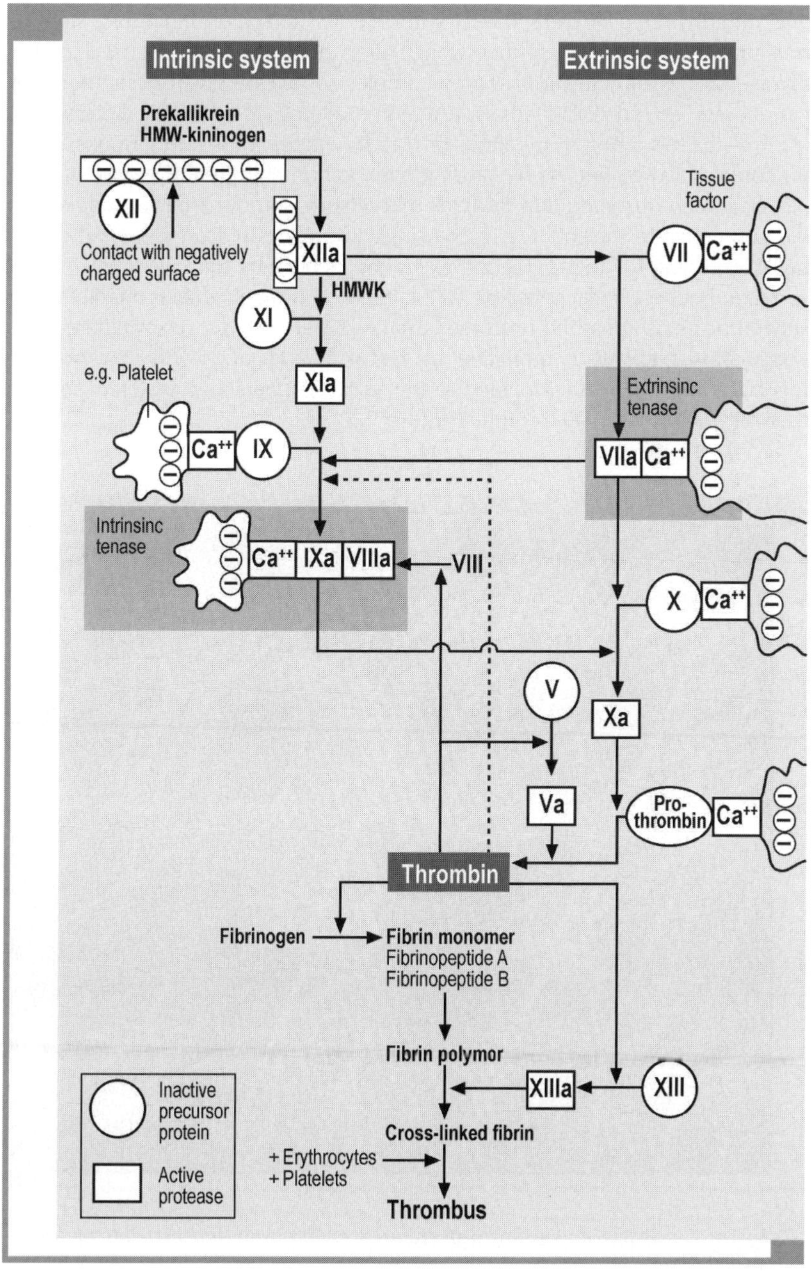
Intrinsic system
Extrinsic system
Prekallikrein
HMW-kininogen
XII
Contact with negatively charged surface
XIIa
HMWK
XI
XIa
e.g. Platelet
Ca++
IX
Intrinsinc tenase
Ca++ IXa VIIIa
VIII
Tissue factor
VII Ca++
Extrinsinc tenase
VIIa Ca++
X Ca++
V
Xa
Va
Pro-thrombin Ca++
Thrombin
Fibrinogen
Fibrin monomer
Fibrinopeptide A
Fibrinopeptide B
Fibrin polymor
XIIIa
XIII
Cross-linked fibrin
+ Erythrocytes
+ Platelets
Thrombus
Inactive precursor protein
Active protease

was demonstrated in experiments with platelet activation inhibitors, such as prostacyclin, which also reduce coagulation activation [19]. In view of the diverse modes of activation, some examples should be given here: mechanical damage of red cells leads to a massive release of adenosin diphosphate (ADP), which is a potent mediator of platelet aggregation. Furthermore, heparin could activate platelets by causing aggregation and granule release [20]. It has also been observed that proteins that adsorb onto an artificial surface can directly generate thrombin [21]. No single protein could be identified as being responsible for this. Evidence exists that thrombus formation on artificial surfaces is caused via adhesion of platelets, a process that is mediated by several proteins adsorbed onto the surface [22]. However, once initiated, the coagulation pathway is amplified by factor V and factor VIII in a positive feedback loop; these factors bind to the surface of activated platelets and are themselves activated by thrombin (**figure 7.5**).

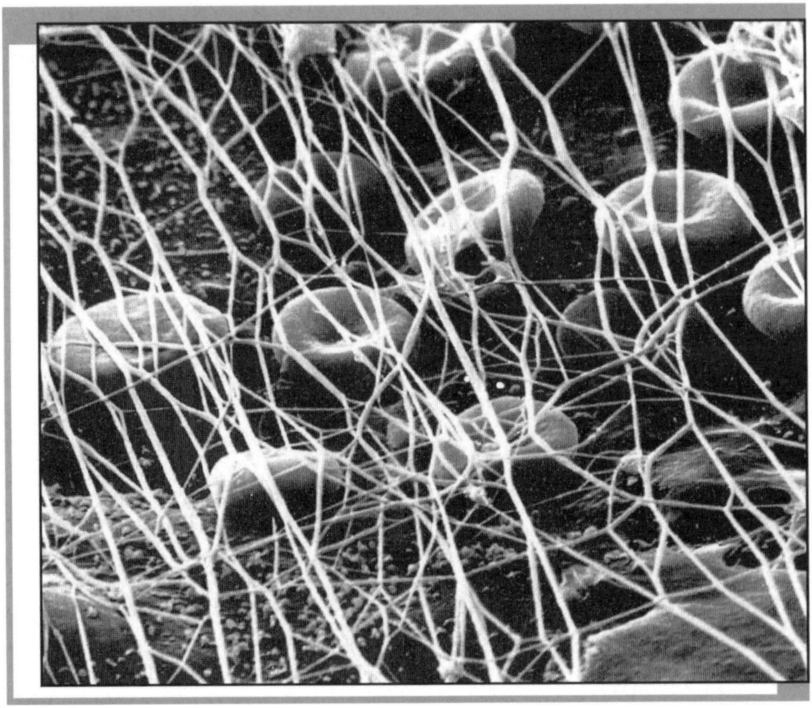

Figure 7.6: Fibrin deposition with trapped erythrocytes and platelets on an artificial surface.

The activation of the coagulation cascade results in the splitting of fibrinogen by thrombin, and involves the generation of fibrinopeptide A and B, which polymerise to form the fibrin polymer that is cross-linked by activated factor XIII (**figure 7.5**). Finally, erythrocytes and platelets are trapped in this fibrin mesh, forming the thrombus (**figure 7.6**).

7.1.3 Main anticoagulatory mechanisms

Anticoagulatory mechanisms of the body that prevent coagulation are (1) inhibition of thrombin formation and other coagulation factors and cofactors, (2) inhibition of platelet function through synthesis of prostaglandin I_2 (PGI_2) by endothelial cells, and (3) inhibition of the fibrinolytic enzyme system. The endothelial cell surface is the major carrier of these defence mechanisms.

In the body, plasmin (a constituent of the fibrinolytic enzyme system) slowly breaks down any fibrin that is formed. Plasmin is produced upon activation of plasminogen by several activators, such as tissue plasmin activator (t-PA), contact system-dependent activator and urokinase-type plasminogen activator (u-PA). These three activator pathways are interrelated: for instance, plasmin arising from the action of t-PA or u-PA activates factor XII and, consequently, the contact phase. Bradykinin develops as a result of contact phase activation, and this is a strong stimulus for t-PA release from endothelial cells. Furthermore, plasmin and kallikrein, another component of the contact phase system, activate u-PA. All these activators are strongly regulated by inhibitors, which are not described here [23].

7.1.4 The role of anticoagulation in biocompatibility

An anticoagulant is infused into the patient's blood during dialysis in order to prevent activation of coagulation. Kolff used hirudin in his first haemodialysis, today heparin and low molecular weight heparin derivatives are state-of-the-art. Investigations with citrate [24] and prostacyclin [25] have also been undertaken in attempts to improve the biocompatibility of extracorporeal systems. However, no anticoagulant can completely avoid activation of the haemostatic system.

7.1.4.1 Heparin / low molecular weight heparins

The naturally occurring glucosaminoglycan heparin (**figure 7.7**) exerts its antithrombotic activity through activation of the potent inhibitor molecule antithrombin III (ATIII). It binds to ATIII over a special pentasaccharide sequence, inducing a conformational change in the molecule. This makes it possible for ATIII to bind and inactivate the clotting factors thrombin, Xa, IXa, XIa and XIIa [28]. Fibrin formation is, consequently, successfully avoided. The anticoagulant activity of heparin is related to its molecular size. Unfractionated heparin is a heterogeneous mixture of molecules with molecular weights

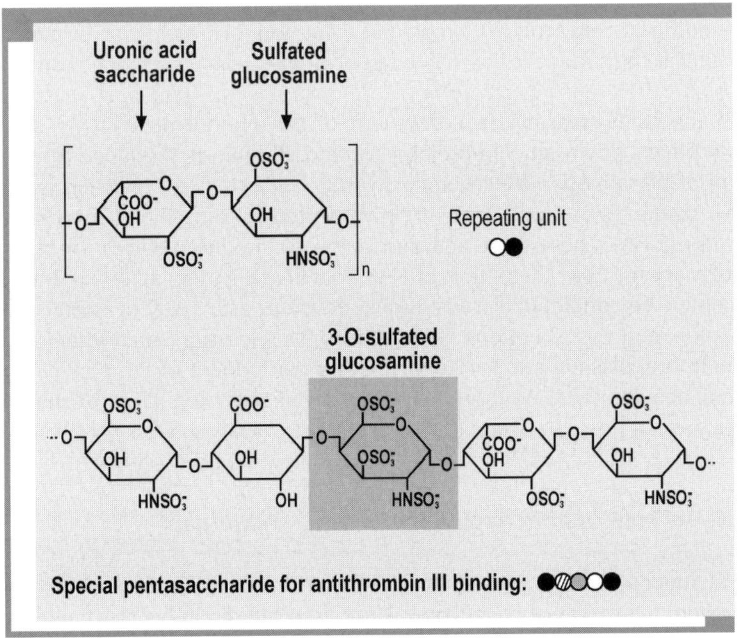

Figure 7.7: ***Chemical structure of heparin.*** *Heparin and low molecular weight heparin (LMWH) are mixtures of sulfated polysaccharide chains with alternating residues of D-glucosamine and uronic acid, the latter being either gluconic acid or iduronic acid (upper formular). In unfractionated heparin, the chains contain an average of 45 saccharide units, while 15 units are the mean length of chains in LMW heparin. The anticoagulation activity is based on binding of a specific pentasaccharide to antithrombin III (lower formular) [26]. 3-0-sulfated glucosamine in the middle of the pentasaccharide is critical for the binding to ATIII [27], but only about 30% of all heparin chains contain this unique sequence [28].*

ranging from 2000 to 40,000, averaging around 15,000 to 18,000. This preparation, together with ATIII, inhibits the clotting factors XIIa, XIa, Xa, IXa and thrombin, but not factor VIIa. Decreasing the molecular weight results in an increase in factor Xa inhibition and a reduction in thrombin inhibition (**figure 7.8**). Low molecular weight heparins (LMWH) are fragments of heparin with mean molecular weights ranging from 4000 to 6500 which are produced by either chemical or enzymatic depolymerisation [28].

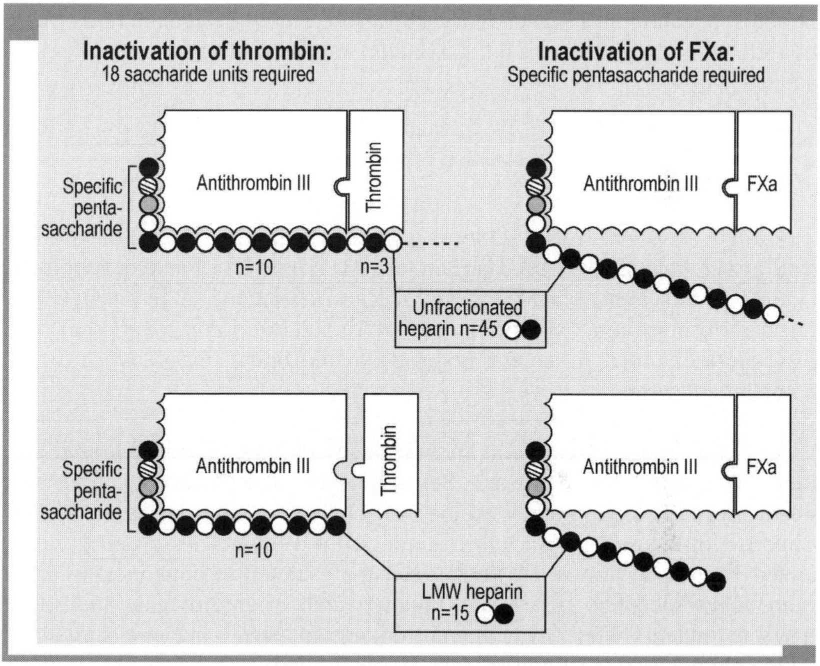

Figure 7.8: Mechanism of anticoagulation by heparin and low molecular weight (LMW) heparin. *Heparin accelerates the binding between ATIII and thrombin by providing a template to which both substances can bind. This template consists of the specific pentasaccharide (**figure 7.7**) plus 10 other saccharide units for the binding of ATIII, as well as 3 saccharide units for the binding of thrombin. Most of the polysaccharide strains are not longer than 15 saccharide units in LMW heparin and, therefore, thrombin cannot be bound and inactivated. However, only the pentapeptide is needed to change the morphology of ATIII so that it can then bind factor Xa (FXa). Therefore, LMW heparins exhibit their anticoagulation activity mainly through the inhibition of FXa (adapted from [28]).*

Despite its importance and widespread use in haemodialysis therapy, unfractionated heparin is implicated in some side effects commonly observed in chronic haemodialysis patients. Examples are hypersensitivity reactions (type I and II), increased bleeding [28], inhibition of platelet function, thrombocytopenia [20], increased levels of circulating triglycerides and release of lipoprotein lipase [29], pruritus and headache. Furthermore, osteoporosis has been associated with the long-term application of unfractionated heparin [29]. Some of these negative effects (not hypersensitivity) can be improved with usage of LMWH. Moreover, LMWH has a much lower affinity for plasma proteins, resulting in a higher bioavailability of the anticoagulant. Doses can be reduced to 2/3 of that of unfractionated heparin and can be prescribed as a bolus [29, 30].

7.1.4.2 Citrate

Citrate chelates divalent cations, such as calcium (Ca^{2+}) and magnesium (Mg^{2+}), with high affinity [24]. Calcium ions are needed for the activation of all clotting factors except factor XII, and calcium chelation is, therefore, a very effective form of anticoagulation. Furthermore, calcium and magnesium ions play important roles in several pathways in the body, one of which is the complement system.

In extracorporeal treatments such as haemodialysis, blood is citrated only during its extracorporeal passage. Because of the interrelation of cations with nearly all physiologic systems in the body, blood calcium levels are replenished by the infusion of calcium chloride at the venous limb distal to the dialyser. The application of citrate is presently restricted to patients who suffer from active bleeding, pericarditis or intercranial haemorrhages, and sometimes to patients who have recently undergone highly invasive surgery or patients who react to heparin with severe thrombocytopenia [31]. Clinical studies reveal that citrate anticoagulation induces less bleeding than anticoagulation with LMWH [32], and less activation of coagulation and thrombus formation than coagulation with LMWH and unfractionated heparin [33]. Studies regarding an improvement in the biocompatibility of the whole system with the use of citrate anticoagulation have yielded conflicting results. In some studies, an attenuation of complement activation with regenerated cellulose and cellulose acetate membranes was observed with the use of citrate compared to heparin [34, 35]. However, another study, measuring the expression of leukocyte surface antigens as a sign of leukocyte activation during dialysis with regenerated cellulose membranes, could not confirm an improvement in system biocompatibility [36].

Citrate anticoagulation is not yet considered suitable for standard haemodialysis treatment. Known pitfalls are the risks of inducing hyper- or hypocalcaemia, hypernatriaemia and metabolic alkalosis in the patient, because Ca^{2+} is difficult to monitor continuously in a cost-effective manner and, therefore, substitution of divalent cations may not be appropriate [37].

7.1.4.3 Prostacyclin

Prostacyclin is the strongest endogenous inhibitor of platelet aggregation. It is liberated from endothelial cells during injury in order to localise platelet aggregation. Synthetic prostacyclin was first used as an anticoagulant in dialysis patients in the early eighties [25]. Its use is restricted to patients with high bleeding risks [38] due to its high expense and because a number of side effects may occur during its use. For example, hypotension secondary to vasodilation, tachycardia, headache, nausea, chest and abdominal pain have all been observed during prostacyclin treatment [31]. Furthermore, although platelet activation is successfully avoided with this substance, activation of the clotting cascade still takes place. This was documented by elevated levels of fibrinopeptide A, a sensitive marker of thrombin generation [19]. It is therefore recommended that prostacyclin application be employed in combination with low dose heparinisation in order to avoid thrombus formation in the extracorporeal circuit [19].

7.2 Complement activation

The complement system is a component of the body's defence system against invading micro-organisms and is activated when blood comes into contact with an artificial surface. In haemodialysis, the dialysis membrane constitutes the main artificial surface. Complement activation increases to its peak value within the first 15 to 30 minutes of treatment, depending on the membrane type, and usually returns to its predialysis level by the end of dialysis. The latter is due to the adsorption of complement products by a large pool of cellular receptors in the blood, as well as by the deposition of proteins on the active site of the dialyser membrane surface. Complement, in synergism with phagocytic cells, produces an acute inflammatory response

Fluid phase proteins		Membrane-bound proteins	
Classical pathway	**MW**	**Regulatory proteins**	**MW**
C1q	400,000	CR1 (CD35)	200,000
C1r	166,000	MCP (CD47)	56,000 / 66,000
C1s	83,000	DAF (CD55)	60,000 – 70,000
C4	200,000	CD59	19,000
C2	102,000		
Alternative pathway	**MW**	**Complement receptors**	**MW**
C3	190,000	CR1 (CD35)	200,000
C5	185,000	CR2 (CD21)	145,000
C6	105,000	CR3 (CD11b)	185,000
C7	95,000	CR4 (CD11c)	150,000
C8	163,000	C1qR	
C9	71,000		
B	90,000		
D	24,000		
Properdin	220,000		
Regulatory proteins	**MW**	**Anaphylatoxin receptors**	**MW**
C1 esterase inhibitor	104,000	C3aR	
C4b binding protein	540,000	C5aR (CD88)	40,000
Factor I	93,000		
Factor H	155,000		

Table 7.1: Factors of the complement system. *The complement system provides a rapid and efficient means of killing invading micro-organisms, but it also presents a potential threat to host cells. Human cells are protected from complement by an array of membrane proteins which inhibit several stages of the complement activation pathway. These include DAF (decay accelerating factor), MCP (membrane cofactor protein), CR1 (complement receptor 1) and CD59, all of which act on the terminal lytic state.*

[39] which may contribute to both acute and chronic clinical consequences (e.g. [40], discussed in chapters 9 and 10).

Complement, like the blood clotting system, is a proteolytic cascade pathway system and consists of almost 30 fluid-phase and cell membrane proteins (**table 7.1**). Two different pathways exist, the classical pathway activated by antigen/antibody complexes, and the alternative pathway that is triggered by the binding of complement factor C3b to a foreign surface. Biologically active end-products of both pathways are (1) the peptide mediators of inflammation, C3a, C4a and C5a (**figure 7.9, 7.10**); (2) C3b, which coats micro-organisms and artificial surfaces and attracts phagocytes by binding to their complement receptors; and (3) the terminal complement components C5b-9 (also termed the terminal complement complex TCC), which form the membrane attack complex (MAC) and lyse foreign cells, but have also an impact on cell activation (**figure 7.11**).

The primary biosynthesis site for 90% of the fluid-phase complement components is the hepatocyte. Monocytes/macrophages, fibroblasts, endothelial cells, leukocytes and adipose tissue (factor D) all belong to the growing list of cells and tissues which also produce complement factors [41]. Craddock et al. were the first to link a well-known side effect of dialysis therapy, i.e. leukopenia, to the action of complement [4], making the generation of activated complement factors one of the most common indicators of bioincompatibility in haemodialysis.

How do foreign surfaces activate the complement cascade?

Complement can be activated by three pathways: the classical pathway, initiated by the binding of immune complexes (explained in more detail in **figure 7.10**); the lectin pathway, which is not mentioned here because it is irrelevant in artificial surface interaction; and the non-specific alternative pathway (explained in **figure 7.9**), which recognises foreign surfaces and was, therefore, long believed to be the only relevant pathway in extracorporeal blood treatment. It is now known, however, that immune complexes and the classical activation pathway are also involved [43].

Cleavage of C5 into C5a and C5b is an important step in complement activation. The role played by the potent anaphylatoxin C5a is explained in more detail below. The development of C5b initiates the assembly of further complement factors (C6, C7, C8 and variable amounts of C9 (n=1-16)) to

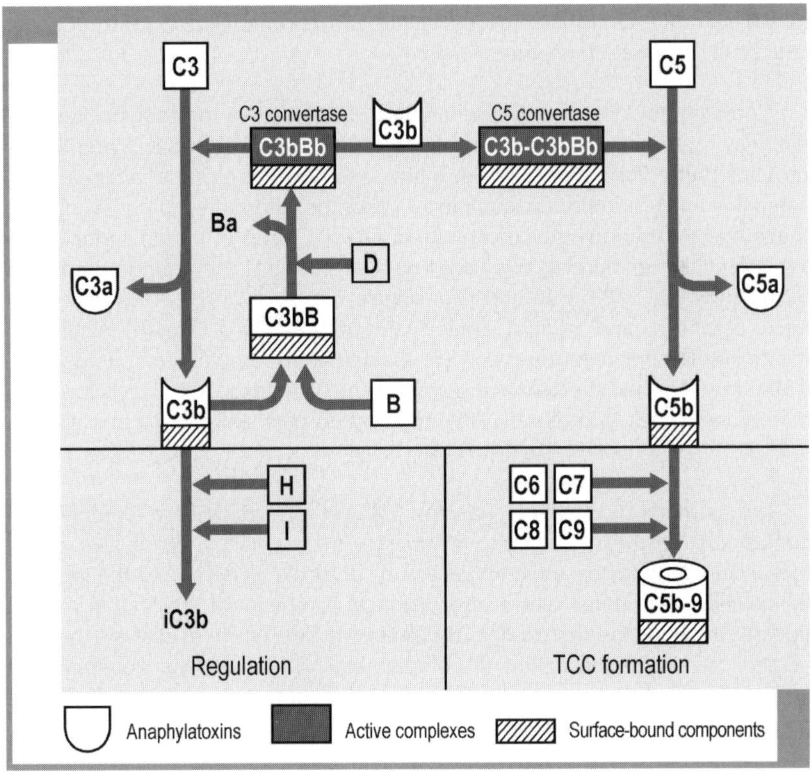

Figure 7.9: Alternative pathway of complement activation. *Initiation phase: the central component is factor C3 which undergoes spontaneous splitting in plasma at a very slow rate (60 ng/ml/min), whereby C3a and C3b develop. Normally C3b has a very short half-live (60 µs) and is hydrolysed and inactivated by the factors H and I. Amplification phase: in the presence of foreign surfaces that expose carbohydrates, C3b attaches to hydroxyl groups (OH^-) or aminogroups (NH_2) of the surface, is then recognised by factor B, cleaved by factor D and more C3 convertase is formed. The breakdown of this is stabilised by its attachment to the surface and factor P (properdin) (see* ***figure 7.10****). The large amounts of C3b produced and covalently bound to the foreign surface act as opsonins (molecules that make the particle they coat more susceptible to engulfment by phagocytic cells). Furthermore, C3b molecules eventually attach to the C3b component of C3 convertase. This C3b-C3bBb complex is the C5 convertase which cleaves C5 into C5a and C5b. The latter attaches to the surface and, together with attached 3b and further complement factors (C6-C9), initiates the formation of the membrane attack complex (MAC) C5b-9, or terminal complement complex (TCC) (explained in* ***figure 7.11****) (adapted from [39, 41]).*

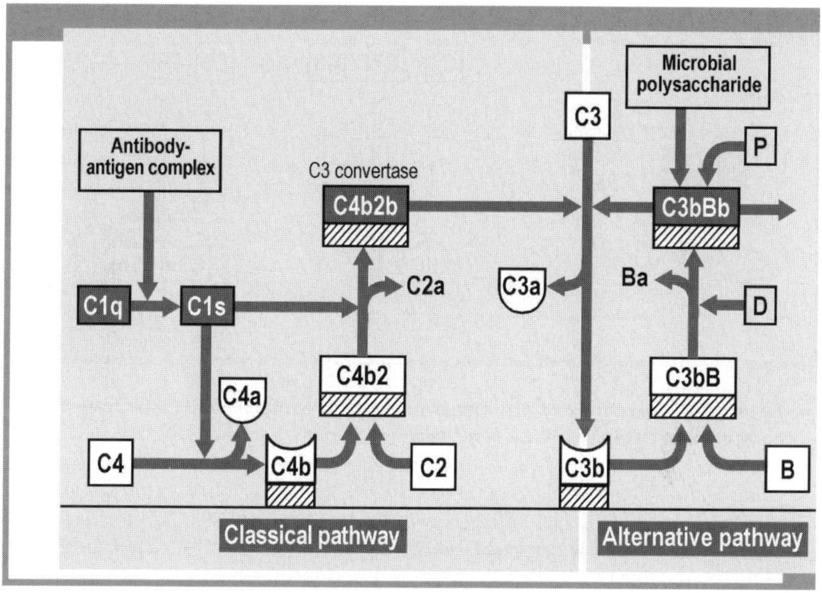

Figure 7.10: Interrelation between classical and alternative complement pathways. *The classical complement pathway is initiated when antibodies (IgG, IgM) attached to a foreign surface (normally micro-organisms) bind the C1q molecule. This binding activates C1s to bind and split C4 into C4a and C4b. C4b covalently binds to the foreign surface and binds C2, making it susceptible to cleavage of C1s. The developing 2b fragment is bound to C4b, constituting the active protease component of the C3 convertase C4b2b of the classical pathway. This enzyme cleaves many molecules of C3 to produce C3b (which binds to the foreign surface) and C3a, a mediator of inflammation. The complete alternative pathway resulting in terminal complement complex formation is presented in* ***figure 7.9.*** *Symbols as in* ***figure 7.9*** *(adapted from [42]).*

form the membrane attack complex (MAC) (**figure 7.11**). This MAC, or terminal complement complex (TCC), forms pores when attached to a foreign cell membrane, e.g. that of a micro-organism , leading to lysis and subsequent cell death. The TCC measurements often reported in the literature refer mainly to the soluble fraction of TCC bound by the scavenger S protein [44].

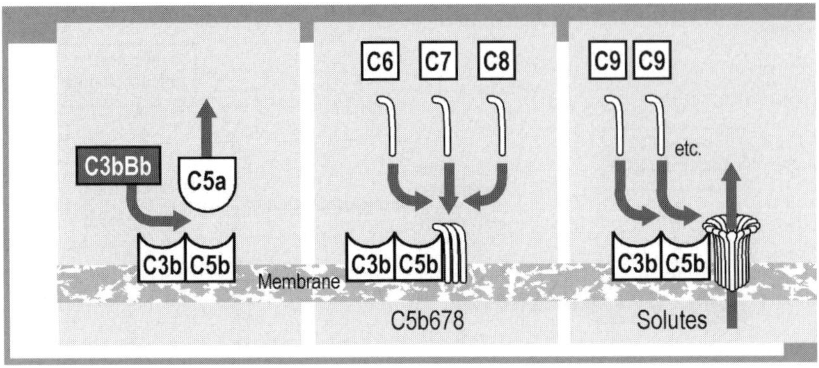

Figure 7.11: Assembly of the membrane attack complex (MAC) or terminal complement complex (TCC). *After recruitment of C3b to the C3bBb enzymatic complex, a C5 convertase is formed, cleaving C5 into C5a and C5b. C5b remains activated and weakly bound to C3b. C6 and later C7 attach to that complex to form C5b67 which interacts with C8 to form C5b678. This structure is capable of penetrating the membrane to which it is attached. After polymerisation with variable amounts of C9 (n=1-16), a transmembrane tubule with a pore radius of about 10 nm is formed [41]. This permits the free exchange of solutes and cell lysis of the micro-organism (adapted from [39 and 41]).*

Why is complement activation a feature of regenerated cellulose membranes?

Membranes made of regenerated cellulose are the strongest complement activators of all dialysis membranes and have, therefore, been well examined regarding this characteristic. These membranes have a considerable number of factor C3b binding sites, i.e. hydroxyl groups, which were thought to be responsible for strong complement activation via the alternative pathway. Today, the initiation process of C3b binding is thought to be only of moderate importance [45]. Associations of C3 with other adsorbed proteins, or protein-electrostatic and protein-hydrophobic surface interactions are suspected of playing a greater role [45]. The strong binding of the positive regulatory factor B and the weak binding of inhibitory factor H are of significance in this context: factor B supports the generation of the C3 convertase (C3Bb), thereby additionally protecting C3b from degradation by factor H; and factor H inhibits the alternative pathway by displacing bound Bb in its binding to C3b, by inhibiting further binding of factor B to C3b and, finally, by serving as a cofactor for the enzymatic degradation of C3b to iC3b by factor I (**figure 7.9**). The number of the complement-enhancing factor B binding sites on regenerated cellulose is approximately 4 times higher than on the less complement-activating cellulose acetate (where most of the hydroxyl groups of cellulose are replaced by acetyl groups) [46]. Furthermore, less inhibitory factor H binds to regenerated cellulose compared to cellulose acetate, also favouring complement activation [46].

Some authors suggest that initial deposition of C3b onto surfaces made of regenerated cellulose is mediated by the classical C3-convertase, C4b2b (**figure 7.10**) [43]. Furthermore, it has been shown that the classical complement cascade is also activated by binding of anti-polysaccharide antibodies to membranes made of regenerated cellulose [43]. A schematic overview of all pathways involved in complement activation by regenerated cellulose is presented in **figure 7.12**.

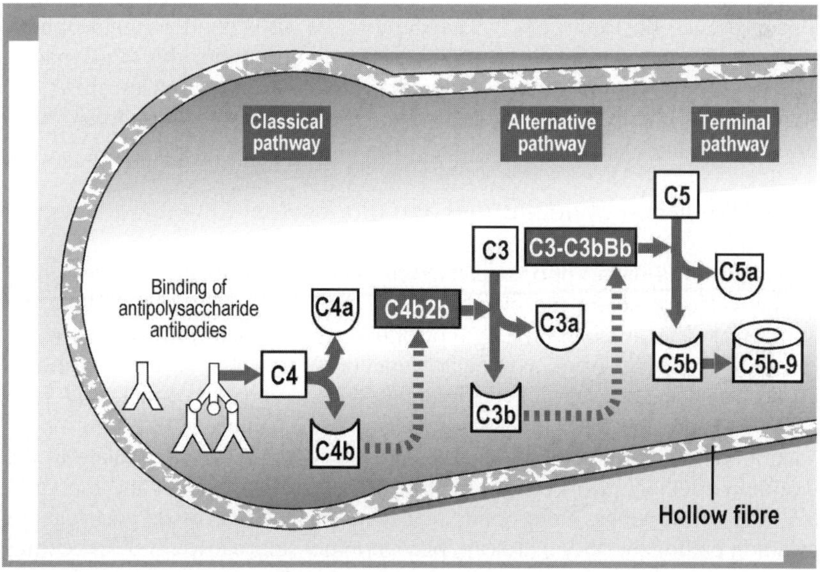

Figure 7.12: Extended model of complement activation by regenerated cellulose. *Evidence exists that regenerated cellulose activates complement via the classical pathway. All steps mentioned above are explained in more detail in **figures 7.9-7.11**. Only the anaphylaxins C3a, C4a and C5a and the final endproduct C5b-9 (TCC) are shown (adapted from [43]).*

7.3 Activation of leukocytes

During haemodialysis, leukocytes are stimulated by complement factors, by contact with foreign surfaces, by bacterial products from contaminated dialysis fluid and/or by the non-physiological environment produced by acetate buffer. An overview of the cells involved in these processes and their terminology is given in **figure 7.13**.

Complement develops its biological effect via ligand-receptor mediated cellular activation with the splitting products C5a and C3a (C4a only plays a minor role). These complement peptides are also called anaphylatoxins because of their ability to (1) stimulate mast cells to release histamine and other vasoactive substances, (2) cause smooth muscle contraction, (3) increase vascular permeability and (4) lead to anaphylactic shock [48]. In addition to their presence on mast cells, C5a receptors are also found on neutrophilic, eosinophilic and basophilic granulocytes and on monocytes and macrophages. Their receptor interaction leads to a variety of responses; these are summarised in **figure 7.14** and discussed in the following in more detail.

7.3.1 Stimulation of neutrophils and monocytes

Circulating polymorphonuclear neutrophils and monocytes are the most common leukocytes in the blood. Due to their phagocytic activity they are also referred to as phagocytes. Neutrophils are the main phagocytes in the blood (eosinophils have a specific function: they phagocytose antibody-coated parasites), while the differentiated macrophages originating from monocytes are the main phagocytic cells in tissue (**figure 7.13**). Neutrophils have a half-life of 6 - 9 hours and about 3000 - 4000 cells/µl circulate in the blood. In addition, pools of these cells exist in the liver, spleen and the capillary bed of the lungs. Neutrophils make up the first line of defence against invading pathogens and, therefore, play an important role when blood comes into contact with foreign surfaces, as in haemodialysis. Monocytes have a longer half-life in the blood of about 17 h, and their blood concentration is about 450 cells/µl. They are not only important as macrophage progenitors, but also for the adaptive immune response: they are essential for the presentation of antigens to lymphoid cells, and secrete a number of immune mediators, such as interleukin-1 (IL-1) and tumor necrosis factor (TNF). Morphologically, neutrophils and monocytes are characterised by their cell nuclei. In neutrophils, the nucleus is multi-lobed, in contrast to monocytes where the nucleus is horseshoe shaped. Phagocytes are filled with similar cytoplasmatic

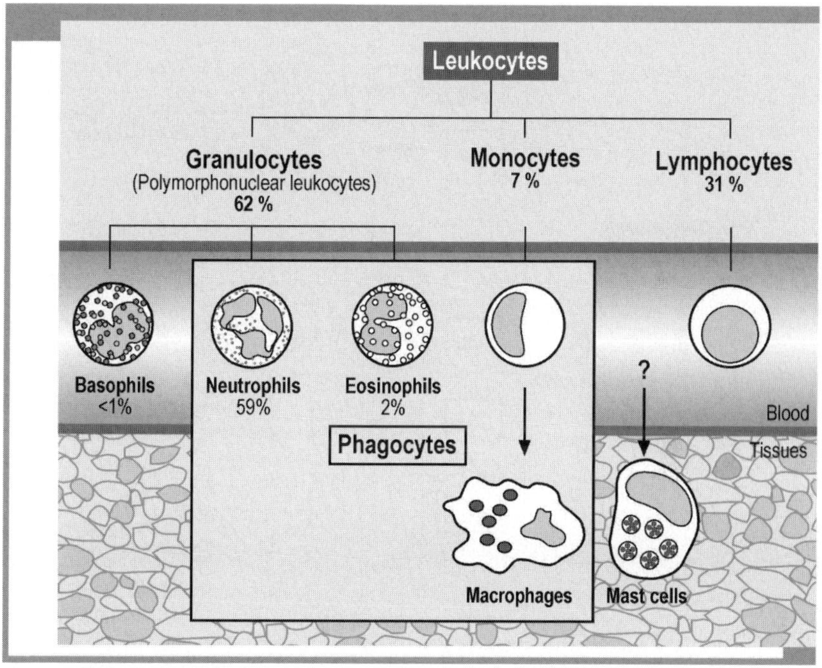

Figure 7.13: Diversification and frequency of leukocytes. *Leukocytes consist of granulocytes (also termed polymorphonuclear leukocytes), monocytes and lymphocytes. The terms polymorphonuclear and granulocyte refer to the irregular shape of granulocyte nuclei and the stainable, dense cytoplasmatic granules, respectively. Monocytes change into macrophages in tissue, where they are the main phagocytic cells of the immune system. Neutrophils are the main phagocytes in the blood, where monocytes and eosinophils also have phagocytic functions. Eosinophils are capable of killing antibody-coated parasites. Mast cells complete their maturation in tissue. It is not clear which cells they derive from. They are important, like basophils, in allergic responses (see allergic reactions). Lymphocytes differentiate into B- and the different T-lymphocytes. They don't phagocytize but are mediators of the specific immune response. With the exception of lymphocytes, all cell types depicted above carry membrane receptors for the anaphylatoxins C3a, C4a or C5a and are, therefore, activated by complement generating membranes. B- and T-lymphocytes bear highly diverse antigen receptors on their surface (adapted from [103]).*

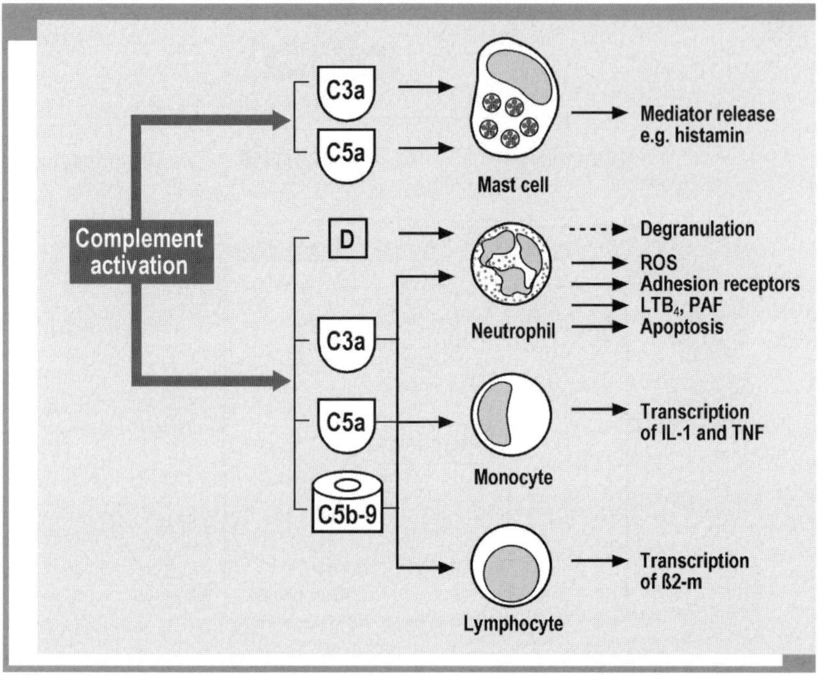

Figure 7.14: Influence of complement products on the function of immune cells. *Products of complement activation, such as the anaphylatoxins C3a and C5a and the membrane attack complex (or terminal complement complex (TCC)), stimulate the various immune cells to release, secrete or express mediators via specific receptors. These mediators induce a number of reactions, which are discussed in more detail in the text. Degranulation of neutrophils is independent of C3a, C5a or TCC but is dependent on complement factor D as this, together with angiogenin, inhibits degranulation. Factor D concentrations increase more during dialysis with complement-activating low-flux membranes than with high-flux membranes, resulting in less lactoferrin release (degranulation product) with the former. High-flux membranes adsorb or filtrate factor D, yielding lower contentrations thereof [48]. The dashed arrow indicates inhibition, activation is indicated by black arrows. C3a and C5a: anaphylatoxins; C5b-9: membrane attack complex (terminal complement complex); ROS: reactive oxygen species;* LTB_4*: leukotriene* B_4*; PAF: platelet-activating factor (adapted from [50])*

Substance	Function
Lysozyme Myeloperoxidase Defensins Bactericidal permeability increasing protein (BPI) Lactoferrin Vitamin B_{12}-binding protein	Destruction of micro-organisms
Elastase Cathepsin N-acetylglucoronidase Collagenase Gelatinase	Lysis and degradation
CR3 (CD11/CD18 complex) Formylated peptide Tumor Necrosis Factor (TNF) CD45 (leukocyte common antigen)	Receptors

Table 7.2: Major constituents of cytoplasmatic granules in neutrophils. *(Adapted from [51]).*

granules whose constituents are released in cases of activation (**table 7.2** for neutrophils). Furthermore, their plasma membranes express a number of receptors for adhesion, chemoattraction, phagocytosis and regulation of these processes. The impact of haemodialysis treatment on the function, structure and even survival of neutrophils and monocytes has been well examined and will be summarised in the following.

How do phagocytic cells react when they come into contact with foreign surfaces?

The primary function of phagocytic cells is the elimination of bacteria and fungi. This requires a number of well-regulated processes, like adherence to the vascular endothelium, migration through the endothelium to the site of infection, phagocytosis of the micro-organism, killing (e.g. by reactive oxygen species) and degradation. All these steps are mediated via ligand/receptor interaction. Foreign materials in the extracorporeal circuit (mainly the dialyser membrane in dialysis) provoke a stimulation of these cells. This may happen either directly, by adsorption of these cells, or indirectly, via mediators induced by the membrane (e.g. complement) or via bacterial products which have passed through the membrane from the dialysis fluid.

Neutrophils and monocytes recognise that the artificial surfaces of the dialysis circuit are foreign. Despite the shear rate induced by the blood flow, some cells may adhere to the surface and become activated. Degranulation occurs, verified by observations of degranulation products (bactericidal enzymes, such as myeloperoxidase, lysozyme, and defensins, see also **table 7.2**). Products like elastase-α_1-antitrypsin are an indication of the cells' attempts to ingest the foreign material (a phenomenon known as frustrated phagocytosis) [51]. In addition, a number of oxidative killing processes are activated which lead in the presence of foreign micro-organisms to their destruction and degradation (**table 7.3**). The production and liberation of superoxide anions (O_2^-, OH, H_2O_2), also termed reactive oxygen species (ROS), is an important process in neutrophil activation which is observed during dialysis; this increases oxidative stress in the patient (described in more detail in section 7.3.2.1).

The activation of phagocytes via mediators, such as complement (which is generated at the foreign surface), is possibly of more clinical importance in haemodialysis than is cell activation by direct adhesion to the membrane (**table 7.4**). Complement proteins induce the expression of adhesion receptors (CD11a/CD18, CD11b/CD18, CD62L) and, consequently, adhesion of phagocytes takes place. Transient leukopenia, the fall of leukocytes shortly after onset of dialysis, is an example of such an effect [4, 62].

Table 7.3: Antimicrobial agents and their function in phagocytic vacuoles. *Microbicidal species are presented in bold letters. O_2^-: superoxide anion; $1O_2$: singlet oxygen; *OH: hydroxyl free radical; H_2O_2: hydrogen peroxide; OCl^-: hypochloride; H_2O: water; NADPH: reduced nicotinamide adenine dinucleotide phosphate; $NADP^+$: oxidised NADPH (adapted from [39]).*

Agent	**Antimicrobial mechanism**
Oxygen-independent	
Defensins Cathepsin G Cationic proteins Bactericidal permeability increasing protein	Membrane damage
Reactive nitrogen intermediates, e.g. nitric oxide Lactoferrin	Complexing iron
Lysozyme Proteolytic enzymes	Splitting of mureinsacculus Degradation
Oxygen-dependent	
$Glc + NADP^{+} \xrightarrow{\text{Glycolysis}} \text{Pentose phosph.} + NADPH$ $NADPH + O_2 \xrightarrow{\text{NADPH oxidase}} NADP^{+} + \mathbf{O_2^{-}}$	O_2 burst and generation of superoxide anion
$2\,O_2^{-} + 2\,H^{+} \xrightarrow{\text{Spontaneous dismutation}} \mathbf{H_2O_2} + {}^{1}\mathbf{O_2}$ $O_2^{-} + H_2O_2 \longrightarrow {}^{*}\mathbf{OH} + OH^{-} + {}^{1}\mathbf{O_2}$	Spontaneous formation of microbicidal agents
$H_2O_2 + Cl^{-} \xrightarrow{\text{Myeloperoxidase}} \mathbf{OCl^{-}} + H_2O$	Myeloperoxidase
$OCl^{-} + H_2O \quad {}^{1}\mathbf{O_2} + \mathbf{Cl^{-}} + H_2O$	Generation of microbicidal agent
$2\,O_2^{-} + 2\,H^{+} \xrightarrow{\text{Superoxide dismutase}} O_2 + H_2O_2$ $2\,H_2O_2 \xrightarrow{\text{Catalase}} 2\,H_2O + O_2$	Protective mechanism used by host and many microbes

Modification of phagocytes	Mechanism	Effect	Ref.
Altered Function	**C5a, C3a, TCC mediated**		
Increased adhesion to endothelium	Enhanced receptor expression of CD11b/CD18, CD11c/CD18	Sequestration of leucocytes in the lung: leukopenia	[51]
Decreased chemotaxis	C5a receptor desensitisation due to chronic C5a generation	Susceptibility to infection?	[52]
Impaired phagocytosis	Elevated intracellular calcium	Susceptibility to infection?	[53]
Increased resting oxygen radical production	Stimulation of resting oxygen radical production	Cell damage, tissue damage?	[54]
Decrease in stimulated oxygen radical production	C5a receptor desensitisation due to chronic C5a generation	Susceptibility to infection?	[54]
Increased degranulation	Liberation of enzymes such as elastase from granules	Susceptibility to infection?	[52]
Disturbed metabolism			
Decreased oxygen consumption and lactate release	Uraemia, malnutrition Iron overload	Susceptibility to infection?	[55, 56] [57]

Modification of phagocytes	Mechanism	Effect	Ref.
Diminished glucose uptake and depressed hexose mono-phosphate activity	Increased intracellular calcium		[53, 55]
	Circulating plasma factors		[56]
Inhibition of glycogen synthase activity	Dialysis treatment		[52]
Apoptosis			
	C3, C5 dependent downregulation of CD14	Susceptibility to infection?	[58, 59]
	Partly mediated by reactive oxygen species		[60]

Table 7.4: Alteration in phagocyte function and metabolism in haemodialysis patients. *Blood interaction with complement-activating materials results in profound and transient leukopenia. The remaining circulating leukocytes are altered in their function [53] and metabolism. The activation of neutrophils by complement results in the production of oxygen radicals and proteases used normally in the destruction of infecting bacteria. It has been speculated that tissue destruction, organ dysfunction and a decreased response to further stimuli may be the consequence if this production is enhanced in the absence of infection [50].*

What happens during haemodialysis-induced leukopenia?

In 1968, Kaplow and Goffinet were the first who reported the transient disappearance of white blood cells from the circulation during haemodialysis [62]. Nearly 10 years later Craddock and colleagues demonstrated an association between complement generation and leukopenia [4]. It is now well accepted that C5a, C3a and the terminal complement complex (TCC or membrane attack complex, MAC) stimulate the expression of receptors on leukocytes. In leukopenia, expression of the adhesion receptors

CD11b/CD18 (also termed as MAC1, macrophage antigen-1, CR3, Mo-1 or OKM-1) and CD11c/CD18 (also termed CR4 or p150/95) on leukocytes is important, as these lead to homotypic aggregation and sequestration in the pulmonary microvasculature [63] (see [64, 65] for reviews on adhesion receptors). Monocytes and granulocytes differ in the kinetics of their receptor expression - monocytes react more slowly than granulocytes [66]. Adhesion is further supported by stiffening of the cytoskeleton of neutrophils via filamentous actin, thus slowing down their passage through the pulmonary capillaries. This process is also induced by C5a modulation [67, 68].

At the nadir of leukopenia, usually 15 minutes after onset of haemodialysis with regenerated cellulose membranes and corresponding to the peak of complement activation, 75-89% of the neutrophils are sequestered in the lung. After about 60 minutes of treatment, leukocyte numbers return to normal and, in some cases, are even higher at the end of treatment. In addition to their release from the pulmonary endothelium, leukocytes are recruited from the marginated pool or from bone marrow stores.

There is evidence that leukosequestration during dialysis with regenerated cellulose membranes is not only a passive phenomenon: enzymes (such as lactoferrin, proteolytic elastase and α-1 proteinase inhibitor) are released from granules [69].

How can the transient character of leukopenia be explained?

A desensitation of neutrophils to stimulation by C5a is partly responsible for the transient character of leukopenia [70]. Whether this is due to a decrease in C5a receptor expression or due to uncoupling of the receptor from its signal transducing pathway, or both, is not yet fully understood. Other influences are (a) the absence of a stimulus which, in cases of infection, boosts migration of the cells through the endothelium, and (b) a temporary downmodulation (shedding) of the selectin CD62L (also termed as LAM-1, leukocyte adhesion molecule-1, L-selectin or Leu-8) on granulocytes [68]. A low CD62L expression can lead to a decrease in leukocyte adhesiveness [66]. Furthermore, CD15s (sialyl-Lewis x molecule) is initially upregulated and later downregulated, and correlates negatively with the number of leukocytes [66].

However, an investigation into the kinetics of complement generation (C3a), expression of CD11b and CD61 integrins on neutrophils and platelets, and the number of neutrophils in the blood found that these do not correlate

[68]. This result strengthens the hypothesis that factors other than complement may also be involved in leukopenia.

Is phagocytic function affected by dialysis-induced leukopenia?

Although leukocyte numbers return to normal after 1 hour of treatment, most of the cells are altered in their function. Their ability to subsequently adhere to endothelial cells is decreased [71] and their response towards activating stimuli is blunted [72]. Phagocyte function is suppressed during dialysis with complement-generating membranes (i.e. membranes made of regenerated cellulose), whereas it remains unaltered with non-complement-generating membranes [72]. Additionally, complement-generating membranes accelerate apoptosis of monocytes, possibly due to a depression of CD14 expression [60]. The same effect was observed with neutrophils, but here a complement factor C3 mechanism was proposed as the cause [59]. Neutrophil apoptosis can also be mediated by reactive oxygen species, especially nitric oxide, or other monocyte products resulting from membrane-monocyte interaction [73]. It has been speculated that the impaired function and accelerated apoptosis of phagocytes may contribute to an increased risk of infection in haemodialysis patients dialysed with complement-generating membranes [72]. An overview of observable effects on phagocyte function and their speculated influence on clinical manifestations is presented in **table 7.4**.

7.3.1.1 Induction of oxidative stress

The term *oxidative stress* in chronic renal failure refers to an increased production of reactive oxygen species (ROS) (**table 7.3**) and other pro-oxidants (carbonyl compounds, homocysteine, transition metals and others) (**table 7.5**) in combination with a decreased antioxidant defence [74]. Dialysis treatment may enhance oxidative stress in chronic renal patients who additionally suffer from a chronic deficiency in the major antioxidant systems [75-77]. This constellation may contribute to atherosclerosis, cardiovascular disease, dialysis-related amyloidosis and anaemia [78-80].

Four main factors are held responsible: (1) uraemia and the comorbid status of the ESRD patient, due to an impairment of the antioxidant control systems (vitamin C and selenium deficiency, reduced intracellular levels of vitamin E, reduced activity of the glutathione system), and due to increased pro-oxidant activity (advanced age, high frequency of diabetes, chronic inflammatory state, uraemic syndrome) [80], (2) antioxidant and trace element (e.g. vitamin C, selenium) losses during treatment, (3) the bioincompatibility of the system, especially of the dialysis membrane and (4) trace amounts of endotoxins entering the blood stream from contaminated dialysis fluid [79, 81]. The bioincompatibility of a membrane in this context refers mainly to its potential for phagocyte activation with subsequent ROS generation [74]. Furthermore, the activation of other leukocytes and platelets can lead to the liberation of haeme-containing proteins and transition metals that can produce ROS or act as catalysts of their reactivity [82]. Uraemic plasma has an inhibitory effect on phagocyte metabolism (mainly that of polymorphonuclear cells) but, surprisingly, these cells show an early deficient responsiveness to stimuli and a high basal activity to generate ROS [83]. The uraemia-induced priming effect on these cells is enhanced by contact with the dialysis membrane, leading to cell hyperreactivity with increased ROS formation [83]. Like inflammation, oxidative stress is related to endothelial dysfunction, as the endothelium is a source and a target of oxidants and also participates in the inflammatory response [80].

One consequence of oxidative stress is the oxidation of polyunsaturated lipids, proteins and sugars, resulting in advanced lipoxidation end-products (ALE), advanced oxidation protein products (AOPP) and advanced glycation end-products (AGE), respectively. Oxidative stress is clinically assessed using these parameters rather than measurements of free radicals as free radicals have a very short half-live [80].

Table 7.5: Main reactive oxygen species (ROS) and other pro-oxidants and their anti-oxidant defences. *ROS can react with other substrates, including lipids, proteins and nucleic acids, to cause damage and form further by-products (e.g. peroxynitrite (O^*_2 with NO^*), hypochlorous acid (H_2O_2 with Cl^-) and lipid hydroxyperoxydes), alkoxyl radicals and organic hydroperoxides (O_2 with polyunsaturated lipids). Free iron, copper ions and the haem-group function as catalysts in ROS formation. Radicals are marked by * (adapted from [74]).*

Pro-oxidant	Anti-oxidant	
	Nonenzymatic	Enzymatic
Reactive oxygen species		
Superoxide radical (O_2*)	Vitamin C	Superoxide dismutase
Oxygen singlet ($^1O_2$)	Vitamin C, uric acid, protein thiols, vitamin E	-
Hydrogen peroxide (H_2O_2)	Vitamin C, protein thiols	Glutathione peroxidase, catalase
Hydroxyl radical (OH*)	Vitamin C, glutathione	-
Lipid hydroperoxides (LOOH)	-	E.g. glutathione peroxidase, glutathione S-transferase
Alkoxyl (LO*) and peroxyl radicals (LOO*)	ß-carotene, albumin thiols and bilirubin	-
Reactive nitrogen species		
Nitric oxide radical (NO*)	Thiols (particularly haemoglobin and albumin), vitamin E	-
Peroxynitrite ($ONOO^-$)	Vitamin C, vitamin E	-
Reactive chlorinated species		
Hypochlorous acid (HClO)	Vitamin C, uric acid, protein thiols (albumin)	-
Free iron	Transferrin	-
Haeme and haeme-containing proteins	Haptoglobin, haemopexin, albumin	-
Copper	Ceruloplasmin, uric acid, albumin	-

7.3.1.2 Stimulation of cytokine generation

Cytokines are polypeptides with molecular weights ranging from 10,000 to 45,000 that are generated by immunocompetent cells in response to infection, inflammation or trauma. They induce cellular responses, even in femto- to picomolar concentrations, distal to their site of secretion by reaction with the appropriate surface receptor of the target cell. Cytokines are sometimes termed "hormones of the immune system" due to their ability to transfer information between cells. However, because this happens in cases of inflammation, they are better considered "the alarm system of the immune system" [84].

Cytokines can be differentiated into five different classes according to their biological properties: (1) pro-inflammatory cytokines, (2) anti-inflammatory cytokines, (3) lymphocyte growth and differentiation factors, (4) haematopoietic colony-stimulating factors, and (5) mesenchymal cell growth factors [85]. In the following, only pro-inflammatory cytokines will be discussed, as these are most relevant in haemodialysis. Pro-inflammatory cytokines are generated mainly by the peripheral blood mononuclear cells (PBMC), comprising monocytes, natural killer cells and T-lymphocytes. Circulating monocytes are most important in this context because these are easily stimulated to release cytokines during haemodialysis treatment. This stimulation occurs by complement activation, by direct interaction with the polymer material, by microbial contamination products, and even by mechanical pumping of blood in the haemodialysis circuit [86].

More than 20 cytokines are produced from PBMC but only a few have been studied intensively in relation to haemodialysis. These are interleukin-1 (IL-1), IL-2, interferon (IFN) α and γ, IL-6, and tumor necrosis factor (TNF).

What are the biological effects of IL-1, IL-6 and TNF?

An overview of the biological effects of the pro-inflammatory cytokines IL-1, IL-6 and TNF is given in **figure 7.15**. Released by stimulated monocytes or macrophages, they initiate, together with other cytokines, the activation of granulocytes, endothelial cells, B-and T-lymphocytes, fibroblasts, bone marrow cells and cells in the brain. All these cells have special functions in the defence against infection or injury. In order to protect, they themselves liberate interleukines, interferons, growth factors, and colony stimulating factors. IL-1 and TNF also trigger the release of neuropeptides in the central nervous sys-

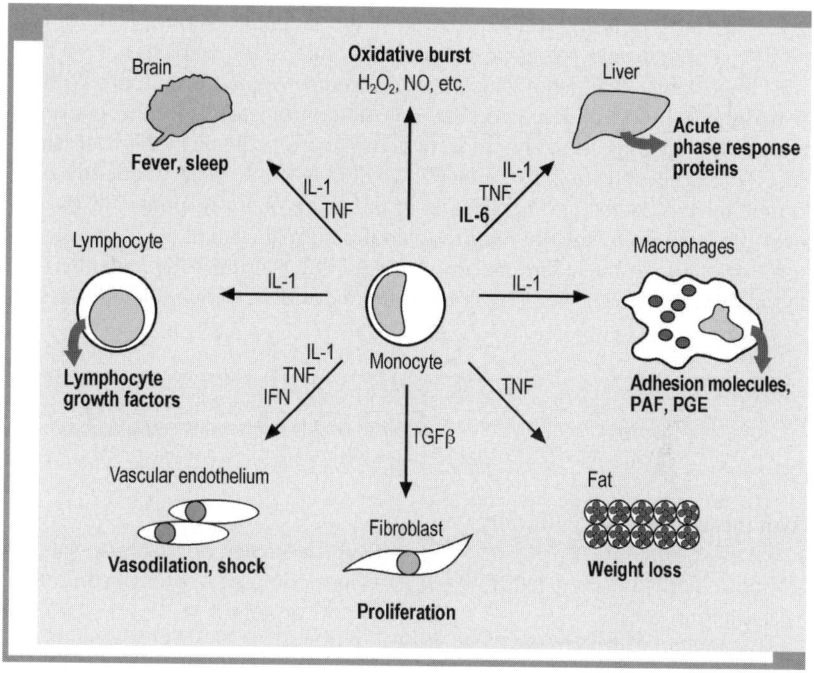

Figure 7.15: Biological effects of pro-inflammatory cytokines. *Stimulated monocytes liberate pro-inflammatory cytokines that activate a number of different cells. These are themselves involved in the immune defence, for example T-lymphocytes, B-lymphocytes and granulocytes (not shown). Furthermore, cells in the hypothalamus are stimulated and fever may be induced as well as tiredness and sleep. Activation of endothelial cells may result in the production of platelet-activating factor (PAF), nitric oxide and prostaglandin E (PGE), all of which lead to vasodilatation and, in high doses, to shock. Acute phase response proteins, such as C-reactive protein (CRP), α_2-macroglobulin and α_2-acid glycoprotein, are liberated in the liver. IL-6, supported by IL-1, is the strongest inducer of CRP. Chronic stimulation of fat cells by TNF may lead to weight loss over time. Fibroblasts are activated to form connective tissue. Oxidative burst may also be induced during activation by cytokines, possibly damaging cells in the absence of bacteria. The interactions shown here are strongly simplified. TGFß: transforming growth factor; IFN: interferon (adapted from [85, 87])*

tem. The most important neuropeptides are adenocorticotropic hormone (ACTH), corticotropin releasing factor and somatostatin [84]. IL-1, TNF and, most importantly, IL-6 (all of which are released by mononuclear cells (PBMC) in peripheral blood and macrophages in tissue) initiate the acute phase response by triggering the generation of acute phase proteins in the liver (**table 7.6**). Among these proteins, C reactive protein (CRP) is most frequently used to monitor the course and magnitude of the acute phase response. Its plasma level increases up to several hundred-fold the normal physiological concentration 8-10 hours after inflammatory stimulus [88]. Plasma CRP and IL-6 concentrations are strong predictors of outcome and cardiovascular disease in

Acute phase protein	Biological function in host defence
High increase in concentration	
C-reactive protein (CRP)	Activates complement for opsonisation
Mannose-binding protein (MBP)	Activates complement for opsonisation
α_1 acid glycoprotein	Transport protein
Serum amyloid A protein (SAP)	?
Moderate increase in concentration	
α_1 proteinase inhibitor	Inhibits bacterial protease activity
α_1 anti-chymotrypsin	Inhibits bacterial protease activity
C3, C9, factor B	Increase complement function
Ceruloplasmin	Oxygen scavanger
Fibrinogen	Coagulation
Angiotensin	Lowers blood pressure
Haptoglobin	Binds haemoglobin
Fibronectin	Cell attachment

Table 7.6: Acute phase proteins*. Acute phase proteins are quickly liberated by hepatocytes in cases of infection and inflammation; they constitute an important part of the innate immune response. CRP recognises and binds to molecular groups on the outer surface of a wide variety of bacteria and fungi in a calcium-dependent manner – these groups are absent in this form on human cells. CRP themself can act as opsonin, but also via binding of complement factors. This opsonisation activates phagocytes to engulf the bacteria. Furthermore, the activation of the complement cascade leads to lysis of the bacteria by the terminal complement complex (TCC, C5b-9) (adapted from [39]).*

end-stage renal disease patients [89, 90], probably because increased IL-6 levels can adversely affect nutritional status and are pro-atherogenic in ESRD patients [90, 91].

Partial insight into the clinical effects of IL-1 and TNF was obtained by direct infusion of the isolated molecules into humans and animals, respectively. The main short-coming of these experiments is that concentrations of the factors used were unphysiologically high. TNF produced hypotension, leukopenia and several metabolic dysfunctions when injected in humans in a concentration of 1 µg/kg body weight (BW). Injected IL-1 (1 ng/kg BW) induced fever and, with increasing doses (100 ng/kg BW), hypotension [84]. Both molecules act synergistically to trigger haemodynamic shock, prostaglandin synthesis and cell toxicity. Effects such as hypotension and shock are mediated by prostaglandin; synthesis of this is triggered by an increase in gene expression of the enzymes cyclooxygenase and phospholipase A_2 [92]. Whereas the cellular metabolism is upregulated by cytokines, and several genes coding for active molecules are increased in their expression, some genes are also suppressed. These include the genes for albumin, lipoprotein lipase, cytochrome P450 and aromatase [85].

How is cytokine generation induced during haemodialysis?

Evidence for the triggering of cytokine release during haemodialysis is found in the increase of plasma IL-1 activity during a single session [94], whereby the rise in activity is dependent on the choice of membrane [95]. A lot of data support the concept that cytokine release during dialysis requires two stimuli. In the first step, complement fragments C5a and C3a, acetate in the dialysis fluid or intrinsic properties of the membrane itself trigger monocytes to increase gene expression of IL-1 and TNF [96, 97]. The mRNA produced is then only translated into the final cytokine if a second trigger is present. This stimulant can be LPS or other bacterial products, or IL-1 itself (**figure 7.16**). Haemodialysis with pyrogen-free dialysis fluid and dialysers containing membranes made of regenerated cellulose serves as a "priming" event for mononuclear cells, inducing IL-1 and TNF transcription. This mRNA formation is detectable even 24 hours later. After LPS stimulation, translation of the IL-1 and TNF proteins occurs [96]. Deppisch et al. proposed the hypothesis of direct monocyte activation by L-fucose, which is present on the surface of cellulosic membranes. After binding of the L-fucose residue to the fucose receptor on the cell surface, cytokines are secreted if a second signal provided by the terminal complement complex (TCC, C5b-9) is present [93]. In summary, cytokine release in haemodialysis is induced (1) by monocyte activation directly on bioincompatible membranes (via L-fucose receptor) in combination with complement factors (TCC, C5b-9), and/or (2) by binding of complement factors (C5a, C3a) to monocyte receptors and subsequent stimulation by dialysis fluid-derived exogenous pyrogenic materials. Thus the detrimental effects of released cytokines can be avoided or minimised by using membranes that do not significantly activate complement in combination with ultrapure dialysis fluid.

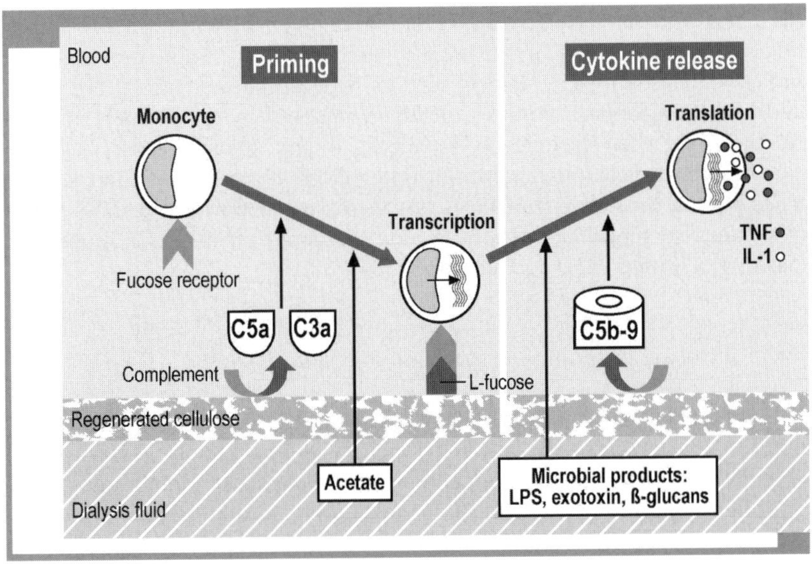

Figure 7.16: Priming and cytokine release of monocytes during haemodialysis. *Circulating monocytes are primed to transcribe the genes for IL-1 and TNF by activated complement factors (C5a, C3a), by membrane contact itself (via receptor - L-fucose interaction) or by acetate in the dialysis fluid. The developing mRNA is only translated if a second signal from ongoing infection or illness is received. This signal (e.g. endotoxin) can come from intestinal tissue, but the most likely source in haemodialysis is the dialysis fluid. Besides bacterial products, IL-1 can induce its own synthesis (i.e. autocrine regulation of its own production). Furthermore, the terminal complement complex (TCC, C5b-9) may also act as a second stimulus (adapted from [84, 93]).*

Which counterregulatory mechanisms play a role in cytokine generation during haemodialysis?

Counterregulatory mechanisms are induced in response to inflammation in order to blunt the response. Nonspecific inhibitors (e.g. lipoproteins, lipids and α_2-macroglobulin) are examples of naturally occurring inhibitors of IL-1, IL-2 and IL-6 [98]. Furthermore, cells that synthesize IL-1 and TNF also produce specific molecules that simultaneously block the action of these cytokines. Measurements have proven this: inhibitory activity was found to be much higher in plasma from haemodialysis patients than in plasma from healthy volunteers (whose cytokine plasma levels were below the detection limit) [99]. IL-1 and TNF initiate their biological effects by binding to their specific receptors expressed on target cells. Preventing this interaction can therefore regulate their action. Soluble TNF receptors exist (proteolytic cleavage products of the cell surface receptors p55 and p75), which bind TNF, thus hampering TNF-cell surface receptor interaction [100]. In contrast, the IL-1 receptor antagonist [IL-1Ra) binds directly to the IL-1 receptors (type I = p80 and type II = p68 receptors) without activating them, blocking IL-1 - IL-1 receptor interaction and, consequently, the biological action of IL-1 [100]. The biological activity of IL-1 and TNF thus results from an interplay between the active molecule, the binding to its cellular receptors, the number and type of receptors expressed by target cells and the inhibitory action of its antagonists.

Evidence now exists that high IL-1Ra levels do not provide sufficient protection against the biological effects of increased IL-1 levels. Rather, they reflect the degree of inflammatory state of haemodialysis patients [101]. Nevertheless, one study reported an improvement in several inflammatory diseases after specific IL-1 receptor blockage [101].

7.3.2 Stimulation of basophilic leukocytes and mast cells

Mast cells and basophilic granulocytes may be stimulated via IgE-dependent reactions during dialysis treatment by anaphylatoxins (C3a, C4a, C5a), by mediators such as histamine releasing factors, and by drugs (morphine, morphine derivatives, codeine, adenocorticotropic hormone (ACTH), calcium ionophores, substance P and other ionophores). Basophils and mast cells carry specific receptors for complement components and may be stimulated to release a number of highly biologically active mediators in cases of complement generation at dialysis membranes (**figure 7.17, table 7.7**). This mechanism is thought to play a role in the development of the first use syndrome [103].

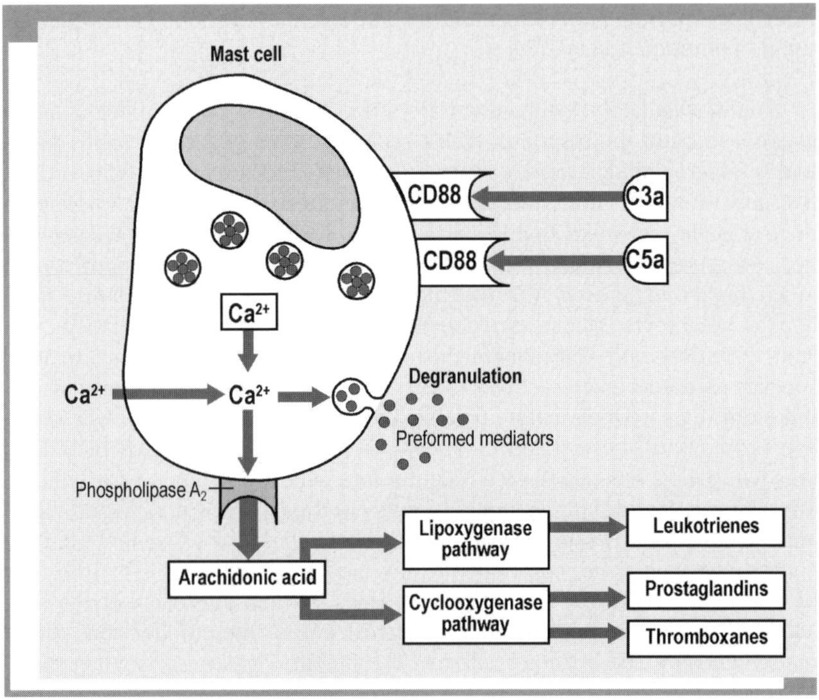

Figure 7.17: Triggering of mast cells by C3a and/or C5a*. There are two different types of mediator release from mast cells following stimulation by the anaphylatoxins C3a, C4a and C5a (C4a not shown here). The first mechanism involves the release of preformed mediators (see* ***table 7.7****) by granules, while arachidonic acid is produced through the activation of phospholipase* A_2 *in the second mechanism. This, in turn, initiates the lipoxygenase and cyclooxygenase pathways, resulting in the release of the mediators leukotrienes, prostaglandins and thromboxanes (see* ***table 7.7****). Calcium ions (*Ca^{2+}*) and cyclic adenosine monophosphate (cAMP) are necessary for these processes (adapted from [39]).*

Furthermore, neutrophils, platelets, alveolar macrophages and monocytes secrete factors when activated which, in turn, stimulate basophils and/or mast cells to release histamine [104]. Three histamine-releasing factors have been identified, with molecular weights of 12 (HRF-1), 14 (HRF-2) and 41 (NAP-2) [105]. Furthermore, cytokines (e.g. IL-1, IL-3 and GM-CSF) can induce histamine release. Elevated histamine levels are observed in many chronic haemodialysis patients and appear to correlate with the incidence of pruritus in some investigations [105].

	Granule release	Effect
	Preformed	
	Histamine	Vasodilation, increased capillary permeability, chemokinesis, bronchoconstriction
	Heparin	Anticoagulation
	Tryptase	C3 activation
	β- glucosaminidase	Off-splitting of glucosamine
	Eosinophil chemotactic factor	Chemotaxis of eosinophils
	Neutrophil chemotactic factor	Chemotaxis of neutrophils
	Platelet-activating factor (PAF)	Mediator release from platelets
Induced by phospholipase A_2 activation and arachidonic acid formation	**Newly synthesised**	
Lipoxygenase pathway	Leukotrienes C4, D4 (SRS-A) and B4	Vasoactivation, broncho-constriction, chemotaxis and/or chemokinesis
Cyclooxygenase pathway	Prostaglandins, thromboxanes	Affect bronchial muscle, platelet aggregation and vasodilation

Table 7.7: Mediators released by triggering of mast cells by C5a and C3a. *(adapted from [39]).*

7.3.3 The role of immune cell stimulation in the generation of ß2-microglobulin

The pathogenesis of ß2-microglobulin (ß2-m) amyloidosis is multifactorial but an involvement of membrane bioincompatibility has been discussed over the last 10 years (e.g. [61]) (**figure 7.18**). ß2-m (MW 11,818) is present on the surface of most nucleated cells as a glycoprotein moiety of HLA class I molecules, and is liberated into plasma by shedding [107]. The main elimination of the protein occurs in the kidney and, therefore, chronic renal failure is associated with high plasma concentrations of ß2-m. These high levels constitute the basic precondition for the deposition of ß2-m in amyloid fibrils, as is detected in patients suffering from dialysis-related amyloidosis. Dialysis, in its intermittent character, cannot totally remove the ß2-m overload, even with high ß2-m removing membranes [106]. In addition, Jahn et al. found increased ß2-m mRNA synthesis and increased surface expression of MHC class I molecules by peripheral blood lymphocytes *in vitro* with regenerated cellulose membranes, but not when polyacrylonitrile or polycarbonate-polyether membranes were used [108]. L-fucose residues, which are present on the surface of regenerated cellulose membranes but not on the surfaces of membranes made from synthetic materials, are held responsible for the activation of this synthesis [109], probably in synergism with the terminal complement complex C5b-9 [110]. Furthermore, there is evidence that proinflammatory cytokines, such as IL-1 and TNFα, (produced during haemodialysis [111]) and lipopolysaccharides (LPS), may enhance ß2-m release by activated cells.

However *in vivo* data did not confirm the *in vitro* findings described above. No difference in gene expression of the ß2-m gene (gene c-fos, GAP-DH gene) could be detected during dialyses with low-flux, regenerated cellulose dialysers and high-flux, polyamide dialysers [112]. In another study, daily *in vivo* ß2-m production was similar in patients dialysed either with a "biocompatible" polyacrylonitrile or with a "bioincompatible" regenerated cellulose membrane [113]. Locatelli et al. also did not find any differences in predialysis ß2-m plasma levels when "bioincompatible", low-flux regenerated cellulose was compared with "biocompatible", low-flux polysulfone dialysis in a prospective multicentre study over 24 months [114]. Therefore, should increased ß2-m mRNA synthesis and ß2-m release from cells really play a role in the development of amyloidosis, then it is only a very minor role. The ß2-m removal ability of membranes (either by adsorption or by filtration) and the use of endotoxin-free, ultrapure dialysis fluid appear to constitute much more important factors [115, 116]. However, bioincompatible membranes may

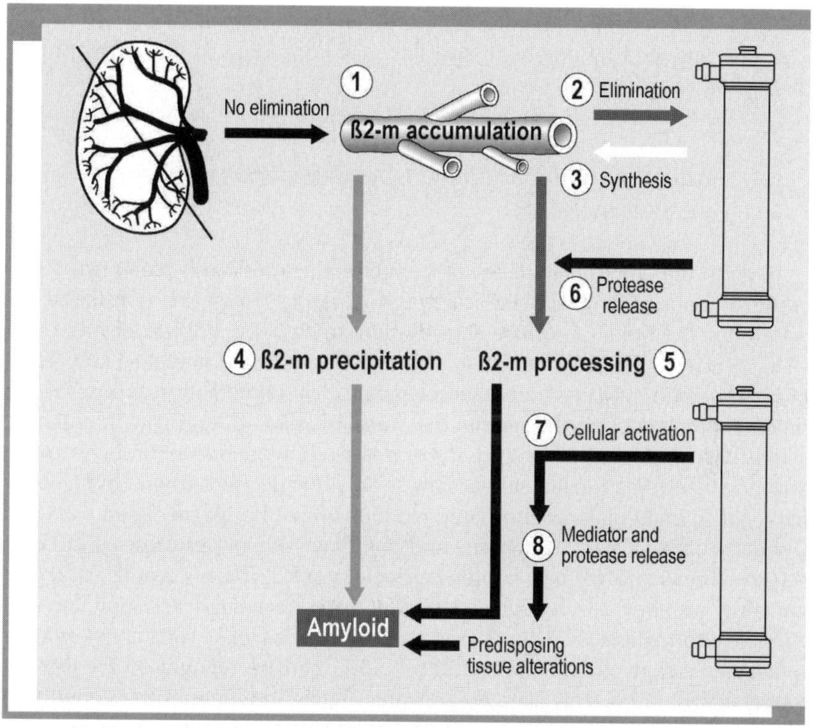

Figure 7.18: Possible role of the dialyser in the pathogenesis of dialysis-related amyloidosis. *(**1**) An increased ß2-m concentration in the blood is a prerequisite for the deposition of ß2-m in amyloid fibrils. It is mainly the consequence of the missing renal elimination which cannot be replaced by (**2**) dialytic removal. (**3**) In addition, an increase in ß2-m synthesis induced by the dialysis membrane in combination with complement fragments, lipopolysaccharide, IL-1, IL-6, TNF and structures on the dialysis membrane itself has also been discussed (indicated by a white arrow). However, the impact of such an increased synthesis on the ß2-m plasma concentrations is considered to be low. (**4**) ß2-m does not simply precipitate in amyloid fibrils (or, if it does, then only to a small extent), but is rather (**5**) processed by proteinases. (**6**) During dialysis, cellular activation - induced by direct membrane contact or complement factors - leads to the liberation of proteases that may induce limited proteolysis of ß2-m. Furthermore, (**7**) tissue cells, especially macrophages, may be activated by mediators released by circulating cells. (**8**) They further release mediators and/or proteases that process ß2-m. The shade of the arrows indicates the importance of the respective factor; black is very important, grey is of minor importance, and white arrows indicate cases of speculated relevance (adapted from [106]).*

induce a systemic inflammatory response, aggravating oxidative stress (which is already induced by uraemia), and this may contribute to the development of amyloidosis [61, 115].

7.3.4 Stimulation of the adaptive (specific) immune system – hypersensitivity

Due to the chronic character of treatment, haemodialysis patients are susceptible to becoming hypersensitive to substances they are constantly exposed to. Examples are hypersensitisation to EtO [3], formaldehyde [117, 118], heparin [119], and even to the buffer substance acetate [120, 121]. Hypersensitivity reactions are characterised by an immediate response of the patient after onset of dialysis in the form of mild to even life-threatening symptoms. These range from pruritis or rhinitis to hypotension, bronchospasm and angio-oedema, up to cardiac arrest. In order to be termed "hypersensitive", these immediate anaphylactic reactions must be IgE-mediated [3, 122]. Chemicals like EtO act as haptens and combine with carrier proteins, such as serum albumin, to form a hapten-carrier complex. These complexes act as antigens, i.e. they are recognised by the immune system as being foreign. Complex formation is a necessary precondition as only substances with a molecular weight greater than 3000 – 5000 can be recognised by the immune system [123]. This allergen activates T-cells and induces the generation of IgE antibodies. In cases of subsequent exposure to these allergens, mast cells and basophils are triggered by IgE to release cytokines (IL-1, IL-3, IL-4, IL-5, IL-6, GM-CSF, IFN, TNF) and mediators of allergy (the latter were described in **table 7.7**). These preformed and newly generated mediators provoke the clinical symptoms described above. It is well known that hypersensitivity can also be induced by other mechanisms [122], but the role of these in dialysis-related reactions is thought to be only slight [123].

Acute phase proteins are released in response to the secretion of IL-1, IL-6 and TNF (**table 7.6**). The plasma concentration of some of these, e.g. CRP, increases up to 100-fold. CRP binds to foreign surfaces in a Ca^{2+}-dependent manner and acts as an opsonin together with complement.

7.4 Activation of the kinin system - anaphylactoid reactions

Negatively charged dialysis membranes are particularly good activators of the kinin-system during haemodialysis [38, 124-128]. These trigger the kinin-cascade via adsorption and activation of factor XII and plasma kallikrein (**figure 7.19**) [129]. The first step of activation has already been described in this work under contact activation and its role in the activation of the clotting cascade during haemodialysis (**figure 7.5**).

The biologically active products of the kinin pathway are the decapeptide kallidin and its cleavage product, the nonapeptide bradykinin. Both are generated from their precursor, high molecular weight kininogen, by kallikrein [130], and both peptides are able to increase cardiac output, cause peripheral vasodilation and a decrease in blood pressure. The last effect is counterbalanced by angiotensin II, a strong vasoconstrictor [131]. The decisive link between the renin-angiotensin and the kinin system is the enzyme angiotensin converting enzyme (ACE): this transforms the precursor angiotensin I into its active form angiotensin II, and inactivates bradykinin by proteolytic cleavage. The consumption of ACE-inhibitors prevents the development of vasoconstrictive angiotensin II and the degradation of bradykinin, resulting in an accumulation of this vasodilator and a decrease in blood pressure. Depending on the extent of bradykinin generation by the particular dialysis membrane, a critical concentration of this mediator can be exceeded and mild to severe anaphylactoid reactions can result [125-129].

The vasodilating effect of bradykinin is mediated by an increased production and release of nitric oxide (NO) by endothelial cells. This short-lived gas is produced by the enzyme NO-synthase and exhibits its vasodilative effect by an increase in cytosolic cGMP in vascular cells of smooth-muscles [130].

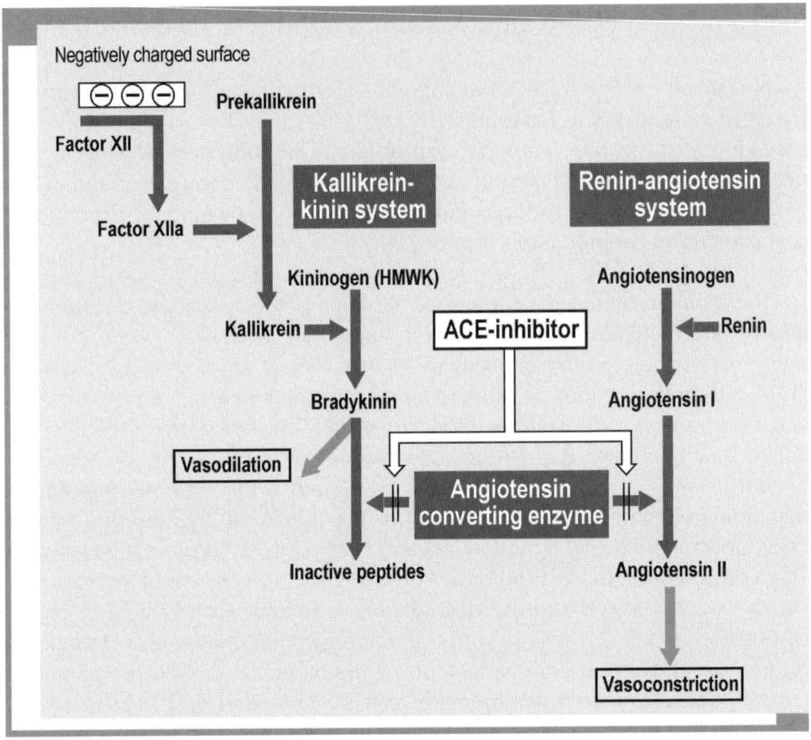

Figure 7.19: Contact activation and generation of bradykinin and angiotensin II. *When blood comes into contact with negatively charged surfaces (e.g. collagen or negatively charged dialysis membranes), the positvely charged factor XII adsorbs onto the surface and undergoes a conformational change. This results in self-activation to factor XIIa. Factor XIIa activates prekallikrein (bound to high molecular weight kininogen (HMWK)) to kallikrein. In a positive feedback-loop, this kallikrein is able to activate more factor XII. Furthermore, it transforms HMWK into bradykinin, which is itself degraded by the angiotensin converting enzyme (ACE). ACE also generates angiotensin II from angiotensin I. When an ACE-inhibitor is applied, the breakdown of the vasodilatative substance bradykinin is prevented and it accumulates. Black arrows indicate activation, grey arrows a biological effect. White arrows mark the action of the ACE-inhibitor (adapted from [130, 131]).*

7.5 Bioincompatibility aspects of advanced glycation and oxidation end-product formation

In uraemic patients, a number of middle molecules accumulate and are modified due to oxidative stress, microinflammation or uraemia per se. These modifications may alter the biological function of the molecules and can play a role in long-term consequences of ESRD, such as amyloidosis and atherosclerosis. ß2-m is an example of one such molecule – this has already been discussed in this chapter. Other examples, which will be described here, are advanced glycation end-products (AGE), advanced lipoxidation end-products (ALE) and advanced oxidation protein products (AOPP).

How are AGE, ALE and AOPP formed?

Proteins, peptides and amino acids which become exposed to glucose or other carbohydrates are finally and irreversibly modified to AGE in a non-enzymatic reaction termed as Maillard reaction (see **figure 7.20** for a more detailed explanation). Early Maillard products, like the Amadori product fructoselysine, are present in significantly higher concentrations in diabetic than in non-diabetic haemodialysis patients, implying that the first steps of AGE formation are under glycaemic control [134]. The irreversible AGE formation, however, appears to be controlled by uraemia-associated processes: diabetic as well as non-diabetic dialysis patients exhibit similar plasma concentrations of the two well-known AGEs, pentosidine and carboxymethyllysine, but levels are up to ten-fold higher in uraemic plasma compared to that of healthy controls [134, 135]. Recently, it was demonstrated that elevated plasma pentosidine concentrations were associated with higher age, inflammation and malnutrition to a statistically significant degree [136].

Proteins are also modified by lipids to become ALE, e.g. by malondialdehyde, which is derived from the oxidation of polyunsaturated fatty acids [135]. Both AGE and ALE are the product of carbonyl amine chemistry, i.e. the reaction between reactive carbonyl compounds (e.g. glyoxal, methylglyoxal, 3-deoxyglucosone, dehydroascorbate or malonedialdehyde) and amino-groups of the protein, peptide or amino acid in question (**figure 7.20**).

Furthermore, proteins, peptides or amino acids can be damaged by reactive oxygen species, such as the superoxide anion, hydrogen peroxide, hydroxyl radicals or hypochlorous acid [137]. In these reactions, amino acid residues (e.g. tyrosine) are oxidised, resulting in the formation of di-tyrosine, protein aggregation, cross-linking and fragmentation. These cross-linked products are designated advanced oxidation products (AOPP) [137].

How does dialysis affect levels of AGE, ALE and AOPP?

Dialysis treatment can influence AGE, ALE and AOPP levels both directly and indirectly by removal of the substances themselves and their precursors, respectively. Observations tend to favour precursor removal rather than end-product removal in that haemodialysis has been shown to have little impact on AGE levels. This is because AGE are linked to plasma proteins (mainly albumin), e.g. 90% pentosidine and N-carboxymethyllysine are protein bound, leaving only the remaining 10% free for removal by haemodialysis – an amount which can be considered negligible [138, 139].

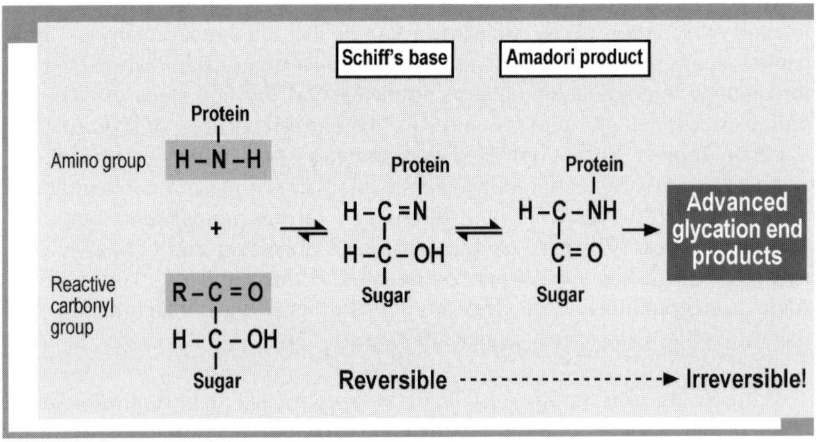

Figure 7.20: Maillard reaction of advanced glycation end-products (AGE) formation. *Amino groups of proteins, peptides or amino acids together with sugar aldehyde groups reversibly form Schiff bases in a non-enzymatic manner. Upon rearrangement, they convert into more stable, slowly-reversible so-called Amadori products [N-(1-deoxyfructosyl)derivatives]. Some Amadori products are further converted into AGE through chemical rearrangement, dehydration and fragmentation reactions – a process which may take months. AGE (e.g. pentosidine, N-carboxymethyllysine, imidazolones) constitute a heterogenous class of structures that tend to polymerise and cross-link [132, 133].*

AOPP consist mainly of aggregated proteins and are, consequently, too large to be removed by haemodialysis (high-molecular weight protein aggregates have molecular weights of around 600,000, low-molecular weight compounds have molecular weights of approx. 80,000) [137]. However, the

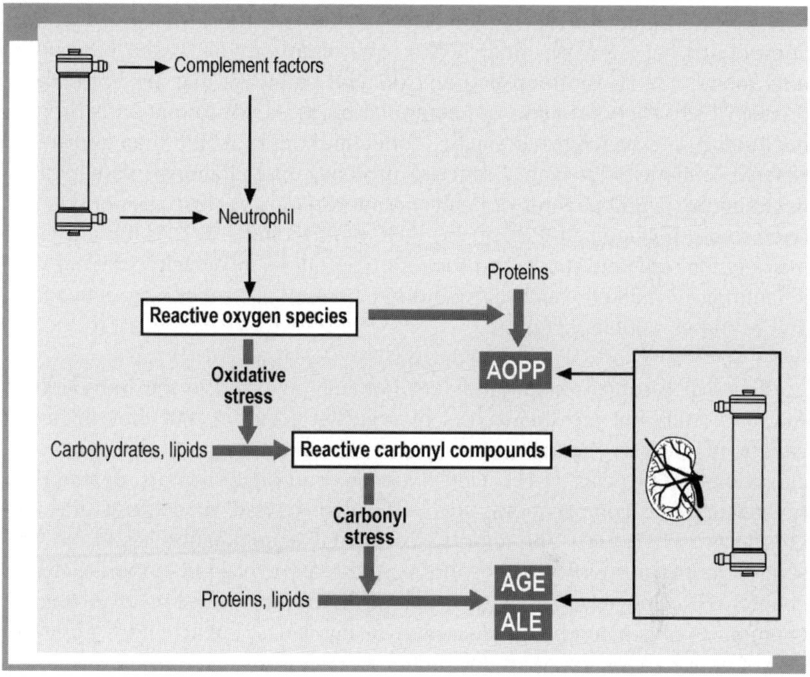

Figure 7.21: Influence of dialyser and membrane bioincompatibility on the formation of advanced glycation end-products (AGE), advanced lipoxidation endproducts (ALE) and advanced oxidation protein products (AOPP). *The formation of AGE and ALE is mainly the result of oxidative and carbonyl stress, together with decreased renal clearance [137]. Uraemia is characterised by an augmented production of oxidants and a decreased level of antioxidants. Furthermore, the haemodialysis treatment itself may result in complement activation, with subsequent neutrophil stimulation or direct cell stimulation leading to the release of reactive oxygen species (**table 7.4**). These reactive oxygen species target proteins, carbohydrates and lipids, which are abundantly present throughout the body. The result is the development of oxidised protein products and various reactive carbonyl compounds that are eventually involved in the formation of AGE and ALE. In addition, non-oxidative processes may also play a role in AGE and ALE formation [141].*

haemodialysis treatment itself may increase oxidative stress and, subsequently, carbonyl stress when complement-generating membranes are used. The consequence is the development of reactive carbonyl compounds, such as glyoxal, methylglyoxal, 3-deoxyglucosone, dehydroascorbate, and malondialdehyde [140] (**figure 7.21**). The accumulation of reactive carbonyl compounds is also a result of the loss of renal excretion - something which is not fully compensated for by haemodialysis (although most reactive carbonyl compounds have a MW under 5000) [140]. Furthermore, reactive carbonyl compounds are also formed by non-oxidative pathways that are not dialysis-related [138]. A contribution of haemodialysis to AOPP formation is proven: haemodialysis patients exhibit higher concentrations of AOPP than undialysed uraemic patients with high C-reactive protein concentrations (marker of inflammation), CAPD patients or healthy controls [137]. A close relationship has been found between AOPP and the AGE pentosidine [137]. AOPP are good markers for oxidative stress, and their concentrations positively correlate with inflammatory markers, such as neopterin (marker for monocyte activation), TNF-α and its soluble receptor.

Reactive carbonyl compounds are not only involved in the formation of ALE and AGE, but are themselves biologically active in that they initiate a variety of cellular responses and thereby induce structural and functional alterations in proteins [141]. Consequently, carbonyl stress is detected in several uraemic complications, such as dialysis-related amyloidosis and atherosclerosis [137, 140]. The importance of AGE accumulation lies in the subsequent numerous biological responses; these are explained in more detail in chapter 10. One example is the role of AGE-modified ß2-m in monocyte chemotaxis and macrophage secretion of cytokines, implicating a contribution of AGE to bone and joint destruction in dialysis-related amyloidosis [142]. Furthermore, AGE and ALE were found to accumulate in aortic elastin, thereby contributing to atherosclerosis [143]. AOPP may also play a role in the development of atherosclerosis [139].

References

1. Gurland HJ, Davison AM, Bonomini V, Falkenhagen D, Hansen S, Kishimoto T, Lysaght MJ, Moran J, Valek A: Definitions and terminology in biocompatibility. Nephrol Dial Transplant 9(Suppl 2): 4-10, 1994

2. Salzman EW: Thrombosis in artificial organs. Transplant Proc 3(4): 1491-1496, 1971

3. Dolovich J, Bell B: Allergy to a product(s) of ethylene oxide gas. Demonstration of IgE and IgG antibodies and hapten specificity. J Allergy Clin Immunol 62(1): 30-32, 1978

4. Craddock PR, Fehr J, Brigham KL, Kronenberg RJ, Jacob HJ: Complement and leukocyte-mediated pulmonary dysfunction in hemodialysis. N Engl J Med 296: 769-774, 1977

5. Craddock PR, Fehr J, Dalmasso AP, Brigham KL, Jacob HS: Hemodialysis leukopenia. Pulmonary vascular leukostasis resulting from complement activation by dialyzer cellophane membranes. J Clin Invest 59(5): 879-888, 1977

6. Henderson LW, Koch KM, Dinarello CA, Shaldon S: Hemodialysis hypotension: the interleukin hypothesis. Blood Purif 1: 3-8, 1983

7. Tielemans C, Madhoun P, Lenaers M, Schandene L, Goldman M, Vanherweghem JL: Anaphylactoid reactions during hemodialysis on AN69 membranes in patients receiving ACE inhibitors. Kidney Int 38: 982-984, 1990

8. Colton CK, Ward RA, Shaldon S: Scientific basis for the assessment of biocompatibility in extracorporeal blood treatment. Nephrol Dial Transplant 9(Suppl 2): 11-17, 1994

9. Lane DA, Bowry SK: The scientific basis for selection of measures of thrombogenicity. Nephrol Dial Transplant 9(Suppl2): 18-28, 1993

10. Addonizio VP, Colman RW: Platelets and extracorporeal circulation. Biomaterials 3: 9-15, 1982

11. Forbes CD: Blood-material interaction: importance of thrombosis in: *Blood-material interaction* edited by Falkenhagen D, Klinkmann H, Piskin E, Opatrný K Glasgow INFA: 56-59, 1998

12. Vroman L, Adams AL, Fischer GC, Munoz PC: Interaction of high molecular weight kininogen, factor XII, and fibrinogen in plasma at interfaces. Blood 55(1): 156-159, 1980

13. Chuang HY, Mohammad SF, Sharma NC, Mason RG: Interaction of human alpha-thrombin with artificial surfaces and reactivity of adsorbed alpha-thrombin. J Biomed Mater Res 14: 467-476, 1980

14. Handin RI: Bleeding and thrombosis in: *Principles of internal medicine* 14th edition, edited by Fauci AS, Braunwald E, Isselbacher KJ, Wilson JD, Martin JB, Kasper DL, Hauser SL, Longo DL, New York McGraw-Hill Companies: 339-345, 1998

15. Weiss C, Jelkmann W: Funktionen des Blutes: Thrombocyten in: *Physiologie des Menschen* 27th edition, edited by Schmidt RF, Thews G Berlin Springer Verlag: 426-433, 1997

16. Holmsen H: Platelet metabolism and activation. Semin Hematol 22(3): 219-240, 1985

17. Spaethe R: Aktivierung und Ablauf des Gerinnungssystems in: *Hämostase, Physiologie, Pathophysiologie, Therapie 1*[st] edition, edited by Spaethe R, Kolde H-J, Baxter Deutschland GmbH: 78-104, 1992

18. Walsh PN: Platelet-mediated trigger mechanisms in the contact phase of blood coagulation. Semin Thromb Haemost 13(1): 86-94, 1987

19. Rylance PB, Gordge MP, Ireland H, Lane DA, Weston MJ: Haemodialysis with prostacyclin (epoprostenol) alone. Proc Eur Dial Transplant Assoc 21: 281-286, 1984

20. Horne MK, Chao ES: Heparin binding to resting and activated platelets. Blood 74(1): 238-243, 1989

21. Rollason G, Sefton MV: Measurement of the rate of thrombin production in human plasma in contact with different materials. J Biomed Mater Res 26: 675-693, 1992

22. Elam JH, Nygren H: Adsorption of coagulation proteins from whole blood on to polymer materials: relation to platelet activation. Biomaterials 13: 3-8, 1992

23. Opatrný K Jr., Vít L, Opatrný K: The fibrinolytic system in blood-material interaction in: *Blood-material interaction,* edited by Falkenhagen D, Klinkmann H, Piskin E, Opatrný K INFA Krems: 65-68, 1998

24. Béguin S, Lindhout T, Hemker HC: The mode of action of heparin in plasma. Thromb Haemost 60(3): 457-462, 1988

25. Turney JH, Fewell MR, Williams LC, Parsons V, Weston MJ: Platelet protection and heparin sparing with prostacyclin during regular dialysis therapy. Lancet 2: 219-222, 1980

26. Rosenberg RD, Lam L: Correlation between structure and function of heparin. Proc Natl Acad Sci USA 76(3): 1218-1222, 1979

27. Atha DH, Lormeau JC, Petitou M, Rosenberg RD, Choay J: Contribution of 3-0 and 6-0-sulfated glucosamine residues in the heparin-induced conformational change in antithrombin III. Biochemistry 26: 6454-6461, 1987

28. Hirsh J, Levine MN: Low molecular weight heparin. Blood 79(1): 1-17, 1992

29. Beijering RJR, Ten Cate H, Nurmohamed MT, Ten Cate JW: Anticoagulants and extracorporeal circuits. Seminars in thrombosis and hemostasis 23 (2): 225-233, 1997

30. Schrader J, Stibbe W, Kandt M, Warneke G, Armstrong V, Müller HJ, Scheller F: Low molecular weight heparin versus standard heparin. A long-term study in hemodialysis and hemofiltration patients. ASAIO Transactions 36: 28-32, 1990

31. Viganó G, Schieppati A, Remuzzi G: Thrombogenesis and anticoagulation in patients undergoing chronic hemodialysis in: *Replacement of renal function,* 4th ed., edited by Jacobs C, Kjellstrand CM, Koch KM, Winchester JF, Dordrecht Kluwer Academic Publishers: 323-332, 1996

32. Flanigan MJ, Von Brecht J, Freeman RM, Lim VS: Reducing the hemorrhagic complications of dialysis. A controlled comparison of low dose heparin and citrate anticoagulation. Am J Kidney Dis 9: 147-153, 1987

33. Hofbauer R, Moser D, Frass M, Oberbauer R, Kaye AD, Wagner O, Kapiotis S, Druml W: Effect of anticoagulation on blood membrane interactions during hemodialysis. Kidney Inter 56: 1578-1583, 1999

34. Böhler J, Schollmeyer P, Dressel B, Dobos G, Hörl WH: Reduction of granulocyte activation during hemodialysis with regional citrate anticoagulation: dissociation of complement activation and neutropenia from neutrophil degranulation. J Am Soc Nephrol 7: 234-241, 1996

35. Wiegmann TB, MacDougall ML, Diederich DA: Dialysis leukopenia, hypoxemia and anaphylatoxin formation: effect of membrane, bath, and citrate anticoagulation. Am J Kidney Dis 11(5): 418-424, 1988

36. Dhondt A, Vanholder R, Waterloos M-A, Glorieux G, De Smet R, Lameire N: Citrate anticoagulation does not correct cuprophane bioincompatibility as evaluated by the expression of leukocyte surface molecules. Nephrol Dial Transplant 13: 1752-1758, 1998

37. Kelleher SP, Schulman G: Severe metabolic alkalosis complicating regional citrate hemodialysis. Am J Kidney Dis 9: 235-236, 1987

38. Matsuda T: Biological responses at non-physiological interfaces and molecular design of biocompatible surfaces. Nephrol Dial Transplant 4(Suppl3): 60-66, 1989

39. Mims C, Playfair J, Roitt I, Wakelin D, Williams R: The innate defenses of the body in: *Medical Microbiology* 2nd edition, edited by Crowe L, London Mosby International Limited: 47-61, 1998

40. Deppisch RM, Beck W, Goehl H, Ritz E: Complement components as uremic toxins and their potential role as mediators of microinflammation. Kidney Int 59(Suppl78): S271-S277, 2001

41. RJ Johnson: Complement activation during extracorporeal therapy: biochemistry, cell biology and clinical relevance. Nephrol Dial Transplant 9 (Suppl.2): 36-45, 1994

42. Mims C, Playfair J, Roitt I, Wakelin D, Williams R: Adaptive responses provide a quantum leap in effective defense in: *Medical Microbiology* 2nd edition, edited by Crowe L, London Mosby International Limited: 63-72, 1998

43. Lhotta K, Würzner R, Kronenberg F, Oppermann M, König P: Rapid activation of the complement system by cuprophane depends on complement component C4: Kidney Int 53: 1044-1051, 1998

44. Deppisch R, Schmitt V, Bommer J, Hänsch GM, Ritz E, Rauterberg EW: Fluid phase generation of terminal complement complex as a novel index of biocompatibility. Kidney Int 37: 696-706, 1990

45. Wettero J, Askendal A, Bengtsson T, Tengvall P: On the binding of complement to solid artificial surfaces in vitro. Biomaterials 23(4): 981-991, 2002

46. Cheung AK, Parker CJ, Wilcox L, Janatova J: Activation of the alternative pathway of complement by cellulosic hemodialysis membranes. Kidney Int 36: 257-265, 1989

47. Janeway CA, Travers P: Basic concepts in immunology in: Immunobiology: The immune system in health and disease. 2nd edition Edinburgh Churchill Livingston: 1.1-1.32, 1996

48. Frank MM, Fries LF: The role of complement in inflammation and phagocytosis. Immunol Today 12: 322-326, 1991

49. Schmaldienst S, Hörl WH: Degranulation of polymorphonuclear leukocytes by dialysis membranes – the mystery clears up? Nephrol Dial Transplant 15: 1909-1910, 2000

50. Hakim RM: Clinical implications of hemodialysis biocompatibility. Kidney Int 44: 484-494, 1993

51. Ward RA: Phagocytic cell function as an index of biocompatibility. Nephrol Dial Transplant 9 (Suppl 2): 46-56, 1994

52. Arnaout MA, Hakim RM, Todd RF, Dana N, Colton HR: Increased expression of an adhesion-promoting surface glycoprotein in the granulocytopenia of hemodialysis. N Engl J Med 312: 457-462, 1985

53. Descamps-Latscha B, Goldfarb B, Nguyen AT, Landais P, London G, Haeffner-Cavaillon N, Jacquot C, Herbelin A, Kazatchkine M: Establishing the relationship between complement activation and stimulation of phagocyte oxidative metabolism in hemodialyzed patients: a randomized prospective study. Nephron 59: 279-285, 1991

54. Haag-Weber M, Hörl WH: Altered cellular host defence in malnutrition and uremia. Contrib Nephrol 98: 105-111, 1992

55. Iijima S, Otsuka F, Hasegawa Y, Koyama A: Hemodialysis neutropenia correlates with a decreased filterability and an increase in the number of cytoplasmatic actin filaments in peripheral blood neutrophils, which is preceded by a decrease in the number of surface expression of L-selectin. Nephron 82(3): 214-220, 1999

56. Boelaert JR, Cantinieaux BF, Hariga CF, Fondu PG: Recombinant erythropoietin reverses polymorphonuclear granulocyte dysfunction in iron-overloaded dialysis patients. Nephrol Dial Transplant 5: 504-507, 1990

57. Haag-Weber M, Hörl WH: Effect of biocompatible membranes on neutrophil function and metabolism. Clin Nephrol 42 (Suppl 1): S31-S36, 1994

58. Vanholder R, van Biesen WV, Ringoir S: Contributing factors to the inhibition of phagocytosis in hemodialyzed patients. Kidney Int 44: 208-214, 1993

59. Rosenkranz AR, Peherstorfer E, Kormoczi GF, Zlabinger GJ, Mayer G, Hörl H, Oberbauer R: Complement-dependent acceleration of apoptosis in neutrophils by dialyzer membranes. Kidney Int 59(Suppl78): S216-220, 2001

60. Carracedo J, Ramírez R, Martin-Malo A, Rodríguez M, Aljama P: The effect of LPS, uraemia, and haemodialysis membrane exposure on CD14 expression in mononuclear cells and its relation to apoptosis. Nephrol Dial Transplant 17: 428-434, 2002

61. Van Ypersele de Strihou C: Are biocompatible membranes superior for hemodialysis therapy? Kidney Int 52(Suppl62): S101-S104, 1997

62. Kaplow LS, Goffinet JA: Profound neutropenia during the early phase of hemodialysis. JAMA 203: 1133-1135, 1968

63. Lundahl J, Hed J, Jacobson SH: Dialysis granulocytopenia is preceded by an increased surface expression of the adhesion-promoting glucoprotein MAC-1. Nephron 61: 163-169, 1992

64. Frenette PS, Wagner DD: Adhesion molecules-Part I. N Engl J Med 334 (23): 1526-1530, 1996

65. Frenette PS, Wagner DD: Adhesion molecules-Part II. N Engl J Med 335 (1): 43-45, 1996

66. Dhondt A, Vanholder R, Lameire N: Hemodialysis-related bioincompatibility and adhesion molecules. Int J Artif Organs 21(9): 501-505, 1998

67. Tabor B, Geissler B, Odell R, Schmidt B, Blumenstein M, Schindhelm K: Dialysis neutropenia: the role of the cytoskeleton. Kidney Int 53(39): 783-789, 1998

68. Rousseau Y, Carreno MP, Poignet JL, Kazatchkine MD, Haeffner-Cavaillon N: Dissociation between complement activation, integrin expression and neutropenia during hemodialysis. Biomaterials 20(20): 1959-1967, 1999

69. Hörl WH, Schaefer RM, Heidland A: Effect of different dialyzers on proteinases and proteinase inhibitors during hemodialysis. J Am Soc Nephrol 5: 320-326, 1985

70. Skubitz KM, Butterfield J, Ma K, Skubitz APN: Changes in neutrophil surface phenotype during hemodialysis. Inflammation 22(6): 559-572, 1998

71. Himmelfarb J, Zaoui P, Hakim R: Modulation of granulocyte LAM-1 and MAC-1 during dialysis-A prospective, randomized controlled trial. Kidney Int 41: 388-395, 1992

72. Coli L, Tumietto F, De Pascalis A, La Manna G, Zanchelli F, Isola E, Perna C, Raimondi C, De Sanctis LB, Marseglia CD, Costigliola P, Stefoni S: Effects of dialysis membrane nature on intradialytic phagocytizing activity. Int J Artif Organs 22(2): 74-80, 1999

73. Nahar N, Shah H, Siu J, Colvin R, Bhaskaran M, Ranjan R, Wagner JD, Singhal PC: Dialysis membrane-induced neutrophil apoptosis is mediated through free radicals. Clin Nephrol 56(1): 52-59, 2001

74. Galli F, Canestrari F, Bellomo G: Pathophysiology of the oxidative stress and its implication in uremia and dialysis in: *Vitamin E-bonded membrane. A further step in dialysis optimization* edited by Ronco C, La Greca G, Contr Nephrol . Basel Karger 127: 1-31, 1999

75. Nguyen-Khoa T, Massy ZA, De Bandt JP, Kebede M, Salama L, Lambrey G, Witko-Sarsat V, Drüeke TB, Lacour B, Thévenin M: Oxidative stress and haemodialysis: role of inflammation and duration of dialysis treatment. Nephrol Dial Transplant 16: 335-340, 2001

76. Weinstein T, Chagnac A, Korzets A, Boaz M, Ori Y, Herman M, Malachi T, Gafter U: Haemolysis in haemodialysis patients: evidence for impaired defence mechanisms against oxidative stress. Nephrol Dial Transplant 15: 883-887, 2000

77. Handelman GJ: Current studies on oxidant stress in dialysis. Blood Purif 21:46–50, 2003

78. Nourooz-Zadeh J: Effect of dialysis on oxidative stress in uraemia. Redox Rep 4 (1-2): 17-22, 1999

79. Morena M, Cristol JP, Canaud B: Why hemodialysis patients are in a pro-oxidant state? What could be done to correct the pro/antioxidant imbalance. Blood Purif 18(3): 191-199, 2000

80. Locatelli F, Canaud B, Eckardt KW, Stenvinkel P, Wanner C, Zoccali C: Oxidative stress in end-stage renal disease: an emerging threat to patient outcome. Nephrol Dial Transplant 18: 1272–1280, 2003

81. Canaud B, Cristol J, Morena M, Leray-Moragues H, Bosc J, Vaussenat F: Imbalance of oxidants and antioxidants in haemodialysis patients. Blood Purif 17(2-3): 99-106, 1999

82. Bonomini M, Sirolli V, Stuard S, Settefrati N: Interactions between platelets and leukocytes during hemodialysis. Artif Organs 23: 23-28, 1999

83. Galli F, Rovidati S, Benedetti S, Canestrari F, Ferraro B, Floridi A, Buoncristiani U: Lipid peroxidation, leukocyte function and apoptosis in hemodialysis patients treated with Vitamin E-modified filters in: *Vitamin E-bonded membrane. A further step in dialysis optimization* edited by Ronco C, La Greca G, Contr Nephrol. Basel Karger 127: 156-171, 1999

84. Dinarello CA: Cytokines: agents provocateurs in hemodialysis? Kidney Int 41: 683-694, 1992

85. Mims C, Playfair J, Roitt I, Wakelin D, Williams R: The cellular basis of adaptive immune responses in: *Medical Microbiology* 2nd edition, edited by Crowe L, London Mosby International Limited: 73-79, 1998

86. Pereira BJG, Dinarello CA: Production of cytokines and cytokine inhibitory proteins in patients on dialysis. Nephrol Dial Transplant 9 (Suppl2): 60-71, 1994

87. Dinarello CA: The role of the interleukin-1-receptor antagonist in blocking inflammation mediated by interleukin-1. N Engl J Med 343(19): 732-734, 2000

88. Schouten WEM, Grooteman MPC, van Houte A-J, Schoorl M, van Limbeck J, Nubé MJ: Effects of dialyser and dialysate on the acute phase reaction in clinical bicarbonate dialysis. Nephrol Dial Transplant 15: 379-384, 2000

89. Stenvinkel P: Inflammatory and atherosklerotic interactions in the depleted uremic patient. Blood Purif 19: 53-61, 2001

90. Stenvinkel P, Barany P, Heimbürger O, Pecoits-Filho R, Lindholm B: Mortality, malnutrition, and atherosclerosis in ESRD: what is the role of interleukin-6? Kidney Int 61 (Suppl 80): S103-S108, 2002

91. Pecoits-Filho R, Lindholm B, Axelsson J, Stenvinkel P: Update on interleukin-6 and its role in chronic renal failure. Nephrol Dial Transplant 18: 1042–1045, 2003

92. Bingel M, Lonnemann G, Koch KM, Dinarello CA, Shaldon S: Plasma interleukin-1 activity during hemodialysis: the influence of dialysis membranes. Nephron 50: 273-276, 1988

93. Deppisch RM, Ritz E, Hänsch GM, Schöls M, Rauterberg EW: Bioincompatibility - perspectives in 1993. Kidney Int 45(Suppl44): S77-S84, 1994

94. Schindler R, Lonnemann G, Shaldon S, Koch K-M, Dinarello CA: Transcription, not synthesis, of interleukin-1 and tumor necrosis factor by complement. Kidney Int 37: 85-93, 1990

95. Luger A, Kovarik J, Stummvoll H-K, Urbanska A, Luger TA: Blood-membrane interaction in hemodialysis leads to increased cytokine production. Kidney Int 32: 84-88, 1987

96. Schindler R, Gelfand JA, Dinarello CA: Recombinant C5a stimulates transcription rather than translation of interleukin-1 (IL-1) and tumor necrosis factor: translational signal provided by lipopolysaccharide or IL-1 itself. Blood 76(8): 1631-1638, 1990

97. Shaldon S, Koch KM, Bingel M, Granolleras C, Deschodt G, Dinarello CA: Modulation of plasma interleukin-1 and its circulating protein inhibitor (CPI) by hemodialysis and hemofiltration (abstract). Kidney Int 31: 245, 1987

98. Dinarello CA, Thompson RC: Blocking IL-1: interleukin 1 receptor antagonist *in vivo* and *in vitro*. Immunology Today 12(11): 404-410, 1991

99. Engelmann H, Aderka D, Rubinstein M, Rotman D, Wallach D: A tumor necrosis factor-binding protein purified to homogeneity from human urine protects cells from tumor necrosis factor toxicity. J Biol Chem 264: 11974-11980, 1989

100. Donati D, Degiannis D, Mazzola E, Gastaldi L, Raskova J, Raska K, Camussi G: Interleukin-1 receptors and receptor antagonist in haemodialysis. Nephrol Dial Transplant 12: 111-118, 1997

101. Dinarello CA: Interleukin-1 and interleukin-1 antagonism. Blood 77(8): 1627-1652, 1991

102. Coppo R, Amore A: Importance of the bradykinin-nitric oxide synthase system in the hypersensitivity reaction of chronic haemodialysis patients. Nephrol Dial Transplant 15: 1288-1290, 2000

103. Hakim RM, Breilatt J, Lazarus JM, Port FK: Complement activation and hypersensitivity reactions to dialysis membranes. N Engl J Med 311: 878-882, 1984

104. Götze O: The potential role of basophilic leukocytes and mast cells. Nephrol Dial Transplant 9(Suppl 2): 57-59, 1994

105. Kaplan AP, Reddigari S, Baeza M, Kuna P: Histamine releasing factors and cytokine-dependent activation of basophils and mast cells. Adv Immunol 50: 237-260, 1991

106. Floege J, Smeby L: Dialysis-related amyloidosis and high-flux membranes in; *Polyamide - The evolution of a synthetic membrane for renal therapy,* edited by Berlyne GM, Giovannetti S, Contrib Nephrol Basel, Karger Vol 96: 124-137, 1992

107. Gejyo F, Arakawa M: Beta2-microglobulin: evidence for a new form of hemodialysis-associated amyloid protein. Kidney Int 33(Suppl24): 30-31, 1988

108. Jahn B, Betz M, Deppisch R, Janssen O, Hansch GM, Ritz E: Stimulation of beta 2-microglobulin synthesis in lymphocytes after exposure to Cuprophan dialyzer membranes. Kidney Int 40(2): 285-90, 1991

109. Meissner C, Deppisch R, Hug F, Schulze M, Ritz E, Ludwig H, Hansch G: L-fucose residues on cellulose-based dialysis membranes: quantification of membrane-associated L-fucose and analysis of specific lectin binding. Glycoconj J 12 (5): 632-638, 1995

110. Schoels M, Jahn B, Hug F, Deppisch R, Ritz E, Hansch GM: Stimulation of mononuclear cells by contact with cuprophan membranes: further increase of beta 2-microglobulin synthesis by activated late complement components. Am J Kidney Dis 21(4): 394-399, 1993

111. Miyata T, Inagi R, Iida Y et al: Involvement of ß2-micorglobulin modified with advanced glycation end products in the pathogenesis of hemodialysis-associated amyloidosis. Induction of human chemotaxis and macrophage secretion of tumor necrosis factor-alpha and interleukin-1. J Clin Invest 93: 521-528, 1994

112. Haufe CC, Eismann U, Deppisch RM, Stein G: Expression of beta2-microglobulin and c-fos mRNA: is there an influence of high-flux or low-flux dialyzer membranes? Kidney Int 78 (Suppl 2001): S177-S181, 2001

113. Van Ypersele de Strihou C, Floege J, Jadoul M, Koch KM : Amyloidosis and its relationship to different dialysers. Nephrol Dial Transplant 9 (Suppl 2): 156-161, 1994

114. Locatelli F, Mastrangelo F, Redaelli B, Ronco C, Marcelli D, La Greca G, Orlandini G and The Italian Cooperative Dialysis Study Group. Effects of different membranes and dialysis technologies on patient treatment tolerance and nutritional parameters. Kidney Int 50(4):1293-302,1996

115. Schiffl H, Fischer R, Lang SM, Mangel E: Clinical manifestation of AB-amyloidosis: effects of biocompatibility and flux. Nephrol Dial Transplant 15: 840-845, 2000

116. Pickett TM, Cruickshank A, Greenwood RN, Taube D, Davenport A: Membrane flux not biocompatibility determines beta-2-microglobulin levels in hemodialysis patients. Blood Purif 20 (2): 161-166, 2002

117. Sandler SG, Sharon R, Bush M, Stroup M, Sabo B: Formaldehyde-related antibodies in hemodialysis patients. Transfusion 19: 682-687, 1979

118. Maurice F, Rivory JP, Larsson PH, Johansson SGO, Bousquet J: Anaphylactic shock caused by formaldehyde in a patient undergoing long-term hemodialysis. J Allergy Clin Immunol 77: 594-597, 1986

119. Rosenzweig P, Gary NE, Gocke DJ, Saidi P, Felton SM, Eisinger RP: Heparin allergy accompanying acute renal failure. Artif Organs 3(1): 78-79, 1979

120. Caravaca F, Pizarro JL, Arrobas M, Cubero JJ, Antona JM, Sanchez E: Hypersensitivity reactions related to acetate dialyzate and cellulose acetate membrane. Nephron 45: 158-159, 1987

121. Papidakis JT, Patrikarea A, Saradi S, Papakostas K, Leondi A, Kravaritis A, Vafladis S: Hypersensitivity reactions during hemodialysis related to the use of acetate dialysate. A case report. Clin Nephrol 35(5): 224-226, 1991

122. Gell PGH, Coombs RRA ed. Clinical aspects of Immunology, 2nd edn. Philadelphia FA Davis, 1969

123. Grammer LC: Hypersensitivity. Nephrol Dial Transplant 9(Suppl2): 29-35, 1994

124. Verresen L, Waer M; Vanrenterghem Y, Michielsen P: Angiotensin-converting-enzyme-inhibitors and anaphylactoid reactions to high-flux membrane dialysis. Lancet 336: 1360-1362, 1990

125. Tielemans C, Madhoun P, Lenaers M, Schandene L, Goldman M, Vanherweghem JL: Anaphylactoid reactions during hemodialysis on AN69 membranes in patients receiving ACE inhibitors. Kidney Int 38: 982-984, 1990

126. Parnes EL, Shapiro WB: Anaphylactoid reactions in hemodialysis patients treated with the AN69 dialyzer. Kidney Int 40(6): 1148-1152, 1991

127. Brunet P, Jaber K, Berland Y, Baz M: Anaphylactoid reactions during hemodialysis and hemofiltration: role of associating AN69 membrane and angiotensin I-converting enzyme inhibitors. Am J Kidney Dis 19: 444-447, 1992

128. Kammerl MC, Schaefer RM, Schweda F, Schreiber M, Riegger GAJ, Krämer BK: Extracorporeal therapy with AN69 membranes in combination with ACE inhibition causing severe anaphylactoid reactions: still a current problem? Clin Nephrol 53(6): 486-488, 2000

129. Kojima S, Harada-Shiba M, Nomura S, Kimura G, Tsushima M, Kuramochi M, Yamamoto A, Omae T: Effect of nafamostat mesilate on bradykinin generation during low-density lipoprotein apheresis using a dextran sulfate cellulose column. Trans Am Soc Artif Intern Organs 37: 644-648, 1991

130. Gavras H, Gavras I: Endothelian function in cardiovascular disease: the role of bradykinin. London, Science Press Limited, 1996

131. Williams GH, Dluhy RG: Diseases of the renal cortex in: *Harrison's principles of internal medicine,* 14th ed., edited by Fauci AS, Martin JB, Braunwald E, Kasper DL, Isselbacher KJ, Hauser SL, Wilson JP, Longo DL, New York, Mc Graso Hill Publishers: 2035-2056, 1998

132. Brownlee M, Cerami A, Vlassara H: Advanced glycosylation end products in tissue and the biochemical basis of diabetic complications. N Engl J Med 318: 1315-1321, 1988

133. Baynes JW, Monnier VM: The Maillard reaction in aging, diabetes and nutrition. Prog Clin Bio Res 304: 1-410, 1989

134. Henle T, Deppisch R, Beck W, Hergesell O, Hänsch GM, Ritz E: Advanced glycated end-products (AGE) during haemodialysis treatment: discrepant results with different methodologies reflecting the heterogeneity of AGE compounds. Nephrol Dial Transplant 14: 1968-1975, 1999

135. Miyata T, Fu MX, Kurokowa K, van Ypersele de Strihou C, Thorpe SR, Baynes JW: Autoxidation products of both carbohydrates and lipids are increased in uremic plasma: Is there oxidative stress in uremia. Kidney Int 54: 1290-1295, 1998

136. Suliman ME, Heimbürger O, Bárány P, Anderstam B, Pecoits-Filho, Ayala ER, Qureshi R, Fehrman-Ekholm I, Lindholm B, Stenvinkel P: Plasma pentosidine is associated with inflammation and malnutrition in end-stage renal Failure patients starting on dialysis therapy. J Am Soc Nephrol 14: 1614-1622, 2003

137. Witko-Sarsat V, Friedlander M, Capeillére-Blandin C, Nguyen-Khoa T, Nguyen AT, Zingraff J, Jungers P, Descamps-Latscha B: Advanced oxidation protein products as a novel marker of oxidative stress in uremia. Kidney Int 49: 1304-1313, 1996

138. Miyata T, van Ypersele de Strihou C, Kurokawa K, Baynes JW: Alterations in nonenzymatic biochemistry in uremia: origin and significance of "carbonyl stress" in long-term uremic complications. Kidney Int 55: 389-399, 1999

139. Miyata T, Ueda Y, Yoshida A, Sugiyama S, Iida Y, Jadoul M, Maeda K, Kurokawa K, van Ypersele de Strihou C: Clearance of pentosidine, an advanced glycation end product, by different modalities of renal replacement therapy. Kidney Int 51: 880-887, 1997

140. Miyata T, Ueda Y, Yamada Y, Izuhara Y, Wada T, Jadoul M, Saito A, Kurokawa K, van Ypersele de Strihou C: Accumulation of carbonyl accelerates the formation of pentosidine, an advanced glycation end product: carbonyl stress in uremia. J Am Soc Nephrol 9: 2349-2356, 1998

141. Miyata T, Saito A, Kurokawa K, van Ypersele de Strihou C: Advanced glycation and lipoxidation end products: reactive carbonyl compounds-related uraemic toxicity. Nephrol Dial Transplant 16 (Suppl 4): 8-11, 2001

142. Miyata T, Iida Y, Ueda Y, Shinzato T, Seo H, Monnier VM, Maeda K, Wada Y: Monocyte/macrophage response to $ß_2$-microglobulin modified with advanced glycation end products. Kidney Int 49: 538-550, 1996

143. Yamamoto Y, Sakata N, Meng J, Sakamoto M, Noma A, Maeda I, Okamoto K, Takebayashi S: Possible involvement of increased glycoxidation and lipid peroxidation of elastin in atherogenesis in haemodialysis patients. Nephrol Dial Transplant 17(4): 630-636, 2002

144. Carreno MP, Rousseau Y, Poignet JL, Jahns G, Cholley B, Kazatchkine MD, Haeffner-Cavaillon N: Dissociation between ß-2 microglobulin and IL-1 production in hemodialyzed patients. Nephrol Dial Transplant 12: 2365-2374, 1997

8. Biocompatibility characteristics of dialysers and haemofilters

The repeated contact of blood with components of the extracorporeal circuit, mainly the dialyser, initiates activation of the immune and thrombogenic systems. Differences between the biological systems of dialysis patients and controls (healthy volunteers, or pre-end stage renal disease (ESRD) patients can be considered an expression of the bio**in**compatibility of the haemodialysis system. Numerous publications regarding biocompatibility of haemodialysers are available in medical databases such as "Medline". However, results relating specific biocompatibility parameters to particular dialysers and haemofilters are not always consistent. One reason for this is the complexity of the human organism and the numerous factors (including methodological inconsistencies) that affect it. A comparison of results from different clinical studies obtained with different patient populations and experimental approaches is, therefore, sometimes fraught with difficulties.

This chapter attempts to provide an overview of the biocompatibility issues pertaining to the most common membranes, dialysers and haemofilters by considering some widely used biocompatibility parameters. Unfortunately, data are not available for all membranes and dialysers. A vast number of papers have been published on the standard product Cuprophan® and the Fresenius Polysulfone®, two of the most widely-used membranes worldwide. However, little can be found in the English literature about membranes used mainly in Asia, primarily Japan, although they may be very popular in that part of the world.

In contrast to the other chapters of this book, the brand names of the membranes or dialysers/haemofilters are used rather than the polymer generic names. This facilitates the evaluation and characterisation of specific membranes from particular manufacturers. A complete list of dialysers, haemofilters and the respective manufacturers is supplied in the appendix.

8.1 Thrombogenicity of dialysers

The thrombogenic potential of a dialyser or haemofilter is strongly dependent on the type of membrane polymer, the design of the device (due to its influence on flow conditions) and its manufacturing quality.

How does the membrane type influence thrombogenicity?

Solely membrane-associated features of thrombogenicity can be investigated by comparing membranes of equal permeability and surface area in identical housings (e.g. minimodules) and under conditions of comparable anticoagulation, ideally using the same blood. Surface free energy, charge, roughness and chemical composition of a dialyser membrane have been identified as being responsible for the variable thrombogenic potential of dialysis membranes [1]. As the extrinsic system of the clotting cascade is activated by negatively charged surfaces, membrane polymers that exhibit an anionic surface (such as polyacrylonitrile membranes PAN, AN69®) could be considered more thrombogenic than more neutral polymers (e.g. polysulfone). In fact, the highest factor XII adsorption and autoactivation to factor XIIa was observed with AN69® membranes *in vitro* [2]. However, activation of the coagulation cascade also depends on other plasma constituents (e.g. high molecular weight kininogen, prekallikrein and plasma inhibitors of factor XIIa) and the action of heparin [2]. High molecular weight kininogen (HMWK), another constituent of the trimolecular complex initiating contact activation, could be eluated in its intact form from used cellulose acetate (Cordis Dow) and regenerated cellulose (Cuprophan® CF 1511, Baxter) dialysers, whereas it was cleaved at PMMA (B2-1.5H, Toray) and polyacrylonitrile (AN69® Filtral 12, Hospal) surfaces, suggesting activation [3]. Moreover, low molecular weight fragments of plasminogen were detected in eluates from AN69® dialysers, indicating that the fibrinolytic system was activated in response to clotting activation. Intact plasminogen was also adsorbed by all other materials tested [3].

Using the *ex vivo* formation of the thrombin-antithrombin III complex (TAT) as a parameter for coagulation activation, a comparison of different membranes revealed that levels were higher with polyacrylonitrile membranes (Asahi PAN and AN69®) than with polysulfone (Fresenius Polysulfone®) and regenerated cellulose (Cuprophan®) [4]. An *in vivo* study also reported these levels to be higher with PMMA than with EVAL® or polysulfone (type not specified) [5]. These findings were confirmed in *ex vivo* recirculation

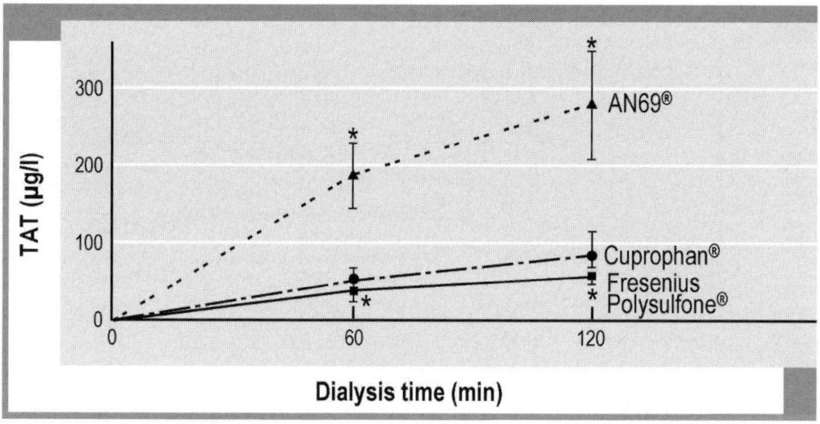

Figure 8.1: Generation of thrombin–antithrombin III (TAT) complex with polysulfone, regenerated cellulose and polyacrylonitrile dialysers during* ex vivo *recirculation. *Blood from healthy donors (equal heparinisation for all dialysers) was recirculated through the commercially available dialysers Nephral 300 (AN69®, 1.3 m², Hospal) (8 parallel experiments with polysulfone), Hemoflow F6HPS (Fresenius Polysulfone®, 1.3 m², Fresenius Medical Care) (8 parallel experiments with AN69® + 5 experiments in parallel with Cuprophan®) and Renak RA-15U (Cuprophan®, 1.5 m², Kawasumi) (5 experiments in parallel to polysulfone). Data are presented as means ± SEM. *statistically significant difference ($p < 0.05$) for AN69® vs. Fresenius Polysulfone® or for AN69® vs. Cuprophan® (adapted from [6]).*

experiments: higher TAT generation was observed with AN69® (Nephral 300, Hospal) than with regenerated cellulose (Cuprophan®, Renak RA-15U, Kawasumi) and polysulfone (Fresenius Polysulfone®, Hemoflow F6HPS) dialysers [6] (**figure 8.1**). A low TAT generation with regenerated cellulose is in agreement with the findings that hydroxyl-bearing surfaces are relatively inert regarding the activation of the intrinsic coagulation pathway: such membranes inhibit the development of the trimolecular complex (high molecular weight kininogen, prekallikrein, factor XII) that is necessary for contact activation [7].

Do positive surface charges also influence membrane thrombogenicity?

Diethylaminoethyl (DEAE)-modified cellulose (Hemophan®), a membrane which is a low-level platelet activator, led to more TAT generation than high-flux polyamide in one *in vivo* study (**figure 8.2**) [8]. This is not the result of

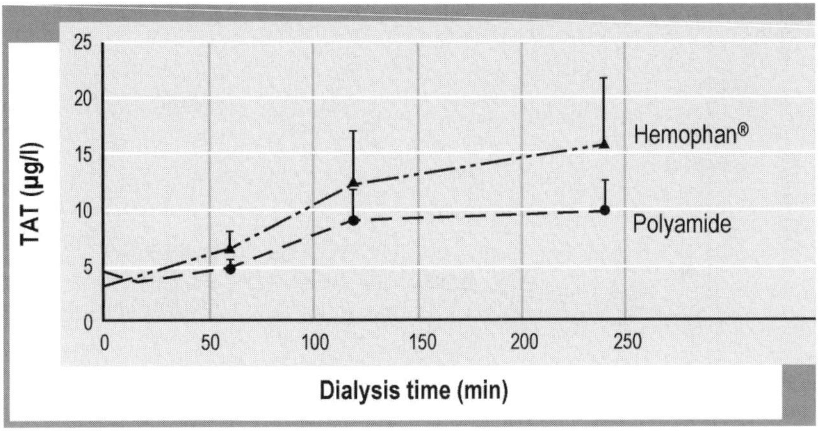

***Figure 8.2: Generation of thrombin–antithrombin III (TAT) complex with polyamide and Hemophan® dialysers* in vivo.** *10 patients were treated under identical conditions with Hemophan® (GFS plus, Gambro) and polyamide (Polyflux 130, Gambro) dialysers. Data are presented as means + SE (adapted from [9]).*

higher contact system activation by DEAE cellulose, but is rather due to the ability of the positive DEAE groups to adsorb negatively-charged heparin from whole blood. This adsorption inactivates heparin and, consequently, sufficient amounts of heparin are not available for anticoagulation. This is normally reflected in an increased heparin consumption for Hemophan® during treatment [10, 11]. However, another *in vivo* investigation failed to find such an increased heparin requirement, and also did not observe any increases in TAT formation with Hemophan® (GFS plus 12, Gambro) compared to low-flux Fresenius Polysulfone® (Hemoflow F6, Fresenius Medical Care) [12].

Another, albeit less reliable, parameter for the assessment of thrombogenicity is the residual blood volume (RBV) in the dialyser after completion of dialysis. This subjective parameter has a number of pitfalls that mostly concern the reproducibility of the method. Although TAT measurements are preferable, RBVs have been reported in the medical literature and some results should, therefore, be discussed here. Under conditions of low heparin dosage, residual blood volumes were found to be higher with Hemophan® dialysers (BL 613 HB, Bellco) than with CA (CA-130, Travenol) and PMMA (B2-1.3 Filtryzer, Toray) dialysers, the last having values similar to Cuprophan® (Hemoflow E3, Fresenius Medical Care) dialysers. Dialysers containing low-flux Fresenius Polysulfone® (Hemoflow F6, Fresenius Medical Care) exhibited lowest residual blood volumes [13]. In another study, higher residual blood volumes were also been reported with Hemophan® when compared to high-flux polyamide (dialyser types not mentioned) [8].

Do membranes and dialysers differ regarding platelet activation?

In contrast to coagulation factors, platelets adhere more to cationic charges and hydrophobic materials [7]. Therefore, it is not surprising that a significant decrease in platelet count of about 9% after 15 min of dialysis was observed with hydrophobic cellulose acetate dialysers (Duo-flux, Cordis Dow), whereas only insignificant decreases were observed with cuprammonium rayon (AM50-Bio, Asahi), Hemophan® (GFS 120 Plus, Gambro), AN69® (Filtral 12, Hospal) and high-flux Fresenius Polysulfone® (F60, Fresenius Medical Care) [14]. In another study, a similar ranking in platelet drop was observed with the same polymers but different dialyser manufacturers: cellulose diacetate (CA 150, Baxter), Hemophan® (Bio-Allegro, Cobe/Organon), cellulose diacetate (Acepal 1500, Hospal) and low-flux Fresenius Polysulfone®

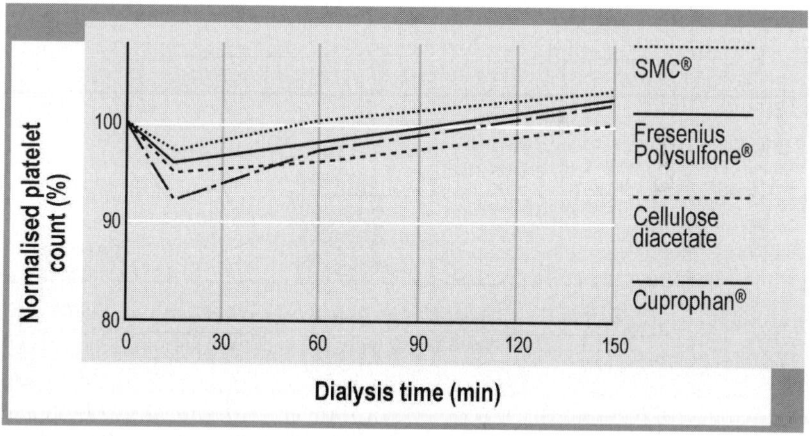

Figure 8.3: Time course of normalised platelet counts during haemodialysis with different membranes. *The following commercially available haemodialysers were used in random order during dialysis with 9 patients: SMC®(type not specified, Baxter), cellulose diacetate (Dicea 1100, Baxter), Cuprophan® (ST 15, Baxter) and Fresenius Polysulfone® (F5 HPS, Fresenius Medical Care). The differences between membranes failed to reach statistical significance with the number of patients treated (adapted from [16]).*

(F6, Fresenius Medical Care) induced platelet losses of 7.7%, 5.0%, 4.4% and 3.8%, respectively [15]. **Figure 8.3** depicts the platelet drop during the time course of a haemodialysis session observed with similar dialysis membranes in a third study [16]. The ranking trend of the different membranes regarding platelet activation is evident, although differences between membranes were not statistically relevant at these low patient numbers.

One reliable parameter for platelet activation is the expression of the glycoprotein GMP-140 at the platelet membrane surface. Highest GMP-140 expression was found with Cuprophan® dialysers (ST-15, Travenol), less expression was observed with cellulose diacetate (CA 110, Nissho) and PMMA dialysers (Filtryzer B 1-1.6H, Toray), and the lowest GMP-140 expression was observed with Fresenius Polysulfone® (Spiraflo HFT 10, Sorin) and AN69® dialysers (Filtral 10, Hospal) (**figure 8.4**) [17]. This ranking for platelet activation was also found for another parameter, the expression of P-selectin on the platelet surface. Expression was highest with Cuprophan® dialysers (ST-15, Travenol), followed by cellulose diacetate (CA 110, Nissho) and triacetate

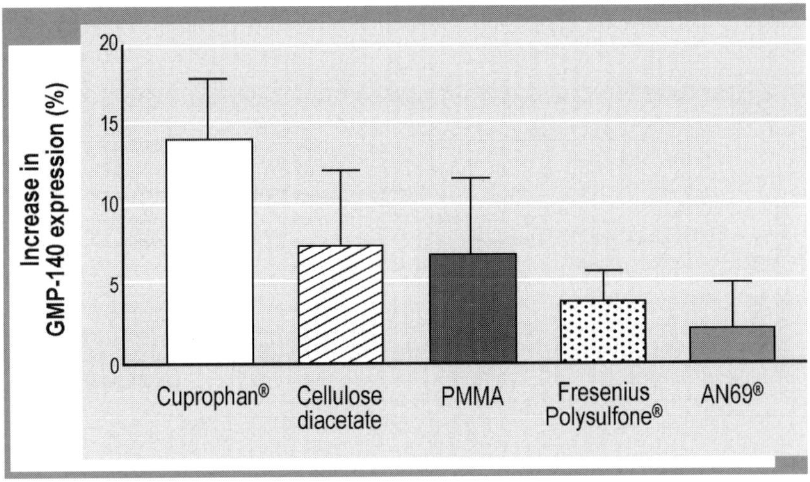

Figure 8.4: Arteriovenous difference in GMP-140 expression with different haemodialysers. *GMP-140 is selectively expressed on platelet membranes after activation. Samples from the arterial and venous blood lines were taken 5 minutes after start of dialysis for flow cytometric analysis. In total, 9 patients were treated with the following membranes and dialysers: Cuprophan® (ST-15, Travenol), cellulose diacetate (CA 110, Nissho), PMMA (Filtryzer B1-1.6 H, Toray), Fresenius Polysulfone® (Spiraflo HFT 10, Sorin) and AN69® (Filtral 10, Hospal). Data are presented as means + SD (adapted from [17]).*

(CT110G, Nissho), and was lowest with Hemophan® (GFS Plus 11, Gambro) and Fresenius Polysulfone® (Spiraflo HFT 10, Sorin) [18]. Although platelets are obviously activated by regenerated cellulose, this activation does not result in or involve activation of the clotting cascade, as is obvious from the previously mentioned investigations into the formation of the TAT complex.

How does design, manufacturing quality and sterilisation mode influence dialyser thrombogenicity?

Haemofilter geometry has to ensure such flow conditions for blood that shear rate, turbulent flow and axial streaming of platelets is kept to a minimum. Under conditions of disturbed flow and low or excessively high blood flow, sustained surface contact results in activation of both platelets and the coagulation cascade. Shear stress is required for the activation of platelets by one of its activators, the von Willebrand factor (vWF), i.e. shear stress must be minimised in order to prevent platelet activation [19]. Consequently, manufacturing quality aspects that concern the lowering of shear stress are also of importance. For example, homogenicity of the inner diameter of fibres is a prerequisite for constant flow conditions; the section of the dialyser header with which blood comes into contact has to be flat and quite smooth; and any damage of the fibres (e.g. in the form of kinks) has to be avoided. Plate dialysers overcome some of the "crushing" problems, but comparisons with hollow-fibre dialysers under controlled conditions did not reveal a benefit regarding thrombogenicity. This is due to other non-manufacturing related factors in plate dialysers, such as flow stagnation and longer blood passage times etc. [20].

Even the method of dialyser sterilisation seems to play a role in thrombogenicity. A lower platelet drop was observed with steam sterilised Fresenius Polysulfone® dialysers compared to the equivalent EtO sterilised dialysers [21].

How reliable are evaluations of thrombogenicity?

Assessment of dialyser thrombogenicity and, especially, the ranking of different dialysers accordingly involves a number of methodological difficulties. The main problem is that dialyser thrombogenicity is dependent on a variety of factors, some of which may have little to do with the dialyser itself or the membrane within. It is well documented that renal failure is associated with mild coagulation disorders often undetected, such as prolonged bleeding time, impaired platelet adhesion and aggregation, defective availability of platelet factor 3 (most important factor for thrombus formation via the intrinsic pathway), poor clot retraction and increased levels of plasma ß-thromboglobulin [22]. Underlying diseases (e.g. infection or atherosclerosis, diabetes), many neoplastic conditions, physical state (e.g. level of exercise taken) and even stress contributes to the activation of the haemostatic system [23]. Furthermore, drugs like aspirin (acetyl salicyl acid) interfere with the haemostatic system and their usage and dosage has to be taken into consideration. The use of erythropoietin is also important: blood viscosity and coagulability are enhanced with use of this drug, resulting in the need for higher heparin doses and, possibly, increased dialyser clotting. The type of anticoagulant also plays an important role: as described earlier (section 7.1.4), the use of heparin, LMWH, prostacyclin or citrate influences thrombogenicity in very different ways. Citrate leads to a marked reduction in thrombus formation compared to heparin and LMWH anticoagulation [24]. Even the presence of an arterial drip chamber influences thrombogenicity: the blood air contact is an important accelerating factor for the activation of the clotting cascade [25].

A number of publications have dealt with theoretical considerations about artificial surfaces and their thrombogenic potential, but biological processes are too complex to easily predict the thrombogenic behaviour from charges, functional groups or other characteristics of current dialysis membranes. Differences between membranes exist, and even between dialysers of different manufacturers containing the same membrane. This has been shown in controlled *ex vivo* or *in vitro* studies using the same blood for all membranes compared. However, the numbers of reports about membranes correlate with their frequency of use in the market, and not necessarily with their thrombogenic behaviour. Therefore, although no published data are available for some membranes, this should not be interpreted as absence of thrombogenic potential per se.

8.2. Complement activation by dialysers

It is accepted today that membranes made of regenerated, unmodified cellulose are the strongest complement activators of all dialysis membranes. This can partly be explained by binding of complement factor C3b to the hydroxyl groups on the membrane surface. In fact, partial substitution of these hydroxyl groups by either acetyl groups (cellulose di- or triacetate), diethylaminoethyl (DEAE) groups (Hemophan®), benzyl groups (SMC®) or coating of the hydroxyl bearing surface with polyethylene glycol (PEG) (PEG grafted regenerated cellulose) resulted in considerable reduction of complement activation compared to unmodified regenerated cellulose (e.g. **figure 8.5**). Surprisingly, the degree of substitution does not necessarily correlate with the degree of complement activation, demonstrating involvement of other factors. For example: in Hemophan®, less than 1% of all hydroxyl groups are modified but complement activation is at least equal to that of cellulose acetate membranes, where about 60% (cellulose diacetate) to 90-100% (cellulose triacetate) of all hydroxyl groups are substituted [28]. Binding of regulatory proteins that downregulate the alternative pathway, such as

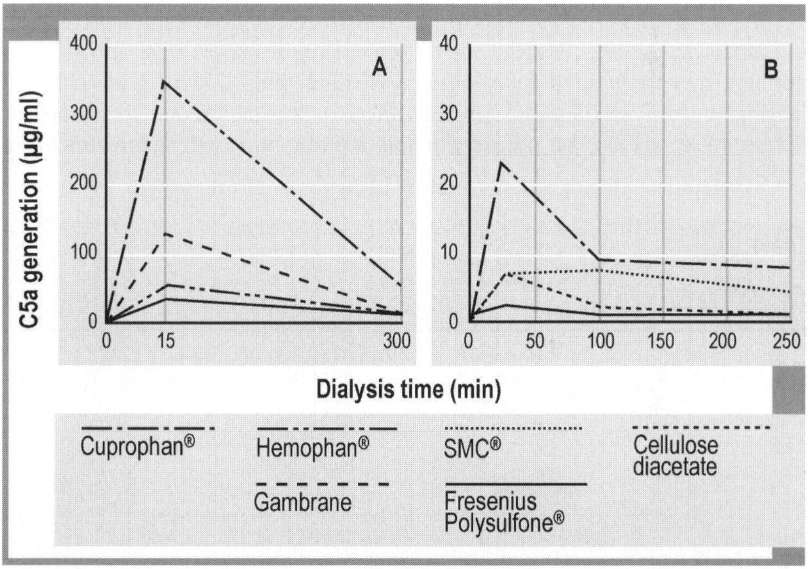

Figure 8.5: C5a generation by cellulosic membranes with different grades and modes of hydroxyl group substitution compared to a synthetic membrane. *Data from two different clinical studies are shown. High-flux Fresenius Polysulfone® (F60, Fresenius Medical Care) was used in the study shown on the left (A), the other dialysers were not specified. On the right (B), the following commercially available haemodialysers were used in random order during dialysis with 9 patients: SMC®(type not specified, Baxter), cellulose diacetate, (Dicea 1100, Baxter), Cuprophan® (ST 15, Baxter) and Fresenius Polysulfone® (F5 HPS, Fresenius Medical Care). The results demonstrate improvement in complement generation by modifying regenerated cellulose (adapted from [16, 26, 27]).*

factor H by Hemophan® [29] or factor D (a rate-limiting enzyme of the alternative pathway) by AN69® [30] and PMMA [31], also plays a role in the extent of complement activation. Factors H and B bind onto cellulose acetate membranes, resulting in an accelerated degradation of surface-bound C3b; neither of these factors bind to regenerated cellulose [32]. However, all measures taken to prevent the interaction of C3 molecules with nucleophilic groups (e.g. hydroxyl or amino groups) on a polymeric surface reduce activation of the alternative pathway. This can be achieved either by avoidance of such groups, as in synthetic membranes, or by masking of such groups, as in the case of the modified cellulosic membranes described above. In order to avoid activation of the classical pathway, IgG, IgM, C1, C2 or C4 complement components should not be adsorbed to the polymeric surface [33].

The parameters mostly used for the assessment of complement activation by haemodialysis membranes are the complement factors C3a and C5a. In addition to its generation, the amount of detectable C3a or C5a in blood leaving the dialyser depends on the ability of the membrane to adsorb or filtrate these factors. The polyacrylonitrile membrane AN69® generates more

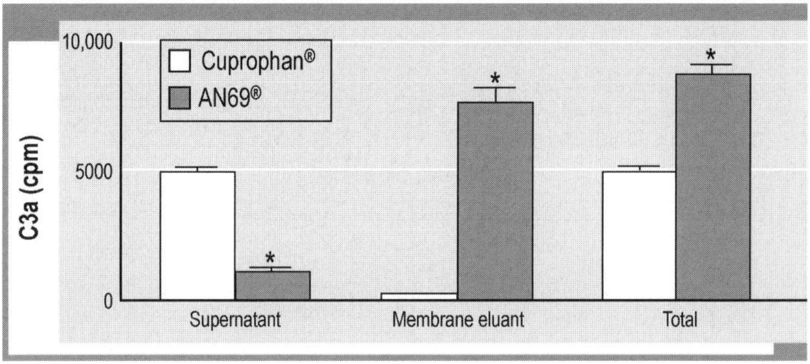

Figure 8.6: Generation and adsorption of complement factor C3a on Cuprophan® and AN69® membranes **in vitro.** *Pieces of Cuprophan® and AN69® membranes were incubated with radiolabeled C3a in C3-depleted serum. Afterwards, proteins in the supernatant as well as those bound to the membrane surface were analysed and quantified by SDS PAGE. More C3a was generated from C3 by AN69® than by Cuprophan® (column pair "total"). However, the protein was almost completely adsorbed to the AN69® membrane, as is evident from the different amounts found in the membrane eluant and the supernatant. Means + SD. *p < 0.001 statistically significant difference between the two membranes (adapted from [34]).*

C3a than regenerated cellulose, but adsorbs it (and C5a) almost completely (**figure 8.6** for C3a) [34]. Furthermore, these anaphylatoxins are eliminated during dialysis by high-flux membranes due to their middle molecular weight (MW C3a: 8900; C5a: 11,000) [35, 36]. This is also the case for the regulatory factor D (MW 23,000). This up-regulator of the alternative complement pathway is eliminated by glomerular filtration in healthy individuals and its concentration is, therefore, markedly elevated in ESRD patients. Factor D removal is negligible with low-flux dialysis but can be significant in haemofiltration [37]. Hence, detectable complement generation may differ between the low-flux and high-flux version of a particular membrane [38]. Furthermore, C3a and C5a binding to receptors of circulating blood cells may also lower the blood concentrations of these anaphylatoxins; here the blood C3a and C5a concentrations may be a patient-specific factor that masks the membrane effect [9]. Therefore, C3a and C5a may not be ideal parameters for detecting small differences between membranes. The terminal complement complex (TCC), sometimes also termed "membrane attack complex" (MAC), may be

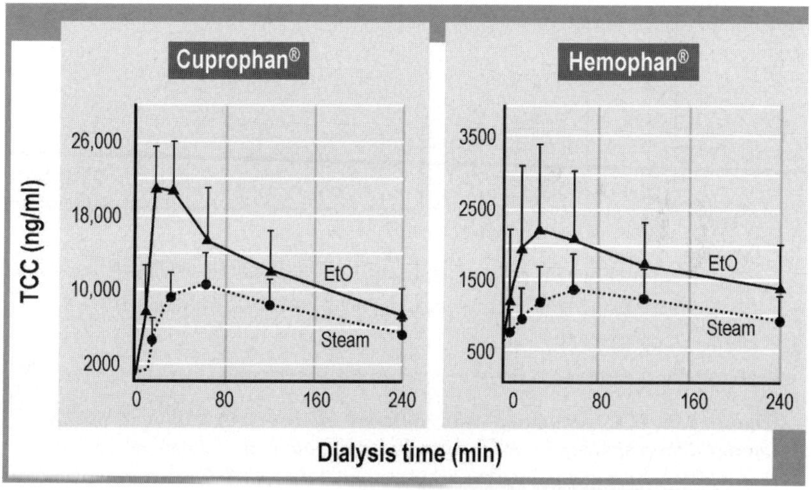

Figure 8.7: Generation of terminal complement complex (TCC) with steam and EtO sterilised Cuprophan® and Hemophan® dialysers. *Data from 5 patients from 2 independent investigations are presented as means + SD. Measurements refer to the dialyser outlet of Cuprophan® steam (GFS 120, Gambro) and EtO (GF 120H, Gambro) sterilised dialysers and Hemophan® steam (GFS Plus 120, Gambro) and EtO (GF Plus 120, Gambro) sterilised dialysers (adapted from [39]).*

of more value in this context [39]. This complex is not adsorbed in considerable amounts by artificial surfaces, and cannot be filtered by high-flux membranes due to its high molecular weight of more than 600,000 [39]. Using this parameter, the influence of dialyser sterilisation method on complement activation could be recognised: EtO sterilised dialysers were found to generate more TCC than their heat sterilised counterparts (**figure 8.7**).

Figure 8.8 presents an overview of TCC generation with different dialysers and treatment modes. Comparing the data for one particular polymer, Fresenius Polysulfone®, TCC generation seems to decrease with increasing membrane permeability and convective treatment mode. A possible explanation is the removal of the regulatory factors D and Ba by high-flux dialysis or haemofiltration, resulting in reduced TCC production [37].

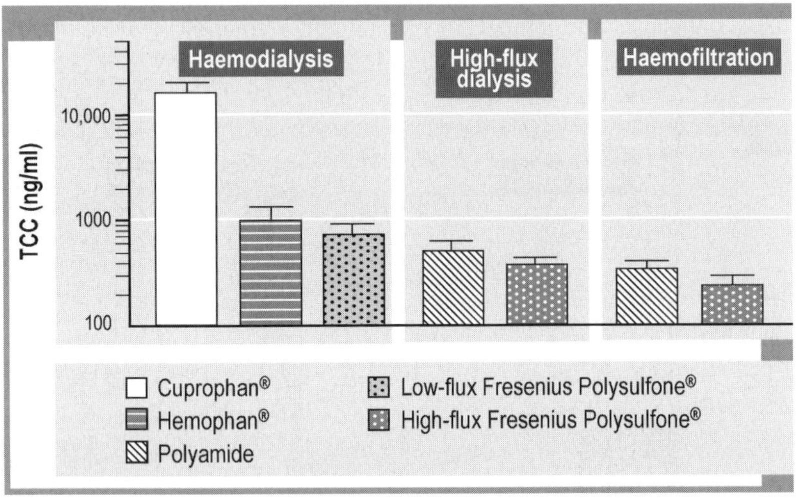

Figure 8.8: TCC generation with different dialysers in different therapy modes. *Maximal arterio-venous differences are presented as mean values + SD. Five patients were studied under identical conditions. HD dialysers: Cuprophan® (GF 120H, Gambro), Hemophan® (GF Plus 120, Gambro) and low-flux Fresenius Polysulfone® (F6, Fresenius Medical Care) – blood flow was 280 ml/min, and all dialysers were EtO sterilised and had a surface area of 1.2 m^2. HFD dialysers: polyamide (Polyflux 130, Gambro) and high-flux Fresenius Polysulfone® (F60, Fresenius Medical Care) – blood flow was 250 ml/min and all dialysers had a surface area of 1.3 m^2. HF filters: polyamide (FH88H, Gambro) and high-flux Fresenius Polysulfone® (HF80, Fresenius Medical Care), 1.8 m^2, blood flow was 500 ml/min (adapted from [39]).*

What are the long-term consequences of complement activation?

Because complement generation peaks 15 to 30 minutes after start of treatment and returns to nearly normal levels by the end of each session, it is of interest whether this effect is relevant or detectable in the long-term perspective. Unfortunately, little data exist on this aspect of complement activation. Predialysis C3a levels were reported to increase slowly over a time period of 1 year in patients treated with the low complement-generating membranes Hemophan® and polyamide [40]. In long-term HD patients (around 8 years on dialysis), the C3 activity is altered in such a way that both the alternative and the classical pathways are suppressed after stimulation. This effect lasts more than 4 hours after the end of a dialysis session, and is more pronounced in sera of patients treated with regenerated cellulose membranes (AM-SD18M, Asahi) than in the sera of those treated with PEG-grafted cellulose (AM-PC15, Asahi) or polyacrylonitrile (PAN-17DX, Asahi) membranes. Therefore, it appears that, due to the chronic high stimulation three times a week, membranes made of regenerated cellulose may induce a suppression of complement activation in the long-term. The mechanism has not been fully elucidated but a contribution of increased levels of the regulatory complement proteins factor H and SP-40,40 has been discussed [41]. This suppression may be beneficial in the respect that it blunts the effect of chronic complement stimulation, but may be of disadvantage in cases when defence against infection is necessary.

8.3. Cell activation by dialysers

Essential functions of polymorphonuclear leukocytes are disturbed in ESRD patients and are additionally influenced by the dialysis procedure, e.g. phagocytosis, oxygen species production, upregulation of specific cell surface receptor proteins and apoptosis. With the exception of polymorphonuclear leukocyte degranulation, complement and, consequently, complement-generating dialysis membranes have the greatest impact on functional alterations of these cells.

8.3.1 Stimulation of neutrophils and monocytes

Leukopenia

The most widely used parameter for the assessment of leukocyte activation is the determination of their disappearance from blood occurring 15 to 30 minutes after the start of haemodialysis. This dialysis-induced leukopenia is mainly induced by the over-expression of receptors (CD11b/CD18, CD15s) on leukocytes, leading to increased adhesiveness and aggregation and subse-

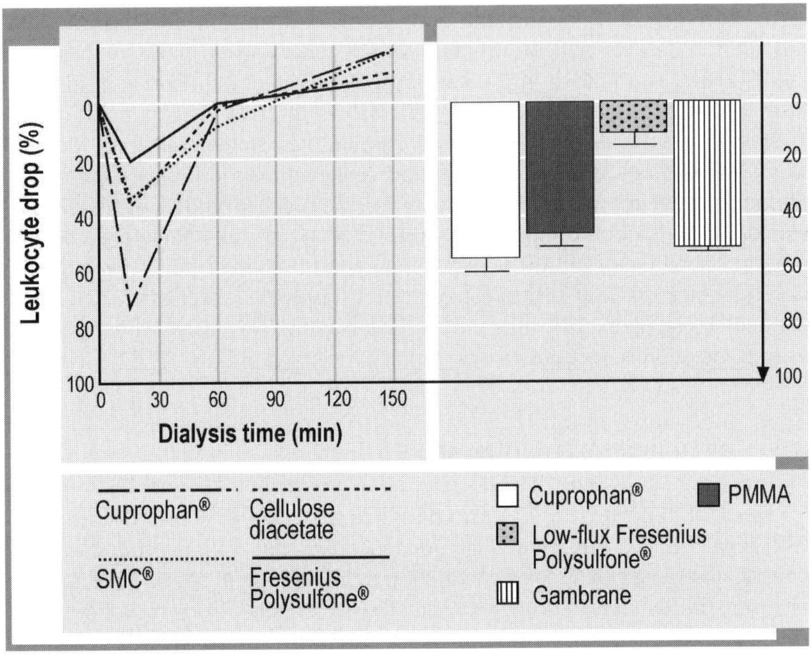

Figure 8.9: Leukopenia with different membranes. *A typical time course for changes in leukocyte numbers during haemodialysis is depicted on the left. Further explanations regarding dialysers and conditions are given in figure 8.3 (adapted from [16]). The right graph depicts the leukocyte drop after 15 min dialysis in a clinical study including 12 patients treated with the following dialysers and membranes: PMMA (Filtryzer B2-1,2H, Toray), low-flux Fresenius Polysulfone®, (Hemoflow F6, Fresenius Medical Care), Gambrane® (flat sheet, LunDia Pro 600, Gambro) and Cuprophan® (flat sheet, LunDia Alpha 600, Gambro). The surface areas of all dialysers were 1.2-1.3 m² (adapted from [43]).*

quent sequestration in the lung. Because these activation processes are mostly complement-mediated, complement activation and leukopenia directly correlate with each other [42]. Therefore, regenerated cellulose membranes cause strongest leukopenia, modified cellulosic membranes cause an intermediate to low drop in leukocyte numbers (depending on the type of modification), and synthetic membranes also induce a moderate to very low drop in leukocyte numbers (depending on the polymer) (e.g. [9, 16, 43]). Examples of leukocyte drops during dialysis with Cuprophan®, cellulose diacetate, SMC® and low-flux Fresenius Polysulfone® haemodialysers are shown on the left of **figure 8.9**. The maximum leukocyte drops for PMMA, low-flux Fresenius Polysulfone® and Gambrane® haemodialysis are presented on the right of **figure 8.9**. Leukocyte drops were similar with polyamide (Polyflux 130, Gambro) and Fresenius Polysulfone® (F60, Fresenius Medical Care) after 15 min; these were approx. 12% in another investigation [9].

Increasing the permeability of regenerated cellulose should, theoretically, result in an increased removal of complement factors and, consequently, an improved biocompatibility with respect to measurable complement generation and leukocyte drop. Surprisingly, this was not the case with RC-HP 400 – a high-performance version of Cuprophan® (production now ceased): this induced the same leukocyte drop as low-flux Cuprophan® [44].

Receptor expression

A deeper insight into mechanisms of cell activation (e.g. those leading to leukopenia) is provided by measuring receptor expression. Upregulation of cell receptors on polymorphonuclear cell surfaces (e.g. CD35, CD11b and CD66b), as well as downmodulation of L-selectin (CD62L) and sialophorin (CD43) have been reported and correlated with the drop in granulocyte numbers during haemodialysis [45]. Increased expression of CD18, CD49 and CD54 and an increase in the activation marker LPS receptor (CD14) have been detected on monocytes after contact with regenerated cellulose [46]. Cell activation by synthetic membranes is low but varies between polymers: CD11b/CD18 expression (CD11b/CD18 is involved in increased cell adhesiveness to the endothelium) and, consequently, leukopenia is lower on neutrophils during EVAL® (KF201 N, Kuraray) than during Fresenius Polysulfone® (BL 634, Bellco) haemodialysis, but CD 15s expression (CD 15s is involved in "rolling" of leukocytes along the endothelium and is important in monocytopenia) is higher with EVAL® than with Fresenius Polysulfone®. These results reveal that the mechanisms of leukocyte activation vary between the different synthetic membranes [47].

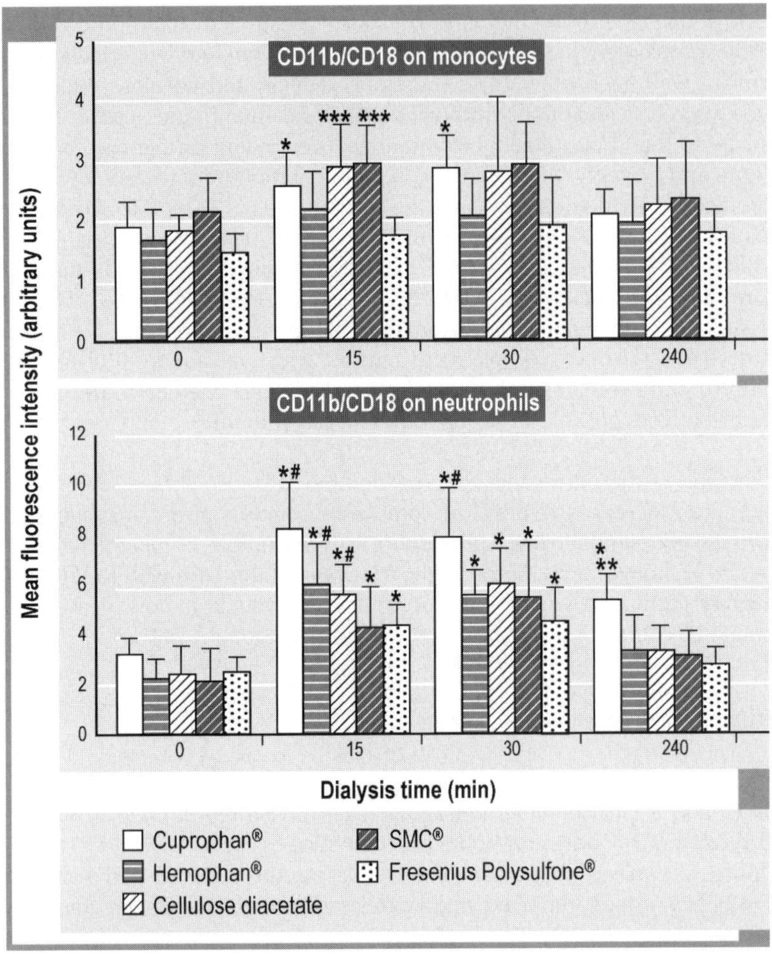

Figure 8.10: Expression of adhesion molecules CD11b/CD18 on monocytes and neutrophils during haemodialysis. *10 patients were treated randomly 6 times with Cuprophan® (Lundia Alpha 600 1.3 m², EtO, Gambro), Hemophan® (NT 1208 G 1.2 m², gamma ray, Bellco), cellulose diacetate (Acepal 1100 G 1,0 m², gamma ray, Hospal), SMC® (NC 1285 G, 1.1 m², gamma ray, Bellco) and Fresenius Polysulfone® (BL 642, 1.1m², EtO, Bellco). Blood samples were drawn from the efferent line at various time points during the sixth treatment. Data are expressed as mean fluorescence intensities + SD. Signs above the columns indicate statistical significance, whereby the comparisons are: versus * predialysis value; ** the four other haemodialysis membranes; # Fresenius Polysulfone® and SMC®; *** Fresenius Polysulfone® (adapted from [48]).*

In accordance with data for leukopenia, significantly higher CD11b/CD18 expression was detected on monocytes and neutrophils when regenerated cellulose (Cuprophan®) as opposed to polysulfone (Fresenius Polysulfone®) was used; expression with modified cellulosic membranes (SMC®, Hemophan®, CDA) held an intermediate position (**figure 8.10**) [48].

Platelet-leukocyte interaction

Platelet-leukocyte interactions are also influenced by haemodialysis membranes. Platelet-monocyte co-aggregates could be detected with Cuprophan® (Lundia alpha 600, Gambro), but not with SMC® (NC 1285 G, Bellco), Hemophan® (NT 1208 G, Bellco), cellulose diacetate (Acepal 1100 G, Hospal) or low-flux Fresenius Polysulfone® (BL 642, Bellco) [48]. In contrast, platelet-neutrophil co-aggregates developed after 15 min and 30 min haemodialysis with Cuprophan®, Hemophan®, cellulose diacetate and Fresenius Polysulfone®, but not with SMC® (same type of dialysers as above) [48].

Foam cell formation

Activation of peripheral monocytes by dialysis membrane - cell contact may contribute to atherosclerosis: first, by increasing oxidative stress and, second, by supporting macrophage-derived foam-cell formation. Accumulation of lipid-loaded foam cells in the subendothelial space is thought to be important in the initiation of atherosclerosis [49]. Foam cells develop by taking up large amounts of oxidised LDL via the macrophage scavenger receptor (SR). Gene expression of SR mRNA is two-fold higher in chronic haemodialysis patients during haemodialysis with regenerated cellulose (cuprammonium rayon AM-SD, Asahi) than in healthy controls or in patients undergoing dialysis with PMMA (B2, Toray) [50].

Apoptosis

Dialysis membranes promote neutrophil apoptosis both directly and indirectly through interaction with monocytes. Reactive oxygen species seem to be strong mediators of this process [51]. In *in vitro* experiments, low-flux cellulose diacetate (CA110, Baxter) induced significantly greater apoptosis than low-flux Fresenius Polysulfone® [51], and Cuprophan® (using pieces of fibres, meaning the outside of the fibres were tested) induced greater apoptosis than polysulfone (manufacturer not specified) [52]. An effect of HD membranes on apoptosis was also found *in vivo* (**figure 8.11**). The percentage of apoptotic mononuclear cells was highest with Hemophan® (GFS 20 Alwall Plus, Gambro) and Cuprophan® (GDE 18, Gambro) dialysers, was moderate with cellulose diacetate (CA 190, Baxter) dialysers, and was relatively low with AN69® (Filtral 16, Hospal) and Fresenius Polysulfone® (HF80, Fresenius Medical Care) dialysers [53]. When seven of these patients were switched from Hemophan® to Fresenius Polysulfone®, apoptosis decreased markedly only after 8 weeks of treatment [53]. In order to eliminate the influence of uraemia, this *in vivo* study was repeated *in vitro* with minimodules of the membranes used and with blood from healthy donors. Interestingly, the results were quite similar, indicating a role of dialysis membrane type (in addition to uraemia) in inducing apoptosis [53].

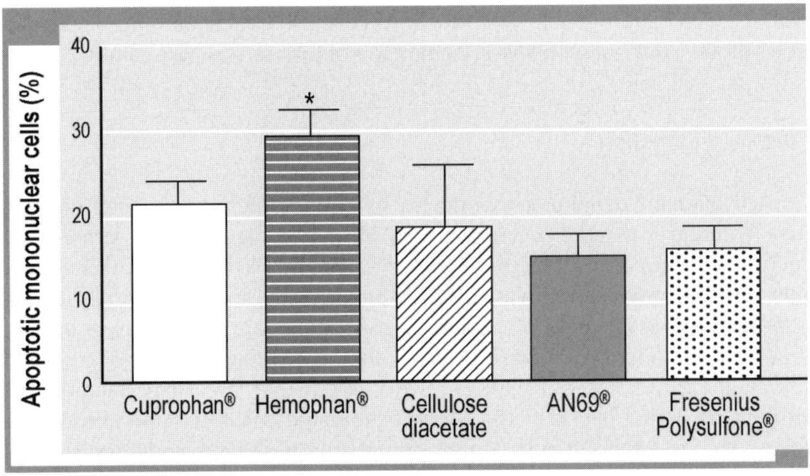

Figure 8.11: Effect of different dialysis membranes on apoptosis of mononuclear cells (MNC). *The type of membrane was unchanged 6 months prior to the study. The following dialysers and patients numbers were tested: Cuprophan® (GFE-18, Gambro), 10 patients; Hemophan® (GFS 20 Plus-Alwall, Gambro), 15 patients; cellulose diacetate (CA190, Baxter), 7 patients; and AN69® (Filtral 16, Hospal), 9 patients. During the study period, bacterial and endotoxin contamination was below the detection limit. Cell apoptosis was measured in circulating MNCs isolated from heparinised blood before the first HD session of the week. Means + SD are shown; * $p < 0.05$ statistically significant different from all other membranes (adapted from [53]).*

An evaluation of the chronic effect of haemodialysis with high-flux polyamide (Polyflux 17, Gambro) and low-flux Hemophan® (GFS Plus 16 or GFS Plus 20) dialysers on T-cell activation markers came to the following result: irrespective of the membrane used, all patients showed a significant elevation of the T-cell activation markers CD69/CD3 and CD25/CD3, as well as a significant decrease in the expression of CD54 (ICAM-1) compared to controls after one year [40].

8.3.1.1 Oxygen species production - Induction of oxidative stress

Dialysis treatment enhances oxidative stress in chronic renal patients who additionally suffer from a chronic deficiency in the major antioxidant systems [54, 55]. Detectable manifestations of this physiological condition are increased plasma levels of protein oxidation products (oxidation of plasma protein-associated thiol groups) in HD patients [56]. Oxidative stress may contribute to atherosclerosis, cardiovascular disease, dialysis-related amyloidosis and anaemia [57, 58]. Four main factors are held responsible: (1) uraemia and the comorbid status of the ESRD patient, (2) antioxidant and trace element losses during treatment, (3) the bioincompatibility of the system, especially of the dialysis membrane and (4) contamination of blood with trace amounts of endotoxins introduced by contaminated dialysis fluid [58, 59].

The highest increase in reactive oxygen species (ROS) production during dialysis was reported with complement-generating membranes (e.g. [48, 45, 60]): Cuprophan® (Lundia alpha 600, Gambro) induced a significant production of reactive oxygen species 15 and 30 min after start of dialysis. A lower production was observed with Hemophan® (NT 1208 G, Bellco), cellulose diacetate (Acepal 1100 G, Hospal) and low-flux Fresenius Polysulfone® (BL 642, Bellco), while increases with SMC® (NC 1285 G, Bellco) were not even statistically significant (**figure 8.12**) [48]. Another clinical study reported low ROS production with AN69® (Crystal 3400, Hospal) and EVAL® (KF 201 N, Kuraray) [47].

As in the case of complement, stimulation of ROS production three times a week by regenerated cellulose membranes leads, over time, to a hyposensitisation against natural stimuli, e.g. bacterial products. ROS production in response to stimulation by endotoxin is suppressed in patients treated with Cuprophan® (GF 120, Gambro), but is normal in patients treated with low-flux Fresenius Polysulfone® (F6, Fresenius Medical Care) or PMMA (B2 1.5 H, Toray) dialysers (e.g. [60, 61]).

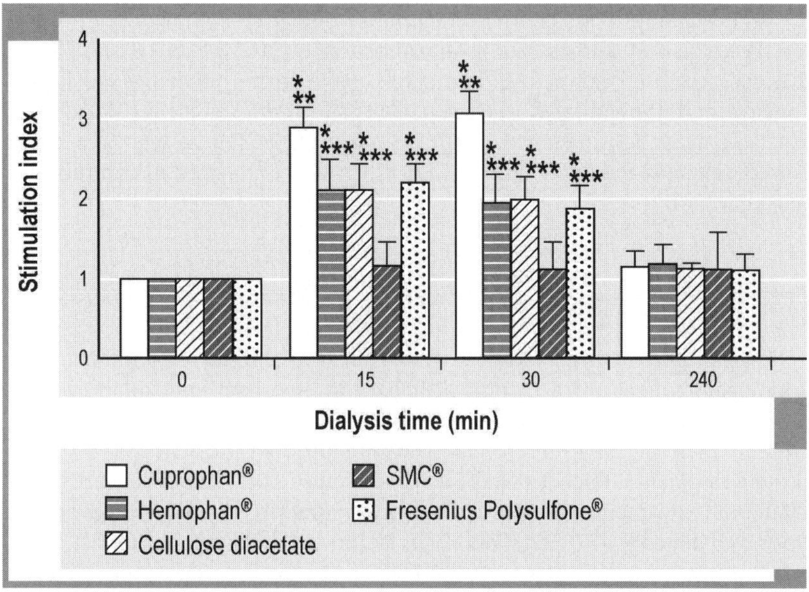

Figure 8.12: Reactive oxygen species (ROS) production by neutrophils during dialysis with different membranes. *Production of ROS is expressed as a stimulation index, defined as x-fold increase over production at time point 0 (means +SD). Ten patients were treated randomly 6 times each with the following membranes/dialysers: Cuprophan® (Lundia Alpha 600, 1.3 m², EtO, Gambro), Hemophan® (NT 1208 G, 1.2 m², gamma ray, Bellco), cellulose diacetate (Acepal 1100 G, 1.0 m², gamma ray, Hospal), SMC® (NC 1285 G, 1.1 m², gamma ray, Bellco) and Fresenius Polysulfone® (BL 642, 1.1 m², EtO, Bellco). The following differences were statistically significant: *vs. predialysis value; **vs. the other four membranes; *** vs. SMC® (adapted from [48]).*

Does the increase of oxidative stress associated with membranes made of regenerated cellulose have an impact on endothelial function?

The higher degree of oxidative stress and the higher leukocyte and platelet activation associated with cellulosic membranes in comparison to modern synthetic membranes might result in endothelial dysfunction [62]. Using decreases in flow-mediated dilatation (FMD) of the brachial artery before and after dialysis as a measure for impaired endothelium function treatment with low-flux polysulfone (Fresenius Polysulfone®, F6 HPS, Fresenius Medical Care) did not significantly affect FMD levels, whereas a significant decrease of about 20% was observed after dialysis with regenerated cellulose (Cuprophan®, Alwall GFS12, Gambro) [63]. The effect with the Cuprophan® membrane was associated with a significant drop in α-tocopherol concentrations (roughly 10%). During polysulfone dialysis, α-tocopherol levels remained stable. One can conclude that the biocompatible polysulfone dialyser caused less vitamin-E consuming oxidative stress and less impairment of endothelial function than the cellulose dialyser [63].

Is the use of a vitamin E-coated dialysis membrane of clinical benefit?

Besides measures targeting improvement of treatment, such as the use of more biocompatible membranes and pyrogen-free dialysis fluid, another approach to reducing the possible deleterious consequences of the pro-oxidant patient status has been followed: supplementation with antioxidant vitamins, such as vitamin E [64]. In addition to oral prescription, some clinical experience has been made with the vitamin E-coated membrane Excebrane: a 10% predialysis increase in plasma vitamin E concentrations (exclusively in HDLs not in LDLs) was observed after a 3-month treatment period with this membrane, whereas plasma levels did not change when conventional biocompatible membranes (AN69®, Fresenius Polysulfone®, PMMA) were used. This effect is believed to be due to the vitamin E sparing effect by the Excebrane membrane [65]. The positive effect of this membrane on vitamin E levels was confirmed in another investigation (increase in predialysis concentrations by 46% after 3 months of treatment) [66]. The ß-carotene content of plasma, and the LDL and HDL level were also around 26% higher than when other biocompatible membranes were used, a finding which can be explained by the secondary protective effect of vitamin E towards ß-carotene [65].

However, no improvement of blood oxidative stress status could be found in this study, which used determinations of thiobarbituric acid-reactive substances and antioxidant defences (e.g. erythrocyte Cu, Zn-superoxide dismutase and plasma and erythrocyte glutathione peroxidase) for assessment [65]. In contrast, another investigation detected an improvement in oxidative stress in the form of a three-fold increase in plasma glutathione concentrations and a slight increase in erythrocyte numbers after three months of treatment [66]. In this study, the improved antioxidant status (increased plasma vitamin E and glutathione peroxidase concentrations) resulted in a tenfold increase in plasma levels of arachidonic acid (one of the most abundant polyunsaturated lipids and a useful marker for lipidperoxidation). Leukocyte function (responsiveness to chemical stimuli) was significantly improved after one month of treatment with Excebrane, and the number of apoptotic mononuclear cells was reduced compared to dialysis with regenerated cellulose [66]. An increase in oxidative markers (e.g. malondialdehyde, advanced glycation end products and 8-hydroxydeoxyguanosine) was prevented with Excebrane but not during dialysis with Terumo polysulfone [67]. Another study used plasma vitamin C levels and ascorbyl free radical (AFR) / vitamin C ratios postdialysis as an index of oxidative stress. After AN69® dialysis, basal vitamin C levels were decreased and the AFR / vitamin C ratio was increased compared to predialysis levels and to dialysis with Excebrane. Both of these oxidative stress parameters remained nearly unchanged compared to predialysis values when the Excebrane membrane was used [68].

Reviewing the available literature, the antioxidant characteristics of Excebrane compared to membranes made from regenerated cellulose are controversial. It seems an interesting new approach to offer a specific and timely protection against oxygen free radicals at their site of generation. However, the efficiency of membrane-associated effects must be compared with other treatment forms, such as oral prescription of vitamin E or other antioxidant therapy (e.g. vitamin C supplementation). A comparison of vitamin E coated membranes with regenerated cellulose plus additional vitamin C infusion (400 mg infused calculated as 200 mg systemic per dialysis) revealed that both approaches had equal positive effects on thiobarbituric acid reacting substances (TBARS, a measure for lipid peroxidation) [69]. The authors argued that vitamin E deficiency is rare in dialysis patients because the vitamin is not removed during dialysis. Lower vitamin E levels may be induced via vitamin C loss, which is considerable (MW 176) during dialysis, and results in less regeneration of vitamin E after dialysis [69]. In their opinion, the therapeutic benefit of vitamin E coated dialysis membranes is comparable with the much more cost-effective additional vitamin C (not vitamin E) prescription.

8.3.1.2 Degranulation of neutrophils

Neutrophil degranulation occurs to some extent during haemodialysis. This is independent of complement activation but influenced by intracellular calcium and two neutrophil degranulation-inhibiting proteins: angiogenin (MW 14,000) [70] and complement factor D (MW 23,000) [71]. Both inhibitors are found to be up to 15-fold elevated in end-stage renal disease patients, protecting against degranulation and, consequently, degranulation products like lactoferrin [71]. Both molecules are removed only in small amounts by highly convective treatments, but some protein-adsorbing membranes, such as PMMA and AN69®, adsorb angiogenin [42] and factor D onto their surfaces [30, 31]. During HD treatments with AN69®, plasma angiogenin and factor D levels decreased by 66% and 37%, respectively, whereas plasma angiogenin concentrations were only reduced by 36% and factor D levels remained unchanged during haemodialysis treatment with high-flux Fresenius Polysulfone® [42]. The removal of inhibitors during AN69® dialysis resulted in more neutrophil degranulation and lactoferrin release than did treatment with Fresenius Polysulfone® [42]. PMMA and Cuprophan® induced more neutrophil degranulation than Hemophan®, high-flux Fresenius Polysulfone® and polyamide in another investigation (**figure 8.13**) [9].

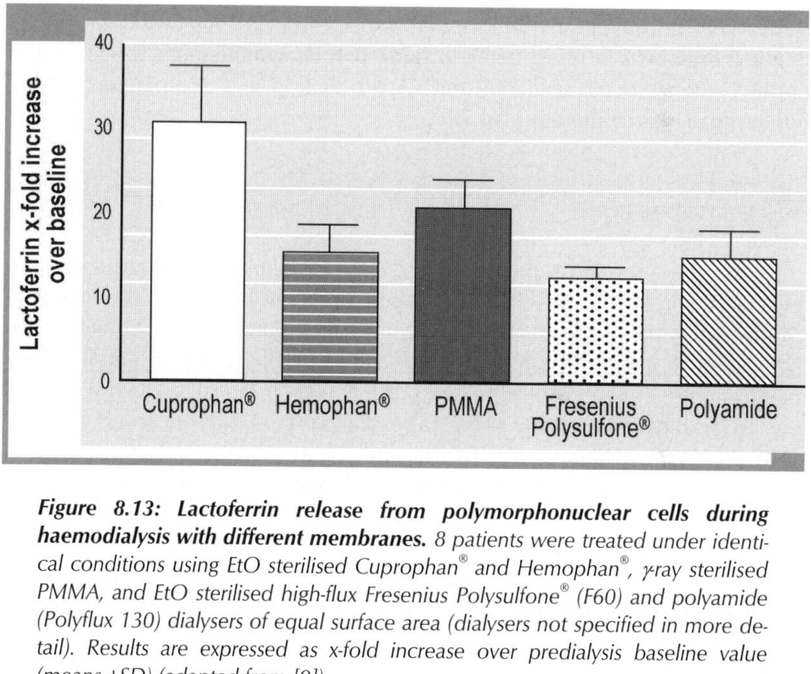

Figure 8.13: Lactoferrin release from polymorphonuclear cells during haemodialysis with different membranes. *8 patients were treated under identical conditions using EtO sterilised Cuprophan® and Hemophan®, γ-ray sterilised PMMA, and EtO sterilised high-flux Fresenius Polysulfone® (F60) and polyamide (Polyflux 130) dialysers of equal surface area (dialysers not specified in more detail). Results are expressed as x-fold increase over predialysis baseline value (means +SD) (adapted from [9]).*

8.3.2 Stimulation of cytokine generation by dialysers

Intracellular cytokine levels

Predialysis intracellular interleukin-1 (IL-1) and TNFα levels are higher in HD patients than in healthy individuals. Furthermore, both cytokines may be transiently generated during dialysis treatment with non-ultrapure dialysis fluid (IL-1 in **figure 8.14**) [72-74, 77]. The same has been described for the soluble receptors IL-1RA and TNFsRp55 [72]. Predialysis IL-1ß and TNFα levels in zymosan-stimulated PBMCs were found to be higher in patients treated with regenerated cellulose than in patients treated with PMMA and healthy volunteers [77]. The membrane factors that are relevant for this cytokine production are explained in more detail in **table 8.1**. As complement is involved in the activation process, cytokine mRNA production and complement activation normally correlate (e.g. [76, 77]).

Plasma cytokine levels

However, a second stimulus is necessary for cytokine protein production and release. In haemodialysis, this is mainly provided by microbial contamination products [84] and, if used, acetate from the dialysis fluid. Therefore, neither higher IL-1 nor TNFα plasma levels could be observed with membranes made of regenerated cellulose when pure, acetate-free dialysis fluid was used (e.g. [85]). In another study using pure dialysis fluid, plasma levels of IL-1β were observed to differ only insignificantly between normal subjects, non-dialysed chronic renal failure patients and haemodialysed patients (figure 8.15) [85]. Therefore, comparison of results from different clinical studies is only meaningful if the purity of the dialysis fluid is similar. In cases of contaminated dialysis fluid, the permeability of a membrane as well as its ability to adsorb microbial products at its outer surface are key factors in cytokine release [86].

The level of circulating cytokines which can be determined with modern methods may also be affected by patient-specific factors, such as residual renal function, different renal and comorbid diseases, drugs and different cellular production. Dialyser-related influencing factors are permeability/clearance, ultrafiltration rate, adsorption of cytokines and stimulation of generation by different materials (e.g. [74, 87]). A comparison of plasma levels of circulating IL-1β, IL-6 and IL-10 measured during haemodialysis over a period of 4 months with high-flux polyamide and low-flux Hemophan® haemodialysers revealed no differences between the membranes [88].

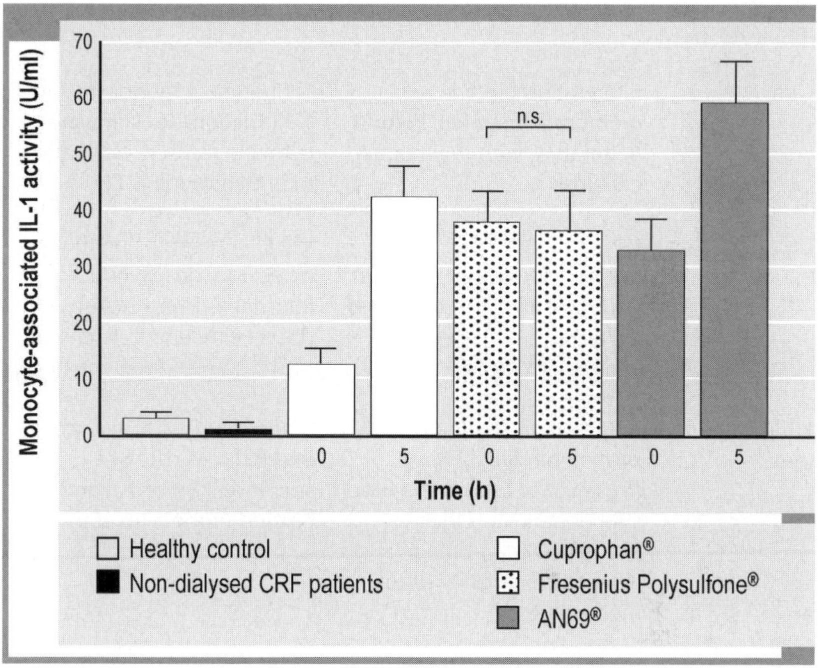

Figure 8.14: Cell-associated IL-1 induced during haemodialysis with different membranes and slightly contaminated dialysis fluid. *Monocyte-associated (intracellular) IL-1 activity was higher before dialysis (t_0) with all membrane types than in healthy volunteers and non-dialysed chronic renal failure (CRF) patients. The levels stayed constant until the end of treatment (t_5) with Fresenius Polysulfone® (F50 or F60, Fresenius Medical Care) but increased with Cuprophan® (Gambro, Hemofrance, Fresenius) and the AN69® (flat sheet, Hospal) membranes. The authors concluded that complement-generating membranes, such as Cuprophan®, transiently generate IL-1 during treatment. The chronic stimulation observed with both high-flux membranes as documented by the particularly high predialysis levels may be the result of dialysis fluid contamination and the transport of such contaminants across the high-flux membranes. This was between 2.5 and 270 EU/ml in this study and may, therefore, induce IL-1 production (adapted from [73]).*

Stimulus	Source/influence of HD membrane	Effect (Reference)
Receptor mediated		
C5a	Generation by the membrane material; highest generation with regenerated cellulose	"Priming" of monocytes via C5a receptor to stimulate cytokine transcription rather than translation [77]
C3a	Generation by the membrane material; highest generation with regenerated cellulose	Via C3a receptor on monocytes; low doses induce internal IL-1 production, high doses stimulate IL-1 release [78]
LBP-LPS complex	LBP: hepatic acute phase protein binding LPS. Presence of LPS on the blood side depends on the permeability and the LPS adsorptive capacity of the membrane.	Binds to mCD14 receptor and induces cytokine secretion by normal and primed monocytes [79]
ß-glucans	In addition to fungi and yeast, these are also present in extracts from cellulose membranes	Induces cytokine production and secretion after binding to ß-glucan receptor [80]
L-fucose	Fucose or fucose-like residues are present in cellulose membranes	Cytokine release after binding to fucose receptors [38]

Stimulus	Source/influence of HD membrane	Effect (reference)
Receptor independent		
C5b-9 (TCC)	Generation by the membrane material; highest generation with regenerated cellulose	Direct monocyte activation with cytokine release and amplification of activation by complement-independent pathways (e.g. via L-fucose) [38]
Exotoxins	From *Pseudomonads* Presence on the blood side depends on the adsorptive capacity of the membrane's outer surface	Direct monocyte activation, independent of complement and receptor binding [81]
Acetate	From the dialysis fluid	Induces IL-1ß production and secretion at 20-40 mmol/l [82]

Table 8.1: Main stimuli of cytokine production and release during haemodialysis *(adapted from [83]).*

Cytokine gene expression

In vitro experiments with isolated monocytes from patients treated with high-flux polyamide and low-flux Hemophan® for at least four months revealed a higher state of cell preactivation in patients treated with Hemophan® than in patients treated with polyamide. Preactivated monocytes secrete high amounts of pro-inflammatory cytokines when exposed to a second stimulus, such as endotoxin [88]. A second study compared gene expression of IL-1ß with different membranes using pure dialysis fluid: as mentioned above, no differences in IL-1ß plasma levels were found between dialysis patients using different membranes, healthy volunteers and non-dialysed chronic renal failure patients (**figure 8.15**), but gene expression of IL-1β was 3-fold higher with regenerated cellulose than with PMMA and polysulfone (**figure 8.16**) [85]. These data clearly demonstrate that gene expression of cytokines, but not necessarily their release from cells, is triggered with regenerated cellulose. Therefore, plasma levels of circulating cytokines may remain stable during treatment (**figure 8.15**).

Do only complement-activating membranes induce cytokine gene expression?

An *in vitro* study with isolated PBMCs from haemodialysis patients recirculated through minimodules containing three membranes with low complement-inducing characteristics revealed highest TNFα mRNA expression by polymorphonuclear cells after their passage through PAN minimodules. The

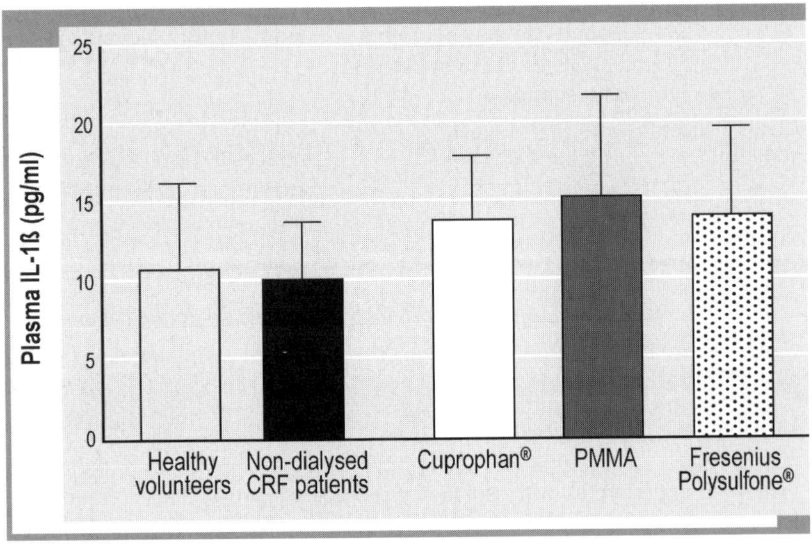

Figure 8.15: Plasma IL-1β levels among different patient groups. *IL-1β was determined directly in plasma (obtained from blood from the venous line of the dialyser) using an enzyme immunoassay for human IL-1β. Samples were collected after 5, 30, 180 and 300 min but measured levels were similar at all time points. No statistically significant differences could be found between the groups. Unfortunately, the dialysers (all of the same surface area 1.2 m²) were not specified in detail in the publication (adapted from [85]).*

membranes tested were PEG-grafted regenerated cellulose, polyacrylonitrile (PAN) and polysulfone (APS®), all three from Asahi and in Asahi housings. Furthermore, highest TNFα release after stimulation with LPS was also detected with the PAN minimodules [89]. This is in accordance with earlier findings that negatively charged surfaces, like that of PAN, promote the expression of mRNAs for some cytokines [90]. *In vitro* experiments confirm the higher intracellular production and extracellular release of IL-1 in MNC exposed to PAN compared to regenerated cellulose in the absence of endotoxin or complement (by using complement depleted plasma). The intrinsic property of the PAN membrane to induce IL-1 production is obviously greater than that of regenerated cellulose. However, PAN binds and clears significantly higher amounts of IL-1 than regenerated cellulose, resulting in lower plasma levels of circulating IL-1 [87].

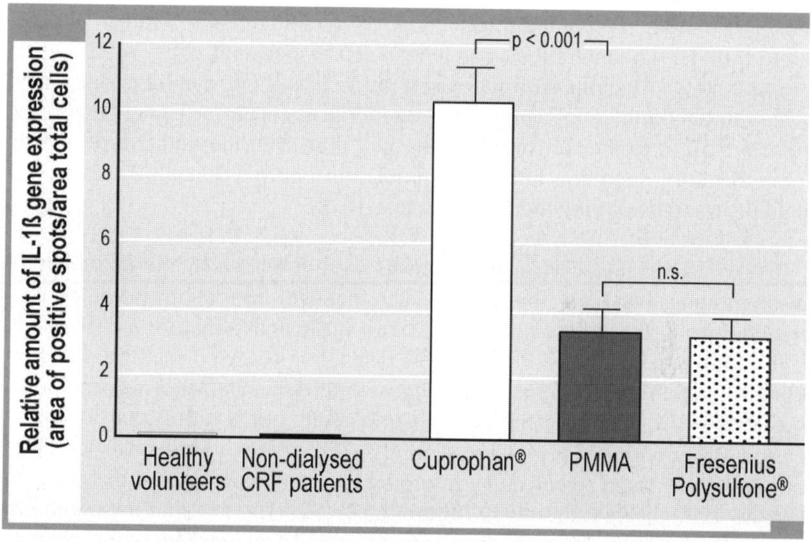

Figure 8.16: Relative amount of IL-1β gene expression in PBMC from healthy volunteers, non dialysed uraemics and HD patients treated with different dialysers. *Maximal accumulation of IL-1β mRNA was observed in blood samples taken from the venous line after 5 min of dialysis. The corresponding samples were then analysed and gene expression was detected by in situ hybridisation. Quantification was undertaken by computer imaging analysis. IL1-ß gene expression could be detected in cells from all HD patients but not in healthy volunteers and non-dialysed uraemics (adapted from [85]).*

How does the type of membrane influence LPS-stimulated IL-1ß secretion?

Intracellular cytokine (e.g. IL-1ß) levels are increased in haemodialysis patients, especially during dialysis with regenerated cellulose (e.g. [73]). This chronic stimulation obviously leads to a suppression of the response to biological stimulants, such as bacterial products. Lipopolysaccharide (LPS)-induced IL-1ß secretion is reduced in patients treated with membranes made of regenerated cellulose compared to healthy controls, non-dialysed chronic renal failure patients and patients dialysed with polyacrylonitrile membranes (data from experiments with isolated PBMC from all patient groups investigated) [91, 92]. This functional change in PBMC response is specific for IL-1ß (it does not happen with TNFα), is haemodialysis membrane dependent and is reversible. Increased prostaglandine E_2 (PGE_2) levels, which suppress IL-1ß secretion, are thought to be responsible due to the following observed effects: when patients dialysed with regenerated cellulose were switched to polyacrylonitrile membranes, total (cell associated means internal and secreted) IL-1ß concentrations remained nearly constant, but the secreted amount after LPS-stimulation increased. In parallel, PGE_2 synthesis decreased with polyacrylonitrile compared to regenerated cellulose. Evidence for the role of PGE_2 is further provided by the fact that, with the addition of a PGE_2 inhibitor, IL-1ß secretion after LPS stimulation improved in PBMC from HD patients treated with regenerated cellulose [91].

New insights into cellular mechanisms were provided by the possibility of distinguishing between the biologically inactive translation product, propeptide proIL-1ß, and the processed, biologically active mature mIL-1ß molecule that is secreted from PBMCs. This distinction revealed that the defect in PBMC function with regenerated cellulose after LPS stimulation is not due to suppressed processing of the proIL-1ß molecule, but is rather due to an impaired ability of the cells to secrete mIL-1ß. This defect is reversible: secretion of mIL-1ß increased significantly, returning to normal levels, after dialysis with low-flux or high-flux polysulfone (**figure 8.17**) [92]. The fact that improvement of mIL-1ß secretion (differences in secreted mIL-1ß being statistically insignificant) was achieved with the biocompatible membrane polysulfone, irrespective of its permeability, excluded the impact of any unknown factor of middle molecular size in these observations.

The higher levels of cell-associated mIL-1ß in HD patients treated with regenerated cellulose compared to polysulfone (second light grey column in **figure 8.17**) represent a state of inflammation that may contribute to inflammatory processes, such as atherogenesis and ß2-m amyloidosis [92]. On the other hand, the suppressed immune response may lead to a higher susceptibility to infection in cases where immune defence is necessary, e.g. during bacterial invasion.

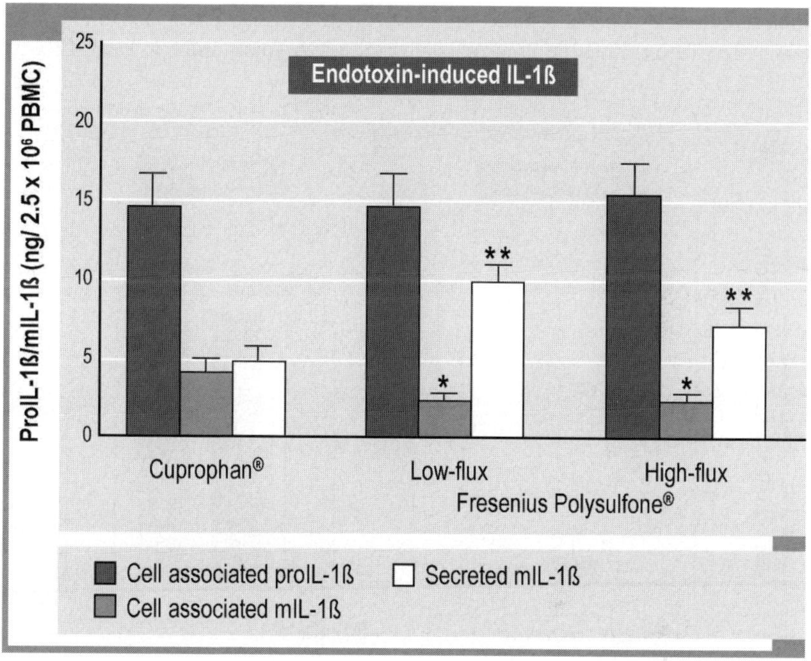

Figure 8.17: Endotoxin-induced prointerleukin (pro)IL-1ß and mature (m)IL-1ß in PBMC of patients dialysed with different membranes. *The following membranes were tested in random order in 8 patients during a study period of 5 weeks for each dialyser : Cuprophan® (GFS 12, 1.3 m², Gambro), low-flux Fresenius Polysulfone® (F6 HPS, 1.3 m², Fresenius Medical Care) and high-flux Fresenius Polysulfone® (F60S, 1.3 m², Fresenius Medical Care). Blood was obtained from the arteriovenous fistula before the start of the HD session that followed the long interdialytic interval. PBMC were isolated from whole blood and incubated with LPS (10 ng/ml) for 18 h. IL-1ß was determined in supernatants (extracellular) and lysed cells (intracellular). Two ELISAs were used, one specific for proIL-1ß, the other for mIL-1ß. No statistically significant differences between the membranes were found for the production of proIL-1ß, but mIL-1ß was accumulated in cells from patients treated with Cuprophan® (* $p < 0.05$ cell associated mIL-1ß significant lower for both polysulfones versus Cuprophan®). This is due to a reduced secretion of the molecule (** $p < 0.05$ secreted mIL-1ß significant higher with both polysulfones versus Cuprophan®) (adapted from [92]).*

Has the defective secretion of IL-1ß with regenerated cellulose also been observed for other cytokines?

Cultured PBMC were analysed from healthy volunteers, non-dialysed chronic renal failure patients and dialysis patients (samples drawn before the dialysis session) treated either with Cuprophan® (Bellco, 1.3 m²) or PMMA (B3.1 3A, Toray) and ultrafiltered dialysis fluid. A small amount of IL-12 was

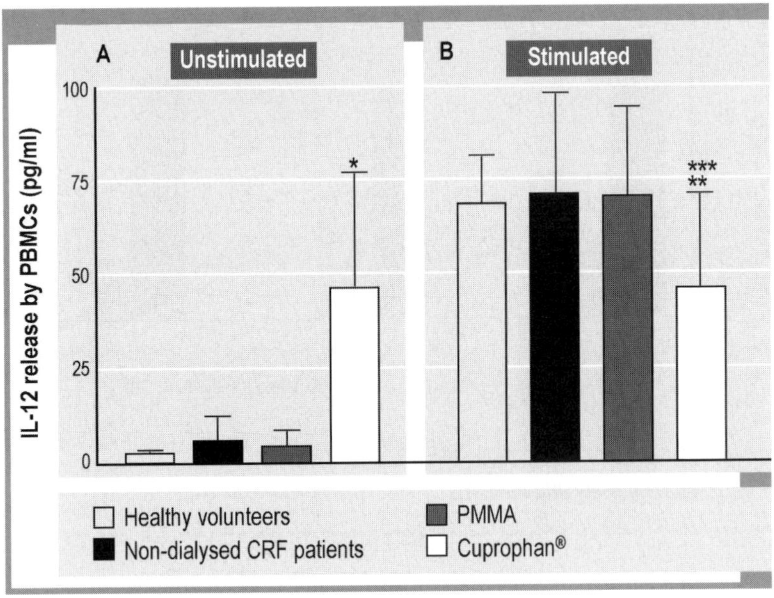

Figure 8.18: Stimulated and unstimulated IL-12 secretion by PBMCs of healthy volunteers, non-dialysed chronic renal failure patients and HD patients. *PMMA (B3.1.3A, 1.3 m², Toray) and Cuprophan® (ETO sterilised, type not specified, 1.3 m², Bellco) dialysers were used for at least one year in the patient groups investigated. Bicarbonate dialysis fluid was ultrafiltered. Samples were taken before a dialysis session. Isolated PBMCs were incubated for 24 h either with or without 10 µg/ml LPS and phythemagglutinin. IL-12 was detected in the supernatants. The left-hand figure (A) shows that unstimulated IL-12 release with Cuprophan® was statistically significantly higher than with all other groups. As shown on the right (B), stimulated IL-12-release with Cuprophan® was statistically significantly lower than in all other groups. * $p < 0.01$ Cuprophan® versus all other groups; ** $p < 0.02$ Cuprophan® versus healthy volunteers; *** $p < 0.05$ Cuprophan® versus PMMA and non-dialysed chronic renal failure patients (adapted from [93]).*

spontaneously released in all groups, but massive release was observed with Cuprophan® (**figure 8.18A**). After stimulation of the PBMCs, either by LPS or by the mitogen phytohemagglutinin, the situation changed: while IL-12 levels in the supernatant remained unaltered compared to unstimulated conditions with PBMC cultures for patients treated with Cuprophan® levels increased significantly in all other patient groups (**figure 8.18B**). IL-12 is produced very early during infection and has an important proinflammatory function in that it activates natural killer cells and T-helper cells. The latter are stimulated by IL-12 to release interferon γ (IFN γ). IFN γ release, both spontaneous and mitogen-stimulated, was also investigated: no differences were observed in the basal spontaneous IFN γ production between the groups. Under mitogen stimulation, IFN γ production was significantly lower with Cuprophan® than in all other groups (**figure 8.19**). These data support the hypothesis that, during

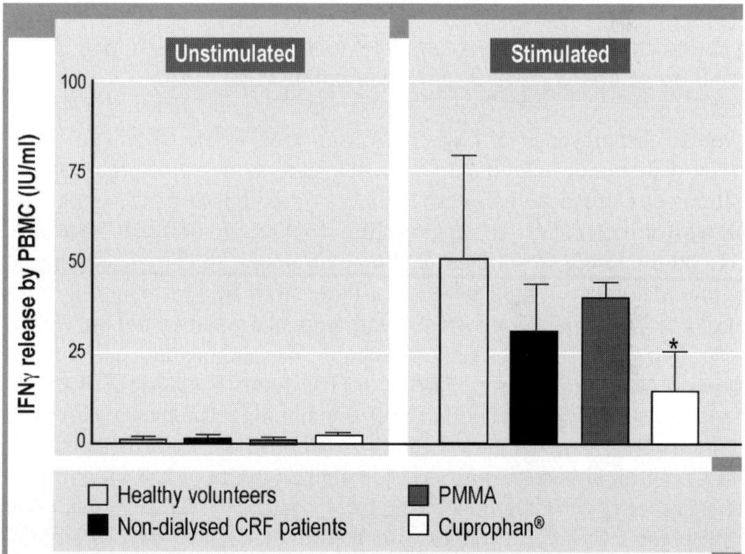

Figure 8.19: Stimulated and unstimulated IFN γ production by PBMCs of healthy volunteers, non-dialysed chronic renal failure patients and HD patients. *Study conditions were described under **figure 8.18.** No statistically significant differences could be observed in the basal IFN γ release between membranes. After stimulation, IFN γ release from PBMCs was statistically significantly higher with all membranes except Cuprophan® compared to unstimulated conditions ($p < 0.01$) – it was statistically significantly lower after Cuprophan® dialysis (*$p < 0.01$ versus all other stimulated probes) (adapted from [93]).*

dialysis with regenerated cellulose, monocytes are activated to release IL-12 and that this chronic stimulation three times a week could, in the long-term, leads to a reduction in the ability of PBMC to produce this cytokine in response to a stimulus. Furthermore, target cells of IL-12, such as T-helper cells, may downregulate their immunologic effects (e.g. IFN γ production) as a consequence of chronic stimulation [93].

This immune abnormality (i.e. activation of cells in their basal state and deficiency upon stimulation), which is observed with regenerated cellulose but not with more biocompatible membranes and not in non-dialysed chronic renal failure patients, may play a role in cell–mediated immunodeficiency of chronic uraemic patients dialysed with regenerated cellulose and their susceptibility to infection (discussed in more detail in chapter 10.6) and neoplastic disease [93].

Can the inflammatory response in HD patients be influenced by cytokine elimination with large-pore dialysis membranes?

Due to the presence of large pores and their ability to adsorb proteins, high-flux dialysers or haemofilters may eliminate some cytokines. Here some limitations of extracorporeal removal have to be kept in mind: cytokines are molecules of molecular size ranging from 15,000 - 30,000 that have a short half-life (in the range of minutes) and may be bound to carrier proteins (such as α_2-macroglobulin) [94]. Therefore, a detectable amount may only be efficiently removed when convective treatments like haemofiltration with high ultrafiltration volumes and highly permeable membranes are perfomed. The adsorption capacity of the membrane for cytokines is probably of more importance. As already mentioned, AN69® membranes (flat sheets, Hospal) are, in contrast to regenerated cellulose (Cuprophan® flat sheets, Membrana/Gambro), able to adsorb considerable amounts of IL-1 *in vitro* [87]. A comparison of *in vitro* haemofiltration for 4 h with high-flux dialysers containing Fresenius Polysulfone®, AN69®, cellulose triacetate and polyamide (dialyser types described in the figure caption) revealed that greatest reductions in TNFα, IL-6 and IL-8 levels were achieved with AN69®. This was caused by adsorption. Adsorption of cytokines was also observed for the other three membranes, but to a much lesser extent. None of the membranes filtered TNFα (**figure 8.20**).

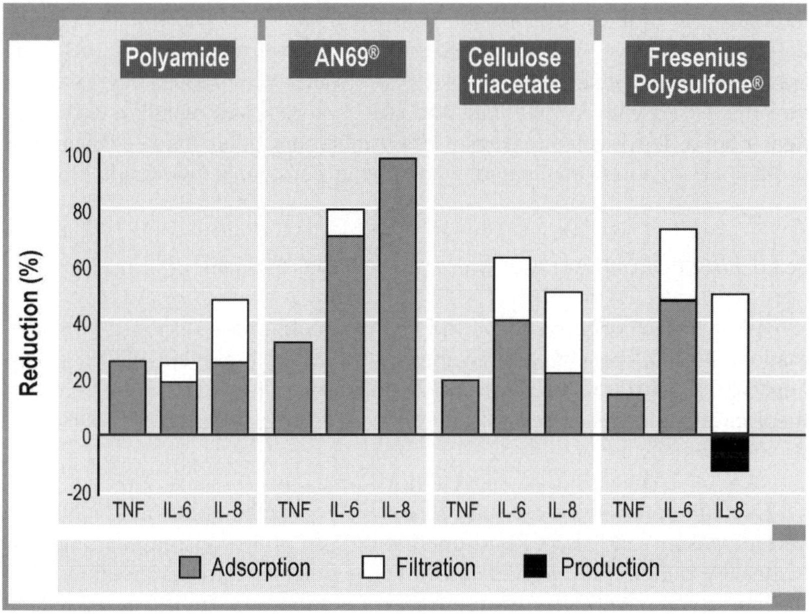

Figure 8.20: Cytokine elimination after 4 h in vitro postdilution haemofiltration (HF) with different high-flux dialysers. *Continuous HF was conducted with heparinised whole blood to which freshly prepared cytokines obtained from venous blood of healthy volunteers after bacterial stimulation were added. The median final concentrations in the test solutions were 76 pg/ml for TNF, 348 ng/ml for IL-6 and 241 ng/ml for IL-8. After a 30 min stabilisation period, HF was started with identical rates of ultrafiltration and substitution (30 ml/min) and a blood flow of 150 ml/min. The following dialysers with a cut-off of 30,000 Dalton (according to the investigators) were investigated: polyamide (Polyflux® L, 1.1 m², Gambro), AN69® (1.3 m², Hospal), cellulose triacetate (CT90, 0.9 m², Baxter) and Fresenius Polysulfone® (F60, 1.2 m², Fresenius Medical Care) (adapted from [95]).*

A recently published study compared the removal and/or induction of pro-inflammatory markers, such as IL-6, CRP and IL-18, and anti-inflammatory markers, such as IL-1Ra and IL-18 binding protein, by low-flux and high-flux dialysis (Fresenius Poysulfone®/F6 and Helixone®/FX100 membranes/dialysers, respectively). In addition, the *Staphylococcus epidermis*-induced production of interferon γ (IFN γ) and IL-18 was determined in whole blood cultures of the low- and high-flux patients, and compared to cultures of healthy volunteers [96]. Ultrafiltered, ultrapure dialysis fluid was used in all treatments in order to exclude the possible influence of bacterial contamination. After 6 weeks, there was no significant difference in plasma levels of all parameters investigated with the exception of IFN γ. Stimulated IFN γ production decreased with low-flux HD and was restored with high-flux dialysis to near normal levels after 6 weeks. IFN γ inhibitors other than IL-18 binding protein are obviously eliminated by the higher permeable membrane [96].

8.3.3 Effect of dialysers on the acute phase reaction

IL-6 is the major regulator of the hepatic acute phase response in inflammation: it stimulates hepatic synthesis of C-reactive protein (CRP), serum amyloid A (SAA) and secretory phospholipase A_2 ($sPLA_2$). Plasma levels of these proteins increase several hundred-fold from baseline 6-10 hours after stimulation [97].

Circulating IL-6 levels are markedly elevated in ESRD patients [53, 98] for several reasons, and also CRP is found to be 5 to 10 fold increased compared to healthy people [99]. In addition to many other factors (reviewed in [99]), haemodialysis membranes obviously also contribute to the increased inflammatory response. This could be demonstrated with isolated mononuclear cells (PBMCs, the main source of IL-6) after membrane contact, and by directly measuring plasma levels of circulating IL-6 at start and end of dialysis [100-102]. Increased plasma levels of acute phase proteins could be detected 8 to 24 hours after dialysis.

Cultured PBMCs from patients dialysed with Cuprophan® spontaneously released more IL-6 than PBMCs from healthy individuals or from patients dialysed with PMMA [102], SMC® (NC 1485, Bellco) or cellulose diacetate (DN 1813-15, Nipro) dialysers [100]. The same effect was observed with the soluble IL-6 receptor, which probably better reflects the biological activity of IL-6 [101]. IL-6 release correlates positively with levels of circulating CRP [97, 100] and haemodialysis patients actually exhibit elevated plasma levels of IL-6 [97, 100], CRP [103] and secretory phospholipase A_2 ($sPLA_2$) [97]. The basic mechanisms behind increases in levels of acute phase proteins are yet not fully understood, but a contribution from dialysis membranes and contaminated dialysis fluid is implicated. For example, IL-6 levels were found to be elevated after the third hour of treatment with cuprammonium rayon membranes (AM-UP-75, Asahi) and correlated with the release of acute phase proteins, albeit with different time schedules [97]. Increased concentrations of CRP and $sPLA_2$ were found 24 hours after start of haemodialysis with cuprammonium rayon (AM-UP-75, Asahi), but neither IL-6 (after 3 hours), CRP nor $sPLA_2$ levels showed marked variation at these time points when Fresenius Polysulfone® (F60S, Fresenius Medical Care) was used [97].

What role does bacterial contamination of dialysis fluid play in the acute phase response?

A recent investigation demonstrated that the use of ultrapure dialysis fluid compared to potentially contaminated (around 95 CFU/ml) dialysis fluid will lower plasma CRP and IL-6 levels in HD patients treated with the F60 (Fresenius Medical Care) dialyser [104]. In another study, the increase in acute phase reactants appeared to be independent of low-level bacterial contamination (median bacterial concentration was 45 (range 0 - 480) CFU/ml; median endotoxin concentration was 0.18 (range 0.05 - 1.13) EU/ml) and solely dependent on the type of membrane used. This was concluded from the finding that there were no differences between the use of ultrapure (bacterial contamination < 1 CFU/ml; endotoxin contamination ≤ 0.03 IU/ml) and contaminated dialysis fluid for a particular membrane [97] (**figure 8.21**). However, bacterial contamination was probably too low to distinguish between membrane effects and others.

Another clinical study supplied evidence for a membrane effect on acute phase response. Plasma CRP levels were compared in patients treated randomly in a cross-over study with dialysers containing polyamide (PF14, Gambro), Gambrane (Pro600 plate, Gambro) and Cuprophan® (Alpha 600, Gambro). Although plasma CRP levels were increased in comparison to healthy individuals (0.14 ± 0.02 mg/dl), levels were found to be highest with Cuprophan® (1.77 ± 0.37 mg/dl), somewhat lower with Gambrane (1.34 ± 0.2 mg/dl) and lowest with polyamide (1.19 ± 0.18 mg/dl). Bacterial contamination of the dialysis fluid was low (20.5 ± 5.8 CFU/ml) in these experiments. However, the authors remarked that they did not exclude the possible influence of varying levels of bacterial contamination in their experimental set-up. The higher CRP levels found with Cuprophan® and Gambrane® may also be influenced by their permeability for small molecular weight bacterial products. Polyamide adsorbs bacterial products at its outer surface. The good results with polyamide dialysers in this study may be due to less complement and cell activation in combination with less permeation of bacterial products from dialysis fluid into the blood [103].

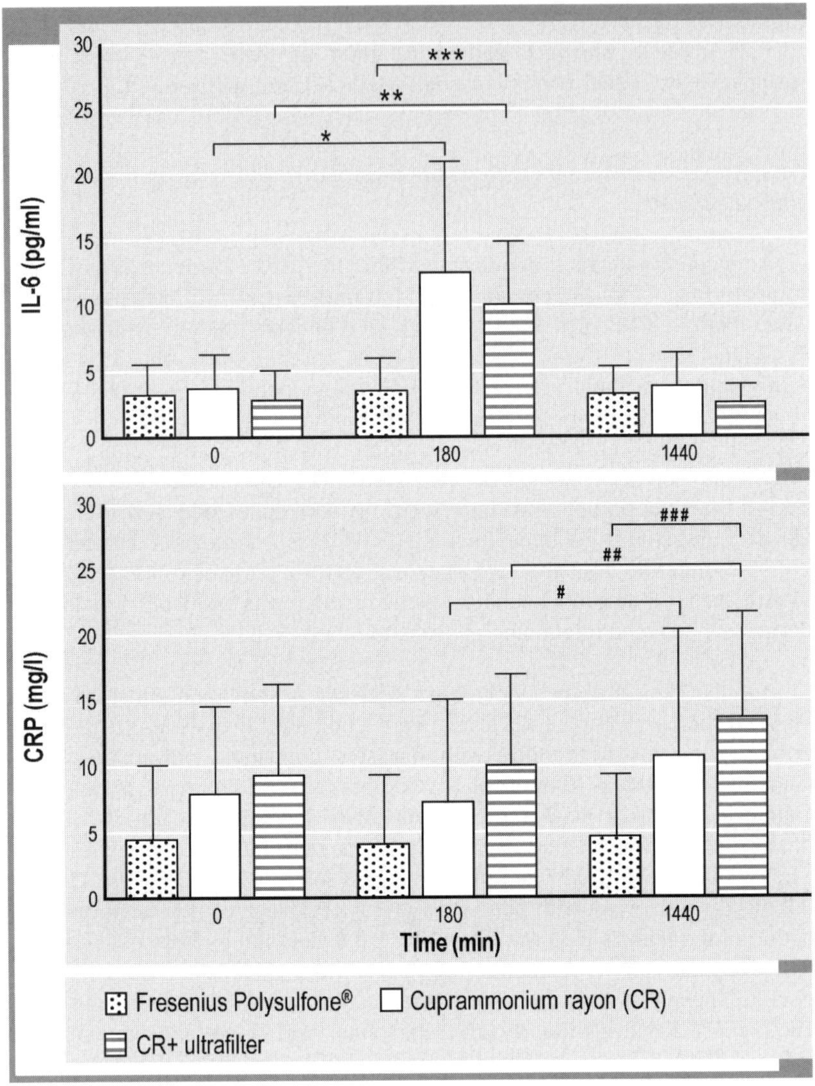

Figure 8.21: IL-6 and CRP release with cuprammonium rayon and Fresenius Polysulfone® dialysers. *With cuprammonium rayon dialysers (AM-UP-75, Asahi), plasma concentration of IL-6 increased to a statistically significant extent (* $p = 0.01$, ** $p < 0.02$) up to the end of haemodialysis treatment (180 min). No such changes could be found with Fresenius Polysulfone® dialysers (F60S, Fresenius Medical Care). The value after 180 min was significantly lower than with cu-*

*prammonium rayon and cuprammonium rayon + ultrafilter (*** $p < 0.02$ difference to cuprammonium rayon). CRP values increased 24 h after both types of cuprammonium rayon dialysis treatment (# $p = 0.01$, ## $p < 0.02$), but not after Fresenius Polysulfone® dialysis. The values for cuprammonium rayon + ultrafilter were significantly different from those for Fresenius Polysulfone® after 1440 min (### $p > 0.002$). The difference between low level contaminated and filtered dialysis fluid during cuprammonium rayon dialysis was not statistically significant (adapted from [97]).*

8.4 Activation of the kinin system by dialysers

The main factor determining activation of the kinin system with subsequent generation of bradykinin is the electronegativity of the dialysis membrane (e.g. [105]). **Table 8.2** provides an overview of the zeta potentials (a parameter for electronegativity) of seven frequently used membranes. As is obvious from these *in vitro* measurements, AN69® and PAN DX are the most electronegative membranes and generate the highest amounts of bradykinin, a mediator of anaphylactoid reactions [105]. When the electronegativity of the polyacrylonitrile (PAN) polymer is reduced to near zero, as in AN69ST, *in vitro* bradykinin generation is reduced 200-fold. This was achieved by coating of the membrane with the polycationic polymer poly(ethyleneimine) [105].

Bradykinin generation with PAN membranes could also be detected *in vivo*, especially in patients under ACE-inhibitor therapy. Bradykinin is normally rapidly degraded in the body by the serine protease kininase II and, therefore, most patients are symptom-free during AN69® and PAN DX dialyses. However, if this enzyme is blocked by ACE inhibitors, plasma levels may increase by over 100-fold and patients may suffer from mild to severe anaphylactoid reactions [106]. Bradykinin levels between 600 and 10,500 fmol/ml were measured in patients suffering from anaphylactoid reactions during AN69® dialysis treatment [107].

The highest bradykinin generation reported was measured *in vivo* in sheep under ACE inhibitor therapy and treated with polyacrylonitrile membranes (AN69®, Filtral 16, Hospal and PAN-85DX, Asahi). Lower generation was observed when a polyacrylonitrile membrane with lower surface electronegativity (SPAN, Membrana - not available on the market) was used [108]. In another study, even symptom-free patients without ACE medication exhibited an approx. 10-fold higher bradykinin generation with AN69® plate dialysers (Biospal 3000S, Hospal) than with Cuprophan® (GFE 18, Gambro), Hemophan® (GFS PLus 16, Gambro) and high-flux Fresenius Polysulfone® (F60,

Fresenius Medical Care) dialysers (**figure 8.22**) [107]. The very low bradykinin generation by high-flux Fresenius Polysulfone® (around 20 fmol/ml; F60, Fresenius Medical Care) and low-flux Hemophan® (around 40 fmol/ml; GFS PLus 16, Gambro) haemodialysers was confirmed also for patients under ACE inhibitor therapy [109].

Membrane	**Zeta potential** (mV)	**Plasma kallikrein** (U/l)	**Bradykinin generation** (fmol/ml)
Polyacrylonitrile AN69®	-70 ± 5	60 ± 15	32,100 (26,500 - 41,200)
Polyacrylonitrile PAN DX	-60 ± 4*	80 ± 20*	28,983 (22,600 - 36,150)*
Polymethyl-metacrylate	-25 ± 2	10 ± 5	130 (50 - 250)
Cellulose triacetate	-20 ± 2	<5	65 (25 - 100)
Cuprophan®	-10 ± 1	<5	78 (25 - 150)
Fresenius Polysulfone®	-5 ± 1	<5	62 (25 - 120)
Polyacrylonitrile AN69ST	-3 ± 1	<5	150 (30 - 450)

**p < 0.001 PAN DX vs. AN69®*

***Table 8.2: Zeta potential (surface electronegativity), plasma kallikrein activity and bradykinin generation with different membranes* in vitro.** *Kallikrein and bradykinin were measured in diluted and undiluted citrated plasma, respectively, after 5 minutes of circulation through minidialysers containing the membranes specified. Values for zeta potential and kallikrein are presented as the mean ± SD of 6 determinations. For bradykinin, mean values of 6 determinations are presented with lower and upper values between parentheses. Plasma kallikrein levels for AN69ST, cellulose triacetate, Cuprophan® and Fresenius Polysulfone® were below the detection limit of the assay (adapted from [105]).*

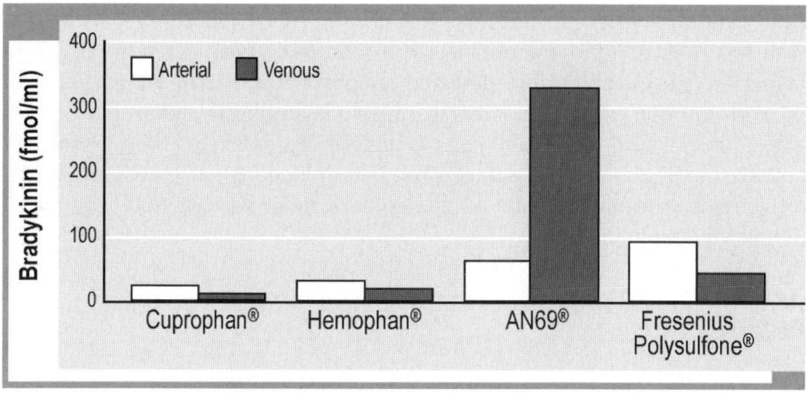

Figure 8.22: Maximum bradykinin generation with different membranes 5 min after onset of haemodialysis. *10 symptom-free patients who were not undergoing ACE inhibitor therapy were treated with the following dialysers: Cuprophan® (GFE 18, Gambro), Hemophan® (GFS Plus 16, Gambro), AN69® (Biospal 3000S, Hospal) and Fresenius Polysulfone® (F60, Fresenius Medical Care). Blood was drawn from the arterial and venous blood lines 5 minutes after the onset of dialysis, and the plasma was then analysed for bradykinin. Even in symptom-free sessions, AN69® provoked a higher bradykinin generation than the other membranes tested. Data are presented as mean (adapted from [107]).*

The other polyacrylonitrile polymer on the market, namely PAN 13 DX (Asahi), led to a higher bradykinin generation than high-flux Fresenius Polysulfone® (F60, Fresenius Medical Care) in patients both on and off ACE inhibitor therapy [110]. In contrast to AN69® dialysers, bradykinin generation is delayed with Asahi PAN membranes. Plasma levels peaked around 10 minutes after initiation of dialysis, not after 5 minutes as in the case of AN69® [110, 111]. Anaphylactoid reactions with high-flux PMMA dialysers in patients undergoing ACE inhibitor therapy have been described in one publication [112]. As can be seen from **table 8.2**, the zeta potential of PMMA is more negative than that of cellulose triacetate, Cuprophan®, Fresenius Polysulfone® or AN69ST. Also plasma kallikrein and bradykinin generation was higher with this membrane than with cellulose triacetate, Cuprophan® and Fresenius Polysulfone®. It has been speculated that this negative charge may be enhanced by special prerinsing procedures or an inadequate pH of the dialysis fluid in such a way that bradykinin generation may occur.

As mentioned earlier, an AN69® type membrane with a reduced surface electronegativity was developed in order to overcome the problem of bradykinin generation. Recently, adverse reactions in ACE inhibitor patients treated with this new AN69ST membrane were reported. These reactions occurred atypically late for bradykinin-mediated anaphylactoid reactions, i.e. between 45 and 150 min of dialysis. Analysis of blood samples revealed that contact activation was also responsible for this undesired side effect [113]. Insufficient coating of the membrane surface probably induced these reactions. An improvement in production should guarantee a more homogenous coating of the membrane in the future [113].

References

1. Tsunoda N, Kokubo K, Sakai K, Fukuda M, Miyazaki M, Hiyoshi T: Surface roughness of cellulose hollow fiber dialysis membranes and platelet adhesion. ASAIO Journal: 418-423, 1999

2. Matata BM, Courtney JM, Sundaram S, Wark S, Bowry SK, Vienken J, Lowe GDO: Determination of contact phase activation by the measurement of the activity of supernatant and membrane surface-adsorbed factor XII (FXII): its relevance as a useful parameter for the *in vitro* assessment of haemodialysis membranes. J Biomed Mater Res 31: 63-70, 1996

3. Cornelius RM, Brash JL: Identification of proteins adsorbed to hemodialyser membranes from heparinized plasma. J Biomater Sci Polymer Edn 4(3): 291-304, 1993

4. Mulvihill J, Crost T, Renaux JL, Cazenave JP: Evaluation of haemodialysis membrane biocompatibility by parallel assessment in an ex vivo model in healthy volunteers. Nephrol Dial Transplant 12: 1968-1973, 1997

5. Ishii Y, Yano S, Kanai H, Maezawa A, Tsuchida A, Wakamatsu R, Naruse T: Evaluation of blood coagulation-fibrinolysis system in patients receiving chronic hemodialysis. Nephron 73: 407-412, 1996

6. Frank RD, Weber J, Dresbach H, Thelen H, Weiss C, Floege J: Role of contact system activation in hemodialyzer-induced thrombogenicity. Kidney Int 60: 1972-1981, 2001

7. Matsuda T: Biological responses at non-physiological interfaces and molecular design of biocompatible surfaces. Nephrol Dial Transplant 4: 60-66, 1989

8. Schultze G, Göhl H, Hollmann S, Sinah P: Formation of thrombin-antithrombin complex using polyamid and cellulosic dialyzers. (Abstract) Int J Artif Organs 14(9): 543, 1991

9. Deppisch R, Betz M, Hänsch GM, Rauterberg EW, Ritz E: Biocompatibility of the polyamide membranes in: *Polyamide – The evolution of a synthetic membrane for renal therapy,* edited by Berlyne GM, Giovannetti S, Basel, Karger, Contrib Nephrol 96: 26-46, 1992

10. Holland FF, Gidden HE, Mason RG, Klein E: Thrombogenicity of heparin-bound DEAE cellulose hemodialysis membranes. ASAIO Journal 1: 24-36, 1978

11. Nakagawa K, Inagaki O, Saian Y, Fujita Y: A study on heparin adsorption in Hemophan membrane dialyzer. Kidney 15: 71, 1992

12. Ward RA, Schmidt B, Gurland HJ: Prevention of blood loss in dialysers with DEAE-cellulose membranes does not require increased doses of heparin. Nephrol Dial Transplant 8: 1140-1145, 1993

13. Debrand-Passard A, Lajous-Petter A, Schmidt R, Herbst R, von Baeyer H, Krause AA, Schiffl H: Thrombogenicity of dialyzer membranes as assessed by residual blood volume and surface morphology at different heparin dosages in: *Improvements in dialysis therapy,* edited by Baldamus CA, Mion C, Shaldon S, Basel, Karger, Contrib Nephrol 74: 2-9, 1989

14. Verbeelen D, Jochmans K, Herman AG, Van der Niepen P, Sennesael J, De Waele M: Evaluation of platelets and hemostasis during hemodialysis with six different membranes. Nephron 59: 567-572, 1991

15. Oosterhuis WP, de Metz M, Wadham A, Daha MR, Go RH: In vivo evaluation of four hemodialysis membranes: biocompatibility and clearances. Dialysis & Transplantation 24(8): 450-458, 1995

16. Hoenich NA, Woffindin C, Stamp S, Roberts SJ, Turnbull J: Synthetically modified cellulose: an alternative to synthetic membranes for use in haemodialysis? Biomaterials 18: 1299-1303, 1997

17. Cases A, Reverter JC, Escolar G, Sanz C, Lopez-Pedret J, Revert L, Ordinas A: Platelet activation on hemodialysis: influence of dialysis membranes. Kidney Int 43(Suppl 41): S217-S220, 1993

18. Cases A, Reverter JC, Escolar G, Sanz C, Sorribes J, Ordinas A: *In vivo* evaluation of platelet activation by different cellulosic membranes. Artif Organs 21(4): 330-334, 1997

19. Kroll MH, Hellums JD, McIntire LV, Schafer AI, Moake JL: Platelets and shear stress. Blood 88(5): 1525-1541, 1996

20. Lins LE, Boberg U, Jacobson SH, Kjellstrand C, Ljungberg B, Skroder R: The influence of dialyzer geometry on blood coagulation and biocompatibility. Clin Nephrol 40(5): 281-285, 1993

21. Müller TF, Seitz M, Eckle I, Lange H, Kolb G: Biocompatibility differences with respect to the dialyzer sterilization method. Nephron 78: 139-142, 1998

22. Rabelink TJ, Zwaginga JJ, Koomans HA, Sixma JJ: Thrombosis and hemostasis in renal disease. Kidney Int 46: 287-296, 1994

23. Fareed J, Bick RL, Hoppenstaedt DA, Bermes EW: Molecular markers of hemostatic activation: applications in the diagnosis of thrombosis and vascular thrombotic disorders. Clin Appl Thrombosis/Hemostasis 1(2): 87-102, 1995

24. Hofbauer R, Moser D, Frass M, Oberbauer R, Kaye A, Wagner O, Kapiotis S, Druml W: Effect of anticoagulation on blood membrane interactions during hemodialysis. Kidney Int 56: 1578-1583, 1999

25. Sperschneider H, Deppisch R, Beck W, Wolf H, Stein G: Impact of membrane choice and blood flow pattern on coagulation and heparin requirement-potential consequences on lipid concentrations. Nephrol Dial Transplant 12: 2638-2646, 1997

26. Vienken J, Diamantoglou, Hahn C, Kamusewitz H, Paul D: Considerations in developmental aspects of biocompatible dialysis membranes. Artif Organs 19 (5): 398-406, 1995

27. Falkenhagen D, Bosch T, Brown GS, Schmidt B, Holtz M, Baurmeister U, Gurland H, Klinkmann H: A clinical study on different cellulosic dialysis membranes. Nephrol Dial Transplant 2(6): 537-545, 1987

28. Schaefer RM, Hörl WH, Gilge U, Konrad G, Heidland A: Biocompatibility profile of the polysulfone 400 membrane in: *Improvement in Dialysis Therapy.* edited by: Baldamus CA, Mion C, Shaldon S. Contrib Nephrol 74 Karger, Basel: 43-51, 1989

29. Rauterberg EW, Ritz E, Schulze H, Rother KO: Limited derivatisation of Cuprophan increases factor H binding and diminishes complement activation. (Abstract) Kidney Int 31: 243, 1987

30. Pascual M, Schifferli JA: Adsorption of complement factor D by polyacrylonitrile membranes. Kidney Int 43: 903-911, 1993

31. Pascual M, Schifferli JA, Pannatier JG, Wauters JP: Removal of complement factor D by adsorption of polymethacrylate dialysis membranes. Nephrol Dial Transplant 8: 1305-1306, 1993

32. Cheung AK, Parker CJ, Wilcox L, Janatova J: Activation of the alternative pathway of complement by cellulosic hemodialysis membranes. Kidney Int 36: 257-265, 1989

33. Deppisch R, Göhl H, Smeby L: Microdomain structure of polymeric surfaces - potential for improving blood treatment procedures. Nephrol Dial Transplant 13: 1354-1359, 1998

34. Cheung AK, Parker CJ, Wilcox L, Janatova J: Activation of complement by hemodialysis membranes: polyacrylonitrile binds more C3a than cuprophan. Kidney Int 37: 1055-1059, 1990

35. Jorstad S, Smeby LC, Balstad T, Wideroe TE: Generation and removal of anaphylatoxins during hemofiltration with five different membranes. Blood Purif 6: 325-335, 1988

36. Falkenhagen D, Brown GS, Boettcher M, Falkenhagen U, Schmidt B, Gurland HJ, Klinkmann H: Permeation of complement factors through high-flux dialyzers and plasma separation membranes in: *Therapeutic plasma exchange and selective plasma separation*, edited by Bambauer R, Malchesky PS, Falkenhagen D, Stuttgart, Schattauer-Verlag: 215-222, 1987

37. Kaiser J, Opperman M, Gotze O, Deppisch R, Göhl H, Asmus G, Rohricht B, von Herrath D, Schaefer K: Significant reduction of factor D and immunosupressive complement fragment Ba by haemofiltration. Blood Purif 13: 314-321, 1995

38. Deppisch R, Ritz E, Hänsch GM, Schöls M, Rauterberg EW: Bioincompatibility-perspectives 1993. Kidney Int 45(Suppl 44): S77-S84, 1994

39. Deppisch R, Schmitt V, Bommer J, Hänsch GM, Ritz E, Rauterberg EW: Fluid phase generation of terminal complement complex as a novel index of biocompatibility. Kidney Int 37: 696-706, 1990

40. Meier P, von Fliedner V, Markert M, van Melle G, Deppisch R, Wauters J-P: One-year immunological evaluation of chronic hemodialysis in end-stage renal disease patients. Blood Purif 18: 128-137, 2000

41. Ohi H, Tamano M, Sudo S: Cellulose membranes suppress complement activation in patients after hemodialysis. Am J Kidney Dis 38(2): 384-389, 2001

42. Hörl WH: Hemodialysis membranes: interleukins, biocompatibility, and middle molecules. J Am Soc Nephrol 13: S62-S71, 2002

43. Klinkmann H, Buscaroli A, Stefoni S: $ß_2$microglobulin and low-flux synthetic dialyzers. Artif Organs 22(7): 585-590, 1998

44. Hoenich NA, Stamp S: Clinical investigation of the role of membrane structure on blood contact and solute transport characteristics of a cellulose membrane. Biomaterials 21: 317-324, 2000

45. Rosenkranz AR, Körmöczi GF, Thalhammer F, Menzel EJ, Hörl WH, Mayer G, Zlabinger GJ: Novel C5-dependent mechanism of neutrophil stimulation by bioincompatible dialyzer membranes. J Am Soc Nephrol 10: 128-135, 1999

46. Carracedo J, Ramírez R, Madueno JA, Soriano S, Rodríguez-Benot A, Rodríguez M, Martín-Malo A, Aljama P: Cell apoptosis and hemodialysis-induced inflammation. Kidney Int 61(Suppl 80): S89-S93, 2002

47. Sirolli V, Ballone E, Amoroso L, Di Liberato L, Di Mascio R, Capelli P, Albertazzi A, Bonomini M. Leukocyte adhesion molecules and leukocyte-platelet interactions during hemodialysis: effects of different synthetic membranes. Int J Artif Organs 22(8): 536-542, 1999

48. Bonomini M, Sirolli V, Settefrati N, Stuard S, Tropea F, Di Liberato L, Tetta C, Albertazzi A: Surface antigen expression and platelet neutrophil interactions in haemodialysis. Blood Purif 17: 107-117, 1999

49. Ross R: The pathogenesis of atherosclerosis: a perspective for the 1990s. Nature 362: 801-809, 1993

50. Konishi Y, Okamura M, Konishi M, Negoro N, Yoshida T, Inoue T, Kanayama Y, Yoshikawa J: Enhanced gene expression of scavanger receptor in peripheral blood monocytes from patients on cuprophane haemodialysis. Nephrol Dial Transplant 12: 1167-1172, 1997

51. Nahar N, Shah H, Siu J, Colvin R, Bhaskaran M, Ranjan R, Wagner JD, Singhal PC: Dialysis membrane-induced neutrophil apoptosis is mediated through free radicals. Clin Nephrol 56(1): 52-59, 2001

52. Rosenkranz AR, Peherstorfer E, Kormoczi GF, Zlabinger GJ, Mayer G, Hörl WH, Oberbauer R: Complement-dependent acceleration of apoptosis in neutrophils by dialyzer membranes. Kidney Int (Suppl2): S216-220, 2001

53. Martín-Malo A, Carracedo J, Ramírez R, Rodríguez-Benot A, Soriano S, Rodríguez M, Aljama P: Effect of uremia and dialysis modality on mononuclear cell apoptosis. J Am Soc Nephrol 11: 936-942, 2000

54. Nguyen-Khoa T, Massy ZA, De Bandt JP, Kebede M, Salama L, Lambrey G, Witko-Sarsat V, Drüeke TB, Lacour B, Thévenin M: Oxidative stress and haemodialysis: role of inflammation and duration of dialysis treatment. Nephrol Dial Transplant 16: 335-340, 2001

55. Weinstein T, Chagnac A, Korzets A, Boaz M, Ori Y, Herman M, Malachi T, Gafter U: Haemolysis in haemodialysis patients: evidence for impaired defense mechanisms against oxidative stress. Nephrol Dial Transplant 15: 883-887, 2000

56. Himmelfarb J, McMonagle E: Manifestations of oxidant stress in uremia. Blood Purif 19: 200-205, 2001

57. Nourooz-Zadeh J: Effect of dialysis on oxidative stress in uremia. Redox Rep 4 (1-2): 17-22, 1999

58. Morena M, Cristol JP, Canaud B: Why hemodialysis patients are in a pro-oxidant state? What could be done to correct the pro/antioxidant imbalance. Blood Purif 18(3): 191-199, 2000

59. Canaud B, Cristol J, Morena M, Leray-Moragues H, Bosc J, Vaussenat F: Imbalance of oxidants and antioxidants in haemodialysis patients. Blood Purif 17(2-3): 99-106, 1999

60. Himmelfarb J, Ault KA, Holbrook D, Leeber DA, Hakim RM: Intradialytic granulocyte reactive oxygen species production: a prospective, crossover trial. J Am Soc Nephrol 4(2): 178-186, 1993

61. Vanholder R, Ringoir S, Dhondt A, Hakim R, Waterloos MA, Van Lantschoot N, Gung A: Phagocytosis in uremic and hemodialysis patients: a prospective and cross sectional study. Kidney Int 39: 320-327, 1991

62. Ritz E, Deppisch R, Steir E, Hansch G. Atherogenesis and cardiac death: are they related to dialysis procedure and biocompatibility? Nephrol Dial Transplant 2: 165-172, 1994

63. Kosch M, Levers A, Fobker M, Barenbrock M, Schaefer RM, Rahn KH, Hausberg M: Dialysis filter type determines the acute effect of haemodialysis on endothelial function and oxidative stress. Nephrol Dial Transplant 18: 1370–1375, 2003

64. Galli F, Canestrari F, Buoncristiani U: Biological effects of oxidant stress in haemodialysis: the possible roles of vitamin E. Blood Purif 17(2-3): 79-94, 1999

65. Bonnefont-Rousselot D, Lehmann E, Jaudon M-C, Delattre J, Perrone B, Rechke J-P: Blood oxidative stress and lipoprotein oxidizability in haemodialysis patients: effect of the use of a vitamin E-coated dialysis membrane. Nephrol Dial Transplant 1: 2020-2028, 2000

66. Galli F, Rovidati S, Chiarantini L, Campus G, Canestrari F, Buoncristiani U: Bioreactivity and biocompatibility of a vitamin E-modified multilayer hemodialysis filter. Kidney Int 54: 580-589, 1998

67. Satoh M, Yamasaki Y, Nagake Y, Kasahara I, Hashimoto M, Nakanishi N, Makino H: Oxidative stress is reduced by the long-term use of vitamin E-coated dialysis filters. Kidney Int 59: 1943-1950, 2001

68. Clermont G, Lecour S, Cabanne JF, Motte G, Guilland JC, Chevet D, Rochette L: Vitamin E-coated dialyzer reduces oxidative stress in hemodialysis patients. Free Radic Bio Med 31(2): 233-241, 2001

69. Eiselt J, Racek J, Trefil L, Opatrný K: Effects of vitamin E-modified dialysis membrane and vitamin C infusion on oxidative stress in hemodialysis patients. Artif Organs 26 (6): 430-436, 2001

70. Fett JW, Strydom DJ, Lobb RR, Alderman EM, Bethune JL, Riordan JF, Vallee BL: Isolation and characterization of angiogenin, an angiogenic protein from human carcinoma cells: Biochemistry 24: 5480-5486, 1985

71. Schmaldienst S, Hörl WH: Degranulation of polymorphonuclear leukocytes by dialysis membranes – the mystery clears up? Nephrol Dial Transplant 15: 1909-1910, 2000

72. Pereira BJG, Shapiro L, King AJ, Falagas ME, Strom JA, Dinarello CA: Plasma levels of IL-1ß, TNFα and their specific inhibitors in undialyzed, chronic renal failure, CAPD, and hemodialysis patients. Kidney Int 45: 890-896, 1994

73. Haeffner-Cavaillon N, Cavaillon JM, Ciancioni C, Bacle F, Delons S, Kazatchkine MD: In vivo induction of interleukin-1 during hemodialysis. Kidney Int 35: 1212-1218, 1989

74. Bingel M, Lonnemann G, Koch KM, Dinarello CA, Shaldon S: Plasma interleukin-1 activity during hemodialysis: the influence of dialysis membranes. Nephron 50: 273-276, 1988

75. Lin YF, Chang DM, Shaio MF, Lu KC, Chyr SH, Li BL, Sheih SD: Cytokine production during hemodialysis: effects of dialytic membrane and complement activation. Am J Nephrol 16: 293-299, 1996

76. Varela MP, Kimmel PL, Phillips TM, Mishkin GJ, Lew SQ, Bosch JP: Biocompatibility of hemodialysis membranes: interrelations between plasma complement and cytokine levels. Blood Purif 19: 370-379, 2001

77. Schindler R, Gelfand JA, Dinarello CA: Recombinant C5a stimulates transcription rather than translation of IL-1 and TNF; translational signal provided by LPS or IL-1 itself. Blood 76: 1631-1638, 1990

78. Haeffner CN, Cavaillon JM, Laude M, Kazatchkine MD: C3a (C3a desArg) induces production and release of interleukin 1 by cultured human monocytes. J Immunol 139: 794-799, 1987

79. Wilde CG, Seilhamer JJ, McGrogan M et al.: Bactericidal/permeability-increasing protein and lipopolysaccharide (LPS)-binding protein. J Biol Chem 269: 17411-17416, 1994

80. Abel G, Czop JK: Stimulation of human monocyte beta glucan receptors by glucan particles induces production of TNF alpha and IL-1 beta. Int J Immunopharmacol 14: 1363-1373, 1992

81. Mahiout A, Lonnemann G, Schulze M, Schindler R, Shaldon S, Koch KM: Low molecular weight, LAL-negative substances from *Pseudomonas* induce cytokines from mononuclear cells. (Abstract) J Am Soc Nephrol 1: 367, 1990

82. Bingel M, Lonnemann G, Koch KM, Dinarello CA, Shaldon S: Enhancement of in-vitro human interleukin-1 production by sodium acetate. Lancet 1: 14-16, 1987

83. Cappelli G, DiFelice A, Perrone S, Ballestri M, Bonucchi D, Savazzi AM, Ciuffreda A, Lusvarghi E: Which level of cytokine production is critical in haemodialysis. Nephrol Dial Transplant 13(Suppl 7): 55-60, 1998

84. Okusawa S, Dinarello CA, Yancey KB, Endres S, Lawley TJ, Frank MM, Burke JF, Gelfand JA: C5a induction of human interleukin 1: Synergistic effect with endotoxin or interferon-γ. J Immunol 139(8): 2635-2640, 1987

85. Qian J, Yu Z, Dai H, Zhang Q, Chen S: Influence of hemodialysis membranes on gene expression and plasma levels of interleukin-1. Artif Organs 19(8): 842-846, 1995

86. Lonnemann G, Behme TC, Lenzner B, Floege J, Schulze M, Colton CK, Koch KM, Shaldon S: Permeability of dialyzer membranes to TNFα-inducing substances derived from water bacteria. Kidney Int 42: 61-68, 1992

87. Lonnemann, G, Koch KM, Shaldon S, Dinarello CA: Studies on the ability of hemodialysis membranes to induce, bind, and clear human interleukin-1. J Lab Clin Med 112: 76-86, 1988

88. Girndt M, Heisel O, Köhler H: Influence of dialysis with polyamide vs haemophan haemodialysers on monokines and complement activation during a 4-month long-term study. Nephrol Dial Transplant 14: 676-682, 1999

89. Kushihata S, Yorioka N, Oda H, Ye XF, Yamakido M: Effects of dialysis membranes on the kinetics of tumor necrosis factor-α production by peripheral mononuclear cells in chronic hemodialysis patients. J Artif Organs 21(7): 384-390, 1998

90. Mahiout A, Courtney JM: Effect of dialyser membranes on extracellular and intracellular granulocyte and monocyte activation in *ex vivo* pyrogen-free conditions. Biomaterials 15: 969-980, 1994

91. Lonnemann G, Barndt I, Kaever V, Haubitz M, Schindler R, Shaldon S, Koch KM: Impaired endotoxin-induced interleukin-1ß secretion, not total production, of mononuclear cells from ESRD patients. Kidney Int 47: 1158-1167, 1995

92. Linnenweber S, Lonnemann G: Effects of dialyzer membrane on interleukin-1ß (IL-1ß) and IL-1ß-converting enzyme in mononuclear cells. Kidney Int 59(Suppl 78): S282-S285, 2001

93. Memoli B, Marzano L, Biseti V, Andreucci M, Guida B: Hemodialysis-related lymphomononuclear release of interleukin-12 in patients with end-stage renal disease. J Am Soc Nephrol 10: 2171-2176, 1999

94. Schindler R, Senf R, Frei U: Influencing the inflammatory response of haemodialysis patients by cytokine elimination using large-pore membranes. Nephrol Dial Transplant 17: 17-19, 2002

95. Bouman CSC, van Olden RW, Stoutenbeek CP: Cytokine filtration and adsorption during pre- and postdilution hemopfiltration in four different membranes. Blood Purif 16: 261-268, 1998

96. Lonnemann G, Novick D, Rubinstein M, Passlick-Deetjen J, Lang D, Dinarello CA: A switch to high-flux Helixone® membranes reverses suppressed interferon-γ production in patients on low-flux dialysis. Blood Purif 21: 225-231, 2003

97. Schouten WEM, Grooteman MPC, van Houte A-J, Schoorl M, van Limbeek J, Nubé MJ: Effects of dialyser and dialysate on the acute phase reaction in clinical bicarbonate dialysis. Nephrol Dial Transplant 15: 379-384, 2000

98. Pecoits-Filho R, Bárány P, Lindholm B, Heimbürger O, Stenvinkel P: Interleukin-6 is an independent predictor of mortality in patients starting dialysis treatment. Nephrol Dial Transplant 17(9): 1684-1688, 2002

99. Wanner C, Metzger T: C-reactive protein a marker for all-cause and cardiovascular mortality in haemodialysis patients. Nephrol Dial Transplant 17(Suppl 8): 29-32, 2002

100. Memoli B, Minutolo R, Bisesti V, Postiglione L, Conti A, Marzano L, Capuano A, Andreucci M, Balletta MM, Guida B, Tetta C: Changes of serum albumin and C-reactive protein are related to changes of interleukin-6 release by peripheral blood mononuclear cells in hemodialysis patients treated with different membranes. Am J Kidney Dis 39(2): 266-273, 2002

101. Memoli B, Postiglione L, Cianciaruso B, Bisesti V, Cimmaruta C, Marzano L, Minutolo R, Cuomo V, Guida B, Andreucci M, Rossi G: Role of different dialysis membranes in the release of interleukin-6-soluble receptor in uremic patients. Kidney Int 58(1): 417-424, 2000

102. Memoli B, Libetta C, Rampino T, Dal Canton A, Conte G, Scala O, Ruocco MR, Andreucci M: Hemodialysis related induction of interleukin-6 production by peripheral blood mononuclear cells. Kidney Int 42: 320-326, 1992

103. Schindler R, Boenisch O, Fischer C, Frei U: Effect of the hemodialysis membrane on the inflammatory reaction *in vivo*. Clin Nephrol 53(6): 452-459, 2000

104. Sitter T, Bergner A, Schiffl H: Dialysate related cytokine induction and response to recombinant human erythropoietin in haemodialysis patients. Nephrol Dial Transplant 15: 1207-1211, 2000

105. Renaux JL, Thomas M, Crost T, Loughraieb N, Vantard G: Activation of the kallikrein-kinin system in hemodialysis: role of membrane electronegativity, blood dilution, and pH. Kidney Int 55(3): 1097-1103, 1999

106. Schaefer RM, Schaefer L, Hörl WH: Anaphylactoid reactions during hemodialysis. Clin Nephrol 42(Suppl 1): S44-S47, 1994

107. Verresen L, Fink E, Lemke HD, Vanrenterghem Y: Bradykinin is a mediator of anaphylactoid reactions during hemodialysis with AN69 membranes. Kidney Int 45: 1497- 1503, 1994

108. Krieter DH, Grude M, Lemke HD, Fink E, Bönner G, Schölkens BA, Schulz E, Müller GA: Anaphylactoid reactions during hemodialysis in sheep are ACE inhibitor dose-dependent and mediated by bradykinin. Kidney Int 53: 1026-1035, 1998

109. Mannstadt M, Touam M, Fink E, Urena P, Hruby M, Zingraff J, Uhlenbusch-Körwer I, Grassman A, Lemke HD, Drüeke T: No generation of bradykinin with a new polyacrilonitrile membrane (SPAN) in haemodialysis patients treated with ACE inhibitors. Nephrol Dial Transplant 10: 1696-1700, 1995

110. Wakasa M, Akizawa T, Kinugasa E, Koshikawa S: Plasma bradykinin levels during hemodialysis with PAN DX and polysulfone membranes with and without concurrent ACE inhibitor. Clin Nephrol 44(Suppl 1): S29-S32, 1995

111. Akizawa T, Kinugasa E, Wakasa M, Kohjiro S, Koiwa F, Koshikawa S: Effect of dialysis membranes and ACE inhibitor on bradykinin levels during hemodialysis. Clin Nephrol 41(4): 241-244, 1994.

112. Schwarzbeck A, Wittenmeier KW, Hällfritsch U, Frank J: Anaphylatoid reactions (AR) associated with PMMA high flux dialyzers (HDF) and ACE- Inhibitors (ACE-I). Nephron 65: 499-500, 1993

113. Des Grottes J-M, Molinaro G, Adam A, Muniz M-C, Nortier J, Thomas M, Tielemans C: A new type of adverse reactions (AR) during hemodialysis (HD) on AN69 hollow fiber dialysers. Solving the problem by a different membrane treatment procedure with polyethylene imine (PEI) (Abstract). J Am Soc Nephrol 13: 579A, 2002

Section D. Clinical experience

9. Acute adverse reactions associated with dialyser choice

This chapter is devoted to a discussion of acute reactions associated with dialyser characteristics, whereby acute reactions are defined as those occurring during and/or shortly after the dialysis session. Dialyser performance is characterised by the diffusive and convective removal of uraemic toxins, and is thus a key determinant of dialysis efficiency. The dialyser performance must then be carefully chosen so as to prevent the occurrence of disequilibrium, especially in children and elderly patients. Furthermore, the biocompatibility of the system is not only affected by the choice of membrane polymer, but also by substances which stem from manufacturing, sterilisation and reprocessing processes. These processes are known to influence the occurrence of acute intra- or postdialysis symptoms (details follow).

A wide range of clinical symptoms may occur during and/or shortly after completion of dialysis. Some of these may be caused by particular characteristics of the dialyser. In general, such acute dialyser reactions are not common, and their incidence has even decreased over the past decades due to progress in large-scale dialyser manufacturing and due to new developments in reprocessing techniques. However, when acute reactions occur, almost any organ can be involved, and symptoms can be mild to life-threatening [1-3]. Primarily, biocompatibility characteristics of the dialyser or haemofilter have been identified as causes of dialyser reactions, but performance characteristics can sometimes (albeit very rarely) be responsible. Knowledge of typical manifestations of acute dialyser reactions, their aetiologies, patient-specific interactions and ways of prevention is necessary for Good Dialysis Practice. In this context, patient observation by experienced staff during treatment and professional documentation and reporting of dialyser reactions are indispensable.

What role does dialyser performance play in dialysis-induced acute clinical symptoms?

High quality industrial dialyser production and dialysis machine technology protect the patient from failures in dialyser performance during treatment. For example, blood leakage is extremely rare in new dialysers, and the blood leak detectors and alarms integrated into the dialysis circuit provide additional protection against blood loss.

However, the choice of dialyser with respect to its clearance properties must suit the particular clinical situation. Furthermore, other parameters of dialysis efficiency have to be considered when choosing fibre polymer type and/or membrane surface area: for example, the achievable blood and dialysis fluid flows, the length of the treatment and the dialysis fluid composition. Membrane surface area is of particular importance regarding the avoidance of extremely rapid solute transfer during the treatment; this results in an excessively fast correction of acidosis, drastic reductions in urea levels and unphysiological electrolyte changes during the treatment, predisposing the patient to dialysis disequilibrium or other adverse effects of disturbed electrolyte balance [4, 5]. When older dialysis machines without automatic ultrafiltration control are used, choosing a dialyser with an inappropriately high hydraulic permeability for a given body weight and/or dialysis efficiency may lead to acute adverse patient reactions, especially in children and in adults with low body weight. For children, the volume of blood in the extracorporeal circuit (consisting of the priming volume of the dialyser (see list in appendix) and the volume of the blood tubing set) should not exceed 8 ml/kg bodyweight or 8-10% of the patient's total blood volume, for example. Failure to adhere to these values can cause hypotension and collapse at the start of treatment, and hypertension after reinfusion of the extracorporeal volume at the end dialysis [6, 7]. Consequently, dialysers used for paediatric haemodialysis are normally $< 1\ m^2$ in surface area. Parallel-plate dialysers have a slightly higher priming volume per unit of membrane surface area than hollow fibre devices [8].

What role does filter biocompatibility play in dialysis-induced acute clinical symptoms?

Today, the term "dialyser reactions" is generally used for a wide spectrum of clinical symptoms that occur during or shortly after dialysis and are associated with the *biocompatibility characteristics* of certain types of dialysers. Here it must be born in mind that the biocompatibility of the whole dialyser is the sum of several variables: the different materials used during production (e.g. membrane polymer, potting compound), and the effects of different manufacturing, sterilisation and, eventually, reprocessing techniques on the natures of these materials.

What role does patient disposition play in dialysis-induced acute clinical symptoms?

A number of patient susceptibility factors may predispose the patient to adverse effects, depending on dialyser or haemofilter biocompatibility characteristics (e.g. sterilisation mode or membrane polymer). Examples of such susceptibility factors are particular types of medication and individual degrees of atopy. Younger age, female gender, some race characteristics (blacks and other minorities) and some causes for ESRD (polycystic renal disease and glomerulonephritis) have been found to be predisposing factors for hypersensitivity and/or anaphylactoid reactions, for example [9, 10]. Therefore, an adverse reaction that occurs in one individual patient during a single dialysis session with a particular dialyser must first be analysed in detail in order to identify the underlying cause and prevent future occurrence. Furthermore, conscientious documentation and reporting of dialyser reactions are indispensable in Good Dialysis Practice; these practices constitute important tools for analysis, therapy and prevention of future reactions – not only for the individual patient, but for the dialysis community as a whole. The more specific or severe a dialyser-induced reaction is, or the greater the number of patients involved, then the higher is the probability that it will be identified and reported [9, 10, 11, 12].

What complicates the reporting of dialyser reactions?

Many symptoms may occur during dialysis. These are mainly associated with the removal of excess fluid, but may also be due to electrolyte imbalances or accompanying illnesses. Dialysis patients are frequently multimorbid, with decreased cardiac function and vascular reactivity. Furthermore, contaminated dialysis fluid, reuse or inadequate dialyser prerinsing may lead to clinical reactions that resemble "pure" dialyser reactions. Consequently, intradialysis symptoms directly attributable to the dialyser must first be recognised as such before their causes can be reported. This requires special education and motivation of the dialysis staff as well time for reporting.

The reporting of dialyser-associated intradialysis symptoms is, however, complicated by differences in perception, staff reaction and the efficiency of the recording system [9-11]. Staff- and patient-reported symptoms may even differ substantially, both for objective symptoms (e.g. hypotension and cramps) and subjective symptoms (e.g. chest pain, back pain and itching). Such discrepancies between staff and patient statements were also found to vary depending on the location of the dialysis centres studied (Chicago, Detroit, Osaka, Rostock, Stockholm) [11].

9.1 Clinical manifestations

Typically, acute dialyser reactions are clinically manifested by their sudden appearance. They usually occur shortly after initiation of dialysis but, in some rare cases, they appear later on in the session or even up to several hours after completion of treatment. The severity of the reactions ranges from mild to life-threatening and symptoms may affect almost any organ system.

Two main subgroups of acute intradialysis reactions have been characterised: Type I and Type II [13, 14] or, alternatively, Type A (anaphylactic) and Type B reactions [15].

The symptomatology of Type A reactions is similar to that of hypersensitivity reactions. These reactions occur either immediately or between 5 and 20-30 (maximum) minutes after dialysis start. Other terms often used for this symptom complex in the observational literature are "first use syndrome", "anaphylactic reactions" or "anaphylactoid reactions", regardless of the cause of the symptoms. Per definition, however, hypersensitivity reactions are only those mediated by preformed antibodies (e.g. IgE) *or* primed cells. Similar reactions with direct complement activation (C3, C5a) but in the absence of specific IgE should, strictly speaking, be termed "anaphylactoid" [16]. Symptoms range from a feeling of warmth (at the fistula site or throughout the body), itching, urticaria, flushing, nausea, chest tightness, dyspnoe to severe reactions, such as abdominal cramps, laryngeal oedema, respiratory and cardiac arrest. In a survey of Type A reactions in 1982/83, the number of such reactions was estimated to be 3.3 and 0.3 per 1000 patients for hollow fibre dialysers and plate dialysers, respectively. According to manufacturers' sales figures, this corresponds to 4.3 and 0.2 reactions, respectively, per 100,000 dialysers sold [9]. In this study, 46.9% of the reactions reported occurred with the first use of a dialyser, but were associated with a 38.5% non-compliance to manufacturers prerinsing recommendations. A review of the incidence of

Type A reactions ten years later (1992 -published in 1999) found much higher numbers: 7 episodes per 1000 patients per year (6 month surveillance of 20,228 patients [10]). This difference in incidence may be due to underreporting, changes in treatment, or other factors that warrant further study. At first, the 1992 study appeared to confirm the suspicion initially aroused that the single or first use of a dialyser was associated with an increased incidence of acute reactions. However, no data were supplied in this study regarding the possible causes of the acute reactions reported, e.g. dialysis fluid bacterial and endotoxin levels, dialysis fluid composition, dialyser sterilisation modes, the dialyser prerinsing practice or the accompanying medication. Therefore, the question of whether first use is associated with an increased risk of acute dialyser reactions remains unanswered, especially when referring to the many clinical reactions reported in association with different reuse practises [12, 17-23], see also **table 12.3**.

Seen clinically, Type B reactions are not anaphylactoid in nature: they usually occur later in the course of a session (approximately 20-30 minutes after dialysis start) and are frequently associated with (often tolerable) chest or back pain. These reactions appear to have almost disappeared over the past years [24].

In addition to Type A and Type B reactions, a number of less acute symptoms are also believed to be associated with dialyser bioincompatibility. Examples are pruritus, hypoxaemia during dialysis, and some postdialysis reactions, such as debility and fatigue. Since the introduction of the "Interleukin Hypothesis" in the early eighties, an additional negative effect of dialyser bioincompatibility on cardiovascular response during dialysis was suspected [25]. However, this has not yet been proven.

Other dialyser reactions that develop later rather than early during treatment are mainly ophthalmologic and otologic in nature (although neurological and even cardiac symptoms have also been reported). Examples are scleritis and iritis ("red eye syndrome"), tinnitus and/or hearing loss, and sometimes even vertigo, headache, confusion, lethargy, paresthesia, ostealgia, myalgia and even cardiac arrest (2 cases). All of these are rare and occurred during or several hours after the use of certain cellulose acetate membranes [12, 26-28]. Finally, after 40 years of dialyser development and the availability of many safe, high-quality dialysers, the dialysis community suffered a deep setback in the year 2001: despite today's high-quality dialyser technology and controls, a number of fatal incidents occurred that were caused by dialyser constituents. Two months after the first announcement of 11 patient deaths in

Spanish hospitals in August 2001, 23 patients were reported to have died in Croatia [29-32] and, somewhat later, 40 in India, 7 in Taiwan, 5 in Germany, 4 in Italy and the USA and 2 in Colombia [29, 30]. All patients were dialysed with the Althane membrane (cellulose acetate) in dialysers from Baxter (series A-15, A-18, AF150, AF180, and AF220). Before death due to shock during treatment or due to cardio-circulatory problems some hours after the treatment [29, 31, 32], the patients exhibited the following symptoms: sweating, nausea, vomiting and, in general, a presyncopal state [33]. The first reports led only to a recall of the batches in question [33], with the first investigations into possible causes conducted in Spain failing to show any causal relationship between the A-18 dialysers used and the fatal outcome [32, 34]. However, the second wave of incidents in Croatia led to a worldwide recall of the dialysers in question [33]. At present, residues of perfluorohydrocarbon [30, 32, 35, 36] and of perfluoroheptane [35] used by Baxter in Ronneby, Sweden, for membrane integrity testing [30, 32] and - as suspected by other authors - probably also for membrane repair [35, 36] is believed to be the cause of the incidents (see chapter 9.2.1.2 for further details).

Table 9.1a and b provides an overview of acute dialyser reactions, their incidence and their clinical manifestations. Possible aetiologies and approaches towards prevention, as far as known to date, are also listed – these will be discussed in the following chapters.

9.2 Aetiology and prevention

The first reactions described in association with specific dialysers were termed "first-use syndrome" and were observed during use of new regenerated cellulose dialysers [55]. This syndrome comprised a broad spectrum of reactions, including hypersensivity, anaphylactoid (e.g. pruritus, urticaria, dyspnoe, chest tightness) and less well-defined adverse reactions of unknown aetiology (e.g. hypotension, fatigue, headache) [24]. Later, similar symptoms were also reported in association with certain dialyser constituents, reused dialysers, other membranes and, particular patient dispositions (see **table 9.1a and b**).

Figure 9.1 summarises the main factors contributing to dialyser reactions, as far as known to date. The provoked symptoms can be roughly related to several different pathophysiological pathways: hypersensitivity reactions, activation of the complement system, bradykinin generation (described in

Acute adverse reactions	Type A	Type B
Incidence	Approx. 5 per 100,000 dialysers sold [24], approx. 3.3 per 1000 patients per year [9], 7 per 1000 patients per year [10]	3-5 per 100 dialysis treatments [24] Disappearing entity
Onset	Immediately or within the first 5 mins of dialysis, onsets up to 20-30 minutes are possible	Within first 60 mins of dialysis
Manifestations	Chest tightness up to cardiac arrest Dyspnoe, angio-oedema, laryngeal oedema up to respiratory arrest Swelling, fullness in mouth and throat Burning, heat sensation Urticaria, itching Rhinorrhea, sneezing, coughing, lacrimation Nausea, vomiting, abdominal cramps	Chest pain, often accompanied by back pain, abating after the first hour of dialysis
Severity	Moderate to severe	Mild to moderate

Acute adverse reactions	Type A	Type B
Aetiology	• EtO hypersensivity: IgE to EtO-altered protein • AN69® membrane-related: increased bradykinin generation • ACE inhibitors: decreased degradation of kinins, substance P • Reuse: reprocessing chemicals?, endotoxins? • Leachable materials used in membrane processing: toxic chemicals? • Regenerated cellulose membranes: complement generation?, thromboxane? • Azide: toxic effect of azide • Contaminated dialysis fluid: endotoxins? • Acetate: adenosine/ thromboxane?	• Complement generation? • Is acetate a necessary co-factor?
Treatment	Stop dialysis immediately Do not return blood Epinephrine Antihistamines Nasal oxygen application, respiratory support if needed	Continue dialysis, no specific treatment

Prevention	• Prerinse the dialyser immediately prior to use according to the stipulations of the manufacturer; this enhances the removal of compounds that may leach from filter materials [37]. • If the AN69® membrane is suspected as being the cause, change to another membrane [37] or, if clinically possible, consider stopping ACE inhibitor therapy. Alternatively, try an alkaline prerinsing of the dialyser [38, 39] or prescribe an AT_1 receptor blocker instead of an ACE inhibitor. • If EtO is suspected as being the cause, change to a gamma-sterilised or steam-sterilised dialysers and tubing systems [37]. • If EtO and AN69® are not likely causes for the reaction, and if the reaction is in an atopic individual, consider changing from acetate to bicarbonate dialysis fluid. • Check endotoxin levels in final dialysis fluid, RO water and bicarbonate concentrates [37]. • Check endotoxin levels in water used for reuse procedures; consider stopping use of bleach or hydrogen peroxide [12] or consider stopping reuse.	• Use a membrane with a low complement-activating potential?

Table 9.1a: Characteristics, aetiology and possible methods of prevention of Type A and B dialyser-associated reactions*.* *Possible contributions of contaminated dialysis fluid, acetate dialysis fluid and patient medication with ACE inhibitors to these symptoms are also indicated. EtO: ethylene oxide; AN69®: dialyser membrane made from polyacrylonitrile.*

	All dialysers			Certain cellulose acetate dialysers	
	Hypoxaemia	**Pruritus**	**Postdialysis fatigue**	**Ophthalmological, otological and other symptoms**	**Deaths reported in year 2001**
Incidence	Common in acetate HD [40, 41], but also found in bicarbonate HD [40, 42]	*Acute pruritus*: a common symptom in HSRs (see type A reactions) *Chronic pruritus:* Common (60 - 90%) in ESRD [43-46], may be aggravated during HD [45]	Common in approx. 50% of patients [47]	1982: 167 patients [26], 1996: 7 patients [27], 2000: 24 patients [28]	Spain: 12 pat.; Croatia: 21 pat. [29, 30]; Taiwan: 7 pat.; Germany: 5 pat.; Italy: 4 pat.; India: 40 pat.; Colombia: 2 pat.; USA: 4 pat. [30]
Onset	First 60-120 min of HD [41, 42, 48]	During HD	After HD	During HD to 24h after HD [26-28]	During HD to some hours after HD
Duration	Approx. 60 - 120 min [41, 42, 48]	Very variable (some hours - whole day)	Some hours	2 - 3 weeks [26]. 3 out of 7 pat. recovered after 1 month, 4 out of 7 pat.: some symptoms persist for the rest of their lives [27]. Chest pain, angio-oedema: some hours; conjunctivitis, headache: 7 days; ostealgia/myalgia: 3 weeks; tinnitus: 6 months [28]	

Mani-festations	*Pa*0_2 drop of approx. 5 - 30 mmHg, symptomatic only in patients with compromised pulmonary and/or cardiovascular function: e g. dyspnoe, angina, arrhythmia, cerebral symptoms [24, 41, 42]	Itching	Washed-out feeling, weakness, fatigue	Common symptoms: *Eyes*: *"red eye symptom"* - conjunctivitis; corneal opacification, pain, vision ↓ *Ears*: tinnitus, earache, hearing ↓ *Other symptoms reported:* *Neurological*: vertigo, headache, confusion, lethargy, paraesthesia *Cardiac*: cardiac arrest (2/7 pat.), chest pain (1/22 pat.)(both in [28]) *Remaining*: fever, nausea, WBC ↑, ostealgia/myalgia (21/22 pat. in [28]), angio-oedema (1/22 pat. in [28])	Shock, cardiac problems [29], pulmonary embolism due to "bubbling" or "foaming" in the blood stream, multiorgan failure [30]
Severity	Mild to severe	Mild to severe	Mild to moderate	Moderate to severe	

	All dialysers			Certain cellulose acetate dialysers	
	Hypoxaemia	**Pruritus**	**Postdialysis fatigue**	**Ophthalmological, otological and other symptoms**	**Deaths reported in year 2001**
Aetiology	*Hypoventilation:* due to loss of CO_2 to the dialysis fluid during acetate dialysis [1, 40]; due to intradialytic alkalosis during bicarbonate dialysis [1]? *Intrapulmonal diffusion block:* Increased alveoloarterial oxygen gradient due to complement activation, leukocyte trapping, mediator release, inflammation at the pulmonary microcirculatory level [40]	*Acute pruritus* may be a manifestation of HSR (see Type A reactions) *Aggravation of chronic pruritus* Complement activation during HD leading to histamine release from mast cells? [45] Are EtO, formaldehyde and acetate contributing factors? [1]	*Excessive fluid removal* *Disequilibrium [49]* *Intradialysis hypoglycemia [50]* *Cytokine generation* induced e.g. via complement activation or contaminated dialysis fluid?	*Leaching of acetylated carbohydrate from hemicellulose because of a change in the sterilisation method.* (Nipro brand NAC series (1982), cellulose acetate capillaries from Toyobo Co. Ltd., chemical material for dialyser production from Toyobo Co. Ltd, Nihon Polyurethane Ind. Ltd. Nihon Iko Co. Ltd., Japan [26]) *Leaching of membrane degradation products from aged cellulose acetate dialysers.* (Dialyser age was 11.5 years, no brand name given in publication [27].) *Noxious substances, allergic process?: due to altered manufacturing or sterilisation methods or unfavourable shipping or storage conditions?* (newly purchased CA 210 dialysers, Nipro, Japan [28])	*Residues of a processing fluid: PF 5070* [30, 32] *Access of PF5070 to the blood during dialysis*: evaporation to gas at normal body temperature when in contact with air in the alveolar space, formation of gas embolies in the pulmonary capillary bloodstream, the pulmonary artery and the right heart.

Treatment	Nasal oxygen	If severe or part of a Type A reaction: antihistamines		Stop dialysis immediately Symptom-oriented therapy	
Prevention	• Bicarborate dialysis fluid with bicarborate levels selected to prevent excessive alkalosis • Use of non-complement-activating membranes [1, 24]	• See prevention of type A reactions • Stop formaldehyde reuse, if itching is associated with reused dialysers [1] • Improvements reported with change to PMMA [46], PSu [46, 51], PAN [52]	• Sodium profiling? [49] • Addition of glucose to the dialysis fluid? [50, 53] • Biocompatible membrane? [54]	• Adherence to dialyser expiry dates • Optimise storaging to minimise membrane degeneration: avoid long storage times, store dialysers under cool and dry conditions.	• Global recall of all Baxter A and AF dialysers (in October 2001, [33]) • Review of the ISO 10993 biocompatibility and cytotoxicity tests [30]

Table 9.1b: Characteristics, aetiology and possible methods of prevention of other acute reactions that are mainly or partially caused by dialysers. *Other possible dialysis-associated causes of these symptoms are also shown. HD: haemodialysis; HSR: hypersensivity reaction; EtO: ethylene oxide; pat: patient; PF 5070: a perfluorohydrocarbon with low vapour pressure which is used for membrane integrity testing and/or repair in 10% of Baxter's Althane dialysers [30, 32, 35,36]; PMMA: polymethylmethacrylate; PSu: polysulfone.*

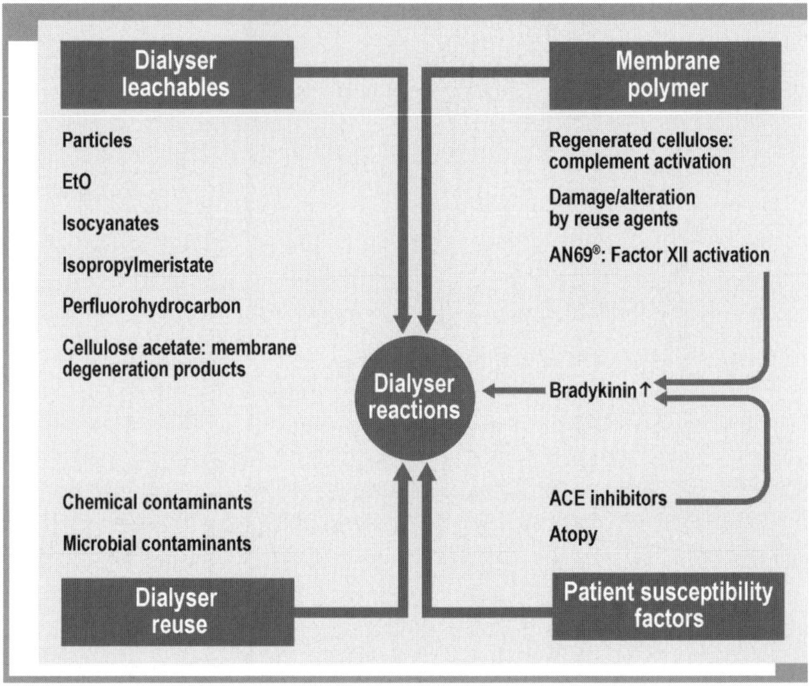

***Figure 9.1: Main factors that induce acute reactions in association with certain dialysers**. Acute dialyser reactions may be caused by leachables from the dialyser constituents, interactions between blood and the membrane polymer (especially in presence of certain patient susceptibility factors, such as medication and atopy) or by chemical or microbial contamination of the dialyser following poor reuse procedures. Reuse factors can also include a disinfectant-related change in membrane polymer structure, leading to increased permeability for endotoxins. EtO: ethylene oxide [9, 11, 12, 23, 56-58].*

detail in section C), other unknown mechanisms and reactions due to leachables (see next paragraph). Acute dialyser reactions associated with reused dialysers are addressed in section E (e.g. reactions to residual disinfectant or endotoxin contamination).

9.2.1 Leachables

From the very beginning of the industrial development of dialysers, an important goal was the production of dialysers with no or negligible release of particles or chemicals during the treatment (so-called "leachables").

In the past, release of particles of sizes mostly between 5 and 200 μm has been reported from haemodialysers [59-61]. These particles constitute a risk of microembolism and allergic reactions in haemodialysis patients. However, no direct connection between dialyser particle release and acute intradialytic symptoms has been reported in recent years, probably because of improved production quality control and because the majority of particles are removed during the recommended dialyser prerinsing procedures (e.g. guideline III.3 of [37]; [59, 60, 62]).

Other leachables cited in the literature originate from the dialyser production/sterilisation process (e.g. sterilisation agents and chemicals used for fibre production testing, particularly membrane integrity testing) or from particular constituents of the dialyser (e.g. potting ground, membrane polymer, packaging solution). These and those rare leachables caused by poor manufacturing standards or membrane degradation (both associated with the certain cellulose acetate dialysers) are listed in **table 9.2**. The procedure used to prerinse the dialyser before treatment may also influence the amount of water-soluble leachables that can gain access to the blood.

9.2.1.1 Ethylene oxide

Of all the leachables possibly present in new dialysers, ethylene oxide (EtO) has been attributed the greatest clinical significance [1, 67]. EtO is a gas capable of killing micro-organisms by the alkylation of the sulphur-containing proteins [68]. It is used to sterilise various medical instruments and supplies (e.g. certain dialysers). Allergic reactions to residual EtO in haemodialysis patients were already described in the seventies [69, 70]. EtO was then the main method of sterilisation for hollow-fibre dialysers. It remained a popular sterilant into the nineties (see **figure 4.1**), although EtO tends to accumulate in the potting compound of hollow fibre dialysers, and sophisticated degassing techniques are necessary to remove it before sale. EtO, when conjugated to human serum albumin (EtO-HSA) [71, 72], can act as allergen: signs of mild, moderate and also severe IgE-mediated hypersensitivity reactions are,

Leachable	Source within dialyser	Symptoms/ other adverse effects	Diagnostic tests	Prevention
EtO	Used in dialyser sterilisation, adsorbed by the potting compound to a significant extent	Anaphylactic reactions	IgE against EtO-HSA (RAST)	Use of EtO-free dialysers and tubings, especially in patients showing otherwise unexplained signs of anaphylactoid reactions, eosinophilia or elevated IgE [37]
MDA	MDA can be released from some aromatic polyurethanes (used as potting compound) following γ irradiation [61] (see chapter 4).	MDA is carcinogenic, mutagenic and toxic, however there is no proof of clinical relevance in ESRD [1, 63].		
Isopropyl-meristate	Core liquid in spinning process	None proven [1]		
Perfluoro-hydrocarbon	Used for membrane integrity testing in 10% of Baxter's Althane dialysers [30]	Fatal incidents because of induced gas embolism		Dialysers were recalled

(1-3)-ß-D-glucan	Cellulose [64-66]	No symptoms proven. However, high levels of (1-3)-ß-D-glucan, measured in ESRD after the use of some dialysers containing membranes made from regenerated cellulose, interfere with diagnostic procedures in patients suffering from deep mycosis and fungal infections ((1-3)-ß-D-glucan is one of the major structural components of fungi) [64-66].	Plasma levels	Avoidance of dialyser membranes made from regenerated cellulose in ESRD patients in which (1-3)-ß-D-glucan levels are used as marker for diagnosis and follow-up of deep mycosis or fungal infections [64-66]
Membrane degeneration products	Membrane polymer (cellulose acetate) contamination with easily degradable hemicellulose [26] Membrane degradation because of polymer age (11-year old cellulose acetate) [27] Other problems in the manufacturing, shipping or storing process [28]	Scleritis, conjunctivitis, impaired vision and hearing, tinnitus, headache, confusion, lethargy, paresthesia, vertigo, myalgia, ostealgia	Gel-permeation chromatography: evaluation of changes in MW of membrane polymer [26, 27] Animal experiment: iv. injection of filter residue solution in rabbits and provocation of "red eye syndrome" and eosinophilic tissue infiltrations [28]	Appropriate shipping and storing of the dialysers Adherence to dialyser expiry dates

Table 9.2: Possible leachables from new dialysers. *EtO: ethylene oxide, MDA: 4,4′ methylene dianiline, RC: regenerated cellulose, MW: molecular weight.*

for example, itching, flushing, bronchospasm and angio-oedema (see **figure 9.2**). Symptoms usually correlate with the presence and with the level of IgE antibodies [71, 73]. Atopic patients were shown to be more at risk of being allergic to EtO than non-atopic patients in one study: here 6% of non-atopic and 55% of atopic patients had EtO-specific IgE antibodies [68]. Furthermore, EtO may also cause allergic reactions in association with other substances, e.g. latex or formaldehyde. The former is used in surgery and the latter is also often employed in dialyser reprocessing [68] (see also **figure 12.3**). Most of

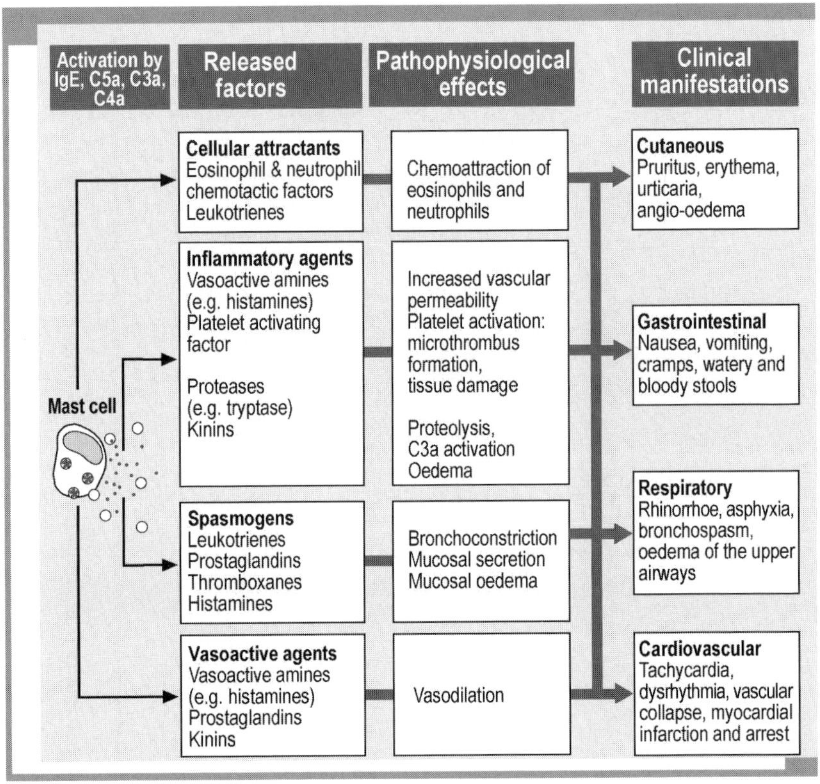

Figure 9.2: Pathophysiology and clinical manifestations of hypersensitivity. *Mast cell and basophil activation occurs via specific IgE or complement components (C5a, C3a, C4a). Released mediators are, for example, cellular attractants, inflammatory agents, vasoactive agents and spasmogens. These induce a number of pathophysiological effects that then contribute to a wide spectrum of clinical manifestations (adapted from [67]).*

the reactions initially reported in the eighties were observed during treatments with regenerated cellulose dialysers (mainly Cuprophan®) and following inadequate dialyser prerinsing (e.g. [74]). Quantitatively speaking, out of 260,000 dialysis treatments in the mid-eighties, 21 severe reactions were reported, including 4 respiratory arrests and 1 death [75]. Another paper reported 5 deaths per year [9]. The composition of the membrane polymer did not appear to play an important role. However, rinsing of the dialyser blood compartment with at least 2 l of saline and of the dialysis fluid compartment by circulation of 500 ml/min of dialysis fluid for 30 min before dialysis was found to reduce residual ethylene oxide to acceptable levels [73]. In the meanwhile, manufacturers have made great efforts to remove residual EtO from dialysers, whereby some also changed the composition and amount of the potting ground to reduce EtO retention. Conscientious dialyser prerinsing is a must in Good Dialysis Practice. Thus significant changes in dialyser production/sterilisation processes, in combination with adherence to stipulated dialyser prerinsing procedures, led to a satisfactory reduction in dialyser levels of EtO residuals and, consequently, to a lower occurrence of EtO reactions [1, 24]. However, although now uncommon, isolated case reports of severe reactions still exist [76]. In cases of patient allergy to EtO, dialysers and blood tubing sets should be chosen that are sterilised by alternative methods. In patients with eosinophilia, the use of steam-sterilised polysulfone dialysers (as opposed to EtO-sterilised devices) seemed to improve intradialytic eosinophil kinetics and led to a reduction of intradialytic hypersensitivity reactions [77]. The recently launched European Best Practice Guidelines for Haemodialysis recommend the use of EtO-free dialysers and tubings in "patients showing otherwise unexplained signs of anaphylactoid reactions, eosinophilia or elevated IgE" (guideline III.4.1 [37]).

9.2.1.2 Other chemical residues

Other residual chemicals measured in extracts from new dialysers during rinsing are isopropylmeristate [61], methanol and freon [61] (all used in hollow-fibre production) and MDA (4,4′-methylene dianiline) (which may be generated from some aromatic polyurethane potting compounds during γ irradiation sterilisation, see chapter 4) [1, 63]. Standard dialyser prerinsing will reduce the already very low levels of eventual residues of these substances further, so that the patient should normally be protected from potentially adverse effects (European Best Practice Guideline III.3 [37]).

However, another leachable residue, the perfluorohydrocarbon PF5070 (made by Minnesota Mining & Manufacturing Co), recently led to more than 50 fatal incidents worldwide [29, 30, 32] (see **table 9.1b**). This processing fluid was used in the production process of Baxter's Althane dialysers at Ronneby, Sweden (representing approximately 10% of Baxter's Althane dialyser production) but is not routinely used in the dialyser manufacturing process in general [78].

PF5070 is a perfluorohydrocarbon with a low vapour pressure that easily forms gas bubbles in the presence of air, a characteristic that made it suitable for the detection [30] and repair [35, 36] of membrane leaks. Therefore it was used in the quality control of Baxter's A and AF cellulose acetate dialyser production [32]. However, residues of this chemical probably remained in some dialysers after completion of production, possibly because of failure in the vacuum fluid evacuation system or inadequate ventilation prior to packaging [30]. Other authors argue that the membrane integrity testing itself was probably not the cause for the retention of PF5070 in the Althane dialysers, but that the subsequent dialyser repair process, only carried out at the Swedish production site in Ronneby, led to a trapping of the substance in only partially sealed capillaries [35, 36]. Thus residues of PF5070 remained in some dialysers and could not be removed by standard dialyser rinsing as the substance is not water soluble. Consequently, this chemical could gain access to the blood during dialysis. As it evaporates at normal body temperature following contact with air in the alveolar space, it might have emulsified the patient's blood, thus creating microbubble aggregates that subsequently plugged pulmonary capillaries and created patchy lung infarction. As a consequence, the oxygen delivery was compromised, inducing severe hypoxaemia with fatal consequences [32]. Such gas embolies were already described in 1976 for dogs injected with some fluorocarbons and breathing room air [79].

A further important leachable is (1-3)-ß-D-glucan. It is a minor component of natural cellulose. Therefore it derives from the cellulose-based materials used in some dialysers. As shown in several publications, dialysis with membranes made from regenerated cellulose (even when coated with vitamin E) led to increased (1-3)-ß-D-glucan levels, especially postdialysis; this was not observed during dialysis with membranes made from cellulose triacetate, polymethylmethacrylate and polysulfone (e.g. [64-66]). An increased level of (1-3)-ß-D-glucan is not known to be associated with any clinical symptoms; however, as (1-3)-ß-D-glucan is one of the major structural components in fungi, high levels of this substance (which has a half-life of about 20 hours) interfere with the use of (1-3)-ß-D-glucan monitoring as a quick and non-invasive diagnostic tool in patients with serious fungal infections [65]. Consequently, such patients should not be treated with dialysers made from regenerated cellulose [65].

9.2.1.3 Membrane degradation products

Certain cellulose acetate membranes may be susceptible to membrane degradation (see **table 9.1b** for details of the particular dialysers), especially if particular changes in production process were undertaken or storage conditions were not appropriate. For example, an unstable membrane polymer structure with leaching of membrane degradation products resulted from a contamination of cellulose acetate with the less stable hemi-cellulose, in combination with a change in sterilisation method to UV radiation. This sterilisation method was applied to the washing baths in the spinning process, and the degree of polymerisation and acetylation of cellulose acetate is labile in UV light [26]. A similar leaching of cellulose acetate degradation products resulted from chain scission or deacetylation of very old cellulose acetate membranes (11.5 years in the 7 reported cases) [27]. While these leachables from certain cellulose acetate dialysers are termed "membrane degradation products" in some studies [26, 27], another report refers to them as "noxious substances" [28]. These leachables mainly induce ophthalmologic symptoms (scleritis, conjunctivitis, decreased vision) and, therefore, the syndrome is often called "red eye syndrome". However, the eye symptoms may also be accompanied by otological dysfunction (tinnitus [26, 28], decreased hearing [27]), severe neurological symptoms [27, 28], ostealgia/myalgia, angio-oedema and chest pain [28]. This stresses the importance of adhering to expiry dates for cellulose acetate dialysers and of storing them under the cool and dry conditions necessary to minimise membrane degradation.

9.2.2 Membrane bioincompatibility

As already pointed out in the previous section, the chemical structure of the membrane surface and the resultant surface electrical charge are key factors determining membrane biocompatibility. Consequently, these factors may also play a role in the genesis of dialyser-related reactions (e.g. [80, 81]). For example, dialyser membranes made from unsubstituted cellulose have many exposed hydroxyl groups on their surface (see **figure 2.4**); these activate the complement cascade in the blood flowing through the dialyser (see

figure 7.12), and this leads to secondary adverse effects, such as leukosequestration [82, 83], stimulation of peripheral blood monocytes (PBMC), and the resultant mediator release shown in **figure 9.2**. Cellulosic membranes in which the hydroxyl groups have been chemically "covered" by either acetate (to form cellulose acetate, cellulose diacetate or cellulose triacetate), a tertiary amino group (to form Hemophan®), a benzyl group (to form SMC® or Polysynthane) or PEG will activate much less complement and induce less neutropenia [24]. Most synthetic membranes (e.g. polysulfone, polycarbonate or polymethylmethacrylate) do not have exposed hydroxyl groups on their surfaces and this is one of the reasons why they induce less complement activation and neutropenia than regenerated cellulose (see **figures 8.5** and **8.6**) [24]. Alternatively, a substantial improvement in neutropenia can be achieved with complement-activating membranes if the membrane in question is also capable of adsorbing the complement fragments, thereby obviating most of their secondary effects. This is the case for polyacrylonitrile, for example [24]. The importance of another polymer characteristic, namely its electric charge, became clear when it was shown that the negatively charged AN69® membrane interferes with the bradykinin system, leading to adverse clinical symptoms. In the following, the association between selected dialyser membrane polymers and those acute dialyser reactions that are mediated via main biochemical pathways (i.e. complement activation and bradykinin release) will be discussed. The various influences of factors such as mediator adsorption/removal by the polymer, additional stimuli (e.g. LPS) and patient susceptibilities (e.g. accompanying diseases, atopy or medication) will also be outlined (see **figure 9.3**).

9.2.2.1 Anaphylactoid reactions

In the past, it was discovered that patients dialysed with new cellulosic membranes suffered more frequently from the so-called "first use syndrome" than those treated with reused dialysers. Furthermore, levels of C5a and C3a were higher during dialysis with new cellulosic dialysers than during treatment with reused cellulosic dialysers. This led to the hypothesis that the generation of complement (C5a and C3a) was responsible for these anaphylactoid reactions [82]. This was supported by the fact that C5a (also called an anaphylatoxin) induces smooth muscle contraction, increases vascular permeability, induces histamine release from mast cells, augments the adherence and autoaggregation of leukocytes, enhances the degranulation of granulocytes, increases the release of proteases and oxygen radicals from granulocytes, and boosts the transcription of cytokines in mononuclear cells [82, 86, 87].

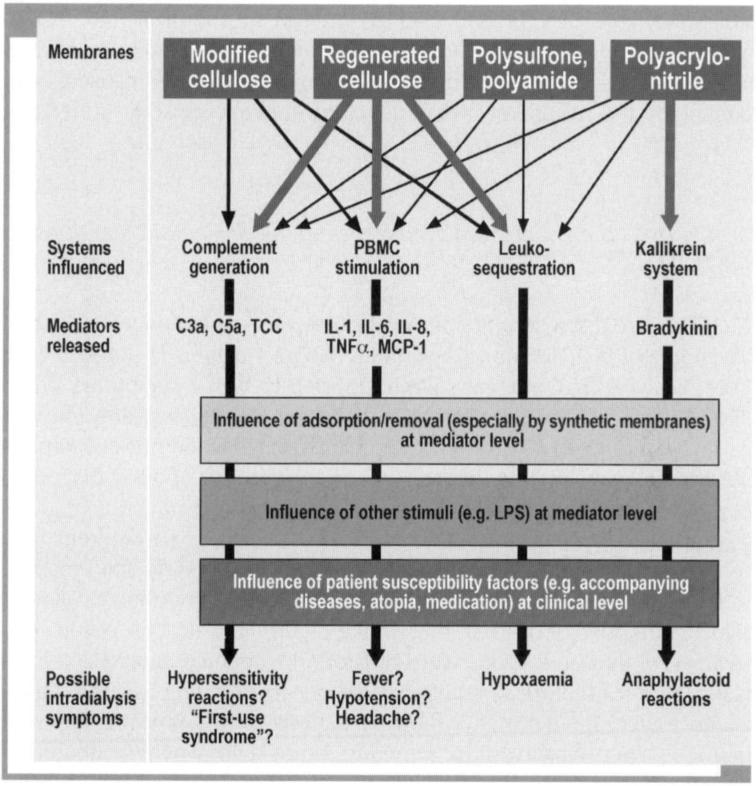

Figure 9.3: Possible contributions of selected dialysis membranes to certain intradialysis symptoms, and modification thereof by other influencing factors. *C3a, C5a: complement factors; IL: interleukin; TNF: tumor necrosis factor; PBMC: peripheral blood mononuclear cells; MCP-1: monocyte chemoattractant protein; TCC: C5b-9 or terminal complement complex. The thickness of the arrows indicates the extent of the various influences (data from [84, 85]).*

Does complement activation really play a role in intradialytic anaphylactoid reactions?

Controlled, prospective studies failed to find differences in the incidence of intradialytic well-being (including anaphylactoid symptoms) between patients dialysed with strong complement-activating regenerated cellulose membranes and the less complement-activating polysulfone and polyacrylonitrile membranes [88-91]. These observations raised doubts about the proposed causal role of C3a and C5a generation in anaphylactoid reactions. However, the possibility remains that complement activation may amplify hypersensitivity reactions due to ethylene oxide or other causes, namely by enhancing the release of histamines, thromboxane or some other mediators [1].

What role does bradykinin generation play in anaphylactoid reactions during dialysis?

In 1990, the first severe anaphylactoid reactions appearing during the first 5-10 minutes of high-flux polyacrylonitrile (AN69®) dialysis in patients simultaneously receiving ACE inhibitors were reported [92]. The symptoms were not mediated by specific antibodies of the Ig-E type (e.g. against ethylene oxide) or via increased levels of C3a or histamine. Symptoms did not develop when the AN69® polyacrylonitrile dialyser was exchanged for another dialyser containing a different type of membrane, or when the ACE-inhibitor medication was stopped in symptomatic patients [93-95]. Initially, two different mechanisms were proposed: a microbial contamination of dialysis fluid leading to endotoxin transfer to the blood by backtransport [96], and the so-called "bradykinin hypothesis" [92]. Facts that spoke against the first proposed mechanism were (a) that endotoxins were not found to induce anaphylactoid reactions [97] and (b) that these reactions also occurred during isolated ultrafiltration with AN69® membranes, where no dialysis fluid is present [98]. AN69® membranes were observed to generate bradykinin when incubated with human blood, and this generation was found to be enhanced by the addition of ACE inhibitors in a dose dependant manner in *in vitro* [99, 100] and *in vivo* animal (sheep) studies [101, 102]. The basic mechanism is described in **figure 7.19**, and the role of the electronegativity of the AN69® membrane compared to other membranes in this process is demonstrated in **table 8.2**.

Bradykinin is responsible for a number of clinical side-effects (**table 9.3**), many of which are related to anaphylaxis. The vasodilating effect of bradykinin results from the increased production and release of nitric oxide (NO). NO is a short-lived gas produced by a specific enzyme, NO synthetase (NOS). It increases cytosolic cGMP in smooth muscle cells, leading to vasodilatation (reviewed in [38]). During dialysis, the negatively charged polyacrylonitrile membrane is known to evoke anaphylactoid reactions both with and without concomitant ACE inhibition [38, 92-94, 98-100, 104-111]. Plasma bradykinin concentrations were higher in patients dialysed with AN69® mem-

Bradykinin	
Effects	**Clinical manifestations**
BK1- receptors	
Contraction and relaxation of smooth muscles	Endotoxic shock
BK2-receptors	
Liberation of factors such as endothelium-derived relaxing factor, prostaglandins	Vasodilatation, tissue perfusion
Relaxation of the vascular muscles	Vasodilatation, tissue perfusion
Augmented vascular permeability	Angioneurotic oedema, inflammatory oedema
Liberation of histamine from mast cells	Angioneurotic oedema, inflammatory oedema
Tissue inflammation	Arthritis, colitis, pancreatitis
Stimulation of sensorial neurons	Pain (blisters, angina, arthopathy)
Stimulation of sympathetic nerve endings	Catecholamine release (arrhythmic stimulus)
Augmented glucose transport across the cell membrane	Augmented insulin sensitivity, improved glucose tolerance
Sensibilisation of the respiratory system	Bronchial constriction, cough, asthma, allergic rhinitis

Table 9.3: Clinical effects of bradykinin, mediated via bradykinin 1 (BK1) and 2 (BK2) receptors *(adapted from [103]).*

branes than in patients dialysed with other membranes, such as Cuprophan® [95], high-flux polysulfone [95, 107], Hemophan® [95] and other polyacrylonitrile membranes with less negative surface charges (SPAN [112], AN69ST [109]) (see **figure 8.22**). Bradykinin values were found to increase steeply after dialysis start with AN69®, reaching peak values after approximately 5 – 15 minutes of treatment [95, 106] (see **figure 9.4**). This predisposes patients treated with AN69® dialysers to acute anaphylactoid reactions, even when not receiving ACE inhibition medication [95, 106]. For example, a value in the dialyser venous effluent of up to 4900 fmol/ml was observed in one patient 5 minutes after dialysis start [106]. This high bradykinin level was associated with clinical symptoms. The reasons why patients who are not on ACE-inhibitor medication are unable to degrade bradykinin during its passage through the pulmonary circulation remain unclear; perhaps the excessive bradykinin generation exceeds the inactivation capacity of the pulmonary circuit. On the other hand, individual intradialytic maximal plasma bradykinin levels up to 2672 fmol/l compared to values ranging approximately from 33 to 125 fmol/l predialysis were observed, but without clinical consequences [108], whereas values around 600 fmol/ml caused symptoms [95]. These

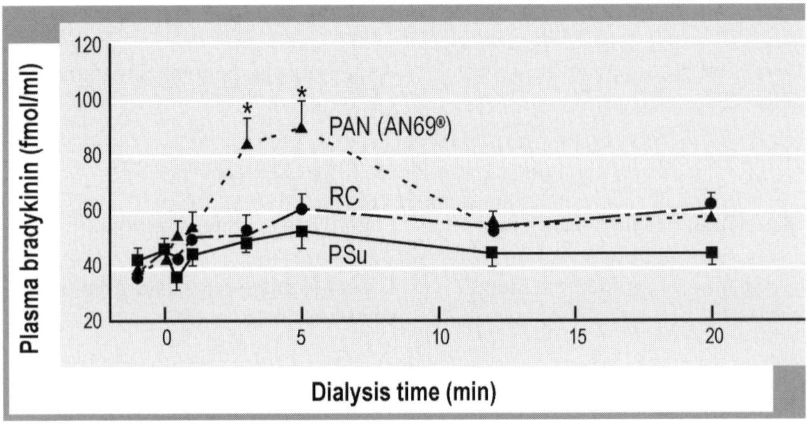

Figure 9.4: Plasma bradykinin concentrations in the venous effluent of various dialysers during the first minutes of dialysis of asymptomatic patients not receiving ACE inhibitor medication. *Results are given as mean values + or - SEM, respectively; $p < 0.05$ for AN69® (Filtral 12, Hospal, 1.3 m^2, n=9) versus other membranes (RC: Cuprophan®, GFE 12, Gambro, 1.3 m^2, n=10; PSu: Fresenius Polysulfone®, F60, Fresenius Medical Care, 1.2 m^2, n=19); all dialysers were EtO sterilised (adapted from [106]).*

observations suggest that the threshold value is difficult to determine individually [108]. In patients taking ACE inhibitors, plasma levels of bradykinin may increase more than 100-fold, increasing the risk of suffering anaphylactoid reactions [106]. Such reactions may range from simple flushing to severe reactions, some of which may require cardiopulmonary resuscitation or other intensive care measures [93, 110]; even one death was reported [93]. The risk of suffering anaphylactoid reactions is five fold higher in patients treated with both AN69® and ACE inhibitors than in patients treated with ACE inhibitors and any other membrane [111]. Recently, two new severe cases of anaphylactoid reactions in patients treated with AN69® and ACE inhibitors were published, one thereof even with the use of an AN69® dialyser in venovenous haemofiltration. These reports serve as a reminder of the potentially lethal combination of AN69® membranes and ACE inhibitor treatment [110]. Recent European Best Practice Guidelines for Haemodialysis stipulate that this combination should be avoided (guideline III.4.3 [37]).

Can membrane-associated bradykinin generation be reduced?

The contact phase activation induced by the electronegativity of dialysis membranes has been shown to be a dilution- and pH-dependent phenomena (see **figure 9.5**). In non-diluted plasma, the kallikrein protease activity is rapidly neutralised by several plasma serine antiproteases, e.g. C1 esterase inhibitor. Dilution of plasma, however, creates a protease-antiprotease imbalance, inhibiting kallikrein neutralisation. During dialysis, plasma dilution with the residual saline rinsing solution is inevitable in the early phase of the treatment, thus predisposing the patient to anaphylactoid reactions shortly after dialysis start. However, kallikrein generation in diluted plasma could be inhibited *in vitro* by maintaining the plasma pH value above 7.4 [39, 109].

These *in vitro* observations may be of clinical relevance. Immediately after the start of dialysis, the pH of the diluted blood can be such as would support bradykinin generation and NOS activation. An Italian, multicentre, retrospective analysis of "hypersensitivity" reactions (not distinguishing between IgE-mediated hypersensitivity and bradykinin-induced anaphylactoid reactions) focused on the question of whether a rinsing procedure which maintains the pH of the diluted blood above 7.4 may prevent such hypersensitivity reactions (HSRs) [113]. HSRs were reported in 54 patients on home dialysis between January 1995 and June 1997. The study confirmed a higher frequency of HSRs in patients using AN69® (72% of the reported HSRs) compared to

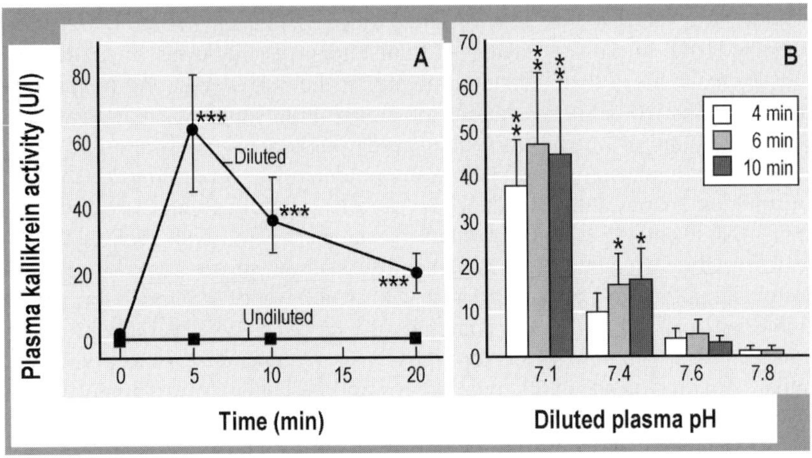

Figure 9.5: Influence of dilution (A) and pH (B) on contact phase activation induced by the AN69® membrane. *Effects of plasma dilution on the kallikrein activity are shown in part A of the figure: measurements were conducted in undiluted (■) and 1/20 diluted (●) plasma after 20 min circulation through AN69® dialysers. Kallikrein activity is shown in part B, as measured in diluted and non diluted plasma equilibrated at four different pH values after 4, 6, 10 minutes circulation through AN69® minidialysers. Data are presented as means ± SD of 6 different plasmas in both figures (***: $p < 0.001$ vs. undiluted plasma; **: $p < 0.01$ for pH 7.1 versus pH 7.4, 7.6, 7.8 at every contact time; *: $p < 0.05$ for pH 7.4 versus pH 7.6 and 7.8 at 6 and 10 min. recirculation times) (adapted from [109]).*

other dialysis membranes, particularly when an ACE-inhibitor was being simultaneously administered (44% of the reported patients). However, the patients with reported HSRs represent only a small percentage of the total number of patients treated with AN69® membranes and/or a combination of AN69® and ACE inhibitors in this study. Two-thirds of the nephrologists did not modify dialyser prescription, but used an alkaline rinsing procedure (BioPrime® with alkaline solution) in an attempt to prevent the acidic change of the patient's diluted blood at the first contact with the membrane. ACE-inhibitor therapy was withdrawn in several cases. However, interestingly, in some cases the combination of AN69® membrane and ACE- inhibitor treatment was kept unchanged, while only the alkaline washing procedure was introduced. A recurrence of HSRs was not observed in any of these cases. The fact remains that the new rinsing procedure prevents anaphylactoid reactions with AN69® membranes.

Not all polyacrylonitrile (PAN) membranes have the same effect on plasma bradykinin levels: levels are very much dependent on the actual membrane surface properties, as these influence both bradykinin generation and bradykinin adsorption [107]. The properties of a membrane surface primarily depend on the blends used to produce a particular PAN membrane. Differences between various PAN membranes were confirmed in animal models, where symptoms were seen during dialysis with the AN69® membrane (both with and without ACE inhibition) and with the PAN DX membrane (in combination with ACE inhibition), but not with the SPAN membrane (even in combination with ACE inhibition) [101]. In a further study, the SPAN membrane did not induce significant bradykinin release or signs of anaphylactoid reactions in a small number of dialysis patients treated simultaneously with ACE inhibitors [112]. However, the SPAN membrane tested was a development product that is now not available on the market.

A step forward in reducing the bradykinin generation by AN69® membranes is also to coat the membrane with a polycationic solution, reducing the surface electronegativity and thus avoiding bradykinin generation, even at low pHs [111]. A 3-year experience using such coated AN69ST plate dialysers (Crystal 4000 series, Hospal, France) at a French dialysis centre was recently published: a total of 10,630 dialysis sessions were performed, and 17 of 56 patients were treated with ACE inhibitors for a total of 3400 dialysis sessions. No anaphylactoid reactions were observed in any patients during the study period, although 3 of the 17 ACE-inhibitor patients had previously suffered from anaphylactoid reactions when dialysed with the original AN69® membrane. However, recently, 1 case-report has appeared concerning an anaphylactoid reaction during dialysis with the AN69ST membrane: this occurred 30 minutes after intradialytic ACE inhibitor medication (standard dose) [114]. Furthermore, 12 unusual adverse reactions were described in 6 patients dialysed with AN69ST membranes: abdominal cramps, diarrhoea, hypotension, vomiting or general malaise occurred late in the course of the haemodialysis session (45-150 min) and quickly resolved when dialysis was stopped [115]. Blood sampling during the reactions in 3 patients revealed contact phase activation leading to the generation of bradykinin. According to the authors, this was probably due to a longitudinal asymmetry of the surface treatment, leaving some areas of the membranes untreated. An improved industrial process should guarantee homogeneous treatment of the AN69ST membrane surface in the future [115]. Prospective studies are necessary to prove the safety of this modified membrane regarding bradykinin generation.

Have clinical effects of bradykinin generation also been observed with other membranes?

One report has been published of anaphylactoid reactions during treatment with high-flux PMMA dialysers and concomitant ACE-inhibitor therapy [116]. Furthermore, anaphylactoid reactions similar to those seen with AN69® membranes have also been reported during low-density lipoprotein apheresis with negatively charged dextrane sulphate columns, incriminating bradykinin as a mediator [117, 118].

Are AT1 receptor blockers a viable alternative for ACE inhibitors when using AN69® membranes?

Finally, another approach towards reducing anaphylactoid reactions (AR) in patients treated with AN69® membranes and concomitant ACE-inhibitor therapy is to exchange the ACE inhibitor for an Angiotensin II type 1 (AT_1) receptor blocker (e.g. losartan, valsartan, candersartan). The AT_1 receptor blocker inhibits the renin-angiotensin-system without influencing bradykinin. In a study involving 96 patients dialysed with AN69® and treated with losartan, only 2 mild ARs occurred. In contrast, 9 of these patients had previously suffered an AR when treated with AN69® in combination with an ACE inhibitor [119]. Another recent case report reported ARs with the combination AN69® membrane and losartan [120]. However, the symptoms in this case occurred rather late during the treatment (approximately one hour after the start), which is uncommon in pure bradykinin-mediated reactions [121]. No ARs occurred during 1188 haemodialysis treatments with AN69® in combination with two other AT_1 receptor blockers, valsartan and candersartan [122]. In summary, it appears that the combination "AN69® membrane and AT_1 receptor blocker therapy" evokes less ARs than the combination "AN69® membrane and ACE inhibitor therapy", but this remains to be proven in larger studies.

9.2.2.2 Dialysis-associated hypoxaemia

Intradialytic hypoxaemia is defined as an arterial partial oxygen pressure (p_aO_2) drop of 5-20 mmHg. This is not usually of clinical significance in patients with normal cardiopulmonary function, however it may be deleterious in patients with pre-existing pulmonary, cardio- or cerebrovascular disease. Patients with compromised cardio-pulmonary function constitute 10-15% (or even more) of the dialysis population. Such patients start dialysis with predialysis paO_2 values below 80 mmHg [40]; an additional 20% loss during dialysis results in oxygen desaturation (decline in sO_2) and may lead to clinical side-effects, such as cardiac arrhythmias, angina and other cerebrovascular events.

Acetate dialysis is the most common cause of dialysis-associated hypoxaemia. The underlying mechanism is based on (a) the loss of bicarbonate into the dialysate in the initial stages of dialysis, (b) the decrease in respiratory quotient during the metabolism of the acetate, and (c) the direct effect of acetate on the respiratory centre (reviewed in [4, 40]). Dialysis-associated hypoxaemia may even develop during bicarbonate dialysis [40], although to a milder degree; this probably results from a decrease in respiratory drive in cases of overcorrection of acidosis, when metabolic alkalosis is created [4, 24, 40, 42].

A contribution of the dialysis membrane to intradialytic hypoxaemia has only been postulated to date. One possibility is that intradialysis complement activation and leukocyte trapping (with resultant mediator release and inflammation at the pulmonary microcirculatory level) cause an increased alveolo-arterial oxygen gradient with a decrease in diffusion capacity [40]. This was first indicated in a prospective, randomised study comparing biocompatible (polyacrylonitrile: AN69®) and bioincompatible (regenerated cellulose: Cuprophan®) membranes, in combination with acetate or bicarbonate dialysis fluid [48]. It was found that the combination "regenerated cellulose membrane and acetate dialysis fluid" yielded the most striking decrease in paO_2, whereas the combination "polyacrylonitrile and bicarbonate dialysis fluid" did not significantly affect paO_2 levels. However, acetate dialysis fluid seemed to be the major influencing factor, as hypoxaemia also occurred in this and other studies when acetate dialysis fluid was used in combination with even biocompatible membranes (i.e. polyacrylonitrile [48], polymethylmethacrylate and polysulfone) (reviewed in [123]). Recently, a small prospective, single blind, randomised study (10 patients) confirmed the disastrous combination of bioincompatible dialysers and acetate dialysis fluid: here the incidence of cardiopulmonary events was analysed under various combinations of dialyser polymers (i.e. cuprammonium rayon, Clirans 101, Terumo; Fresenius Polysulfone®, Hemoflow F60, Fresenius Medical Care) and buffer contents of the dialysis fluid (bicarbonate dialysis fluid, acetate and bicarbonate dialysis fluid) [41].

Studies of mechanically ventilated intensive care patients dialysed with cuprammonium rayon dialysers (AM-50, Asahi) and bicarbonate dialysis fluid (35 mEq/l) confirmed the occurrence of neutropenia with a nadir 15 minutes after dialysis start, but found no cases of hypoventilation or hypoxaemia and an unchanged ventilation pattern during dialysis [124-126]. Furthermore, a recent study suggested varying susceptibility to complement activation with different dialysis membranes: it revealed (a) that the kinetics of complement generation (C3a) were dissociated from those of adhesion molecule upregulation, early neutrophil margination and decrease in $pa0_2$ during the first 30 minutes of haemodialysis, (b) that the results were similar with all three types of dialysis membranes examined in combination with bicarbonate dialysis fluid (i.e. regenerated cellulose (Cuprophan®, E3, Fresenius Medical Care), cellulose acetate (Acepal 1300, Hospal) and Fresenius Polysulfone® (F6 HPS, Fresenius Medical Care)) and (c) that complement activation varied distinctly between the patients studied [127]. Finally, using biocompatible low-flux polysulfone (F6, Fresesnius Medical Care) compared to bioincompatible regenerated cellulose membranes did not lead to statistically significant differences in the occurrence of postdialysis hypoxaemia [128]. These data strengthen the hypothesis that factors other than complement are involved in the triggering of dialysis-related neutropenia and hypoxaemia. The level of contribution of dialyser bioincompatibility to dialysis-associated hypoxaemia is, therefore, still a subject of debate, and the suspicion arises that this contribution was perhaps overestimated in the past.

9.2.2.3 Cardiovascular and other intra- and postdialytic reactions

During dialysis, a number of acute symptoms may occur that differ from the hypersensitivity and anaphylactoid reactions already discussed. Some of these can be very serious. Examples are cardiovascular side effects, such as hypotension and arrhythmias. In addition, fever, muscle cramps, headache, nausea, pruritus and fatigue during dialysis, as well as fatigue and lack of energy after dialysis are frequent problems, and numerous causal factors have been acclaimed. However, symptom-reporting in dialysis is complicated by individual perception, staff reactions and the nature of the reporting procedure, so ethnic and cultural differences must be taken into consideration when analysing haemodynamic differences and prescription-related elements of symptoms [11]. The question of relevance here is whether differences in dialyser characteristics (i.e. their particular blood-membrane interactions) influence the occurrence of the intradialytic and postdialytic symptoms listed above. However, it is important to bear in mind that all these symptoms may also be induced by factors other than the dialyser, such as treatment prescription and patient comorbidity; these may even overrule any membrane effect.

In this context, **figure 7.16** provides an overview of the role of the dialysis membrane in cytokine generation, whereby the membrane has both a direct and an indirect influence on cytokine levels (the latter through complement activation). The figure also points out the contribution of dialysis fluid bacterial contamination to cytokine generation [88, 87, 129-131] (see **table 8.1** for more details). Interleukin-1 (IL-1) and tumor necrosis factor (TNF)-α were shown to induce fever and hypotension when injected to humans ([132] and reviewed in [85]). A vast number of studies have demonstrated that membrane-induced complement activation and the release of cytokines, prostaglandins and oxygen free radicals varies between membranes and is also subject to various influencing factors (see chapter 8 for more details). It was shown that synthetic membranes (e.g. polysulfone [41, 87-89, 91, 133-136], polymethylmethacrylate [134, 137] and polyacrylonitrile [48, 89, 90, 129, 138, 139]) exert a more positive influence on biochemical and cellular phenomena associated with the blood-membrane contact than regenerated cellulose (reviewed in [40, 81, 84, 85, 123, 131, 140]). These factors certainly make a contribution to numerous *chronic* dialysis-associated diseases (see following chapter), but do they actually affect the incidence of intradialytic acute symptoms? Although the "Interleukin Hypothesis", first proposed in the early eighties, suggests that the release of proinflammatory cytokines acts as an underlying pathophysiologic event in haemodialysis-associated acute manifestations, such as fever and hypotension [25, 141], this was not reflected in the results of corresponding clinical studies [41, 88-91, 142-145] (see **table 9.4**).

Cardiovascular reactions

The course of systolic, diastolic and mean blood pressure during dialysis was found to be similar for cellulosic and synthetic membranes [41, 88, 90, 91, 143, 146, 147]. This was also found to hold true for heart rate [88, 91, 143, 145], total peripheral resistance [90], the number of intradialytic hypotensive episodes [41, 88-91, 143, 145, 147] and so-called dialysis-related symptoms, such as headache [88, 89, 143, 147], nausea, muscle cramps and pruritus [88, 89, 147]. The two main groups of membranes compared were regenerated cellulose (Cuprophan® and cuprammonium rayon) versus polycarbonate (Gambrane®), polyamide, DEAE cellulose (Hemophan®), polyacrylonitrile (AN69®), and high or low-flux polysulfone (Fresenius Polysulfone®). In

Reports	Study design/ treatment mode	Number of patients	Number of dialyses/ length of study	Membrane tested	Biochemical parameters		Other parameters measured	Clinical symptoms
					Complement	Leukocyte count		
Schohn et al., 1986 [142]	Prospective HD	8		PC, CU	C3, CH50: ⇓⇓ CU ⇓ PC C5a: ⇑ CU ⇔ PC	⇓⇓⇓ CU ⇓ PC	Hypoxaemia observed with CU not observed with PC PAP ⇑ with CU PVR ⇑ with CU	
Skroeder et al., 1990 [143]	Randomised, controlled HD	23	92	PA, HE, CU			Syst. BP⇔ Diast. BP ⇔ HR ⇔	Hypotensive episodes ⇔ Headache, muscle cramps, pruritus, nausea, chest pain, dyspnoe, back pain ⇔
Bergamo collaborative dialysis study group, 1991 [88]	Multi-centre, randomised, double-blind, controlled HD	428	856	PSu, CU	C3a ⇑⇑⇑ CU ⇑ PSu (ven. side of HD circuit) C3a ⇑⇑⇑ CU ⇔ PSu (art. side of HD circuit)		Syst. BP⇔ Diast. BP ⇔ HR ⇔	Hypotensive episodes ⇔ Headache, pruritus, nausea, muscle cramps, well being ⇔

Collins et al., 1993 [89]	Prospective, randomised, cross-over HD	35	6 months	PAN, CU	C3a: ⇑⇑⇑ CU ⇔ PAN	⇓⇓⇓ CU ⇔ PAN	No hypoxaemia with CU and PAN	Hypotensive episodes ⇔ Headache, pruritus, nausea, muscle cramps, well being ⇔
Skroeder et al., 1994 [91]	Prospective, crossover HD	20	234	HE, PA, CU	C3a: ⇑⇑⇑ CU ⇑⇑ HE ⇑ PA	⇓⇓⇓ CU ⇓ HE, PA	Syst. BP⇔ Diast. BP ⇔ HR⇔	Hypotensive episodes ⇔ Headache, pruritus ⇔
Aakhus et al., 1994 [90]	Randomised double blind, crossover HD	8	16	PAN, CU		⇓⇓ CU ⇔ PAN	MAP⇔ Cardiac index ⇔ Stroke index ⇔ TPR ⇔ HR ⇔	Hypotensive episodes ⇔
Locatelli et al., 1996 [145]	Prospective, randomised HD/HDF	380	2 years	LF/ HF PSu, CU		⇓⇓ CU ⇔ PSu	Syst. BP⇔ Diast. BP ⇔	Hypotensive episodes ⇔

Reports	Study design/ treatment mode	Number of patients	Number of dialyses/ length of study	Membrane tested	Biochemical parameters		Other parameters measured	Clinical symptoms
					Complement	Leukocyte count		
Munger et al., 2000 [41]	Prospective, single blind, randomised HD/acetate HD/Bic	10	40	PSu, CR		⇓⇓ CR (Bic/Acetate) ⇓ PSu (Acetate) ⇔ PSu (Bic)	MAP⇔ *Hypoxaemia* mean nadir, mean decreament PSu/Bic versus CR/Bic ⇔ PSu/acetate versus CR/acetate ⇔ Number of desaturation events PSu versus CR ⇔ Duration ⇓ with PSu/Bic compared to CR/Acetate *Ventricular ectopy* ⇔ *Supraventricular ectopy* ⇔ *Silent ischemia* Number ⇔ Intensity ⇓ PSu versus CR	Hypotensive episodes ⇔

Table 9.4: Membrane biocompatibility and intradialytic symptoms in chronic renal failure. *HD: haemodialysis; HDF: haemodiafiltration; Bic: bicarbonate dialysis fluid; Acetate: Acetate dialysis fluid; CU: Cuprophan®; HE: Hemophan®; PAN: polyacrylonitrile (AN69®); PC: polycarbonate (Gambrane®); PA: polyamide; PSu: Fresenius Polysulfone®; PAP: pulmonary artery pressure; PVR: pulmonary vascular resistance; CR: cuprammonium rayon; HF: high-flux; LF: low-flux; MAP: mean arterial pressure; syst. BP: sytolic blood pressure; diast. BP: diastolic blood pressure; PAP: pulmonary artery pressure; PWP: pulmonary wedge pressure; TPR: total peripheral resistance; ⇔ unchanged; ⇓ slight, ⇓⇓ medium, ⇓⇓⇓ strong decrease; ⇑ slight, ⇑⇑ medium, ⇑⇑⇑ strong increase.*

a recent study, no differences were also found in the number of ventricular and supraventricular ectopy and silent ischemia. However, in this study, the intensity of silent ischemia was significantly reduced for polysulfone (Fresenius Polysulfone®, Hemoflow F60, Fresenius Medical Care) versus cuprammonium rayon (Clirans 101, Terumo) [41].

Other symptoms

No differences in intra- and postdialytic symptoms could be detected between regenerated cellulose (Cuprophan®), DEAE cellulose (Hemophan®) and polyamide; the symptoms studied were headache, muscle cramps, nausea, chest pain, back pain, dyspnoe and pruritus [143]. Postdialysis fatigue is another common symptom among dialysis patients (e.g. 50% in [47]): excessive ultrafiltration, intradialytic disequilibrium, intradialytic hypoglycaemia, depression and antihypertensive treatment seem to be important contributing factors (reviewed in [47, 49, 50, 148]). Release of somnogenic cytokines in response to blood-membrane interactions (especially TNF-α and, to a smaller extent, IL-1β) has also been shown to be higher predialysis and to rise more during dialysis in patients suffering from postdialysis fatigue [54]. However, no difference was found between regenerated cellulose and polymethylmethacrylate dialysers in patients with postdialysis fatigue [47, 149], even when TNF-α levels increased by an average of 18.3% with regenerated cellulose membranes and only by 2.4% with membranes made of polymethylmethacrylate [149].

References

1. Salem M, Ivanovich PT, Ing TS, Daugirdas JT: Adverse effects of dialysers manifesting during the dialysis session. Nephrol Dial Transplant 9(Suppl 2): 127-137, 1994

2. Lemke HD: Hypersensitivity reactions during haemodialysis: The choice of methods and assays. Nephrol Dial Transplant 9(Suppl 2): 120-125, 1994

3. Salem MM, Brennan JF: Anaphylactoid reactions in dialysis patients: pathogenesis and Management. Seminars in Dialysis 8(4): 212-219, 1995

4. Grassmann A, Uhlenbusch-Körwer I, Bonnie-Schorn E, Vienken J: Correction of acidosis in hemodialysis in *Composition and management of hemodialysis fluids*, edited by Vienken J, Pabst Science Publishers, Lengerich: 60-89, 2000

5. Grassmann A, Uhlenbusch-Körwer I, Bonnie-Schorn E, Vienken J: Elektrolytes in *Composition and management of hemodialysis fluids*, edited by Vienken J, Pabst Science Publishers, Lengerich: 100-159, 2000

6. Schärer K, Müller Wiefel DE: Dialyse im Kindesalter in *Blutreinigungsverfahren*, 5th ed., edited by Franz HE and Hörl WH, Thieme, Stuttgart: 390-406, 1997

7. Mendley SR, Fine RN, Tejani A: Dialysis in infants and children in *Handbook of dialysis*, third ed., edited by Daugirdas JT, and Ing TS, Little Brown and Company: 562-579, 2001

8. Hoenich NA, Woffindin C, Ronco C: Haemodialyzers and associated devices in *Replacement of renal function*, 2nd ed., edited by AM Davison, JS Cameron, JP Grünfeld, Kerr DNS, E Ritz, CG Winearls, Oxford University Press: 188-229, 1996

9. Villarroel F, Ciarkowski AA: A survey on hypersensitivity reactions in hemodialysis. J Artif Organs 9(3): 231-238, 1985

10. Bright RA, Torrence ME, Daley WR, McClellan WM: Preliminary survey of the occurrence of anaphylactoid reactions during haemodialysis. (Letter) Nephrol Dial Transplant 14(3): 799-800, 1999

11. Levin NW, Zasuwa G: Relationship between dialyser type and signs and symptoms. Nephrol Dial Transpl 8(Suppl2): 30-39, 1993

12. Arduino MJ: CDC investigations of non-infectious outbreaks of adverse events in hemodialysis facilities, 1979-1999. Semin Dial 13(2): 86-91, 2000

13. Gotch FA, Keen ML: Care of the patient on hemodialysis, edited by Cogan MG, Garovoy MR, Churchill Livingstone, New York: 73, 1985

14. Henderson LW, Cheung AK, Chenoweth DE: Choosing a membrane. Am J Kidney Dis 3(1): 5-20, 1983

15. Daugirdas JT, Ing TS: First-use reactions during hemodialysis: a definition of subtypes. Kidney Int 33(Suppl 24): S37-S43, 1988

16. Gurland HJ, Davison AM, Bonomini V, Falkenhagen D, Hansen S, Kishimoto T, Lysaght MJ, Moran J, Valek A: Definitions and terminology in biocompatibility. Nephrol Dial Transplant 9(Suppl 2): 4-10, 1994

17. Miller GB, Wilber J: Update: acute allergic reactions associated with reprocessed hemodialyzers - United States, 1989-1990. Dialysis and Transplant 20(11): 692-694, 1991

18. Rudnick JR, Arduino MJ, Bland LA, Cusick L, McAllister SK, Aguero SM, Jarvis WR: An outbreak of pyrogenic reactions in chronic hemodialysis patients associated with hemodialyzer reuse. Artif Organs 19(4): 289-294, 1995

19. Ng YY, Yang AH, Wong KC, Lan HY, Hung TL, Kerr PG, Huang TP: Dialyzer reuse: interaction between dialyzer membrane, disinfectant (formalin) and blood during dialyzer reprocessing. Artif Organs 20(1): 53-55, 1996

20. Klinkmann H, Grassmann A, Vienken J: Dilemma of membrane biocompatibility and reuse. Artif Organs 20(5): 426-432, 1996

21. Sodemann K, Lubrich-Birkner I, Berger O, Mahiout A: Identification of oxidized protein and bradykinin generation in dialyzer reuse with polysulphone membranes: Abstract ISN Sydney, 1997

22. Vinhas J, Pinto dos Santos J: Haemodialyser reuse: facts and fiction. Nephrol Dial Transplant 15: 5-8, 2000

23. Roth VR, Jarvis WR: Outbreaks of infection and/or pyrogenic reactions in dialysis patients. Semin Dial 13(2): 92-96, 2000

24. Bregman H, Daugirdas JT, Ing TS: Complications during dialysis in *Handbook of Dialysis*, third ed., edited by Daugirdas JT, Blake PG and Ing TS, Lippincott Williams and Wilkins, Philadelphia: 148-168, 2001

25. Henderson LW, Koch KM, Dinarello CA, Shaldon S: Hemodialysis hypotension: The interleukin-1 hypothesis. Blood Purif 1:3-8, 1983

26. Oba T, Tsuji A, Nakamura A, Shintani H, Mizumachi S, Kikushi H, Kaniwa M, Kojima S, Kanotha K, Kawasaki Y, Furuya T, Matsumoto K, Tobe M: Migration of acetylated hemicellulose from capillary hemodialyzer to blood causing scleritis and /or iritis. Artif Organs 8(4): 429-435, 1984

27. Hutter JC, Kuehnert MJ, Wallis RR, Lucas AD, Sen S, Jarvis WR: Acute onset of decreased vision and hearing traced to hemodialysis treatment with aged dialyzers. JAMA 283(16): 2128-2134, 2000

28. Averbukh Z, Modai D, Sandbank J, Berman S, Cohn M, Galperin E, Cohen N, Dishi V, Weissgarten J: Red eye Syndome: clinical and experimental experience in a new aspect of diffuse eosinophilic infiltration. Artif Org 25(6): 437-440, 2001

29. Kovac C: US company at centre of dialysis scare. BMJ 323: 956, 2001

30. Murphy B: Causal link seals Baxter dialyser crisis. Clinica 983: 1-2, 2001

31. Garcia Lopez FJ, Anchuela OT, Lopez-Abente G: Sudden death related to a brand of diacetate cellulose dialysers. (Abstract) J Am Soc Nephrol 13(9): 579A, 2002

32. Canaud B: Performance liquid test as a cause for sudden deaths of dialysis patients: perfluorohydrocarbon, a previously unrecognized hazard for dialysis patients. Nephrol Dial Transplant 17: 545–548, 2002

33. Bosch X: Baxter withdraws dialyser after 12 patients die. BMJ (News) 324: 529, 2001

34. Excerpt of TÜV report concerning the deaths in Spain from october 9, 2001.

35. Shaldon S, Koch KM: Understanding the epidemic of deaths associated with the use of the Althane dialyzer. Artif Organs 26(10): 894-895, 2002

36. Shaldon S, Koch KM: Dialyzer repair: A disastrous exercise in cost effectiveness. ASAIO J 48(5): 453-454, 2002

37. Kessler M, Canaud B, Pedrini LA, Tattersall J, ter Wee PM, Vanholder R, Wanner C: European Best Practice Guidelines for Haemodialysis (part 1). Nephrol Dial Transplant 17(Suppl 7): 1-107, 2002

38. Coppo R, Amore A: Importance of the bradykinin-nitric oxide synthase system in the hypertensivity reactions in haemodialysis patients. Nephrol Dial Transplant 15(9): 1288-1290, 2000

39. Coppo R, Amore A, Cirina P, Scelfo B, Giacchino F, Comune L, Atti M, Renaux LR: Bradykinin and nitric oxide generation by dialysis membranes can be blunted by alkaline rinsing solutions. Kidney Int 58(2): 881-888, 2000

40. De Broe M: Haemodialysis-induced hypoxaemia. Nephrol Dial Transplant 9(Suppl 2): 173-175, 1994

41. Munger MA, Ateshkadi A, Cheung AK, Flaharty KK, Stoddard GJ, Marshall EH: Cardiopulmonal events during hemodialysis: effects of dialysis membranes and dialysate buffers. Am J Kidney Dis 36(1): 130-139, 2000

42. Nielsen AL, Jensen HAE, Hegbrandt J, Brinkenfeldt H, Thunedborg P: Oxygen status during haemodialysis. The Cord Group. Acta Anaesethesiol Scand 39(Suppl 109): 195-200, 1995

43. Merkus MP, Jager KJ, Dekker FW, de Haan RJ, Boeschoten EW, Krediet RT: Physical symptoms and quality of life in patients on chronic dialysis: results of The Netherlands Cooperative Study on Adequacy of Dialysis (NECOSAD). Nephrol Dial Transplant 14(5): 1163-1170, 1999

44. Virga G, Mastrosimone S, Amici G, Munaretto G, Gastaldon F, Bonadonna A: Symptoms in hemodialysis patients and their relationship with biochemical and demographic parameters. Int J Artif Organs 21(12): 788-93, 1998

45. Schwartz IF, Iaina A: Uraemic pruritus. Nephrol Dial Transplant 14: 834-839, 1999

46. Kato A, Takita T, Furuhashi M, Takahashi T, Watanabe T, Maruyama Y, Hishida A: Polymethylmethacrylate efficacy in reduction of renal itching in hemodialysis patients: crossover study and role of tumor necrosis factor -α. Artif Organs 25(6): 441-447, 2001

47. Sklar AH, Riesenberg LA, Silber AK, Ahmed W, Ali A: Postdialysis fatigue. Am J Kidney Dis 28(5): 732-736, 1996

48. De Backer WA, Verpooten GA, Borgonjon DJ, Vermeire PA, Lins RR, De Broe ME: Hypoxemia during hemodialysis: effects of different membranes and dialysate compositions. Kidney Int 23: 738-743, 1983

49. Sadowsky RH, Allred EN, Jabs K: Sodium modeling ameliorates intradialytic symptoms in young dialysis patients. J Am Soc Nephrol 4(5): 1192-1198, 1993

50. Leski M, Niethammer T, Wyss T: Glucose-enriched dialysate and tolerance to maintenance hemodialysis. Nephron 24: 271-273, 1979

51. Kato A, Hamada M, Maruyama T, Maruyama Y, Hishida A: Pruritus and hydration state of stratum corneum in hemodialysis patients. Am J Nephrol 20: 437-442, 2000

52. Dimkovic N, Djukanovic L, Radmilovic A, Bojic P, Juloski T: Uremic pruritus and cell mast cells. Nephron 61: 5-9, 1992

53. Raju SF, White AR, Barnes TT, Smith PP, Kirchner KA: Improvement in disequilibrium symptoms during dialysis with low glucose dialysate. Clin Nephrol 18: 126-129, 1982

54. Dreisbach AW, Hendrickson T, Beezhold D, Riesenberg LA, Sklar AH: Elevated levels of tumor necrosis factor alpha in postdialysis fatigue. Int J Artif Organs 21(2): 83-86, 1998

55. Ing TS, Daugirdas JT, Popli S, Gandhi VC: First-use syndrome with cuprammonium cellulose dialyzers. Int J Artif Organs 6: 235-239, 1983

56. Bonnie-Schorn E, Grassmann A, Uhlenbusch-Körwer I, Weber C, Vienken J: Water quality control in reprocessing practices in *Water quality in hemodialysis*, edited by Vienken J, Pabst Science Publishers, Lengerich: 80-86, 1998

57. Bonnie-Schorn E, Grassmann A, Uhlenbusch-Körwer I, Weber C, Vienken J: Clinical consequences of poor water and dialysis fluid quality in *Water quality in hemodialysis*, edited by Vienken J, Pabst Science Publishers, Lengerich: 50-79, 1998

58. Brunet P, Berland Y: Water quality and complications of haemodialysis. Nephrol Dial Transplant 15(5): 578-580, 2000

59. Hoenich NA, Thompson J, McCabe J, Appleton DR: Particle release from hemodialyzers. Int J Artif Organs 13(12): 803-808, 1990

60. Inagaki H, Hamazaki T, Kuroda H, Yano S: Foreign particles contaminating hemodialyzers and methods of removing them by rinsing. Nephron 46: 343-346, 1987

61. Ronco C, Ghezzi PM, Hoenich NA, Delfino P: Membranes and filters for hemodialysis, Database 2001 page 55, CD ROM Karger, ISBN 3-8055-7062-7, 2001

62. Haemodialysis adequacy workgroup: National Kidney Foundation DOQI™: clinical practice guidelines for hemodialysis adequacy, 2000 update. Am J Kidney Dis 37(Suppl 1): S7-S64, 2001

63. Grammer LC, Harris KE, Shaughnessy MA, Dolovich J, Patterson R, Evans S: Antibodies to toluene diisocyanate in patients with and without dialysis anaphylaxis. Artif Organs 15(1): 2-4,1991

64. Kato A, Takita T, Furuhashi M, Takahashi T, Maruyama Y, Hishida A: Elevation of blood (1-->3)-beta-D-glucan concentrations in hemodialysis patients. Nephron 89(1): 15-19, 2001

65. Kanda H, Hamasaki K, Kanda Y, Kitamura T, Fujita T, Yamamoto K, Mimura T: Influence of various hemodialysis membranes on the plasma (1-->3)-beta-D-glucan level. Kidney Int 60(1): 319-321, 2001

66. Oishi T, Ohara M, Watanabe Y, Yamaguchi K, Kojima C, Mochizicki T: Influence of various dialysis membranes on plasma (1->3)-beta-D-glucan. (Abstract) ASN (SU-PO874), 2003

67. Grammer LC: Hypersensivity. Nephrol Dial Transplant 9(Suppl 2): 29-35, 1994

68. Puerello D'Ambrosio F, Savica V, Gangemi S, Ricciardi L, Bagnato GF, Santoro D, Cuzzocrea S, Bellinghieri G: Ethylene oxid allergy in hemodialysis patients. Nephrol Dial Transplant 12: 1461-1463, 1997

69. Dolovich J, Bell B: Allergy to a product(s) of ethylene oxide gas: demonstration of IgE and IgG antibodies and hapten specificity. J Allergy Clin Immunol 62(1): 30-32, 1978

70. Poothullil J, Shimizu A, Day RP, Dolovich J: Anaphylaxis from the product(s) of ethylene oxide gas. Ann Intern Med 82(1): 58-60, 1975

71. Grammer LC, Patterson R: IgE against ethylene oxide-altered human serum albumin (ETO-HSA) as an etiologic agent in allergic reactions of hemodialysis patients. Artif Organs 11(2):97-99, 1987

72. Lemke HD, Heidland A, Schaefer RM: Hypertensivity reactions during haemodialysis: role of complement fragments and ethylene oxide antibodies. Nephrol Dial Transplant 5(4): 264-269, 1990

73. Bommer J, Ritz E: Ethylene oxide (ETO) as a major cause of anaphylactoid reactions in dialysis. Artif Organs 11(2): 111-117, 1987

74. Popli S, Ing TS, Daugirdas JT, Kheirbek AO, Viol GW, Vilbar RM, Gandhi VC: Severe anaphylactic reactions to cuprophan capillary dialysers. J Artif Organs 6(3): 312-315, 1982

75. Daugirdas JT, Ing TS, Roxe DM, Ivanovich PT, Krumlowsky F, Popli S, McLaughlin MM: Severe anaphylactoid reactions to cuprammonium cellulose hemodialysers. Arch Intern Med 145, 489-494, 1985

76. Kraske GK, Shinaberger JH, Klaustermeyer WB: Severe hypersensivity reaction during hemodialysis. Ann Allergy Asthma Immunol 78(2): 217-220, 1997

77. Santoro A, Ferrari G, Francioso A, Zuchelli P, Duranti E, Sasdelli M, Rosati A, Salvadori M, Sanna GM, Briganti M, Fusaroli M, Lindner G, Stefani A, Borgatti P, Badiali F, Mignani R, Cagnoli L, Aucella F, Stallone C, Massazza M, Borghi M, Gualandris L, Modoni S, Grandone E, Margaglione M, Scatizzi L, Orlandini G: Ethylene-oxide and steam-sterilized polysulfone membrane in dialysis patients with eosinophilia. Int J Artif Organs 19(6): 329-335, 1996

78. Wolfgang Kummerle: Comment on Dr Canaud's editorial. (Letter) Nephrol Dial Transplant 17: 2034-2035, 2002

79. Sass DJ, Van Dyke RA, Wood EH, Johnson SA, Didisheim P: Gas embolism due to intravenous FC 80 liquid fluorocarbon. J Appl Physiol 40(5): 745-751, 1976

80. Pertosa G, Grandaliano G, Gesualdo L, Schena FP: Clinical relevance of cytokine production in hemodialysis. Kidney Int 58(Suppl 76): S104-S111, 2000

81. Hakim RM: Clinical implications of biocompatibility in blood purification membranes. Nephrol Dial Transplant 15(Suppl 2): 16-20, 2000

82. Hakim R, Breillatt J, Lazarus JM, Port FK: Complement activation and hypertensitivity reactions to dialysis membranes. N Engl J Med 311: 878-82, 1984

83. Craddock PR, Fehr J, Dalmasso AP, Brigham KL, Jakob HS: Hemodialysis leukopenia: pulmonary vascular leukostasis resulting from complement activation by dialyzer cellophane membranes. J Clin Invest 59: 879-888, 1977

84. Clark WR, Hamburger RJ, Lysaght MJ: Effect of membrane composition and structure on solute removal and biocompatibility in hemodialysis. Kidney Int 56: 2005-2015, 1999

85. Gesualdo L, Pertosa G, Grandaliano G, Schena FP: Cytokines and biocompatibility. Nephrol Dial Transplant 13: 1622-1626, 1998

86. Chenoweth DE: The properties of human C5a anaphylatoxin. The significance of C5a formation during hemodialysis. Contrib Nephrol 59: 51-71, 1987

87. Schindler R, Lonnemann G, Shaldon S, Koch KM, Dinarello CA: Transcription, not synthesis of Interleukin-1 and tumor necrosis factor by complement. Kidney Int 37: 85-93, 1990

88. Bergamo Collaborative Dialysis Study Group (Mingardi G, Rota S, Orlandini G, Misiani R, Bernareggi S, Facci O, Marchesi D; Bonetti L, Schieppati A, Benigni A, Piccinelli A, Gualandris L, Licini R, Mangili A; Mecca G, Poletti E, Tiraboschi G, Grassi C, Bracchi O, Pedroni G, Metarangelis A, Lorenz M, Ondei P, Pedrini L, Cozzi G, Faranna P, Borghi M, Vendramin G, Massazza M, Rusconi L, Guiliano P): Acute intradialytic well-being: results of a clinical trial comparing polysulphone with cuprophan. Kidney Int 40: 714-719, 1991

89. Collins DM, Lambert MB, Oliverio M, Schwab SJ: Tolerance of hemodialysis: a randomized, prospective trial of high-flux versus conventional high efficiency hemodialysis. J Am Soc Nephrol 4(2): 148-54, 1993

90. Aakhus S, Bjoernstad K, Jørstad S: Systemic cardiovascular response in hemodialysis without and with ultrafiltration with membranes with high and low biocompatibility. Blood Purif 13(5): 229-240, 1995

91. Skroeder NR, Jacobson SH, Lins LE, Kjellstrand CM: Acute symptoms during and between hemodialysis: the relative role of speed, duration, and biocompatibility of dialysis. Artif Organs 18(12): 880-887, 1994

92. Tielemans C, Madhoun P, Lenaers M, Schandene L, Goldman M, Vanherweghem JL: Anaphylactoid reactions during hemodialysis on AN69 membranes in patients receiving ACE inhibitors. Kidney Int 38: 982-984, 1990

93. Parnes EL, Shapiro WB: Anaphylactoid reactions in hemodialysis patients treated with the AN69 dialyzer. Kidney Int 40(6): 1148-1152, 1991

94. Brunet P, Jaber K, Berland Y, Baz M: Anaphylactoid reactions during hemodialysis and hemofiltration: role of associating AN69 membrane and angiotensin I-converting enzyme inhibitors. Am J Kidney Dis 19(5): 444-447, 1992

95. Verresen L, Fink E, Lemke HD, Vanrenterghem Y: Bradykinin is a mediator of anaphylactoid reactions during hemodialysis with AN69 membanes. Kidney Int 45: 1497-1503, 1994

96. Verresen L, Waer M, Vanreterghem Y, Michielsen P: Angiotensin-converting-enzyme-inhibitors and anaphylactoid reactions to high-flux membrane dialysis. Lancet 336: 1360-1362, 1990

97. Dinarello CA: ACE inhibitors and anaphylactoid reactions to high-flux membrane dialysis. (Letter) Lancet 337: 370, 1991

98. Jadoul M, Struyven J, Stragier A, Van Ypersele de Strihou C: Angiotensin-converting-enzyme-inhibitors and anaphylactoid reactions to high-flux membrane dialysis. (Letter) Lancet 337: 112, 1991

99. Fink E, Lemke HD, Verresen L, Shimamoto K: Kinin generation by hemodialysis membranes as a possible cause of anaphylactic reactions. Brazilian J Med Biol Res 27(8): 1975-1983, 1994

100. Lemke HD, Fink E: Accumulation of bradykinin formed by the AN69- or PAN 17DX-membrane is due to the presence of an ACE inhibitor in vitro. (Abstract) J Am Soc Nephrol 3: 376, 1992

101. Krieter DH, Grude M, Lemke HD, Fink E, Bönner G, Schölkens BA, Schulz E, Müller A: Anaphylactoid reactions during hemodialysis in sheep are ACE inhibitor dose-dependant and mediated by bradykinin. Kidney Int 53: 1026-1035, 1998

102. Krieter DH, Fink E, Bönner G, You HM, Eisenhauer T: Anaphylactoid reactions during haemodialysis in sheep are associated with bradykinin release. Nephrol Dial Transplant 10: 509-513,1995

103. Gavras H, Gavras I: Endothelian function in cardiovascular disease: the role of bradykinin, Science Press limited, London: 1996, deutsche Übersetzung: 9-57, 1998

104. Lazarus JM, Owen WF: Role of bioincompatibility in dialysis morbidity and mortality. Am J Kidney Dis 24(6): 1019-1032, 1994

105. Koch KM: Clinical relevance of biocompatibility. Nephrol Dial Transplant 9(Suppl 2): 126, 1994

106. Schaefer RM, Fink E, Schaefer L, Barkhausen R, Kulzer P, Heidland A: Role of bradykinin in anaphylactoid reactions during hemodialysis with AN69 membranes. Am J Nephrol 13(6): 473-477, 1993

107. Wakasa M, Akizawa T, Kinugasa E, Koshikawa S: Plasma bradykinin levels during hemodialysis with PAN DX and polysulfone membranes with and without concurrent ACE inhibitor. Clin Nephrol 44(Suppl 1): S29-S32, 1995

108. Van der Niepen P, Sennesael JJ, Verbeelen DL: Kinin kinetics during different dialysis protocols with AN69 dialyser in ACEI-treated patients. Nephrol Dial Transplant 10(9): 1689-1695, 1995

109. Renaux JL, Thomas M, Crost T, Loughraieb N, Vantard G: Activation of the kallikrein-kinin system in hemodialysis: role of membrane electronegativity, blood dilution, and pH. Kidney Int 55: 1097-1103, 1999

110. Kammerl MC, Schaefer RM, Schweda F, Schreibner M, Riegger GAJ, Krämer BK: Extracorporal therapy with AN69 membranes in combination with

ACE inhibition causing severe anaphylactoid reactions: still a current problem? Clin Nephrol 53(6): 486-488, 2000

111. Maheut H, Lacour F: Using AN69 ST membranes: a dialysis center experience. (Letter) Nephrol Dial Transpl 16: 1519-1520, 2001

112. Mannstadt M, Touam M, Fink E, Hruby M, Zingraff J, Uhlenbusch-Körwer I, Grassmann A, Lemke HD, Drüeke T: No generation of bradykinin with a new polyacrylonitrile membrane (SPAN) in haemodialysis patients treated with ACE inhibitors. Nephrol Dial Transplant 10: 1696-1700, 1995

113. Amore A, Pertosa G, Guarnieri F, Atti M, Schena FP, Coppo R: Use of alkaline rinsing solution to prevent hypersensitivity reactions during hemodialysis: data from a multicentre retrospective analysis. J Nephrol 12(6): 383-389, 1999

114. Peces R: Anaphylactoid reaction induced by ACEI during haemodialysis with surface-treated AN69 membrane. (Letter) Nephrol Dial Transplant 17(10): 1859-1860, 2002

115. Grottes JM, Molinaro G, Adam A, Muniz MC, Nortier J, Thomas M, Tielemans C: A new type of adverse reactions (AR) during hemodialysis (HD) on AN69 hollow fiber dialysers. Solving the problem by a different membrane treatment procedure with polyethylene imine (PEI). (Abstract) J Am Soc Nephrol 13: A579, 2002

116. Schwarzbeck A, Wittenmeier KW, Hällfritsch U, Frank J: Anaphylatoid reactions (AR) associated with PMMA high flux dialyzers (HDF) and ACE- Inhibitors (ACE-I). Nephron 65: 499-500, 1993

117. Kojima S, Harada-Shiba M, Nomura S, Kimura G, Tsushima M, Kuramochi M, Yamamoto A, Omae T: Effect of nafamostat mesilate on bradykinin generation during low-density lipoprotein apheresis using a dextran sulfate cellulose column. Trans Am Soc Artif Int Org 37: 644-648, 1991

118. Olbricht CJ, Schauman D, Fischer D: Anaphylactoid reactions, LDL-apheresis with dextrane sulfate, and ACE inhibitors. (Letter) Lancet 340: 908-909, 1992

119. Saracho R, Martin-Malo A, Martinez I, Aljama P, Montenegro J: Evaluation of the losartan in haemodialysis (ELHE) Study. Kidney Int 54(Suppl 68): S125-S129, 1998

120. John B, Anijeet HKI; Ahmad R: Anaphylactic reaction during haemodialysis on AN69 membrane in a patient receiving angiotensin II receptor antagonist. (Letter) Nephrol Dial Transplant 16(9): 1955-1956, 2001

121. Krieter DH, Canaud B: Anaphylactic reaction during haemodialysis on AN69 membrane in a patient receiving angiotensin II receptor antagonist. (Letter) Nephrol Dial Transplant 17: 943-944, 2002

122. Tepel M, van der Giet M, Zidek W: Efficacy and tolerability of angiotensin II type1 receptor antagonists in dialysis patients using AN69 dialysis membranes. Kidney Blood Press Res 24(1): 71-74, 2001

123. Lemke HD, Grassmann A, Vienken J, Shaldon S: Biocompatibility - clinical aspects in *Replacement of renal function*, 2nd ed., edited by AM Davison, JS Cameron, JP Grünfeld, Kerr DNS, E Ritz, CG Winearls, Oxford University Press: 734-749, 1996

124. Huang CC, Lin MC, Yang CT, Lan RS, Tsai VH, Tsao TCY: Oxygen, arterial blood gases and ventilation are unchanged during dialysis in patients receiving pressure support ventilation. Respir Med 92(3): 534-540, 1998

125. Tsai YH, Huang CC, Lin MC, Chen NH, Chang YJ, Lee CH: Arterial oxygenation is unchanged during hemodialysis in patients mechanically ventilated in assist-control mode. J Formos Med Assoc 97(2): 90-96, 1998

126. Huang CC, Tsai YH, Lin MC, Yang CT, Hsieh MJ, Lan RS: Respiratory drive and pulmonary mechanics during haemodialysis with ultrafiltration in ventilated patients. Anaesth Intens Care 25(5): 464-470, 1998

127. Rousseau Y, Carreno MP, Poignet JL, Kazatchkine MD, Haeffner-Cavaillon N: Dissociation between complement activation, intergrin expression and neutropenia during hemodialysis. Biomaterials 20(20): 1959-1967, 1999

128. Dhakal MP, Kallay MC, Shelly MA, Talley TE: Post-hemodialysis hypoxemia occurs with both biocompatible and bioincompatiible dialyzers. Dial Transplant 28(11): 666-672, 1999

129. Haeffner-Cavaillon N, Cavaillon JM, Ciancioni CH, Bacle F, Delons S, Kazatchkine MD: In vivo induction of interleukin-1 during hemodialysis. Kidney Int 35: 1212-1218, 1989

130. Kushihata S, Yorioka N, Oda H, Ye XF, Yamakido M: Effects of dialysis membranes on the kinetics of tumor necrosis factor-α production by peripheral mononuclear cells in chronic hemodialysis patients. Int J Artif Organs 21(7): 384-390, 1998

131. Pereira BJG: Cytokine production in patients on dialysis. Blood Purif 13: 135-146, 1995

132. Michie HR, Manogue KR, Spriggs DR, Revaugh A, O'Dwyer S, Dinarello CA, Cerami A, Wolff SM, Wilmore DW: Detection of circulating tumor necrosis factor after endotoxin administration. N Engl J Med 318(23): 1481-1486, 1988

133. Bingel M, Lonnemann G, Koch KM, Dinarello CA, Shaldon S: Plasma interleukin-1 activity during hemodialysis: the influence of dialysis membranes. Nephron 50: 273-276, 1988

134. Qian Z, Yu Z, Dai H, Zhang Q, Chen S: Influence of hemodialysis membrane on gene expression and plasma levels of interleukin-1ß. Artif Organs 19(8): 842-846, 1995

135. Mandolfo S, Tetta C, David S, Gervasio R, Ognibene D, Wratten ML, Tessore E, Imbasciati E: *In vitro* and *in vivo* biocompatibility of substituted cellulose and synthetic membranes. Int J Artif Organs 20(11): 603-609, 1997

136. Bonomini M, Sirolli V, Settefrati N, Stuard S, Tropea F, Di Liberto L, Tetta C, Albertazzi A: Surface antigen expression and platelet neutrophil interactions in haemodialysis. Blood Purif 17(2-3): 107-117, 1999

137. Lin YF, Chang DM, Shaio MF, Lu KC, Chyr SH, Li Bl, Sheih SD: Cytokine production during hemodialysis: effects of dialytic membrane and complement activation. Am J Nephrol 16(4): 293-299, 1996

138. Lonnemann G, Koch KM, Shaldon S, Dinarello CA: Studies on the ability of hemodialysis membranes to induce, bind, and clear human interleukin. J Lab Clin Med 112(1): 76-86, 1988

139. Lonnemann G , Barndt I, Kaefer V, Haubitz M, Schindler R, Shaldon S, Koch KM: Impaired endotoxin induced interleukin-1ß secretion, not total production, of mononuclear cells from ESRD patients. Kidney Int 47: 1158-1167, 1995

140. Coli L, Tumietto F, De Pascalis A, La Manna G, Zanchelli F, Isola E, Perna C, Raimondi C, De Sanctis LB, Marseglia CD, Costigliola P, Stefoni S: Effects of dialysis membrane nature on intradialytic phagocytizing activity. Int J Artif Organs 22(2): 74-80, 1999

141. Shaldon S, Deschodt G, Branger B, Granolleras C, Baldamus CA, Koch KM, Lysaght M, Dinarello C: Haemodialysis hypotension: the interleukin hypothesis restated. Proc EDTA-ERA 22: 229-243, 1985

142. Schohn DC, Jahn, HA, Eber M, Hauptmann G: Biocompatibility and hemodynamic studies during polycarbonate versus cuprophane membrane dialysis. Blood Purif 4: 102-111, 1986

143. Skroeder NR, Jacobson SH, Lins LE, Kjellstrand CM: Biocompatibility of dialysis membranes is of no importance for objective or subjective symptoms during or after hemodialysis. Trans Am Soc Artif Intern Organs 36: M637-M639, 1990

144. Locatelli F: Influence of membranes on morbidity. Nephrol Dial Transplant 11(Suppl 2): 116-120, 1996

145. Locatelli F, Mastrangelo F, Redaelli B, Ronco C, Marcelli D, La Greca G, Orlandini G: Effects of different membranes and dialysis technologies on patient treatment tolerance and nutritional parameters. Kidney Int 50: 1293-1302, 1996

146. Davenport A, Davison AM, Will EJ: Membrane biocompatibility: Effects on cardiovascular stability in patients on hemofiltration. Kidney Int 43(Suppl 41): S230-S243, 1993

147. Brunet P, Saingra Y, Leonetti F, Vacher-Coponat H, Ramananarivo P, Berland Y: Tolerance of haemodialysis: a randomized cross-over trial of 5-h versus 4-h treatment time. Nephrol Dial Transplant 11(Suppl 8): 46-51, 1996

148. Sklar A, Newman N, Scott R, Semenyuk L, Schultz J, Fiacco V: Identification of factors responsible for postdialysis fatigue. Am J Kidney Dis 34(3): 464-470 1999

149. Sklar AH, Beezhold DH, Newman N, Hendrickson T, Dreisbach AW: Postdialysis fatigue: lack of effect of a biocompatible membrane. Am J Kidney Dis. 31(6): 1007-1010, 1998

10. Possible contributions of dialyser characteristics to long-term problems in ESRD

In this chapter, the possible contributions of both dialyser performance (as discussed in section B) and bioincompatibility (as discussed in section C) to long-term problems in ESRD will be discussed. Dialyser performance characteristics define the diffusive and convective removal of uraemic toxins and, therefore, determine together with other important parameters, such as blood and dialysis fluid flow as well as treatment lenght and intervals, the dose of dialysis that a patient receives. Dialysis dose is known to strongly correlate with patient morbidity and survival [1-16]. Consequently, recommendations for dialysis adequacy have been formulated on the basis of dialysis dose quantification for small solutes by national and international committees, e.g. minimum equilibrated eKt/V ≥ 1.0 (or single-pool spKt/V ≥ 1.2) and/or urea reduction rate ≥ 65% by the National Kidney Foundation's Dialysis Outcome Quality Initiative (NKF-DOQI™) [17], the Renal Association in the UK [18] and the Canadian Society of Nephrology [19], or eKt/V ≥ 1.2 (spKt/V ≥ 1.4) according to the European Best Practice Guidelines for Haemodialysis (EBP guideline II.1.3 [20]). The actual method of determination of Kt/V (i.e. either eKt/V or spKt/V) is clearly of clinical importance here.

However, the performance characteristics of a dialyser are defined in part by its permeability or adsorptive capacity for middle molecules, such as ß2-microglobulin (e.g. [21-24] and chapter 5). Furthermore, dialysers also differ in their abilities to absorb endotoxins from the blood (e.g. [25-32]). Consequently dialyser performance characteristics exert an influence on particular diseases common in ESRD. Chronic inflammatory state and amyloidosis are examples of such diseases. High-flux dialysers may also remove putative inhibitors of erythropoiesis (e.g. [33, 34]), lipoprotein lipase A (e.g. [35-38]) and homocysteine metabolism (e.g. [39, 40]) during the treatment, influencing renal anaemia and atherosclerotic risk factors (i.e. hyperhomocysteinaemia and hyperlipidaemia). Therefore, first recommendations that take the need for enhanced middle molecule removal in achieving haemodialysis adequacy into account have recently been launched: e.g. the use of synthetic high-flux membranes, the addition of a convective component, the increase of treatment time and/or frequency in association with high-flux dialysis (European Best Practice Guideline II.2.2 [20]). Finally, dialysers and haemofilters are permeable to essential nutrients, such as amino acids or vitamins, and thus may influence the nutritional state of the patient.

On the other hand, the bioincompatibility of a dialyser has an impact on immune modulation in such a way that complement activation and cytokine release are induced (e.g. [41-48] and chapters 7 and 8). Therefore, dialyser bioincompatibility contributes to the chronic inflammatory state in ESRD, as well as to oxidative and carbonyl stress. This contribution of bioincompatibility is achieved through various, partially interrelated, pathophysiological pathways.

All the above-mentioned mechanisms are believed to promote atherosclerosis and to partially contribute to malnutrition, renal anaemia, loss of residual renal function, susceptibility to infection, pruritus, disturbed peripheral nerve function and amyloidosis. They are, therefore, the main focus of attention in both this chapter and current Good Dialysis Practice in general. **Figure 10.1** offers an overview of these diseases and their sometimes common pathophysiological origins.

10.1 Pathophysiological pathways common to various diseases

In ESRD, the presence of an inflammatory state with a multi-factor genesis is common [32, 49-53]. In addition, there is evidence of augmented oxidative stress resulting from an accumulation of several pro-oxidants, i.e. various low molecular weight proteins (< 3000), carbonyls and homocysteines [54]. Oxidation of carbohydrates and lipids leads to the formation of reactive carbonyl compounds (RCOs); this also indirectly results in carbonyl stress as the advanced glycation and lipidoxidation of proteins form advanced glycation end products (AGE) and advanced lipidoxidation end products (ALE), respectively [55]. These three conditions, inflammation, oxidative stress and carbonyl stress, can be considered common steps in the pathophysiological pathways of various diseases, and are interrelated in the sense that they often amplify

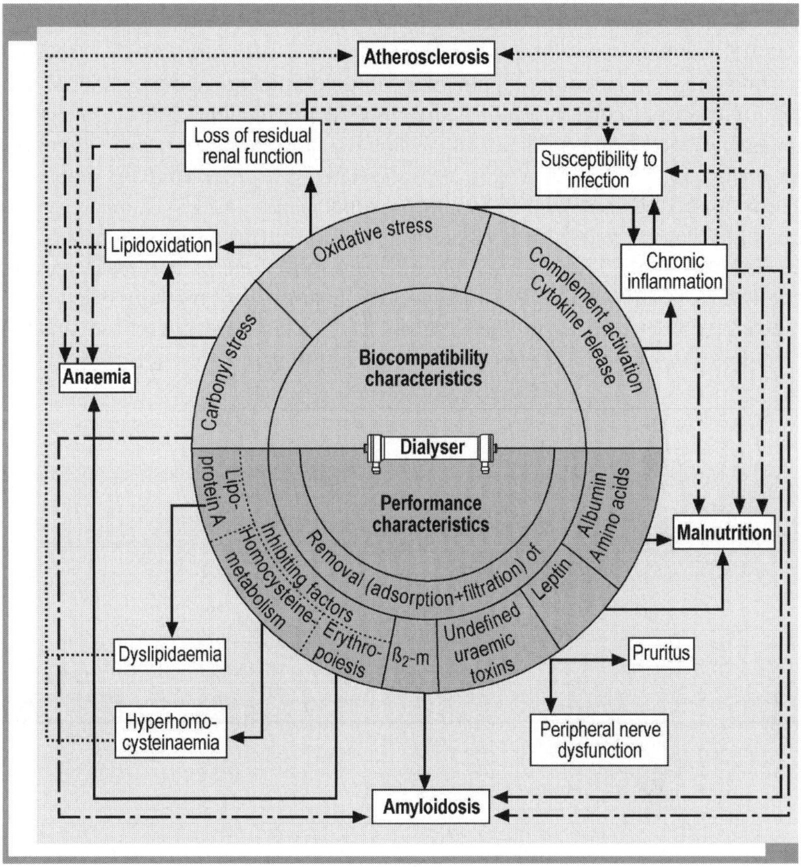

Figure 10.1: *Possible contributions of dialyser and haemofilter performance and biocompatibility to major clinical problems in ESRD and interrelations thereof. Black arrows show direct contributions, grew or dotted arrows indicate secondary effects and/or interrelations.*

each other. The consequence is an increased influence on many of the diseases mentioned in **figure 10.1** and discussed in detail in sections 2 - 9 of this chapter.

10.1.1 Chronic inflammatory state

Inflammation has been identified as an epidemiological important risk factor for cardiovascular disease in the general population [56-59]. In dialysis patients, it is a strong predictor of cardiovascular and the so-called "all-cause" mortality [50, 51, 60-69], and is also correlated with morbidity, as measured in days of hospitalisation [70]. In chronic renal failure and ESRD, inflammation not only plays a role in atherosclerosis [71-75], but also in malnutrition [61, 62, 64, 71, 76-80] and anaemia [81-85]. The term "microinflammatory state" evolved from the finding that increases in inflammatory markers (such as C-reactive protein (CRP) and interleukin-6 (IL-6)), which were even too small to have any obvious clinical effects, predicted future vascular events [86].

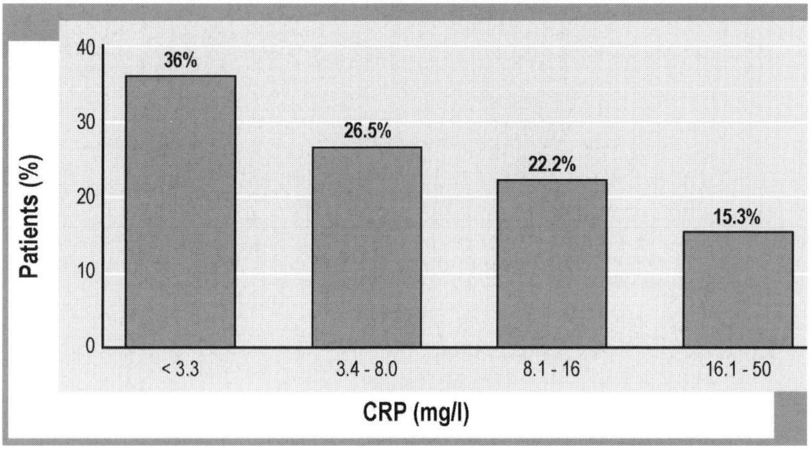

Figure 10.2: Presence of microinflammation in ESRD. *Levels of C-reactive protein (CRP) were measured in blood samples taken routinely from 72 dialysis patients on long-term dialysis (at least 1 year ESRD) and treated with low-flux polysulfone dialysers (F5/F6, Fresenius Medical Care). Data from patients diagnosed with bacterial or viral infections or with other known chronic inflammatory diseases (e.g. vasculitis, lupus erythemathodes, hepatitis) were not included. In 62.5% of the patients, CRP values were below the level of clinical relevance, defined as 8.0 mg/l for the assay used (CRP levels were below the detection limit (< 3.3 mg/l) in 36% of the patients, and between 3.4 and 8.0 mg/l in 26.5% of the patients). However, elevated CRP levels were measured in 37.5% of the patients: levels were slightly elevated in 22.2% and very elevated in 15.3% thereof (adapted from [32]).*

Causes of chronic inflammation in ESRD	
Not associated with the dialysis treatment	**Associated with the dialysis treatment**
Individual reactivity to inflammatory stimuli	
Inflammatory diseases e.g. • underlying nephropathy • previous therapy	
Unrecognised persistent infections e.g. • Chlamydia pneumoniae • Cytomegalie, herpes, hepatitis • Dental or gingival infections	(Un)recognised (persistent) infections • Graft-, fistula,- catheter infections
Chronic heart failure • "Leaky gut" syndrome	
Atherosclerotic disease • Plaque disruption and release of cytokines from activated monocytes	
Protein malnutrition	

Uraemic state per se
• Reduced removal of cytokines
• Accumulation of end products of advanced glycation and lipid oxidation
• Accumulation of reactive carbonyl compounds
• Oxidative stress
• Hyper-/dyslipidaemia
	Bioincompatibility of the system
	• Direct membrane effect
	• Exposure to bacterial or other cytokine-inducing substances
	  • from contaminated dialysate via backfiltration and/or backdiffusion
	  • from poor reuse practices

Table 10.1: Main factors contributing to chronic inflammation in ESRD.

Microinflammation is common in dialysis patients [32, 49-53, 69] (see **figure 10.2**). A recent review of various studies on microimflammation in dialysis patients reports prevalences of between 35 and 65% in the patients examined [87]. The occurrence and the degree of microinflammation may also vary with time, i.e. it may be intermittent and of varying intensity in character, rather than a continuous, constant feature in all patients [88]. The cause of chronic inflammation is likely to be multifactorial (see **table 10.1**). In addition to those infections that are clinically apparent, hidden infections also play a role [73, 75, 89, 90]. Several other factors may promote inflammation in uraemia as well, e.g. increased oxidative stress, the accumulation of reactive carbonyl compounds and advanced glycation and lipidoxidation end products, and protein malnutrition [55, 91-100]. Finally, the dialysis treatment also involves repeated exposure to stimuli, which can promote inflammation, such as the use of non-ultrapure dialysis fluid or bioincompatible material (reviewed in [5, 47, 48, 101, 102]).

The question of interest here is whether the dialyser itself (and especially the membrane) has any effect on the microinflammatory state of the dialysis patient. Possible direct membrane effects are membrane-associated complement activation and cytokine release, and membrane permeability for bacterial substances from the dialysis fluid. The possible individual and synergistic contributions of these factors to the microinflammatory state of dialysis patients will be addressed in the following.

Does membrane permeability for bacterial fragments influence the microinflammatory state in dialysis patients?

In order to answer this question, we first have to consider the different permeabilities of the various dialyser membranes to substances of bacterial origin that can be present in the dialysis fluid. As reviewed in previous works [31, 32], both *in vitro* and *in vivo* studies have provided evidence that all membranes are permeable to cytokine inducing substances (CIS) of bacterial origin that have molecular weights lower than 5000 [32] (e.g. peptidoglycans, endotoxin fragments, some outer membrane proteins) (e.g. [25-30]). However, the ability of a membrane to inhibit transfer of such CIS from the dialysis fluid to the blood varies substantially from membrane to membrane, whereby the adsorptive capacity of the membrane, rather than pore size, is decisive for the retention of CIS and proteins [25, 32, 103, 104], as shown in **table 10.2**.

Dialyser	UF-coefficient (ml/h·mmHg)	Membrane	Lipid A adsorbed onto the membrane (µg/m²)	LPS adsorbed onto the membrane (ng/m²)
F4	2.8	Low-flux polysulfone	38.8 ± 8.1	360 ± 42
E3 (Cuprophan®)	5.8	Regenerated cellulose	4.5 ± 3.4	91 ± 29
Acepal 1300	8.0	Cellulose acetate	10.7 ± 2.3	162 ± 38
Altraflux	15.0	Cellulose acetate	11.0 ± 1.3	90 ± 42
Filtral 12 (AN69®)	32.0	Polyacryl-onitrile	12.8 ± 4.7	109 ± 84
F60	40.0	High-flux polysulfone	55.5 ± 7.1	567 ± 80
Polyflux 110	42.0	Polyamide	61.1 ± 10.8	352 ± 123

Table 10.2: Dialysis membranes have different adsorption capacities for bacterial fragments. *The adsorption capacities of 7 dialysis membranes are shown for lipid A from E. coli and LPS from P. aeruginosa, as measured by the limulus amoebocyte lysate (LAL) test after incubation with 1 l of water spiked with 100 ng/ml and 1 ng/ml, respectively (adapted from [30]).*

Three mechanisms contribute to the pyrogen retention capacity of a membrane. First, hydrophobic interactions between the dialysis membrane and lipophilic LAL-reactive material prevail in the adsorption process. Therefore, hydrophobic membranes, such as polysulfone and polyamide, reveal a high binding capacity for the bacterial product lipid A. On the other hand, adsorption is insignificant with hydrophilic materials, such as regenerated cellulose, cellulose acetate or AN69® [30]. However, hydrophilic membranes are able to bind LPS, although to a lesser extent than hydrophobic membranes, indicating that other factors may be also involved in the adsorption processes [30]. Second, among other parameters, the membrane thickness determines the diffusive resistance of the dialyser membrane [103]. Diffusion is an important transport mechanism for CIS. Therefore, a thicker membrane will be less permeable for CIS than a thinner one. Low-flux cellulosic membranes are only 6-8 μm thick, whereas synthetic membranes are approximately 35-50 μm in thickness. Synthetic membranes consist of a thin, skin-like surface on the blood side of the hollow fibre that is supported by a thick sponge-like structure. Coming from the dialysis fluid side, the CIS first enter the support structure; here adsorption is particularly effective. A third mechanism involved in the pyrogen retention capacity of a membrane is the formation of a second layer of plasma proteins on the blood side of the dialyser membrane. This so-called "protein coating" affects the transport of CIS from the dialysis fluid to the blood. Membranes differ in their susceptibility to protein coating and/or the effect thereof on CIS transfer: protein coating of polysulfone (F40, Fresenius Medical Care) with 10% plasma was much more pronounced than with a modified cellulose triacetate (Sureflux FB 70E, Nissho) membrane, and could successfully avoid CIS transfer as measured by IL-1 generation [104]. Polyethersulfone (DIAPES® HF800 membrane) was also shown to attenuate passage of CISs from moderately contaminated dialysis fluid (50 EU/ml) *in vitro* when whole blood was used [105, 106]. However, high challenge doses induced a higher IL-1β and TNF-α production after 30 minutes for the DIAPES® membrane compared to polysulfone, although the absence of detectable differences after 60 minutes between the membranes is an issue of academic interest as the acute biological effects of the cytokines would already be manifest at the earlier time point [106]. Furthermore, two recent *in vitro* studies comparing the permeability of different high-flux and low-flux dialysers to bacterial pyrogens confirmed that the Fresenius Polysulfone® and Helixone® membranes (F60S, FX60, F6HPS) as well as membranes made from Polyamide S™ (Polyflux 14S, Polyflux 14L) are a safer barrier for pyrogen transfer from the dialysis fluid compartment into the saline-filled blood compartment than the DIAPES® membrane (BSL814SD in one study and BLS814G, BLS 517SD and BLS 517G in the second study) [107, 108] (see **figure 10.3**). Parameters measured in these studies after challenge with purified *E.coli* or *Pseudomonas aeruginosa* LPS and filtrates from *Stenothrophomonas maltophilia* cultures were IL-6, IL-1β, TNF-α production, IL-1 receptor antagonist- inducing activity and limulus amoebocyte lysate test (LAL) reactivity. However, the observed differences between membranes may not be as large when a protein layer is formed onto the membrane under *in vivo* dialysis conditions.

In addition to the above three membrane-associated factors, it is of interest that the endotoxin retention capacity of a membrane may differ even between manufacturers. For example, Fresenius Polysulfone® (F60) showed a much lower permeability for endotoxin *in vitro* than another polysulfone dialyser (PN 1913®, Primus 1350® Renal Systems (now Minntech)) [28]. However, in another study, Fresenius Polysulfone® (F60S) did not differ from Asahi Polysulfone® (APS 650) regarding passage of CIS [109].

Considering that the CIS retention capacities of different dialysers vary so much, one would expect this to be reflected by differences in the microinflammatory state of patients treated with different kinds of dialysers. But has this actually been observed? In studies addressing this, the peripheral blood mononuclear cell (PBMC) content of interleukin-1 receptor antagonist (IL-1Ra) is often used as a marker for monocyte activation. One of the first studies showed that monocyte activation dropped significantly in patients dialysed with low-flux regenerated cellulose dialysers when the moderately contaminated dialysis fluid was filtered through a Fresenius Polysulfone® high-flux membrane (F80) [110]. In a second study using similar dialysis fluid quality, monocyte activation was shown to be significantly less in patients treated with Fresenius Polysulfone® (F60) than in patients treated with regenerated cellulose membranes (see **figure 10.4**). This long-term clinical study also revealed that CRP values in patients treated with Fresenius Polysulfone® did not change when the dialysis fluid was ultrafiltered; this reflects the good CIS retention of Fresenius Polysulfone®. However, about one third of all the patients studied had elevated CRP values (CRP > 8 mg/l) [32] (see **figure 10.5**). At the same time, the *in vivo* effects of different dialyser membranes on the inflammatory state were compared using moderately contaminated dialysis fluid [52]. In this crossover study, the patients were treated with 3 different dialysers for 8 weeks each, namely polyamide (PF14 (hollow fibre), Gambro), polycarbonate-polyether (Pro 600 (plate), Gambro) and regenerated cellulose (Alpha 600 (plate), Gambro). Both plasma CRP and IL-1Ra levels were significantly lower when patients were dialysed with polyamide compared to regenerated cellulose. The levels of both of these laboratory markers were also lower for polycarbonate compared to regenerated cellulose, but differences did not attain statistical significance (see **figure 10.6**). Taken together, the results of these studies suggest that the use of moderately contaminated dialysis fluid in combination with a pyrogen-permeable dialyser membrane causes not only cytokine induction, but also contributes to elevated CRP plasma values in haemodialysis patients.

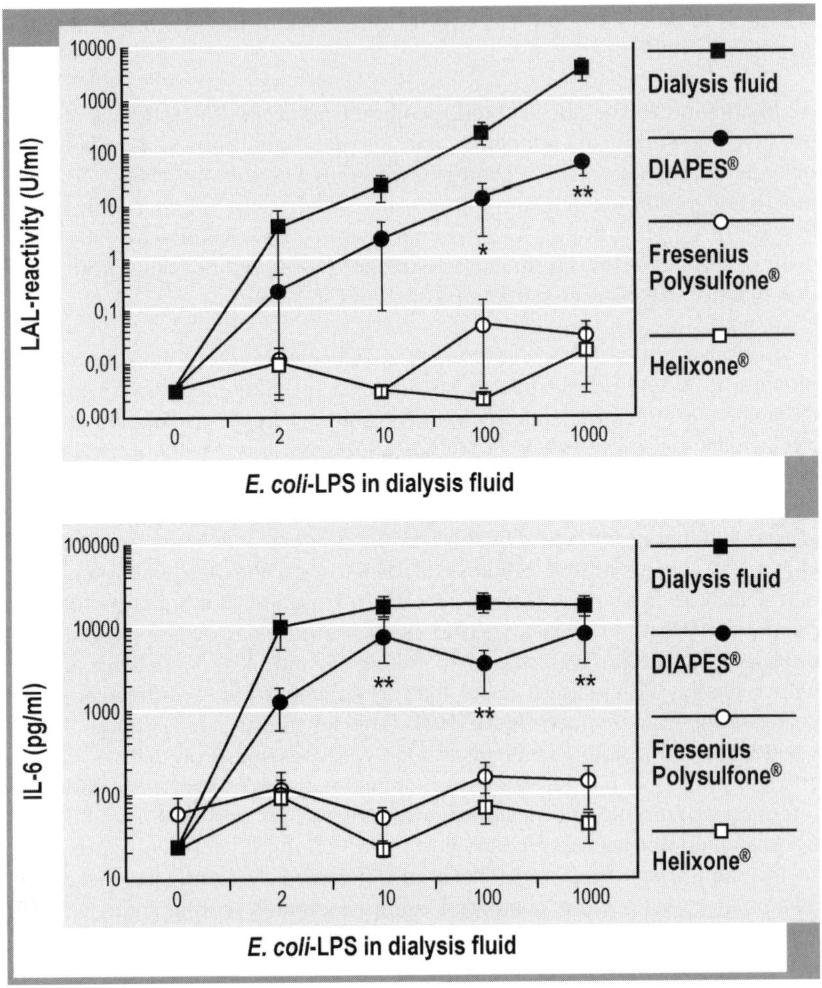

Figure 10.3: In vitro differences in the permeability of selected high-flux membranes for bacterialy pyrogens, as measured using (A) the LAL test and (B) cytokine induction. *The membranes tested were made from polysulfone (Fresenius Polysulfone® (F60S) and Helixone® (FX60), both from Fresenius Medical Care) and polyethersulfone (Diapes® (BLS 814 SD) from Bellco). Both dialysis fluid and blood compartments of the dialysers were filled with sterile saline solution at the start of the experiment. After initiation of circulation, the challenge doses of* E. coli *lipopolysaccharide (LPS) in the dialysis fluid were increased every 30 minutes. After 30 minutes of recirculation, samples from the blood cir-*

cuit were taken for analysis of pyrogen content, as measured via limulus amoebocyte lysate (LAL) reactivity (n = 7; the results are depicted in ***figure 10.3A****) and as measured by production of the cytokine Interleukin-6 (IL-6) in peripheral blood mononuclear cells (PBMCs) (n = 10; results given in* ***figure 10.3B****). The results of this experimental setting demonstrate the significantly smaller pyrogen permeability and subsequent cytokine induction with the use of the two polysulfone membranes compared to the polyethersulfone membrane, especially at higher dialysis fluid contaminations.*p < 0.05, **p < 0.01 (adapted from [107]).*

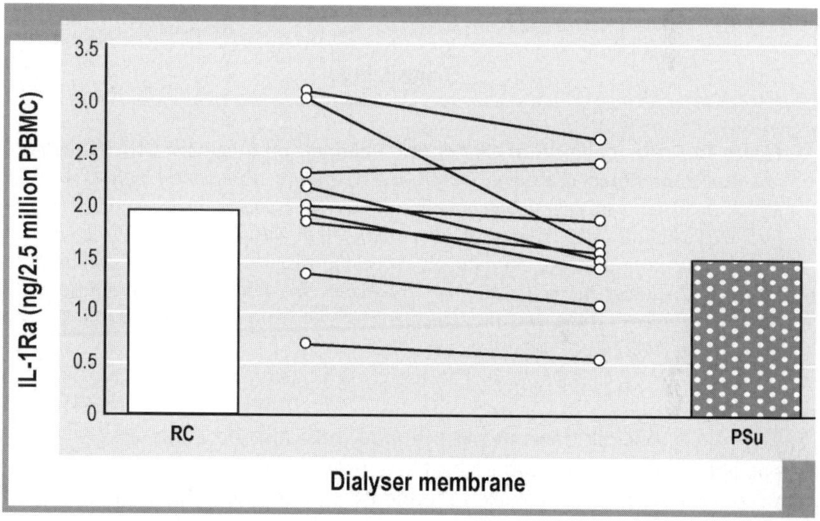

Figure 10.4: Cytokine-induction during dialysis with non-ultrafiltered dialysis fluid is influenced by the removal characteristics of the dialyser for cytokines. *IL-1Ra in PBMCs (ng/2.5 million PBMC), which represents monocyte activation, was shown to be significantly less in patients treated with Fresenius Polysulfone® (F60)(PSu) than in patients treated with regenerated cellulose (RC) membranes when non-filtered dialysis fluid was used (contamination: CFU: 159/ml, endotoxin: 0.18 EU/ml). This crossover study involving 10 stable haemodialysis patients lasted 6 weeks for each dialyser. Symbols represent the mean of 3 - 6 measurements. Horizontal columns indicate the group means (p < 0.013) (adapted from [32]).*

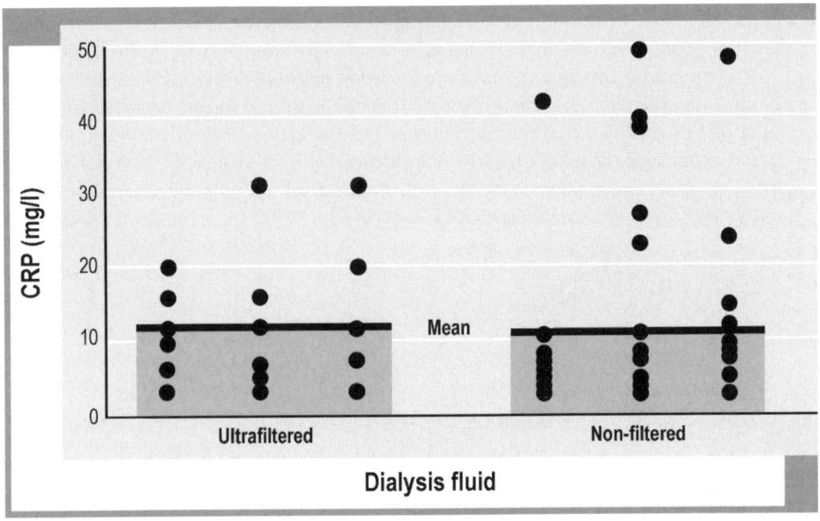

Figure 10.5: Plasma levels of CRP in ESRD patients on long-term dialysis with low-flux polysulfone dialysers. *During the 12-month observation period, the ESRD patients were all treated with low-flux polysulfone dialysers (F5, F6, Fresenius Medical Care). Dialysis fluid contamination was about 94 CFU/ml. This dialysis fluid was used for 54 patients, while the dialysis fluid was ultrafiltered (Diasafe®, Fresenius Medical Care) for 18 patients. The horizontal bars represent the group means. There was no significant difference in CPR levels (mg/l) between these two groups (adapted from [32]).*

The role of backfiltration in this scenario must also be taken into account, as was shown in various studies by Panichi et al. [53, 111, 112]. They compared IL-1Ra and IL-1ß values in patients treated with haemodiafiltration (HDF) with and without backfiltration. Here backfiltration could be avoided by using a special double chamber haemodiafiltration technique consisting of a haemofilter (highly permeable polysulfone HFT 05, Bellco) to perform ultrafiltration and a low-flux dialyser for diffusive solute transport (Hemophan®, NC2085, Bellco). A highly permeable polysulfone dialyser was used (BLS 672, Bellco) for the standard HDF with backfiltration. The endotoxin concentration of the dialysis fluid was comparable in both experimental settings (LAL: 0.13-0.18 EU/ml). Levels of IL-1Ra and IL-1ß increased significantly ($p < 0.002$) from baseline in the treatments involving backfiltration, but did not increase in patients treated with HDF in the absence of backfiltration [111]. These *in vivo* data demonstrate the need to use ultrapure dialysis fluid when employing

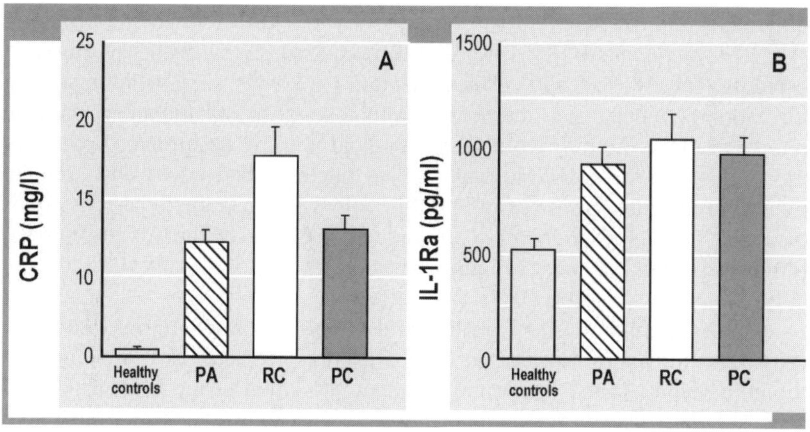

***Figure 10.6**: **Effects of different dialyser membranes and non-filtered dialysis fluid on patient inflammatory state** **in vivo**. In this crossover study, 21 patients were subsequently treated with 3 different dialysers for 8 weeks each. The dialysers were polyamide (PF14 hollow fibre, Gambro), polycarbonate-polyether (Pro 600 plate, Gambro) and regenerated cellulose (Alpha 600 plate, Gambro). The dialysis fluid was moderately contaminated (20.5 ± 5.8 CFU/ml, range 0 - 100 CFU/ml). Mean plasma CRP levels and whole blood content of IL-1Ra are shown in figures A and B, respectively ($p < 0.05$ for RC versus PA in both figures). Mean CRP levels in all haemodialysis patients were higher than in healthy controls (i.e. 16.3 ± 2.3 mg/l as opposed to 1.4 ± 0.2 mg/l, $p < 0.0001$) (adapted from [52]).*

high-flux dialysers if dialysis-associated inflammatory reactions are to be avoided.

Does membrane biocompatibility influence the microinflammatory state in dialysis patients?

As shown in chapters 7 and 8, dialyser membranes induce complement, neutrophil and monocyte activation to varying extent. This means that levels of potential inflammatory factors, such as C3a, C5a, IL-1, IL-6, TNF, factor D and granulocyte inhibiting peptide II, differ according to the membrane used. Synthetic, grafted cellulosic and cellulose acetate membranes exert a less negative influence on biocompatibility parameters (e.g. complement activation, cytokine production/adsorption and monocyte and neutrophil activation) than regenerated cellulose. This has been shown in numerous studies for polymethylmethacrylate [113-115], polysulfone [114, 116-121], polyamide [122], polyacrylonitrile [25, 117], polycarbonate [116], synthetically modified cellulose (SMC®) [123] and cellulose acetate [113, 119, 123]. When assessing the biocompatibility of a membrane with respect to inflammatory markers, one has to take the purity of the dialysis fluid and the adsorptive capacity of the membrane for e.g. biologically active bacterial derivatives and complement into account (reviewed in [41-48]). This is because bacterial substances may pass the dialysis membrane and induce activation of the immune system (discussed in the previous paragraph).

A pure membrane effect on IL-6 and CRP levels was demonstrated in a crossover study with polysulfone (F60, Fresenius Medical Care) and cuprammonium rayon (AM-UP-75, Asahi) dialysers, the latter having been used with both standard dialysis fluid (mean endotoxin content of 0.18 IU/ml (range 0.05 - 1.13 IU/ml)) and ultrafiltered dialysis fluid (mean endotoxin content of 0.06 IU/ml (range 0.05 - 0.19 IU/ml)). In this study, filtering of the standard dialysis fluid did not influence the increase in CRP observed only with cuprammonium rayon dialysers 24 hours after dialysis treatment (**figure 8.21**) [120]. Recently, dialyser membranes were shown to affect plasma levels of both CRP and albumin (this was probably affected secondary to CRP and is taken as a parameter for nutrition in ESRD) [123]. In this study, patients who were routinely dialysed with regenerated cellulose dialysers (RC, Bellco) were subsequently switched to SMC® dialysers (NC 1485, Bellco) and then to cellulose diacetate (DN 1813, Nipro) for a period of six months each using ultrafiltered dialysis fluid. For both membranes made of modified cellulose, CRP values dropped and albumin values rose during the observation period (see **figure 10.7**). These data suggest that biocompatibility characteristics of the membrane do contribute to the inflammatory syndrome in ESRD.

Is there a synergistic effect of membrane permeability to bacterial substances and membrane bioincompatibility on the inflammatory state in dialysis patients?

Several *in vitro* studies show a synergistic effect of dialyser membrane bioincompatibility and bacterial products (e.g. LPS) on cytokine levels in dialysis patients; inflammatory reactions are thus promoted in the presence of both factors ([124, 125] and reviewed in [42]). Obviously two steps are required for IL-1 and IL-1Ra production: mRNA transcription, induced by membrane contact, is followed by LPS-induced translation. In addition, cellular and plasmatic components of whole blood interact with bacterial CIS, altering their pyrogenic activity [126].

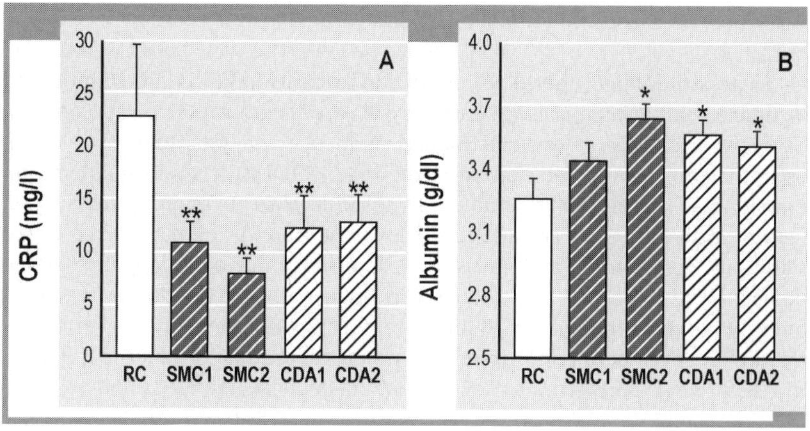

***Figure 10.7**: **Effect of various dialyser membranes on CRP and albumin levels**. The membranes, which were used consecutively in 18 patients on standard haemodialysis, were regenerated cellulose (RC), followed by synthetically modified cellulose (SMC®) and, finally, cellulose diacetate (CDA). Plasma levels of CRP and albumin measured 3 and 6 months after the switch to the respective modified cellulosic membranes are shown (SMC®1/CDA1 and SMC®2/CDA2, respectively). Compared to RC, CRP levels declined and albumin levels rose after 3 and 6 months treatment with the SMC® membrane and with the CDA membrane (*$p < 0.05$ versus RC, **$p < 0.01$ versus RC) (adapted from [123]).*

10.1.2 Oxidative stress

Oxidative stress is defined as the tissue damage resulting from an imbalance between an increased production of reactive oxygen species (ROS) and other pro-oxidants, and a decreased anti-oxidant defence (see **table 7.5**). Generation of oxidative compounds is physiologically relevant in, for example, inflammation and tissue repair processes. Consequently, it plays an important role in the defence mechanisms against microorganisms or tumor cells, as well as in tissue healing or remodelling. However, an increased, maladaptive stimulation of oxidative processes may be chronically present in uraemia, contributing to cell and tissue injury in ESRD patients (reviewed in [127-130]).

What are the causes of oxidative stress?

Factors that affect the total pool of pro-oxidants in ESRD are summarised in **figure 10.8**. Uraemia is associated with an accumulation of several pro-oxidants, e.g. various low and middle molecular weight proteins (< 3000), carbonyl compounds and homocysteine [54, 129, 130, 132, 133]. Therefore, uraemia per se, the multimorbid status of ESRD patients and the dialysis procedure itself all enhance oxidative stress in ESRD [54, 95, 129, 131]. Other significant contributory factors are the presence of inflammation, anti-oxidant deficiency (e.g. due to anti-oxidant and trace metal losses during the treatment), the bioincompatibility of the system (especially the dialysis membrane) and trace amounts of endotoxins from non-ultrapure dialysis fluid [54, 91, 93, 95, 129, 134]. Furthermore, several pharmaceutical agents commonly pre-

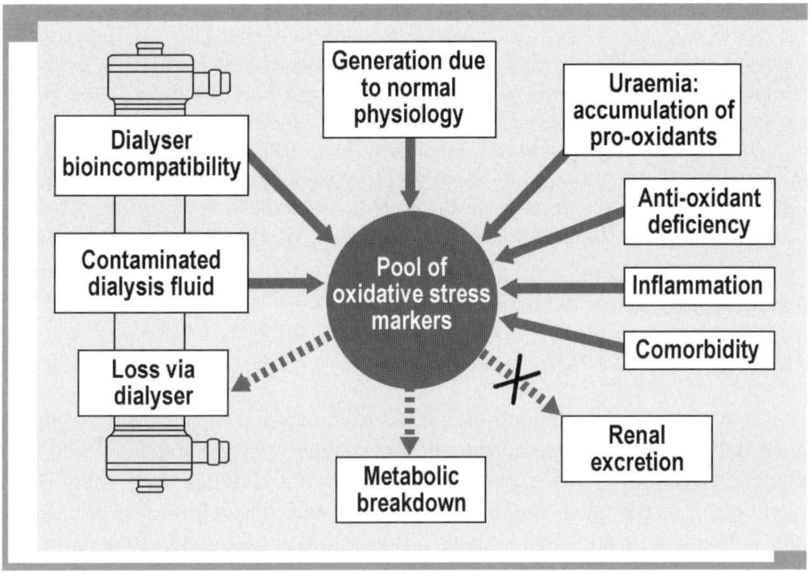

Figure 10.8: Factors influencing the total pool of pro-oxidants in ESRD. *Dialysis-associated factors (i.e. bioincompatibility, microbial contamination of dialysis fluid and loss via dialyser) and patient-associated factors (i.e. uraemia per se, anti-oxidant deficiency, anuria, inflammation and other co-morbid conditions, as well as generation and breakdown due to normal physiology) influence the degree of oxidative stress in ESRD patients. Continuous arrows represent factors which enhance the level of pro-oxidants; dashed arrows refer to factors which reduce the level of pro-oxidants (adapted from [95]).*

scribed for dialysis patients may modulate patient susceptibility to oxidation: heparin promotes the oxidation of albumin or lipoprotein when bound to these substances; intravenously supplied iron may play a role in lipid peroxidation damage (reviewed in 127, 128, 135]; and even erythropoietin has been found to enhance the superoxide anion of fMLP (N-formyl-methionyl-leucyl-phenylanaline)-stimulated peripheral mononuclear cells (reviewed in [136]).

What are the biological effects of oxidative stress?

The key relationships between oxidative stress and inflammation, leading to an amplified inflammatory response, are demonstrated in **figure 10.9**. Oxidative stress and its biological effects are therefore of pathological relevance in many diseases [96, 129, 138], especially those having an inflammatory component [129, 138]. The atherogenic effects of oxidative stress that particularly involve a disturbed endothelian function (reviewed in chapter 7.3.2.1) and the generation of oxidised low-density lipoproteins have been observed in patients undergoing dialysis treatment ([68, 139-141] and reviewed in [54, 94, 95, 129, 135, 138]). Furthermore, oxidative stress plays a role in dialysis-associated amyloidosis, malnutrition and anaemia [129, 135, 142].

How can the degree and the consequences of oxidative stress be measured?

The term "oxidative stress" generally expresses the outcome of oxidative damage to biologically important molecules. As ROS have a very short half-life of often only a few seconds, oxidative stress is usually measured by the detection of various modified macromolecules in plasma that were generated from ROS, e.g. molecules from lipid peroxidation (such as malonaldehyde and F2-isoprotanes), advanced lipid oxidation products, specific anti-oxidised LDL antibodies or molecules from protein oxidation (such as advanced oxidation end products (AOPPs)) [95, 129, 136]. In addition, evaluation of enzymatic or non-enzymatic anti-oxidant systems, and of levels of inflammatory proteins may help to define the individual degree of oxidative stress [129]. Levels of such markers are significantly increased in haemodialysis patients compared to healthy controls [95, 143, 129, 130]. However, a direct evaluation of the possible clinical impact of dialyser characteristics on oxidative stress is not possible in many clinical studies comparing dialyser membranes.

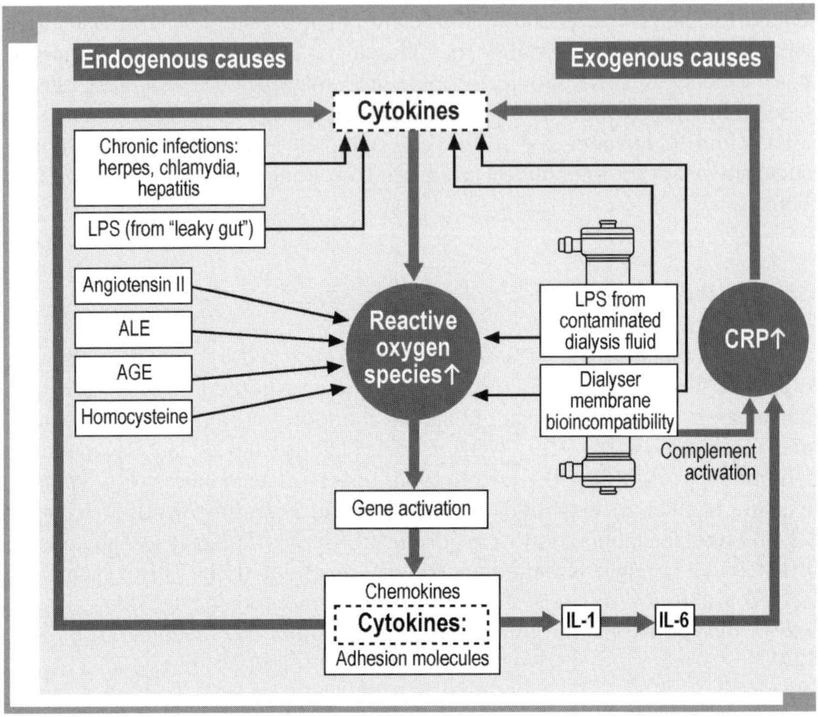

Figure 10.9: Key pathways of interplay between oxidative stress and inflammation leading to an amplified inflammatory response. *Various endogenous and exogenous factors lead to increased oxidative stress via cytokine stimulation. Typical endogenous factors are persistent chronic infections (e.g. chlamydia, herpes and hepatitis), LPS from an eventually "leaky gut", and elevated levels of pro-oxidants (e.g. angiotensin II, advanced glycation and lipid oxidation end products (AGE/ALE)). Exogenous factors are, infections of the vascular access (e.g. fistulas, grafts and dialysis catheters) and dialysis-associated factors (e.g. dialyser bioincompatibility and endotoxin (LPS) transfer from contaminated dialysis fluid (DF)). Oxidative stress, in turn, leads to gene activation for the production of chemokines, cytokines and adhesion molecules, via activation of nuclear transcription factors. Especially the cytokines (e.g. interleukin 1 and 6 (IL-1, IL-6) induce augmented production of C-reactive protein (CRP) and, thus, amplify the inflammatory response (thick arrows) (adapted from [137]).*

This is because direct parameters of oxidative stress are not measured, and we are forced to rely on indirect markers, such as markers of inflammation or of endothelial malfunction [129]. Therefore, oxidative stress is indirectly assessed in those chapters of this work dealing with the chronic inflammatory syndrome in ESRD and ESRD-associated diseases (atherosclerosis, anaemia, malnutrition, lipid disorders and homocysteine accumulation). Here, only the clinical impact of the anti-oxidant therapy will be discussed.

How can oxidative stress be reduced?

Two main approaches have been proposed for the prevention/reduction of oxidative stress in HD patients. One recommends the use of biocompatible dialysers (e.g. [128, 129, 144], guideline III.1 in [20]) (see chapter 8 and **table 8.1**) in combination with ultrapure dialysis fluid (e.g. [31, 129] and guideline IV.1 in [20]). The other recommends administration of anti-oxidants to anti-oxidant deficient patients. This could be achieved by oral or intradialytic supplementation. Important anti-oxidants in plasma include vitamins C and E, uric acid and albumin (reviewed in [127]). Therefore, attempts to improve patient prognosis with anti-oxidative therapy have been made. In addition to supplementation with anti-oxidants such as vitamin C, supplementation with vitamin E has especially been tested in clinical studies. However, even the anti-oxidant acetylcysteine has recently been given in ESRD in an attempt to reduce oxidative stress [145].

The role of vitamin E as anti-oxidant

Vitamin E is a lipo-soluble vitamin formed by eight chemical compounds divided into two classes, called tocopherols and tocotrienols, with different biological activities. Of these, α-tocopherol is most active. Vitamin E is stored in adipose tissue, liver and muscles, and is transported in plasma by lipoproteins to the cells, where it is exchanged with that in the cell membrane through HDL cholesterol. At its main site in the cell membrane, it is the most effective chain-breaking anti-oxidant, protecting membrane phospholipids from oxidative damage. Therefore, it essentially contributes to the stability of all cell membranes and protects the cell structures from damage caused by oxygen free radicals or the products of lipid peroxidation. For example, vitamin E influences cell proliferation and cell signalling, promotes neurological function, stimulates the immune system, prevents erythrocyte haemolysis and reduces lipid peroxidation [146]. One study reported that vitamin E levels were not reduced in haemodialysis patients and did not change during standard dialysis [147]. However, cases of relative vitamin E deficiency in that predialysis vitamin E/triglyceride ratios were reduced have also been detected [141]. Lower vitamin E levels were found in predialysis patients suffering from malnutrition than in well nourished patients, and these low levels were also associated with an increased carotid intima-media area, a marker for the degree of atherosclerosis [71].

In standard procedures, vitamin E is administered orally. In ESRD patients, however, oxidative stress is thought to be at its highest during the haemodialysis treatment itself, because the pro-oxidant effects of the bioincompatibility of the materials used add to the pro-oxidant effects of the uraemic environment. Therefore, dialysers containing membranes coated with vitamin E have been developed with the aim of reducing the oxidative burst induced by the dialysis treatment itself (see chapter 2.1.3). The binding between vitamin E and the membrane polymer is very tight in these membranes, and *in vitro* studies failed to show a transfer of the membrane-bound vitamin E to the plasma [148, 149]. The function of the vitamin E bound to these membranes is not, therefore, that of a plasma vitamin supplement, but is rather that of a "bioreactor" which immediately reduces the amount of reactive oxygen species induced during treatment [148]. Nevertheless, while some studies indeed reported unchanged vitamin E levels with the use of such dialysers [150, 151], others measured increases in levels in plasma [140, 141, 149, 152], high density lipoproteins (HDLs) [140] and erythrocytes [149, 152]. A proposed explanation is that an exchange of reducing equivalents with the anti-oxidant network of the patient blood, together with the *in situ* scavenging of reactive species on the membrane surface, may permit a saving of the endogenous vitamin E pool. The final result would be an accumulation of this anti-oxidant in the lipophilic compartment [149].

Does oral vitamin E administration influence clinical outcome in the general population?

Some earlier papers reported a reduced risk of cardiovascular death and non-fatal myocardial infarction in patients treated with vitamin E (CHAOS (Cambridge Heart Anti-Oxidant Study) [153]). However, several recently-conducted large-scale studies on the progression of atherosclerosis and the corresponding clinical outcome that involved tens of thousands of patients with coronary and/or cerebrovascular disease failed to find any benefit of oral vitamin E administration during a 3-5 year follow-up time [154-160]. The studies in question were, for example, HOPE (Heart Prevention Outcome), GIZZI, SECURE (Study to Evaluate Carotide Ultrasound changes in patients treated with Ramipril and vitamin E), and HPS (Heart Protection Outcome Study).

Does oral vitamin E administration, the use of vitamin F-coated membranes or the intake of acetylcysteine influence clinical outcome in ESRD?

Only one study was published to date that addressed supplementation with oral vitamin E and clinical outcome in ESRD patients, namely SPACE (Secondary Prevention with Anti-oxidants of Cardiovascular disease in End-stage renal disease). In this study, ingestion of 800 IU/day of vitamin E resulted in a reduced incidence of cardiovascular end-points (e.g. unstable angina, myocardial infarction, ischaemic stroke, progressive peripheral vascular disease) in almost 200 patients with prevalent cardiovascular disease. However, this ingestion did not have any significant effects on total mortality or mortality from cardiovascular disease alone, the latter being in accordance with the results of the multiple studies for the general population cited above [161]. The authors interpret their data as resulting from the especially high cardiovascular risk profile of ESRD patients, and compare their results to the findings of the CHAOS study in which vitamin E supplementation reduced the rate of cardiovascular deaths in another high-risk group for cardiovascular problems, i.e. in non-ESRD patients with angiographically proven cardiovascular disease [153]. Another study on the effect of oral supplementation with vitamin E in combination with selenium and lipoic acid on clinical outcome, namely DOSS (Dialysis Oxidant Stress Study (DOSS), is expected to be finished in 2003 [128].

Up to now, no studies have been published concerning patient morbidity and/or mortality with the use of vitamin E-coated membranes.

Recently, the influence of acetylcysteine, a thiol-containing anti-oxidant was tested in a prospective, randomised placebo-controlled study in 134 haemodialysis patients [145]. The primary end points defined were; cardiac events (fatal or nonfatal myocardial infarction, cardiovascular diseases death, need for cardiovascular angioplasty or coronary bypass surgery), ischaemic stroke, or peripheral vascular disease (need of angioplasty or amputation). Secondary endpoints were: each of the component outcomes, total and cardiovascular mortality. After a median follow-up time of 14.5 months the number of primary endpoints was significantly reduced in the group treated with acetylcyteine (28%) compared to the placebo group (47%) (relative risk 0.60

(95% CI 0.38 to 0.95), p = 0.03). No significant differences in the secondary end points or total mortality were detected. These results suggest a positive influence of an oral intake of acetylcysteine on composite cardiovascular endpoints in ESRD.

Does oral vitamin E administration or the use of vitamin E-coated membranes influence clinical factors that correlate with clinical outcome in ESRD?

Many studies on supplementation with vitamin E in ESRD patients deal with measurements of clinical or laboratory parameters that are known to correlate with clinical outcome, e.g. degree of atherosclerosis, endothelial function, levels of lipids or their modified forms induced via lipid peroxidation (e.g. [134, 141, 150, 162-165]). Two small studies investigated the possible benefits of vitamin E-modified dialysers on atherosclerosis compared to the use of membranes made from regenerated cellulose under the same conditions. In one study, the percentage increase of the aortic calcification index was significantly lower after 2 years treatment with vitamin E-modified membranes [150]. In the other study, the intima-media thickness decreased after one year observation in the group treated with the vitamin E-bonded membrane, but the prevalence of atherosclerotic plaques remained unchanged [165]. In both studies, some of the patients were previously treated with biocompatible synthetic membranes (polysulfone or polymethymethacrylate). This complicates interpretation of the results because the potential benefit of the vitamin E-modified membrane shown here may not only be due to the special vitamin E-mediated anti-oxidant effect – it may also be due to differences in biocompatibility between the membranes tested. Bioincompatibility of membranes made from regenerated cellulose may have caused an increase in oxidative stress during hemodialysis in patients treated with these membranes, and thus promoted endothelian dysfunction. This negative influence of bioincompatible membranes on oxidative stress and endothelian function was confirmed in two further studies: endothelial function, estimated as flow-mediated vasodilatation of the brachial artery, was preserved in patients treated with dialysers made from polysulfone [134, 162] or vitamin E-modified membranes [162, 164], whereas it was not when regenerated cellulose was used [134, 164]. Triglyceride levels remained stable with the use of vitamin E modified dialysers [141], but the fraction of polyunsaturated fatty acids [141] and levels of high-density lipoprotein cholesterol increased [163].

Regarding oral vitamin E supplementation, studies concerning another target of oxidative stress, namely erythropoiesis and erythrocyte survival, found that a reduction in oxidative stress appears to slightly improve the response to erythropoietin [139, 166-168]. However, use of vitamin E-modified dialysers (Clirans EE-N, Terumo [169]; SF170E, Nipro [170]) did not lead to changes in haemoglobin or erythropoietin dosage when compared to polysulfone (Clirans PS, Terumo [169]; HF80LS, Fresenius Medical Care [170]). When vitamin E bonded dialysers (Clirans EE, Terumo) were compared to dialysers made from regenerated cellulose (C15NL, Terumo), haemoglobin levels and erythropoietin dosage remained unchanged in one study [171], but erythropoietin dosage increased with the use of dialysers made from regenerated cellulose in another study [165]. However, in the latter study, patients treated with regenerated cellulose had lower ferritin levels at start and were previously partially treated with biocompatible synthetic membranes (polysulfone, polymethylmethacrylate). Other vitamin E-modified dialysers (E15NL (low-flux) and EE15NL (high-flux), also both from Terumo) showed an erythropoietin sparing effect compared to low-flux cellulosic dialysers (C15 NL, Terumo). However, this was probably mediated by a reduction in dialyser clotting – a comparison of the vitamin E-modified membrane with high-flux polysulfone (F60, Fresenius Medical Care) did not reveal any such differences [172].

Are laboratory markers of oxidative stress influenced by vitamin E supplementation or the use of vitamin E-modified membranes?

Multiple publications exist concerning the influence of oral vitamin E supplementation or the use of dialysers coated with vitamin E on various blood parameters that are considered markers for increased oxidative stress in dialysis patients (e.g. [140, 141, 148-150, 164, 171, 173-175]), and on the effect of vitamin E on membrane biocompatibility [175-178]. When analysing the results of such studies, one must be aware that membrane biocompatibility itself also influences oxidative stress (see **figure 10.9**).

Looking at parameters which indicate intradialytic oxidative burst (e.g. levels of low molecular weight, oxidised lipoproteins (ox-LDL), malondialdehyde (MDA, a product of lipid peroxidation) [147] and superoxide anions), the following results were found when vitamin E-modified dialysers were compared with dialysers containing regenerated cellulose (RC). (1) The intradialytic increase in ox-LDL levels observed with RC was prevented [140, 164], reduced in magnitude [162, 171, 175, 179] or unaffected [150] when vitamin E-modified dialysers were used. (2) MDA levels decreased with the vitamin E -

coated membranes [150, 175, 179]. (3) Superoxide anion production was lower with vitamin E-coated membranes than with RC [175]. When vitamin E-coated cellulosic membranes were compared to polyacrylonitrile (AN69®), higher levels of ascorbyl free radicals were found using the synthetic membrane [151]. A comparison of vitamin E-coated cellulosic membranes (Clirans® EE-N, Terumo) with polysulfone (Clirans® PS, Terumo) revealed no difference in serum MDA levels between the membranes for non-diabetic patients, while these levels in the diabetic ESRD patients decreased significantly when they were treated with the vitamin E-modified membrane and not when treated with polysulfone [169]. However, the data in this study were not corrected for solute concentration during dialysis, so the reported differences between membranes may be misleading [174]. A negative side effect of treatment with the vitamin E-coated membranes was pointed out in this study: total cholesterol levels rose significantly in all patients [169]. Other studies comparing levels of different reactive oxygen species (ROS) with the use of various membranes showed a deleterious effect of regenerated cellulose on anti-oxidant activity. Less negative effects on different ROS were observed with the other membranes. Roughly summarised, cellulose diacetate provided an intermediate protection from oxidative stress, while a slightly better protection was supplied by polymethylmethacrylate, polyacrylonitrile and the combination of Hemophan® and polysulfone; MDA levels decreased with all membranes tested [144, 180, 181]. A recent study reported that switching from cellulose acetate to low-flux polysulfone improved protein oxidation status over an observation period of one year [182]. Red blood cells were found to be more susceptible to oxidative stress when dialysers made from regenerated cellulose were used compared to such made from cellulose triacetate (Sureflux 130L, Nipro) or polysulfone (F6HPS Fresenius Medical Care) [183].

Membranes which are more biocompatible than regenerated cellulose seem to offer some protection against oxidative stress per se. Therefore, many of the above-cited studies which compare vitamin E-coated dialysers with regenerated cellulose (e.g. [140, 149, 162, 164, 171, 175, 179]) are difficult to interpret in terms of a vitamin E effect: the anti-oxidant influences of vitamin E and good biocompatibility are not discernible (e.g. [183-185]).

Should anti-oxidative therapy be recommended for ESRD patients?

In view of the largely negative results with anti-oxidant trials in the general population and the only few positive results in ESRD [145, 153], it is difficult to gauge the benefit of anti-oxidative therapy in ESRD and to formulate recommendations. Multiple questions remain unanswered (reviewed in [128, 186]), such as, in the clinical trials done so far, were the right anti-oxidants chosen? Were the right parameters followed up? Was the anti-oxidant dosage appropriate? Were the patients chosen appropriately, or early enough, or treated and observed long enough? Whereas the oral intake of 800 IU vitamin E (as reported in the SPACE study [153]) or of 600 mg of acetylcysteine [145] appears safe (reviewed in [129, 186]), one must also take the potential dangers of anti-oxidative therapy into account: vitamin E administration blunts the protective rise in high density lipoprotein (HDL) 2 cholesterol when lipid-reducing therapy is given [187], and excessive supplementation with vitamin C may result in hyperoxalaemia and thereby contribute to vascular disease in ESRD [188].

The partially conflicting data, the multiple origin of oxidative stress in ESRD [91] (see also **figures 10.8** and **10.9**), and the lack of evidence regarding improved morbidity and mortality mean that further larger studies are necessary [128, 129, 186]. Such studies should also supply evidence that vitamin E-modified cellulosic membranes have a satisfying biocompatibility and long-term clinical outcome, being at least comparable with standard, biocompatible, synthetic membranes.

10.1.3 Carbonyl stress

Carbohydrates, lipids and amino acids are abundantly present in the human body and are the precursors of the reactive carbonyl compounds (RCOs) formed by the oxidation of carbohydrates and lipids (see **figure 7.21**). RCOs indirectly lead to advanced glycation or lipidoxidation of proteins, thereby forming advanced glycation (AGE) or lipidoxidation (ALE) end products, respectively [55, 189]. AGE-modified proteins are thought to play a role in normal tissue remodelling, but their accumulation may lead to tissue damage [190].

Chronic uraemia is associated with increased modification of proteins by RCOs. This so-called "carbonyl stress" leads to a rise in plasma [191] and tissue contents of AGEs and ALEs and may have deleterious biological effects, as shown in **table 10.3** (reviewed in [55, 189]). Consequently, carbonyl stress has been linked to several clinical complications commonly found in ESRD, such as the atherosclerotic and inflammatory state in uraemia and dialysis-associated amyloidosis ([192] and reviewed in [98, 189]). Recent immunohistochemical and chemical analyses indicate that the ß2-microglobulin amyloid deposited in amyloidosis is modified by carbonyl stress [55, 92, 97]. Incubation of human synovial fibroblasts with AGE-modified ß2-m induces degradation of this AGE-modified protein and increases monocyte chemoattractant protein-1 mRNA and protein expression. This expression is possibly involved in the inflammatory processes associated with dialysis-related amyloidosis [193]. Furthermore, carbonyl stress may be linked to atherosclerosis: not only were AGEs and ALEs found in vascular lesions of aged subjects, diabetic patients and patients who had carotid artery interventions, but AGEs and ALEs may also activate the inflammatory response in uraemia (see **figure 10.9**) (reviewed in [55]).

Biological effects of RCO, AGE and ALE	
RCO	• Structural alteration of matrix proteins • Resistance to the action of calcitriol • Vascular endothelial growth factor production from endothelial and mesothelial cells • Cell apoptosis • Intracellular signalling
AGE / ALE	• Chemotaxis of monocytes • Inflammatory cytokine secretion from macrophages • Collagenase secretion from synovial cells • Osteoclast-induced bone resorption • Proliferation of vascular smooth muscle cells • Aggregation of platelets • Altered intracellular signalling

Table 10.3: Biological effects of reactive carbonyl compounds (RCO), advanced glycation end products (AGE) and advanced lipid oxidation end products (ALE) *(adapted from [55]).*

What role does the dialyser play in uraemia-associated carbonyl stress?

The genesis of carbonyl stress in uraemia is not completely understood. Two mechanisms should be considered: first, carbonyl stress may result from an increased generation of RCOs, for example via oxidative stress; second, it may derive from a decreased clearance or detoxification of RCOs, via depletion of thiols in ESRD [55, 136, 194]. The choice of dialyser may influence both mechanisms: dialyser performance characteristics can affect the removal of RCOs or RCO precursors and the dialyser biocompatibility characteristics may modulate RCO and, thus, oxidative stress.

Markers for the quantification of carbonyl stress in uraemia are pentosidine, a fluorescent cross-link, and carboxymethyllysine. These are frequently used as glucoxidation markers for AGE in proteins, although other less well-examined AGE compounds are sometimes preferred [195]. Free pentosidine has a low molecular weight (379), but approximately 95% is albumin-bound. Removal of this protein-bound fraction by dialysis should be negligible or very low [190, 196]. Speaking quantitatively, up to tenfold higher plasma pentosidine levels have been measured in dialysis patients compared to healthy controls [195, 196].

During a single haemodialysis session with regenerated cellulose membranes, 80% of the free pentosidine was removed, followed by a rebound to predialysis values 24 hours postdialysis [197]. These results for regenerated cellulose were confirmed in another study, which also found that the percentage reduction in free pentosidine during haemodialysis was independent of the membrane polymer tested. These were polyacrylonitrile (PAN: AN69®, Hospal), polymethylmethacrylate (PMMA: Toray), regenerated cellulose (RC: Asahi) and two brands of high-flux polysulfone (PSu: Fresenius Medical Care, and Asahi) [198]. However, in this study, the predialysis levels of both free and protein-bound pentosidine were significantly lower in the patient groups treated with the two different high-flux PSu membranes (see **figure 10.10**). The authors carefully excluded the potential influence of residual renal function on this effect, and even found this reduction in predialysis levels confirmed when patients were switched from PAN to PSu and again back to PAN, i.e. predialysis pentosidine levels decreased while using PSu, and re-increased when PAN membranes were used again. This effect cannot be explained by the pentosidine filtration characteristics of the membrane because pentosidine removal and predialysis levels did not differ between the two high-flux membranes PAN and PMMA and the low-flux cellulosic membrane. The authors speculate that this pentosidine-lowering effect of high-flux polysulfone may be due to either (A) the specific removal of carbonyl precursors derived from carbohydrates by this polymer or (B) a decrease in oxidative stress and, secondary to this, in carbonyl stress. On the other hand and independent of the membrane used (high-flux polysulfone, high-flux polymethylmethacrylate, and cellulose acetate), the pentosidine-levels diminished significantly ($p < 0.001$) 3 and 6 months after a switch from standard to ultrapure dialysis fluid in a recent study [199]. This indicates an additional influence of dialysis fluid quality on carbonyl stress.

The hypothesis that circulating AGEs may promote the inflammatory status of ESRD patients was not confirmed in a clinical study searching for a relationship between AGE and the incidence of diseases: levels of total serum fluorescent AGEs (AGE-fl) did not correlate with the incidence of vascular disease, diabetes, levels of C-reactive protein or the use of high-flux dialysers

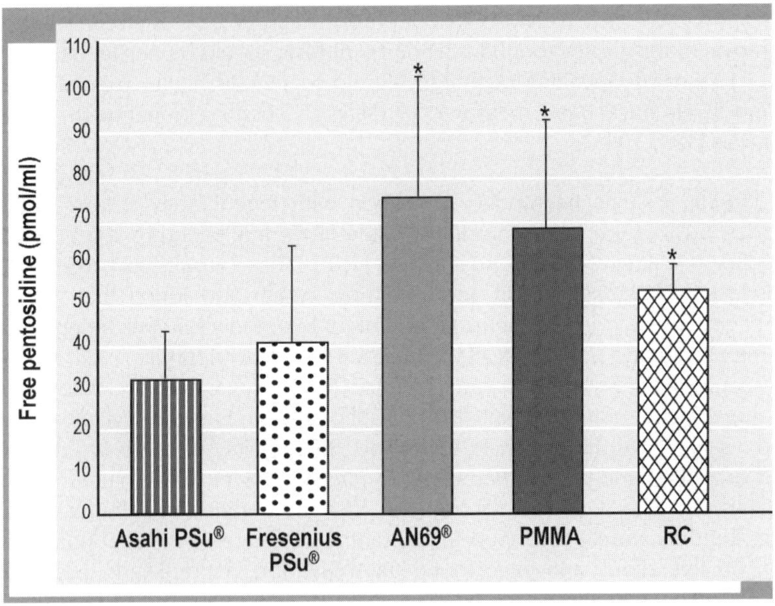

Figure 10.10: Predialysis pentosidine levels in five membrane groups. *Both free and protein-bound pentosidine levels were significantly lower predialysis in the group treated with the two high-flux polysulfones (PSu: Asahi Polysulfone® (Asahi); Fresenius Polysulfone® (Fresenius Medical Care). The other membranes tested were polyacrylonitrile (AN69®, Hospal), polymethylmethacrylate (PMMA: Toray) and regenerated cellulose (RC: Asahi); *$p < 0.01$ versus Asahi PSu® and Fresenius PSu® groups (adapted from [198]).*

(defined as having an ultrafiltration coefficient > 20 ml/h/mmHg) [191]. Thus, even though carbonyl stress is linked to ß2-m amyloidosis and atherosclerosis, further clinical studies are needed to explore the potential contributions of specific dialyser characteristics to carbonyl stress.

10.2 Malnutrition

Malnutrition has been identified as a major predictor of morbidity and mortality in ESRD [3, 13, 62, 64, 70, 200-206]. It was shown to be a direct cause of death in 5% of the patients in a recent study (n=128, follow up 36 months) [64].

Malnutrition in various degrees is a common problem in haemodialysis patients [64, 77, 79, 200, 206-212]: prevalence values of about 65% were reported in recent studies [64, 77], and values in the ranges 18 - 56% and 23 - 73% were cited by others (reviewed in [201] and [64], respectively). Analysis of the nutritional status of the first 1000 patients randomised in the HEMO study sponsored by the American National Institute of Health [213] revealed that 29% had hypoalbuminaemia, and that dietary intake, protein intake and protein catabolic rate were all below the National Kidney Foundation Kidney Disease Outcomes Quality Initiative (NKF-K/DOQI™) guidelines in 76%, 61% and 52% of patients, respectively [211]. Malnutrition is often already present at dialysis start, e.g. in 39% of 206 patients in one study [79].

Various anthropometric and laboratory parameters are employed to assess malnutrition. A low percentage of ideal body weight or low body mass index was found in 10 - 30%, a low triceps skinfold thickness in 20 - 60%, a low arm muscle circumference in 0 - 44%, a low serum albumin concentration in 13 - 70% and a low transferrin level in 30 - 60% of patients with persistent malnutrition (reviewed in [207]). Lean body mass, body fat mass measured by dual-energy X-ray absorptiometry, hand grip strength and subjective global assessment are further means of assessing malnutrition [79]. The predictive value of each of these parameters concerning outcome varies, depending mainly on sex and the prevalence of co-morbid factors, such as diabetes, cardiovascular disease and, especially, inflammation [79].

There are multiple causes for malnutrition in ESRD patients. Major factors in many patients are anorexia, poor nutrition and the protein catabolic factors associated with uraemia – in particular the presence of a chronic inflammatory state and the catabolic effects of the dialysis procedure itself (see **table**

10.4). Because of the major impact of inflammation on survival of patients with persistent malnutrition, even a division of malnutrition into two different subtypes has been proposed: "type I" for patients with malnutrition which is predominately not inflammatory-related (e.g. low protein and energy intake due to uraemic anorexia, inadequate dialysis, physical inactivity etc.), and "type II" for patients with malnutrition which mainly results from inflammatory stimuli [77]. Disturbed synthesis or catabolism of proteins or a combination of both may cause malnutrition; whereas nutritional variables mainly affect synthesis (e.g. of albumin), inflammatory stimuli primarily cause increased albumin catabolism [78].

What role does dialysis play in the genesis of malnutrition in ESRD?

The dialysis treatment itself is an overall catabolic event [217-219], as pointed out already in **table 10.4**. The performance characteristics of the dialyser membrane may allow amino acid and even, under certain circumstances, protein loss [207, 220-222], while the biocompatibility characteristics of the membrane may [214, 223] or may not [224] influence protein breakdown during the treatment. In addition, the use of non-biocompatible membranes or contaminated dialysis fluid can stimulate chronic inflammation, and so promote malnutrition. Therefore, the question arises of whether the choice of dialyser (and especially its membrane) plays a clinically identifiable role in the incidence and degree of malnutrition in ESRD patients.

To what extent does dialyser or haemofilter performance influence amino acid and albumin loss and markers of nutrition during haemodialysis?

During haemodialysis, average losses of free amino acids into the dialysis fluid were reported to be in the range of 6 - 13 g/dialysis (as summarised in section 5.4.1). Peptide and protein losses in the ranges 2 - 3 g and 1 - 2 g per treatment, respectively, have also been observed [225]. The analysis of studies measuring protein losses during dialysis conducted in chapter 5 came to the conclusion that albumin losses with most commercially available dialysers are generally < 1 g per session, with some exceptions.

Factors contributing to malnutrition in ESRD		
Anorexia and poor nutrition	**Protein catabolism**	
	associated with uraemia	**associated with the dialysis procedure**
Uraemic toxicity (underdialysis) Unpalatable diets Gastrointestinal disorders Medication Chronic inflammation, infection, sepsis Increased leptin levels? Psycho-social factors: Poverty Loneliness Depression Dialysis-associated factors: Cardiovascular instability Nausea, vomiting Postdialysis fatigue	Uraemic toxicity (underdialysis) Metabolic acidosis Endocrine abnormalities: Hyperparathyroidism Anaemia, Low IGF-1 Insulin resistance Decreased gluconeogenesis and glucagon synthesis Amino acid abnormalities Chronic inflammation Infection, sepsis Heart failure Plasma volume expansion Physical inactivity	Loss of amino acids and peptides: (9-13 g/dialysis) Loss of protein: *1-2 g/session*: due to loss into dialysate with single use in HD *0.5-1.5 g/session*: due to blood loss *Up to several g/session:* depending on reuse number and method With the use of protein permeable membranes in HF and HDF Blood-membrane contact: With bioincompatible membranes, protein breakdown corresponding to 15-20 g protein/dialysis Complement activation Cytokine release Dialysis fluid: Endotoxin transfer Cytokine release Acetate dialysis fluid

Table 10.4: Genesis of malnutrition in ESRD. *HF: haemofiltration; HD: haemodialysis; IGF-1: insulin-like growth-factor 1 (adapted from [207, 214, 215, 216]).*

Amino acid losses differ slightly among different membranes, e.g. per treatment losses of 8.9 ± 2.8 g for high-flux polysulfone, 6.1 ± 1.5 g for polymethylmethacrylate and 7.1 ± 2.6 g for regenerated cellulose have been reported [226]. These small differences may be due to variations in dialyser surface area and blood flow rates and are probably biologically insignificant [207]. An amino acid loss of 12 ± 2 g/dialysis was recorded for polyacrylonitrile in one study [222]; a comparison of amino acid losses with this membrane with those lost from polysulfone and regenerated cellulose membranes of equal surface area and under conditions of equal blood flow revealed that protein losses for polyacrylonitrile were much higher (6.1 ± 2.3 g/session) than for polysulfone and regenerated cellulose (3.8 ± 1.3, $p < 0.05$ and 3.7 ± 1.3 g/session, $p < 0.01$, respectively) [221]. After 6 months follow-up, the higher amino acid loss observed with polyacrylonitrile compared to regenerated cellulose in this study did not lead to any change in parameters representing malnutrition (i.e. serum levels of total protein, albumin and transferrin; arm muscle circumference; triceps skinfold and relative weight) [221]. However, in a different study, where amino acids where supplemented during haemodialysis (creating a net positive balance and preventing a reduction in plasma concentrations), increases in albumin levels, transferrin levels and the protein catabolic rate were observed (dialyser: polyacrylonitrile 1.7 m^2, not specified further) [222]. This indicates that the intradialytic amino acid losses otherwise present may contribute to malnutrition, especially in patients of poor nutritional status (assuming that the positive balance effect is not the decisive factor).

Albumin losses are generally negligible (i.e. < 1 g/session) during single-use haemodialysis [227] (see chapter 5.4.1). High albumin losses were reported only in association with bleach reuse of cellulose triacetate (4.24 g/dialysis) and some older polysulfone dialysers (20 g/dialysis); the latter have now been replaced by polysulfone dialysers with much lower protein losses, e.g. only 1.15 g/dialysis after 19 reuses (see chapter 12 for details).

In the recently published HEMO study relating nutritional parameters to membrane flux in 1846 patients, high-flux dialysis had favourable associations with calf and arm circumference, as well as with daily protein intake [228].

Thus, in summary, there are some differences in amino acid and albumin losses during the haemodialysis treatment depending on the dialyser membranes used. However, up to now, the few data relating amino acid or protein losses during first use of a dialyser in haemodialysis to laboratory or clinical parameters of malnutrition did not show a membrane effect [78, 221]. On the other hand, high-flux dialysis seems to positively influence nutritional parameters compared to low-flux dialysis [228].

To what extent does dialyser and haemofilter performance influence amino acid and albumin loss and markers of nutrition during haemofiltration or haemodiafiltration?

In therapy modes involving high filtration volumes, such as haemofiltration (HF) and haemodiafiltration (HDF), amino acid and albumin losses may become more pronounced than in haemodialysis (reviewed in chapter 5.4). This would be undesirable, especially in patients with a poor nutritional status [225, 229]. On the other hand, some uraemic toxins are albumin-bound and, therefore, a certain albumin removal during the treatment might be considered positive from this point of view ([47, 225, 230, 231] and reviewed in [232]). There are few recommendations for maximal albumin losses per treatment: these specify maximum losses of 5 [233, 234] or 8-10 g per session [229].

Specific measurements for albumin loss in HF and HDF are rare in the scientific literature, appearing only in congress abstracts [235, 236] and few papers [231, 234, 237, 238]. These reported losses vary from 1 to about 19 g/session: e.g. 18.9 ± 3.5 g with a polyacrylonitrile membrane (Asahi) in off-line HDF (20 litre fluid replacement) [237]; 10 g with Superflux and HDF100S® (two polysulfone membranes from Fresenius Medical Care) [234]; 8 g with Althane® (a cellulose diacetate membrane previously produced by Althin) [234]; 3.99 ± 1.81 g [234] or 5.7 ± 0.4 g [231] with DIAPES® HF800 (a highly permeable polyethersulfone membrane from Membrana) in high-volume on-line HDF; 1 - 3 g [235] or 1.0 ± 0.4 g [238] with Polyflux® (a polyamide/PES/PVP alloy from Gambro); and 2 g with HF80 [234] or 3.5 ± 0.4 g with HF 80S [231](a polysulfone from Fresenius Medical Care). A recently published comparison of albumin loss in pre- and post-dilution haemofiltration using three different synthetic high-flux dialysers showed similar values of 1.7 g/session for polyamide (Polyflux 17S, Gambro) and Fresenius Polysulfone® (Helixone®, FX80, Fresenius Medical Care), but significantly higher losses of 8.6 g/session for polyethersulfone (DIAPES®, Syntra 160, Baxter) in the post-dilution mode ($p < 0.004$) [236]. In the pre-dilution mode, albumin loss was lowest with Fresenius Polysulfone® (0.4 g/session), intermediate during polyamide treatment (1.2 g/session), and highest for polyethersulfone (3.3 g/session). A recent study comparing 8 different high-flux dialysers at 3 different ultrafiltration rates found a decrease in albumin loss after the first 30 minutes of treatment and an exponential increase of albumin loss with augmenting ultrafiltratrion volumes for all dialysers [238]. The tested dialysers differed drastically in the amount of albumin lost per dialysis treatment (0.4 to 7 g at maximal ultrafiltration rates) whereby even different potein losses were found for dialysers containing membranes made from the same polymer. For dialysers made from polysulfone, for example, albumin loss ranged from 0.4 - 2 g/session with Helixone® (FX60, Fresenius Medical Care), from 0.6 - 3.8 g/session with Asahi Polysulfone® (APS 650S, Asahi), and from to 2 - 8 g/session with Toraysulfone® (BS-1.3U, Toray) (see **figure 5.21**). However, these losses did not have a significant impact on albumin levels measured before and after each treatment. The study design did not accommodate a long-term observation of albumin levels with use of the different dialysers. However, albumin loss can be reduced by changes in the HDF method: "programmed filtration" [239] or "pressure-controlled push/pull HDF" [237] reduced the loss of albumin (the latter by approximately 66%).

The corresponding clinical studies did not, however, observe deterioration in nutritional state of the patients. This was also not seen by Canaud et al. analysing data from 13 years of on-line HDF using high-flux polysulfone dialysers (HF80, Fresenius Medical Care) - the parameters analysed were nPCR, plasma albumin, plasma prealbumin and lean body mass [24]. Also Maduell et al. found no deterioration in nutritional status after changing 37 patients from conventional HDF to high-flux HDF using high-flux polysulfone, cellulose triacetate and polyacrylonitrile (AN69®) dialysers and following their progress for 12 months [21]. In a prospective, randomised study, Wizemann et al. found no differences in nutritional parameters (i.e. body weight, skinfold thickness, nPCR, plasma albumin and transferrin) between low-flux haemodialysis (using low-flux polysulfone (F8) from Fresenius Medical Care) and on-line HDF (using two high-flux polysulfone (F80-S) filters from Fresenius Medical Care) [22].

In summary, there are marked differences in albumin loss in HF and HDF depending on the membrane used. However, only the results of a few clinical studies have been published to date, so a recommendation regarding which membranes are best in this respect cannot be given. This is especially difficult to formulate as recommendations regarding acceptable albumin losses per treatment are not available, and a balance between albumin loss and ß2-m removal has to be taken into consideration (see chapter 5). The few clinical studies available on nutritional state in HF and HDF do not find a deterioration of nutritional parameters despite the possible augmented albumin loss in these treatments. A prospective multicentre Italian study has recently been launched to further investigate this matter [240].

To what extent does membrane biocompatibility influence the nutritional status of ESRD patients?

A balance between protein synthesis and catabolism is mandatory for adequate nutrition. The loss of amino acids, peptides and proteins during haemodialysis, together with poor nutrition, may lead to a reduced availability of amino acids and peptides which is possibly of significance in protein synthesis [78]. Another key mechanism in malnutrition in ESRD patients is protein catabolism. This is related to the inflammatory state of the patients [78] and this, in turn, is possibly influenced by dialyser biocompatibility, among other things. In the early nineties, Gutierrez et al. found that amino acids were released from the leg tissues (muscles) of normal subjects, corresponding to a protein breakdown of 15 - 20 g, when they were subjected to sham dialysis with regenerated cellulose dialysers (i.e. the *in vivo* circulation of blood through a dialyser but without circulating dialysis fluid) [223]. This was not the case when more biocompatible dialysers (polyacrylonitrile and polysulfone) were used [223, 241]. It was then hypothesised that bioincompatible membranes, such as regenerated cellulose, induce monocyte activation and cytokine release via direct membrane contact and complement activation (although other factors, such as endotoxin crossing the membrane, can also stimulate these processes) and that this is associated with lower albumin levels and, consequently, poorer nutritional status [62, 64, 73, 76, 208, 242]. One indicator for dialysis-associated cytokine production, namely the production of interleukin-1 receptor antagonist by peripheral blood mononuclear cells, was found to correlate with several nutritional parameters in patients treated with reprocessed cellulosic dialysers (i.e. body-mass index and anthropometry-derived arm muscle area) [242]. Among the different cytokines, generation of interleukin-6 (IL-6) also appears to play an important role in mediating malnutrition [76, 80]: increased levels of IL-6 do not only predict hypoalbuminaemia [62, 73, 76], but also promote weight loss in ESRD patients [76] and are associated with various other markers of nutrition in cross-sectional studies (reviewed in [80]). IL-6 levels were increased with the use of dialysers containing regenerated cellulose membranes [76, 115, 123].

However, the designs of the various clinical studies investigating the influence of membrane biocompatibility on nutrition in ESRD patients vary to a high degree and, as shown in **table 10.5**, the results of these studies are conflicting. Follow-up times range from 3 dialysis sessions [243] to 24 months [245], and patient numbers vary from 17 [243] to 483 [245]. Usually membranes made of regenerated cellulose (RC) were tested against membranes

Authors/ date of publication/ study design	Membranes/ dialysers tested	Patient number/ follow-up time	Parameters observed/ results	Remarks
Docci et al. 1992 [243] Prospective, randomised	RC (Bl 610 H, Bellco) vs. Hf-PSu (BL 624, Bellco)	n=17 3 dialysis treatments	Prealbumin ⇓ 24h postdialysis with RC ($p < 0.01$)	Dialysis fluid not tested for endotoxins
Parker et al. 1996 [244] Prospective, randomised	RC (T175, Terumo) vs. PMMA (B2-1.5, Toray)	n=159 18 months	Serum albumin ⇔ PCR ⇔ IGF-1 ⇑ and prealbumin ⇑ Body weight ⇑ with PMMA ($p < 0.05$)	Mean Kt/V higher with PMMA than with RC (1.37 ± 0.25 vs. 1.24 ± 0.27, $p < 0.01$), patients all relatively new to HD treatment, all have low albumin levels (3.5 g/dl)

Locatelli et al. 1996 [245] Prospective, randomised	RC vs. Lf-PSu, Hf-PSu (dialysers not further specified)	RC-HD n=182 Lf-PSu HD n=201 Hf-PSu HD n=51 Hf-PSu HDF n=50 24 months	Serum albumin, transferrin, PCR, sub-scapular skinfold, triceps skinfold, mid-arm circumference, body weight: no difference between the groups	Serum albumin at enrolment onto HD: 4.2 ± 0.4 g/dl
Tayeb et al. 2000 [210] Prospective	RC (C-121; T-150, Terumo) vs. Lf-PSu (F8, Fresenius Medical Care)	n=28 3 months	Serum albumin ⇑ with Lf-PSu ($p < 0.002$) both in diabetic and non-diabetic patients PCR ⇑ with Lf-PSu ($p < 0.065$)	All patients have low serum albumin at start of observation (3.3 g/dl)
Memoli et al. 2002 [123] Prospective, crossover	RC (Bellco) SMC® (NC 1485, Bellco) CDA (DN 1813-15, Bellco)	n=18 6 months for each dialyser	IL-6 release by cultured PBMCs ⇓ with the use of SMC® and CDA ($p < 0.05$) vs. RC CRP ⇓ with the use of SMC® and CDA ($p < 0.05$), Albumin ⇑ with the use of SMC® and CDA ($p < 0.05$) vs. RC	All patients have low serum albumin at start of observation (3.25 g/dl)

Table 10.5: Studies investigating the influence of membrane choice on nutritional state. *RC: regenerated cellulose; PMMA: polymethylmethacrylate; Lf-PSu: low-flux polysulfone; Hf-PSu: high-flux polysulfone; CDA: cellulose diacetate; SMC®: benzyl cellulose; IL-6: interleukin-6; PBMC: peripheral blood mononuclear cells; IGF-1: insulin-like growths factor 1; PCR: protein catabolic rate; ⇓: decrease; ⇑: increase; ⇔: no change.*

made from low- and/or high-flux polysulfone (PSu) [210, 243, 245], polymethylmethacrylate (PMMA) [244] or synthetically modified cellulose (benzyl cellulose (SMC®), cellulose diacetate (CDA)) [123]. Locatelli et al. failed to find any membrane influence (RC versus low-flux and high-flux PSu) on laboratory or anthropometic parameters of nutrition during two years of follow-up of a large number of mainly well-nourished ESRD patients (mean serum albumin of 4.2 ± 0.4 g/dl and protein catabolic rate (PCR) of > 1g/kg/day) [245]. On the other hand, although Parker et al. also did not observe any correlation between membrane biocompatibility and serum albumin levels and PCR when comparing RC with PMMA in the same year, they did find an increase in insulin-like growth-factor-1, prealbumin and body weight when the synthetic membrane was used [244]. Unfortunately, the mean Kt/V was higher in the PMMA group than in the RC group, making interpretation of the results somewhat difficult [209, 244]. In two recent studies with smaller patient numbers, one comparing SMC® and CDA with RC [123] and one testing low-flux PSu and RC [210], the following changes in plasma levels compared to treatment times with RC were observed: (A) serum albumin levels rose with all three comparison membranes (SMC®, CDA and low-flux PSu); (B) PCR levels increased when PSu was used [210]; and (C) levels of CRP and the release of interleukin-6 from peripheral blood mononuclear cells decreased with SMC® and CDA [123] (see also **figure 10.7**). It is interesting that in all studies showing a membrane effect on nutritional parameters (i.e. [123, 210, 244]), patients had low albumin values and were enrolled in the respective studies soon after initiation of dialysis. These patients are, therefore, possibly predisposed to an amelioration of their poor nutritional state simply by the initiation of chronic renal replacement therapy [246].

In summary, the use of a more biocompatible membrane than RC has been shown to positively influence laboratory parameters related to nutrition (i.e. PCR and serum prealbumin, albumin and CRP levels) in selected patients (i.e. those with low albumin values and who only recently started renal replacement therapy with haemodialysis); even an increase in body weight has been reported with the use of a biocompatible membrane in one study. Further studies are needed to confirm the effect of membrane biocompatibility on malnutrition for the dialysis population in general.

10.3 Renal anaemia

Renal anaemia is a major contributor to morbidity and mortality in ESRD patients; it reduces patient quality of life, exercise tolerance and cognitive and cardiovascular functions (reviewed in [247-253]). There are multiple causes: erythropoietin (EPO) deficiency, chronic blood loss, haemolysis, disturbed iron resorption and iron metabolism, folat or vitamin B_{12} deficiency, aluminium toxicity, bone marrow fibrosis, hyperparathyroidism, malnutrition and presence of inflammation or infection. All of these contribute to renal anaemia and inadequate response to EPO therapy [84, 85, 247, 254]. However, therapeutic strategies, such as anaemia management (e.g. erythropoietin and iron supplementation) and ensuring dialysis adequacy, can help correct renal anaemia in ESRD [247, 251, 252, 254-257]. These findings have led to today's guidelines for anaemia management in ESRD (e.g. [258, 259]).

Is renal anaemia affected by the choice of dialyser?

In an early study relating improved erythropoietin response and anaemia control to dialysis adequacy, the increase of dialysis dose was achieved by a 30 minute longer dialysis treatment and, additionally, by switching patients from a low-flux cellulose acetate dialyser (MCA 160, Althin) to a high-flux polysulfone dialyser (F80, Fresenius Medical Care) [255]. This led to the question of whether the choice of dialyser membrane (in particular, its permeability or biocompatibility characteristics) contributed - at least partially – to the resulting improved response to erythropoietin. The results of key clinical studies that addressed this question are partially conflicting (see **table 10.6**); these will be discussed below.

Is renal anaemia affected by dialyser permeability?

Augmented dialyser permeability can improve the removal of larger putative uraemia-associated inhibitors of erythropoiesis, as shown *in vitro* for the high-flux PMMA BKF dialyser [33, 34]. The improvement in anaemia observed in ESRD patients after starting CAPD and in haemodialysis patients after being switched to CAPD also supports the hypothesised existence of such "erythropoiesis-inhibiting middle molecules" that are better cleared by CAPD than by haemodialysis (reviewed in [269]). However, a recent crossover clinical study comparing low-flux and high-flux polysulfone (F7HPS vs. F60, both from

Study/ year/ design	Dialysis mode/ dialysers compared	Patient number	Follow-up time	Influence on parameters important for anaemia management	Influence on renal anaemia
	HD vs. HD				
Villaverde et al. 1999 [260] Prospective	HD: RC, low-flux CA vs. high-flux PSu (HF 80, Fresenius Medical Care)	31		*Kt/V*: similar in both groups *Erythropoietin*: 14% less EPO required	Target Hct of 35% was achieved
Usberti et al. 1999 [168] Prospective	HD: RC, CA, PMMA, PAN vs. vitamin E modified membrane	11 RC: 6; CA: 3 PMMA: 1 PAN: 1	1 month	*Erythropoietin* : EPO dose unchanged	Hb, Hct unchanged
Locatelli et al. 2000 [261] Randomised, controlled	HD: RC vs. PMMA (BKF-PMMA, Toray)	84	12 weeks	*Kt/V* not different between the groups and stable during observation period; *Ferritin/ transferrin* not different between the groups and stable during observation period; *Iron therapy* more frequent in the RC group than in the PMMA group (77 vs. 54%), but dosage not changed during study; *EPO therapy* more frequent in the RC group than in the PMMA group (82 vs. 74%), but mean *Epo doses* remained equal in both groups during the study.	Hb, Hct and erythrocyte counts increased in both groups (treatment effect?). Differences between the groups concerning these parameters were not statistically significant.

Cortes et al. 2001 [262] Controlled	HD: RC vs. PAN (AN69®, Hospal)	25	5 months	*Kt/V* not different between the groups and stable during observation period; *EPO* dosage stable in both groups	Significant increase in Hct in the PAN group after 2 months
Opartrný et al. 2002 [263] Prospective, randomised, crossover	HD: Low-flux PSu vs. high-flux PSu (F7 HPS vs. F60, both Fresenius Medical Care)	25	8 weeks	*Iron, ferritin, transferrin saturation, aluminium, PTH, CRP, albumin, residual dialyser blood volume, EPO plasma level* and *EPO therapy*: no difference between the groups and during the study	No correlation between Hct and membrane used
Godino et al. 2002 [264] Prospective, register data	HD: Switch from low-flux PSu (at least 6 months) to high-flux PSu (all PSus from Fresenius Medical Care)	892	6 months for each membrane	*Kt/V* and *ferritin* higher during high-flux than during low-flux HD (Kt/V: 1.50 ± 0.29 vs.1.46 ± 0.25, $p = 0.002$; ferritin: 396 ± 284 vs. 366 ± 268 µg/dl, $p < 0.001$); *EPO dose*: no difference after the switch from low-flux to high-flux HD	Hb increase after the switch from low-flux to high-flux HD (11.55 ± 1.41 vs. 11.88 ± 1.43, $p < 0.001$)
Richardson et al. 2003 [170] Randomised, controlled	HD: CTA (SF170F, Nipro) vs. PSu (HF80LS, Fresenius Medical Care)	211 CTA: 103 PSu: 108	7 months	*Iron, ferritin, percentage of hypochromic red blood cells, PTH, CRP, albumin, EPO therapy*: no difference between the groups	No correlation between Hb and membrane used

Study/ year/ design	Dialysis mode/ dialysers compared	Patient number	Follow-up time	Influence on parameters important for anaemia management	Influence on renal anaemia
	AFB/HDF vs. HD/HDF				
Schrader-v.d. Meer et al. 1998 [265] Randomised, controlled	AFB with PAN (AN69®, 1.0 m^2, Hospal) vs. HD with PAN (AN69®, 1.2 m^2 Hospal)	11 AFB 9 HD	12 months	*Erythropoietin*: no change of EPO dose in either group	Hb levels: no change in either group
Maduell et al. 1999 [21] Prospective	Conventional HDF (1-3 l/h) vs. on-line HDF (3-9 l/h); dialysers not changed when switched to on-line HDF: high-flux PSu: n = 17, PAN (AN69®) n = 8, CTA: n = 3	37	12 months	*Erythropoietin: significant decrease in dose after 3 months*	Significant increase in Hb and Hct after 4 months
Ward et al. 2000 [266] Prospective, randomised	On-line HDF with PA (Polyflux 1.7 m^2, Gambro) vs. high-flux HD with PA (Polyflux 1.4 m^2, Gambro)	24 HDF 21 HD	12 months	*Erythropoietin:* increase of EPO dose in both groups	Hb, Hct: no change in either group

Wizemann et al. 2000 [22] Prospective, controlled	On-line HDF with high-flux PSu (F80s) vs. HD with low-flux PSu (F6), both Fresenius Medical Care)	23 HDF 21 HD	24 months	*Erythropoietin* (used in 40% of patients in the HDF group and 42% of patients in the HD group): no change of EPO dose in either group	Hct: no change in either group
Eiselt et al. 2000 [267] Randomised, controlled	AFB with PAN (AN69®, Hospal) vs. low-flux HD ("cellulosic" or PSu, not further specified)	10 AFB, 10 HD	12 months	*Erythropoietin*: reduction in EPO-dose with AFB	Hb, Hct: no change in either group
Basile et al. 2001 [268] Prospective, crossover	AFB with PAN (AN69®, 1.2 m^2, Hospal) vs. dialysis with cellulose acetate (1.4 m^2, Baxter)	10	6 months	*Iron, ferritin, transferrin saturation:* no difference between the groups and during the study *Erythropoietin:* no EPO therapy in any patient	Hct, Hb, reticulocytes: no difference between the groups and during the study

Table 10.6: Studies addressing the influence of dialyser membranes and dialysis modality on renal anaemia, and important parameters for anaemia management. *CA: cellulose acetate; PA: polyamide; PAN: polyacrylonitrile; PMMA: polymethylmethacrylate; PSu: polysulfone; RC: regenerated cellulose; HD: haemodialysis; AFB: acetate free biofiltration; HDF: haemodiafiltration; Hb: haemoglobin; Hct: haematocrit; PTH: parathyroidhormone; CRP: C-reactive protein; EPO: erythropoietin.*

Fresenius Medical Care) did not show a membrane effect on EPO dose or haematocrit after 8 weeks observation time [263]. Data from the European Clinical Dialysis Database (EuCliD®) show an increase in haemoglobin from 11.55 ± 1.41 to 11.88 ± 1.43 g/l in 892 patients evaluated for haemoglobin/erythropoietin outcome after shifting from at least 6 months of low-flux haemodialysis with polysulfone (PS 400, Fresenius Medical Care) to high-flux membranes (Fresenius Polysulfone® or Helixone® (58.3% of the patients), both from Fresenius Medical Care) [264]. Erythropoietin dose remained stable during treatment with both types of dialysers but, after the shift from low-flux to high-flux dialysis, Kt/V increased from 1.46 ± 0.25 to 1.50 ± 0.29 ($p = 0.002$), and ferritin levels rose from 366 ± 268 to 396 ± 284 µg/dl ($p < 0.001$); both of these factors might also have contributed to the rise of haemoglobin reported. Analysis of only those patients in the database where no significant changes were made in iron management, EPO dosage or dose of dialysis, showed that there was only a borderline statistically significant increase in haemoglobin, i.e. from 11.4 ± 0.9 to 11.8 ± 0.9 g/l ($p = 0.055$). Even increasing convective solute transport by acetate-free biofiltration (AFB) or on-line haemodiafiltration (HDF) using high-flux dialysers did not change EPO dosage or renal anaemia in 4 out of 6 studies (i.e. in [22, 265, 266, 268], but not in [21, 267]). Factors other than membrane permeability or convective transport could possibly explain the results of the 2 studies showing an improvement in anaemia and EPO dose: in one of these studies, EPO dose was less in the AFB group than in the HD group already at the start of the study, before declining during the follow-up time [267]; and Kt/V was increased by 15% after changing from conventional HDF to on-line HDF in the other study [21].

Is renal anaemia affected by dialyser biocompatibility?

Less cytokines are released when membranes are used that are not made exclusively from regenerated cellulose (i.e. more biocompatible membranes). This biocompatibility aspect is thought to play a role in erythropoietin response (see **figure 10.11** and [83, 247, 269]). In two separate studies, comparison of the synthetic, biocompatible membranes high-flux polysulfone [260] and polyacrylonitrile [262] with regenerated cellulose resulted in an ameliorated response to EPO and an increase in haematocrit, respectively, after several months observation time. On the other hand, Locatelli et al. [261] did not find significantly higher haemoglobin levels with polymethylmethacrylate compared to regenerated cellulose, although a rising trend in haemoglobin was present in the PMMA group during the short 8-week observation period. Also Basile et al. failed to find any differences in EPO dosage and renal anaemia when comparing AFB using polyacrylonitrile membranes with haemodialysis using low-flux cellulose acetate membranes over a 6 month interval [268], and Richardson et al. did not detect differences in EPO dosage or renal anaemia when comparing mid-flux polysulfone with mid-flux cellulose triacetate dialysis membranes [170].

Red blood cell susceptibility to oxidative stress may also be considered a measure of dialyser biocompatibility, as this possibly reduces red blood cell longevity in haemodialysis patients. Dialysers containing regenerated cellulose (i.e. NT 1375 S, Bellco) were found to increase red blood cell susceptibility for oxidative stress via neutrophil activation and oxygen-free radical production. This was not observed when cellulose triacetate (Sureflux 130-L, Nipro) and low-flux polysulfone (F6HPS, Fresenius Medical Care) dialysers were used [183]. In another study, switching 11 patients (most of whom were dialysed

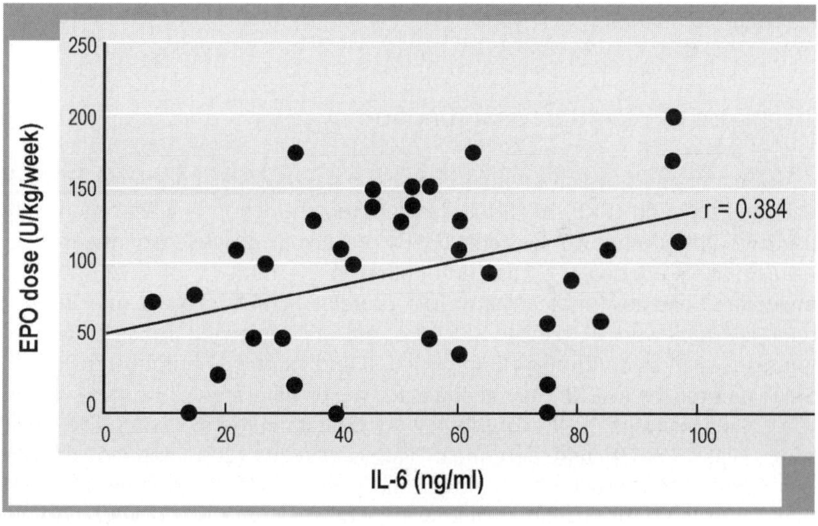

Figure 10.11: Interleukin-6 levels and EPO doses in dialysis patients. *Interleukin-6 (IL-6) levels in the supernatants of peripheral blood mononuclear cells before start of a midweek dialysis treatment with regenerated cellulose (n = 29) and polysulfone membranes (n = 5) in 34 tested patients are plotted against the respective patient erythropoietin (EPO) doses. No major cause for erythropoietin (EPO) resistance was identified in the patients tested. The IL-6 and EPO dose levels were found to correlate to a certain degree (r = correlation coefficient, p = 0.039) (adapted from [82]).*

with cellulosic dialysers, i.e. 6 with regenerated cellulose, 3 with cellulose acetate, and one each with PMMA and AN69®) to a vitamin E-modified membrane (Clirans E, Terumo), resulted in a reduction of markers for oxidative stress, but not in an improvement in renal anaemia. Only after an additional i.v. application of the anti-oxidant reduced glutathione, did the patients' haemoglobin and haematocrit values improve, allowing EPO dose to be reduced [168].

It appears therefore that, in contrast to dialysis dose (which seems to have a clear influence on renal anaemia [247, 255, 256, 270, 271]), the role of dialyser permeability and biocompatibility in renal anaemia remains unclear. To date, the removal of putative inhibitors of erythropoiesis via increased dialyser permeability has not been shown to play a very important, clinically identifiable role. Data concerning biocompatibility are even more conflicting: whereas some studies indicate a positive influence of synthetic dialysers on EPO-dosage and renal anaemia [260, 262], this was not confirmed in other investigations [261, 268]. Further larger, controlled studies are needed to elucidate the matter.

10.4 Loss of residual renal function

In recent years, much attention has been paid to the importance of residual renal function (RRF) in ESRD. Residual renal function is a term generally used for any glomerular filtration (GFR) present in dialysis patients. It influences dialysis adequacy by its contribution to the removal of small, "middle molecules" and low molecular weight proteins; it also plays a role in fluid removal (reviewed in [272]). RRF also reflects remaining renal endocrine functions such as erythropoietin production and vitamin D homeostasis [272]. Small differences in RRF may account for major differences in quality of live [273]: for example, RRF contributes to overall nutritional status in both haemodialysis [274] and peritoneal dialysis patients [275]. Indeed, it even correlated with mortality in peritoneal dialysis: the CANUSA study revealed that every 0.5 ml/min higher GFR was associated with a 9% lower risk of death [275, 276].

RRF normally declines continuously after enrolment in chronic haemodialysis treatment. Two theories exist concerning the underlying mechanisms. The first theory pinpoints the removal of solutes or nitrogenous compounds that act as osmotic agents promoting continued urine output, even in damaged kidneys: the efficient removal of these substances by dialysis may reduce the osmotic drive that supports RRF [277]. In the second theory, reduced renal perfusion by ultrafiltration-induced transient hypotension during dialysis is blamed for the further decrease in GFR [278]. Irrespective of the cause, the positive influence of RRF on patient morbidity and mortality means that it is important to identify factors that preserve or prolong RRF in ESRD patients. Factors that have been identified to date are peritoneal dialysis, higher serum calcium, intake of ACE inhibitors and calcium channel blockers [272], and use of ultrapure dialysis fluid [279].

Use of biocompatible dialyser membranes has also been discussed as a means of slowing down the loss of RRF. Bioincompatible membranes activate complement and leukocytes, and products of these activations have direct and indirect vasoconstrictive properties that can exacerbate renal ischaemia. Furthermore, some complement and leukocyte products have deleterious effects on tubular and glomerular cells [280]. Several small retrospective studies conducted between 1993 and 1995 showed that biocompatible, synthetic membranes (i.e. polysulfone and polyacrylonitrile) were associated with a slower decline in RRF than Cuprophan® [281-283], whereas this effect was not found in one study [284]. Two larger studies performed later (20 patients, prospective design [280]; 50 patients, retrospective design [285]) documented the more positive influence of Fresenius Polysulfone® (F60 [280], F80 [285]) on prolonging RRF compared to cellulose acetate (Baxter CA 130 [280], CA 110 [285]) (see **figure 10.12**). When the decline of RRF in 175 patients treated with high-flux biocompatible membranes (e.g. polysulfone and polyacrylonitrile), was compared to the decline of RRF in 300 CAPD patients (in whom RRF is known to be usually better preserved than in patients treated with haemodialysis), no difference was found between the groups within the follow-up period of 48 months [286]. However, dialysis was initiated rather late in this study (urea clearance < 5 ml/min for both modalities), which makes it diffcult to identify possible long-term effects of the different treatment modalities on the decline of RRF. A recent retrospective analysis of 4000 patients from the United States Renal Data System (USRDS) Dialysis and Mortality Study (DMMS) wave 2 [272] did not show any difference in RRF between the group of patients treated with synthetic or modified cellulosic membranes (together 81% of patients) and the group treated with regenerated cellulose membranes (19% of patients). Comparison of high-flux synthetic dialysers with all other dialyser membranes also didn't yield statistically significant differences in RRF loss. This appears to speak against the positive influence of biocompatible, synthetic dialyser membranes on RRF found in the other studies cited above (i.e. in comparison to regenerated cellulose [281-283] or modified cellulose [280, 285]). However, the percentage of patients treated with regenerated cellulose membranes in this study may have been too low to detect a difference between the two groups. In addition, dialysers were regularly reused and subsequent induced membrane changes might mask any sharp distinctions between low- and high-flux membranes.

In summary, studies addressing the influence of membrane biocompatibility on RRF provide some evidence for prolonged RRF with the use of synthetic membranes [280-283, 285, 286]. The ongoing Membrane Permeability Study (MPO) should provide further insight into this subject, as only new ESRD patients will be enrolled and treated with either low-flux or high-flux membranes [287].

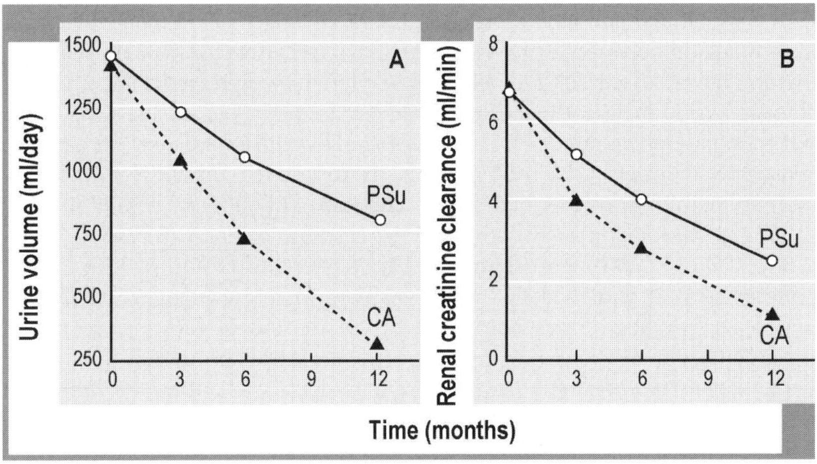

Figure 10.12: Decline in residual renal function (RRF) after onset of haemodialysis with polysulfone and cellulose acetate dialysers. *Decline in RRF as indicated by decreases in (A) daily urine volume (ml/day) and (B) renal creatinine clearance (ml/min) is shown for various times within a 12-month observation period. Values for patients treated with polysulfone (PSu) (F60, Fresenius Polysulfone®) were over twice those measured for patients treated with cellulose acetate (CA) (CA 130, Baxter) (adapted from [280]).*

10.5 Atherosclerosis

Cardio-, cerebro- and peripheral vascular complications due to accelerated atherosclerosis are clear causes of morbidity in patients with ESRD (see **figure 10.13**) [13, 288, 289]. The onset of the atherosclerotic process lies definitively in the period prior to ESRD, resulting in an already increased atherosclerotic burden at onset of dialysis therapy [290-292]. This partially explains the high prevalence of atherosclerotic disease sites in maintenance dialysis patients, even at young ages [293].

Atherosclerosis is a multifactorial disease that develops over a time period of several years or even decades. Apart from the traditional risk factors and the commonly increased atherosclerotic burden at dialysis start, several uraemia- and dialysis-related risk factors also exist in dialysis patients (see **figure 10.14**). In particular, the presence of a chronic inflammatory process, an atherogenic lipid profile, increased oxidative stress and hyperhomocysteinaemia lead to an acute phase reaction (see **table 10.1**) which, via a chronic systemic inflammatory response, accelerates atherosclerosis [65, 133]. Therefore, atherosclerosis is especially associated with the presence of inflammation in ESRD [71-75], although other co-morbid states (e.g. diabetes, malnutrition or hyperparathyroidism) also play roles [71, 294, 295].

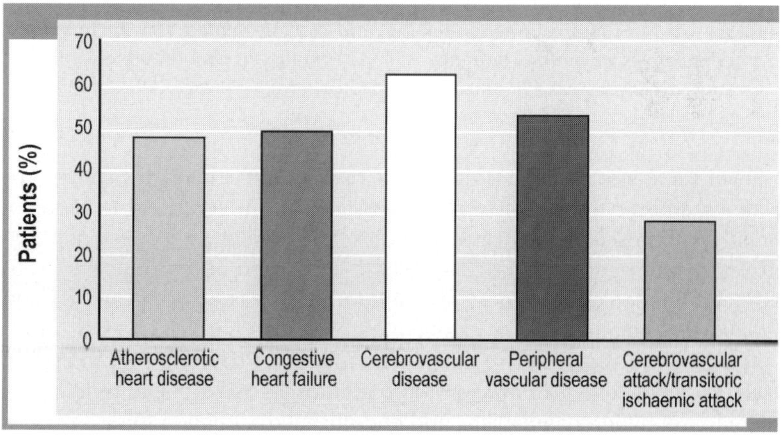

Figure 10.13: Percent of ESRD patients with vascular disease and associated cardiac problems. *Data are taken from the 2002 USRDS report and refer to patients on dialysis on December 31st, 1998, having started ESRD replacement therapy at least 9 months beforehand (adapted from [13]).*

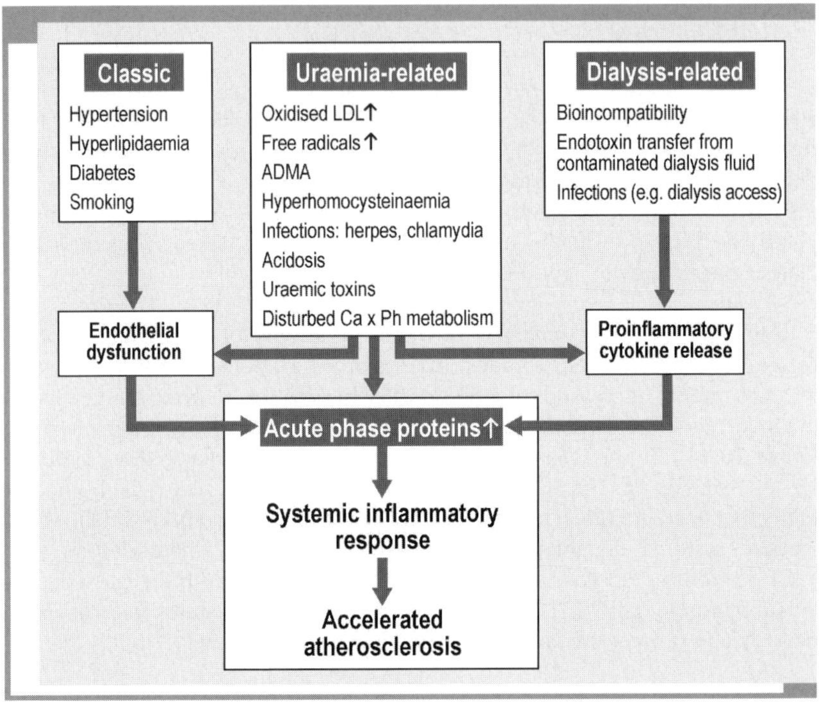

Figure 10.14: Classic, uraemia-related and dialysis-related risk factors for atherosclerosis in dialysis patients. *ADMA: asymmetric dimethylarginine; LDL: low density lipoprotein. Ph: phosphate (adapted from [65] and [74])*

Several parameters that are at least partially influenced by dialyser performance and biocompatibility characteristics have been found to be associated with atherosclerosis in clinical studies. For example, Kt/V was negatively correlated with peripheral vascular disease [295], and both C-reactive protein (CRP) and interleukin-6 (IL-6) were found to be associated with carotid intima-media thickness, a marker for carotid atherosclerosis [74]. IL-6 was also found to predict the progress of this atherosclerosis [73]. Proposed mechanisms via which cytokines (e.g. IL-6) may promote atherosclerosis are lipid modification, generation of hypercoagulability, and endothelial dysfunction [65].

However, despite the possible contribution of dialyser characteristics to several atherosclerotic risk factors (i.e. inflammatory state, oxidative stress, dyslipidaemia and homocysteine levels, as discussed in chapters 10.1.1,

10.1.2, 10.5.1 and 10.5.2, respectively), it is difficult to isolate pure dialyser-related effects of atherosclerosis or atherosclerosis-induced morbidity. This is because of the multifactorial genesis of atherosclerosis and its role in different diseases, e.g. cardiovascular, cerebrovascular and peripheral vascular problems. While several studies relate cardiovascular mortality to dialyser characteristics [10, 206, 296-299] (see chapter 11), only few clinical studies relate dialyser characteristics to atherosclerosis-induced morbidity: Koda et al. compared the incidence of cardiovascular disease in patients who were switched from low-flux cellulosic membranes (i.e. regenerated cellulose (77.4%), cellulose acetate (19.9%) and others (2.7%)) to high-flux dialysers (i.e. polymethylmethacrylate (32.4%), polyacrylonitrile (AN69®) (17.2%), polysulfone (16.7%), cellulose triacetate (28.6%), polyester-polymer-alloy (3.4%) and others (1.7%)) [297]. However, the study design did not allow a differentiation between biocompatibility characteristics [300]. The authors found a slightly higher incidence of cardiovascular disease with the cellulosic membranes, but this was not statistically significant [297]. In the recently published Hemodialysis Outcome (HEMO) study, patients were treated either with low-flux (n = 925) or high-flux dialysers (n = 921 patients) for a mean follow-up time of 4.48 years [206]. In total, 17 different low-flux dialysers and 8 different high-flux dialysers were employed. The low-flux dialysers were mostly polysulfone (F8, Fresenius Medical Care, 46%) or cellulose acetate (CA210, Baxter, 43%). No regenerated cellulose dialysers were used. Nearly all the high-flux dialysers were made from polysulfone (F80, Fresenius Medical Care, 43%) or cellulose triacetate (CT190, Baxter, 48%). No differences were found in the primary outcome, death for any cause, and in the major secondary outcomes, e.g. first hospitalisation for cardiac reasons. However, reductions (unadjusted $p < 0.05$) in the case of high-flux dialysis were found in the risk of death for cardiac complications and in the combined outcome of first hospitalisation for cardiac reasons or death due to cardiac complications. The weak results of this study have been intensively discussed worldwide [301-308]; major points of criticism refer to the design: (a) exclusion of very old patients, resulting in a lower mean age (57.6 ± 14.0 years) than the normal population of dialysis patients; (b) less malnourished patients due to exclusion of patients with a serum albumin less than 2.6 g/l; (c) exclusion of patients with body weight in excess of 80 kg; (d) a long history of dialysis (3.7 years) before entering the study; (e) the use of high-flux dialysers in already approximately 60% of the patients before entering the study; and (f) the acceptance of dialyser reuse, which possibly interferes with the membrane permeability in such a way that a sharp distinction between low-flux and high-flux membranes is compromised. All these factors might have prevented the detection of clear beneficial effects of high-flux.

Thus, even though there are some indications that dialyser characteristics influence major factors contributing to atherosclerosis in ESRD (e.g. inflammatory state, oxidative stress, dyslipidaemia and homocysteine), the few clinical studies which searched for a relationship between atherosclerosis-induced morbidity and dialyser characteristics conducted to date failed to find a statistically significant effect [297], or found only weak beneficial effects for high-flux dialysis [206].

10.5.1 Plasma lipids

The prevalence of dyslipidaemia is very high in ESRD patients [294, 309-315]. Typical findings are: variable increases in serum triglycerides together with low levels of high density lipoprotein (HDL) cholesterol; elevated levels of low density lipoprotein (LDL), especially in diabetics; and accumulations of partially metabolised triglyceride-enriched very low density lipoproteins (VLDL-remnants) and intermediate density lipoproteins (IDL). These changes in lipid profile are mainly due to a defective triglyceride-rich lipoprotein catabolism in ESRD, secondary to a reduced activity of lipolytic enzymes, such as lipoprotein lipase (LPL) or hepatic triglyceride lipase (HTGL) [294, 309]. LPL is bound to the luminal surface of capillary endothelial cells where it can be released into the blood stream by heparin. Proposed underlying mechanisms for the reduced lipolytic activity in ESRD are (A) a depletion of LPL stores by repeated administration of heparin and (B) the presence of increased levels of apolipoprotein C3 or cytokines, both of which also inhibit LPL activity (reviewed in [316-319]).

Although the absolute levels of total cholesterol and triglycerides in serum of ESRD patients are not extremely high, the pattern of dyslipidaemia is clearly atherogenic. This is especially the case in ESRD patients because lipoprotein(a) (Lp(a)) levels are also elevated (see **table 10.7**). Lp(a) is composed of an apolipoprotein(a) (apo(a)) linked to an LDL particle, and is an independent cardiovascular risk factor in ESRD [315, 320, 321]. The apo(a) isoform size can also predict cardiovascular complications [71, 322]. Furthermore, cross sectional data show that the presence of coronary heart disease in ESRD is associated with smoking, hypertension, smaller apo(a) phenotypes, higher LDL values, lower levels of HDL and higher apo B and fibrinogen values (reviewed in [310] and [323]). Increased intima–media thickness of the carotid and femoral arteries was shown to be associated with elevated IDL levels [294]. Lipid-reducing therapy reduces both ischaemic cardiac events

Parameter	Atherogenicity	Plasma concentrations in haemodialysis patients
Chylomicra	-	↔
Chylomicron remnants	+	↑
VLDL	-	↑
VLDL remnants/ IDL	++	↑
LDL	+++	↓↔
HDL	protective	↓
Lp(a)	++	↑

Table 10.7: Atherogenicity of lipids, some of their metabolic intermediate products (remnants) and lipoprotein a (Lp(a)) and common changes of plasma levels in haemodialysis patients. *VLDL: very low density lipoproteins; LDL: low density lipoprotein; HDL: high density lipoprotein; IDL intermediate density lipoproteins; the degree of atherogenicity is graded from none (-) to very strong (+++); ↔ : no change compared to normal level; ↑ : increased compared to normal level; ↓ : decreased compared to normal level (adapted from [309]).*

and mortality in patients without renal disease [324] and reviewed in [310] but is, although recommended by specialists [311, 325], not yet standard treatment in ESRD. However, first recent reports confirm the safety and the positive effect of lipid-reducing therapy on mortality in ESRD [326, 327]. This is reflected in the recently published European Best Practice Guidelines: these recommend lipid reducing therapy for haemodialysis patients with dyslipidaemia (guideline VII.2 [20]).

In this context, any possible effect of dialyser membranes on serum lipid levels gains importance. Membrane biocompatibility could, for example, influence the lipid profile by differential release of cytokines and other inflammatory markers. Increased membrane permeability of high-flux dialysers could improve convective transport of larger solutes and, consequently, the removal of e.g. circulating lipoprotein inhibitors, such as apolipoprotein C3 and pre β-HDL (reviewed in [35-38, 319]). However, the results of different studies addressing this issue are conflicting (for details see **table 10.8**). Earlier smaller studies, mostly with short follow-up times, showed an amelioration in predialysis or intradialysis lipid profiles with high-flux dialysis using polysulfone [35, 316, 317, 328, 329], polyamide [36] and cellulose triacetate [328] compared to low-flux dialysis with unmodified [35, 316, 317, 329] and modified cellulosic membranes (cellulose acetate in [328]). Later, this was confirmed in a prospective, crossover study of 27 patients comparing high-flux polysulfone with low-flux cellulosic dialysers and having a follow-up time of 3 months [330]. Also, recently, more evidence was supplied in a study comparing high-flux dialysis using cellulose triacetate and the Helixone® membrane with low-flux dialysis using polysulfone in 30 patients [38]. In this study, the use of the Helixone® membrane additionally reduced the level of oxidised LDL. Data from the European Clinical Dialysis Database (EuCliD®) confirmed this effect: a switch from low-flux polysulfone (PS 400, Fresenius Medical Care) to high-flux polysulfone (Fresenius Polysulfone® (41.7%) or Helixone® (58.3%), both from Fresenius Medical Care) led to significant reductions in total cholesterol ($p < 0.001$), and in LDL cholesterol ($p = 0.001$), as well to a significant increase in HDL cholesterol ($p = 0.006$) in the 1046 patients enrolled (see **figure 10.15**) [264]. However, other studies did not show any benefit of high-flux dialysers when the following membranes were tested: high-flux polysulfone [173, 319], low-flux polysulfone [173, 319], Hemophan® [173], polyacrylonitrile [332] and cellulose diacetate [332]. Data for low-flux dialysers are also conflicting: whereas Goldberg et al. [317] did not find a positive influence of low-flux polysulfone on the lipid profile of 14 patients tested, switching 6 patients from regenerated cellulose to low-flux polysulfone improved the lipid profile in a study by Kimak et al. [331]. Other low-flux dialysers were also tested: for example, when using two cellulose acetate dialysers with different clearances of higher molecular weight substances (sieving coefficient for ß2-microglobulin negligible in one), the better removal of higher molecular weight substances was associated with an improvement of intradialytic lipid parameters, but did not influence predialysis levels [318].

In the face of the conflicting results presented above together with other evidence- based therapeutic approaches for treating disturbances in lipid status (such as life style changes or lipid lowering therapy (EBP guidelines VII 2.6-2.10 [20]), a general recommendation for dialyser selection with the aim of improving lipid status in ESRD is difficult to make. Nevertheless, there are some indications for the use of certain dialysers in future for the treatment of ESRD patients with disturbed lipid profil, i.e. the improvements in lipid profiles found with the use of high-flux membranes, predominately with high-flux polysulfone but also with high-flux polyamide and high-flux cellulose triacetate [35, 36, 38, 264, 316, 328-330]. However, the actual reason for the improvements seen with these high-flux membranes still remains unclear: possibilities include the removal of lipoprotein lipase inhibitors, good biocompatibility, or a combination of these or even other factors. Because of the heparin-induced reduction in lipolytic activity in ESRD patients, different heparinisation modes may also contribute to the conflicts in the results presented; this deserves further investigation. A reduction in the dose of heparin (unfractionated and fractionated) administered during treatment also appeared to improve lipid profiles (e.g. [173, 333]).

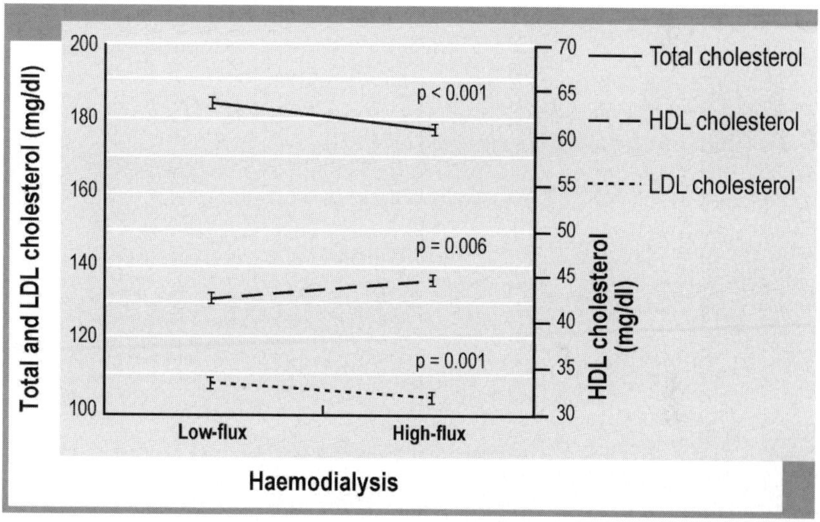

Figure 10.15: Effect of high-flux dialysis on lipid profile. *High-flux dialysis (Fresenius Polysulfone® or Helixone®, both Fresenius Medical Care) significantly decreased total cholesterol ($p < 0.001$) and LDL cholesterol ($p = 0.001$) and increased HDL cholesterol ($p = 0.006$) in 1046 patients previously treated with low-flux polysulfone (PS 400, Fresenius Medical Care) (adapted from [264]).*

Study/ year/ design	Dialysers compared	Patient numbers	Follow-up time	Changes in lipid profile
Josephson et al., 1992 [328]	High-flux PSu (F80, Fresenius Medical Care) and CTA (CT190G, Baxter) CA (CA110, Baxter)	18 (2 PSu/16 CTA) 16 (CA)	One predialysis value	Triglycerides: ⇔ (PSu/CTA), ⇑ (CA) HDL: ⇔ (PSu/CTA), ⇓ (CA)
Seres et al. 1993 [35]	High-flux PSu Saponified cellulose ester (SCE)	10 (PSu) 9 (SCE)	one pre- to postdialysis value	Triglycerides: ⇓ (PSu), ⇔ (SCE) HDL: ⇑ (PSu), ⇔ (SCE)
Blankestijn et al. 1995 [316] Controlled, prospective	High-flux PSu RC	14 (PSu) 14 (RC)	6 weeks	Triglycerides: ⇓ (PSu), ⇔ (RC) HDL: ⇑ (PSu), ⇔ (RC)
Docci et al. 1995 [329]	High-flux PSu RC	13 (PSu) 13 (RC)	One predialysis value	HDL cholesterol ⇑, Apo A ⇑ for PSu compared to RC
Goldberg et al. 1996 [317] Randomised, crossover	Low-flux PSu (F8, Fresenius Medical Care) High-flux PSu (F80, Fresenius Medical Care) RC (Terumo 220)	7 high-flux PSu/RC 8 RC/high-flux PSu 7 RC/ low-flux PSu 7 low-flux PSu/RC	One month with each membrane	Triglycerides ⇓, cholesterol ⇓ only for high-flux PSu compared to RC No differences between low-flux PSu and RC

De Precigout et al. 1996 [36]	High-flux PA RC	6	4 months	Triglycerides ⇓, total cholesterol ⇓, Apo B ⇓, Apo C3 ⇓, HDL ⇑, HDL-cholesterol ⇑, PL activity ⇑ for PA compared to RC
Tanaka H. et al. 1997 [330] Prospective, crossover	High-flux PSu (wet-type PS-1.3UW, Fresenius Medical Care) RC (Clirans15), vitamin E-coated RC (Clirans EE 15NL), both Terumo	27	3 months with each membrane	HDL ⇓, HDL2-triglycerides ⇓, HDL2-PL ⇓ for vit E-coated RC compared to RC; Total cholesterol ⇓, HDL-cholesterol ⇓, Apo B ⇓, Apo C3 ⇓ for low-flux PSu compared to RC ✶
Kimak et al. 1998 [331] Prospective, crossover	RC (E-3, Fresenius Medical Care) Low-flux PSu (F6, Fresenius Medical Care)	6	6 months with each membrane	Triglycerides ⇓, total cholesterol ⇓, LDL cholesterol ⇓, HDL cholesterol ⇑, Apo A1 ⇑ for low-flux PSu compared to RC
Ingram et al. 1998 [318] Randomised, crossover	Low-flux CA (Altranova 140, Althin), siev. coeff. for ß2m: 0.6, urea clear 193ml/min Low-flux CA (CA210, Baxter), siev. coeff for ß2m: negligible, urea clear 247 ml/min	16	4 dialysis sessions with each membrane	*Intradialytic changes*: Total cholesterol, Apo A1, Apo B: no difference between the membranes; rise in triglycerides: attenuated by AN140; HDL ⇑, Apo E ⇑, total Apo C3 ⇔ with AN140 *Predialysis lipid levels:* no difference between the membranes

Study/ year/ design	Dialysers compared	Patient numbers	Follow-up time	Changes in lipid profile
Cianciolo et al. 2000 [173] Prospective	HE, high-flux PSu, low-flux PSu	32 HE 26 HF- PSu 28 LF- PSu	18 months	Triglycerides, total cholesterol, HDL cholesterol, LDL cholesterol, Apo's, Lp(a): no difference between the membranes
House et al. 2000 [319] Prospective, randomised	High-flux PSu (F80 Fresenius Medical Care), low-flux PSu (F8 Fresenius Medical Care)	24	3 months	Triglycerides, total cholesterol, LDL cholesterol, HDL cholesterol, Lp(a): no difference between the membranes
Ottosson et al. 2001 [332] Prospective, randomised	Low-flux CDA (FB 170T, Nissho), high-flux PAN (Nephral 4000, Hospal)l	23 CDA 19 PAN	3 months	Triglycerides, total cholesterol, HDL cholesterol, LDL cholesterol, Apo A1, Apo A2, Apo B, Apo C3, Apo E, Lp(a), Apo A and Apo B containing Lps: no difference between the membranes

Wanner et al. 2002 [38] Prospective, cross over	Low-flux Psu (F7HPS, Fresenius Medical Care) High-flux CTA (CT210 G, Baxter) Helixone® (FX 100, Fresenius Medical Care)	30	6 weeks	High-flux membranes significantly reduced levels of triglycerides, RPL cholesterol and Apo C3 compared to low-flux membranes ($p < 0.005$-0.001). Helixone® additionally reduced ox LDL ($p < 0.001$).
Godino et al. 2002 [264] Prospective, register data	HD: Switch from low-flux PSu (at least 6 months) to high-flux PSu (all PSus from Fresenius Medical Care)	1046	6 months for each membrane type	Total cholesterol ⇓ ($p < 0.001$), HDL cholesterol ⇑ ($p = 0.006$), LDL cholesterol ⇓ ($p = 0.001$) after switch from low-flux to high-flux dialysis

Table 10.8**: **Results of studies investigating the influence of membrane choice on lipid profiles in ESRD. *CA: cellulose acetate; CDA: cellulose diacetate; CTA: cellulose triacetate; CE: saponified cellulose ester; HE Hemophan®; PA: polyamide; PAN: polyacrylonitrile; PSu: polysulfone; RC: regenerated cellulose; HDL: high density lipoprotein; LDL: low density protein; RPL: remnant lipoprotein; VLDL: very low density protein; Apo: apolipoprotein; PL: plasma lipase; Lp: lipoprotein; ⇑: increase; ⇓: decrease; ⇔: constant; ✶: similar effect as seen in patients treated with HMG-coA reductase inhibitors.*

10.5.2 Homocysteine

Elevated homocysteine levels have been increasingly recognised as an important independent risk factor for vascular disease, both in the general population [334-337] as well as in patients with impaired renal function and ESRD [338-342]. Hyperhomocysteinaemia also predicts cardiovascular outcome in ESRD patients [341, 342]. It is present in 85 - 100% of dialysis patients [181, 339, 340, 343-353] and, while the normal upper plasma total homocysteine values in healthy subjects are around 12 µmol/l [354], values in these patients range from 20 to 50 µmol/l [354]. Evidence is growing that shows that hyperhomocyteinaemia exerts its toxic effects by oxidative stress-induced endothelial dysfunction (reviewed in [348, 351]).

Homocysteine is a sulfhydryl amino acid, resulting from demethylation of the essential amino acid methionine. Homocysteine can be remethylated to methionine or transsulfurated to cysteine [344, 351]. The different pathways of homocysteine metabolism are shown in **figure 10.16**, as are the additional substances required as precursors, co-factors or substrates (e.g. folate, vitamin B_6 and B_{12}).

Which pathophysiological mechanisms influence plasma homocysteine levels in ESRD?

The exact pathophysiological mechanism behind the reduced clearance of homocysteine from plasma in ESRD is unclear [355]. Loss of elimination as a result of a decreased renal clearance seems unlikely, as the urinary excretion of homocysteine is negligible in healthy subjects (reviewed in [344, 351]) and the normal kidney parenchyma, according to newer investigations and in contrast to earlier belief [355, 356], does not seem to contribute to homocysteine metabolism to a significant extent [357]. However, the presence of increased intermediate products of homocysteine metabolism in ESRD patients, especially products of transsulfuration, indicate that homocysteine metabolism is altered in ESRD [39, 358]. Studies have shown that low levels of folate, vitamin B6 and/or B12 were found in patients with elevated levels of homocysteine and vascular complications [340]. Therefore, in order to optimise homocysteine metabolism in ESRD, substitution therapies with the different vitamins or combinations thereof have been conducted. These reduce homocysteine levels significantly, but often don't normalise them [340, 344, 347-350]. Generally, a mean total homocysteine reduction about 30% is obtained, with exceptions reporting decreases of 60-70% (reviewed in [354]).

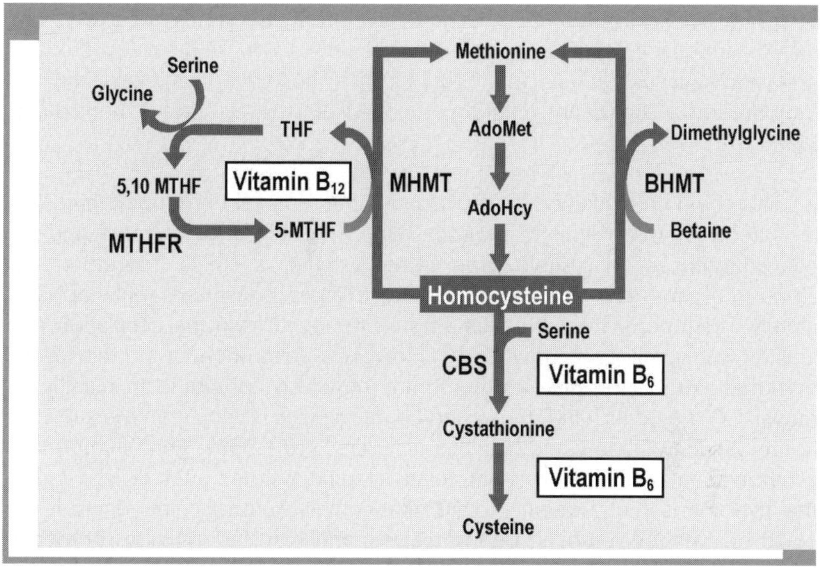

Figure 10.16: Homocysteine metabolism. *Homocysteine results from the demethylisation of methionine. During its metabolism, it can be remethylated to methionine or transsulfurated to cysteine. There are two different remethylation pathways: one requires vitamin* B_{12} *as a co-factor and 5-methyltetrahydrofolate (5-MTHF), a folic acid metabolite, as methyl donor; the other requires betaine as methyldonor. The transsulfuration pathway consists of two irreversible, vitamin* B_6*-dependant reactions. AdoMet: S-adenosylmethionine; AdoHcy: S-adenosylhomocysteine; THF: tetrahydrofolate; 5-MTHF: 5-methyltetrahydrofolate; MTHFR: 5,10-methylene-tetrahydrofolate-reductase; MHMT: methyltetrahydrofolate-homocysteine methyltransferase; BHMT: betaine-homocysteine methyltransferase; CBS: cystathionine ß-synthase (adapted from [351]).*

Does haemodialysis treatment contribute to homocysteine removal in ESRD?

Haemodialysis itself is thought to influence homocysteine levels either by removal of non-protein-bound, free homocysteine, or by elimination of putative "inhibitors" of homocysteine metabolism. Due to its molecular weight of only 268 or lower [351], free homocysteine is eliminated by both low- and high-flux membranes to similar extents. This was reflected by similar predialysis free homocysteine levels in studies comparing high-flux polysulfone and polyacrylonitrile with low-flux polysulfone and cellulose acetate over periods of several weeks [319, 332]. The intradialytic reduction rates correlated with dialysis adequacy (Kt/V) and were roughly 30% [319, 359] for low-flux and 40% for high-flux dialysis ($p < 0.02$) [319] - however, this effect did not translate into a significant difference in predialysis levels after 3 months [40, 319].

This could be explained by the fact that the removal of homocysteine during haemodialysis is limited: homocysteine is mostly protein-bound and the concentration of dialysable, free homocysteine is small. Therefore, the amount of homocysteine removable by dialysis constitutes only approximately a few percent of the total amount removed from the circulation of a healthy individual every day [359]. However, adsorption of protein-bound homocysteine by the dialyser membrane may also contribute to dialytic removal. On the other hand, the observed differences in reduction rates of total homocysteine with low and high-flux dialysers [319, 359] in combination with a rebound of total homocysteine levels starting 8 hours after dialysis led to the hypothesis that uraemic toxins that inhibit homocysteine degradation could possibly be removed during dialysis, and that this facilitates homocysteine degradation, especially after dialysis [359]. This hypothesis is supported by the results of two different studies, representing two alternative ways to increase removal of such putative inhibitors of homocysteine degradation, i.e. via an increase in dialysis frequency or via an enhanced removal of uraemic toxins by an alternative dialyser design. Nocturnal dialysis (6 - 7 nights/week) using Polyamide S™ (a PA/Polyarylether-sulfone/PVP alloy from Gambro, here Polyflux S 17/21) decreased total homocysteine levels significantly compared to standard dialysis (12.7 versus 20.0 µmol/l, $p < 0.05$) and reduced the prevalence of mild to moderate hyperhomocysteinaemia (> 12.0 µmol/l) (57% versus 94%, $p = 0.002$) [353]. Alternatively, haemodialysis with the so-called "Superflux" dialysers (F500S, polysulfone from Fresenius Medical Care and Tricea 150G, cellulose triacetate from Baxter) with enhanced convective transport of higher molecular weight substances (sieving coefficients for ß2-microglobulin 0.9 and 0.8, respectively) achieved a significant decrease in predialysis total homocysteine levels after 12 weeks compared to standard high-flux polysulfone dialysers (F60, Fresenius Medical Care, sieving coefficient for ß2-microglobulin 0.65) [351]. Studies comparing levels of homocysteine and reactive oxygen species with the use of different membranes showed a deleterious effect of regenerated cellulose on anti-oxidant activity, an intermediate protection from oxidative stress for cellulose diacetate and a better protection for polymethylmethacrylate, polyacrylonitrile and the combination of DEAE cellulose and polysulfone (paired filtration device) [144, 180, 181]. The lowest plasma homocysteine values both before and after dialysis were measured in patients treated with paired filtration and the combination of DEAE cellulose and polysulfone [144].

In summary, preliminary studies suggest that, in addition to standard supplementation with vitamins (i.e. with folate, vitamin B_6 and/or B_{12}), increases in dialysis adequacy in the form of either augmented dialysis frequency or the use of very highly permeable dialysers may contribute to reducing homocysteine levels in ESRD patients. However, larger studies are needed to confirm these first results.

10.6 Susceptibility to infection

As already shown in this chapter and in chapters 7 and 8, the immune system of uraemic patients is characterised by a disturbance in the interacting networks: the physiological equilibrium between anti- and pro-oxidant, anti- and pro-inflammatory, anti- and proaptotic and of inhibitory and stimulating factors is out of balance. There is evidence that ESRD patients present an increased susceptibility to infections: among haemodialysis patients, infection accounted for 12% of the deaths and an average of 7.6 bacteremic episodes per 100 patient years (0.076 per year), of which 48% were associated with access infections [360]. Several factors contribute to this increased susceptibility for infections: breakdown of protective barriers (e.g. suboptimal fistula/graft punction techniques for blood access), presence of dialysis catheters, affinity of bacteria for foreign materials (e.g. dialysis catheters or vascular grafts), uraemic toxin retention, deficiency and resistance to vitamin D, carriership of pathological or multiresistent germs, and malnutrition (reviewed in [361]). Furthermore, the dialysis treatment itself contributes to unphysiological activities of immune cells; these are mainly mediated by dialyser bioincompatibility and/or the use of contaminated dialysis fluid [362-366].

Does dialyser choice influence parameters of infection in ESRD?

The possible negative effects of repeated cytokine induction by regenerated cellulose on the immune function of patients have already been discussed (chapter 8.3.2). The metabolic response to phagocytosis stimuli is also lower in patients dialysed with regenerated cellulose than in those dialysed with polysulfone [367]. In addition, high-flux dialysis with polysulfone (Helixone®, Fresenius Medical Care) was recently shown to restore suppressed whole blood production of interferon-γ in 12 ESRD patients previously dialysed with low-flux polysulfone (F6, Fresenius Medical Care) [368]. To date, three clinical studies looked for a relationship between susceptibility to infection and dialyser characteristics. The incidence of infections in patients dialysed with high-flux membranes was compared to the incidence in patients treated with a mix of biocompatible and bioincompatible low-flux membranes [297, 369] or with regenerated cellulose alone [370]. No significant differences in incidence of infections [297, 369] or in the days of hospital admissions [370] were found in these studies. One of these studies was prospective, comparing polymethylmethacrylate, cellulose triacetate, polyacrylonitrile and polysulfone with regenerated cellulose and cellulose acetate [297]; the other two were retrospective, one comparing polysulfone, PAN (AN69®) and polymethylmethacrylate with DEAE cellulose, cellulose acetate and regenerated cellulose [369], and the other comparing high-flux polysulfone with regenerated cellulosic membranes [370]. However, in one retrospective study primarily focusing on mortality, the relative adjusted risk of death due to infections was reduced by 31% with the use of synthetic or modified cellulosic membranes compared to regenerated cellulose [298] (see chapter 11 for more details). In the recently published HEMO study, which includes 1846 patients, 23.1% of deaths were due to infections; there were 1698 infection-related hopitalisations, giving an annual rate of 35% [371]; and there was no difference in first hospitalisation rate, in death rate due to infection, in composite infectious outcomes, in major classes of infections or in infection-free survival between patients treated with low or high-flux dialysis. Bioincompatible dialysers made from regenerated cellulose were excluded; it is therefore not possible to draw conclusions from the HEMO study about their effect on infections. Additionally, reuse of dialysers up to 20 times was permitted in this study; this possibly influenced the performance characteristics of the dialysers, thereby affecting the results [372]. Furthermore, the design of the HEMO study favoured a selection of patients who already had a relatively long history of dialysis before entering the study (3.7 years), and excluded patients with advanced age, with severe comorbidities and with severe access problems. As all of these conditions are more common in the average dialysis population, it cannot be ruled out that some patients, in particular patients with these characteristics, could benefit from high-flux dialysis (discussed in [302-308]).

One may conclude that further studies are needed to elucidate the role of dialyser performance and/or biocompatibility in ESRD patient susceptibility to infections. One such ongoing study is, for example, the European multicenter Membrane Permeability Outcome study (MPO) in which only new dialysis patients will be enrolled and dialyser reuse is not permitted [287].

10.7 Amyloidosis

Dialysis-related amyloidosis, or ß2-microglobulin (ß2-m) amyloidosis, is a serious complication in ESRD patients. The clinical features are dominated by the carpal tunnel syndrome and by chronic invalidating arthralgias developing to destructive arthropathies. Other complications include bone fractures, spinal cord compression and, in the case of visceral manifestations, gastroenteral bleeding and perforations (see **table 10.9**) [373, 374]. Symptoms result from the accumulation of ß2-m amyloid deposits within synovial membranes, tendons, periarticular structures, at the end of long bones, within intervertebral disks and in the visceral tract [375, 376]. Systemic ß2-m amyloid deposits may even be found in the heart, lungs, medium-sized blood vessels and also subcutaneously [374].

Although a few cases of ß2-m amyloidosis have been reported even before dialysis start, clinical symptoms usually don't appear before 5 years of haemodialysis treatment; they then increase progressively to be present in nearly all patients after 20 years of treatment [373]. The histological prevalence of dialysis-related amyloidosis (bone or synovial biopsies) is much greater than suspected on the basis of clinical symptoms: one third of the patients are affected after 4 years of haemodialysis, over 90% after 7 years and almost 100% after over 10 years [373]. In addition to time since dialysis start, patient age at dialysis start has also been established as a risk factor for amyloidosis, i.e. older age at dialysis start predisposes to earlier manifestation

Clinical features of ß2-m amyloidosis
• Carpal tunnel syndrome
• Chronic arthralgias (usually starting in the shoulder)
• Decreased joint mobility
• Periarticular soft-tissue swelling
• Pathological fractures (especially in hip region)
• Spinal cord compressions
• Gastrointestinal bleeding / perforation
• Subcutaneous amyloid mass (rare)

Table 10.9: Clinical features of ß2-m amyloidosis *(adapted from [373, 374]).*

of ß2-m amyloidosis [373, 377, 378]. Furthermore, the purity of the dialysis fluid [48, 379-381] and/or the choice of dialyser membrane used in haemodialysis [48, 373-375, 377, 382-385] have been reported to influence the clinical signs of ß2-microglobulin amyloidosis. In order to analyse the influence of dialyser characteristics on clinical signs of ß2-m amyloidosis, it is useful to first review its pathogenesis.

The pathogenesis of ß2-m amyloidosis is not yet completely understood, but several phases of development can be defined. (1) The declining kidney function leads to a retention of ß2-microglobulin (ß2-m), normally eliminated via the kidney. This results in high ß2-m plasma levels of approximately 20 - 40 mg/l and higher in ESRD patients compared to 1 - 2 mg/l in healthy subjects [48]. The ß2-m is deposited in the synovial tissue of joints, in cartilage, and in bones. (2) Unique fibrils, which predominantly consist of ß2-m, are formed at the site of deposition. This deposition and fibril formation occurs in the absence of ß2-m amyloid modification by advanced glycation end products (AGEs), and also in the absence of a local inflammatory response. (3) Later, AGEs modify ß2-m and induce a local inflammatory response by attracting macrophages by chemotaxis and by stimulating these cells to release proinflammatory cytokines. Unmodified ß2-m itself also induces inflammatory activities. The severity of this local inflammation seems to determine the degree of destruction in tissues and bones (reviewed in [48, 374]) (see also **figure 7.18** for details).

What role does the dialyser play in the development of ß2-m amyloidosis?

Systemic and local factors involved in the pathogenesis of ß2-m amyloidosis can be isolated; these are listed in **table 10.10**. It is obvious that several of these factors can be influenced by dialyser performance and/or biocompatibility characteristics: performance characteristics determine ß2-m removal abilities and retention capacities for cytokine-inducing substances, while biocompatibility characteristics influence the inflammatory state and oxidative as well as carbonyl stress. Because biocompatible high-flux dialysers are mostly compared with less biocompatible low-flux dialysers in clinical studies, and because the bacterial quality of the dialysis fluid is not always mentioned in these studies, it is difficult to assign the reported effect on clinical symptoms strictly to either performance, biocompatibility or bacterial product retention characteristics of the dialysers tested [48, 385]. Therefore, the results of clinical studies concerning ß2-m amyloidosis will be discussed according to the following four main subject groups: (1) low-flux versus high-flux dialysis, (2) haemodiafiltration/haemofiltration versus haemodialysis, (3) dialyser biocompatibility and (4) bacterial contamination of the dialysis fluid.

Mechanisms potentially involved in the pathogenesis of ß2-m amyloidosis

Systemic factors

- High precursor (ß2-m) concentration in the circulation
- Proteolytic changes in ß2-m
- Complex formation of circulating ß2-m
- Modification of ß2-m by AGE or AOPP
- Inflammatory state induced by uraemia or dialysis-related factors (dialyser bioincompatibility, endotoxin transfer from contaminated dialysis fluid leading to complement activation, cytokine release and formation of reactive oxygen species)
- Secondary hyperparathyroidism?

Local factors

- Local generation and/or degradation of precursor molecules and of native or modified ß2-m (AGE, AOPP)
- Crystal deposits (aluminium, iron, calcium apatite, calcium oxalate)?
- Local microinflammatory state (role of AGE-ß2-m, AGE-collagen?)?
- Focal modification of collagen
- Globin chains, immunoglobulin light chains
- Changes in amyloid components (glucosaminoglycans (heparin sulfate))
- Disturbed interaction between proteinases and proteinase inhibitors (α2-macroglobulin)
- Ubiquitin

Table 10.10: Mechanisms possibly involved in the pathogenesis of ß2-m amyloidosis. *AGE: advanced glycation end products, AOPP: advanced oxidation protein products (adapted from [374]).*

Low-flux versus high-flux haemodialysis

Dialyser/haemofilter performance characteristics determine ß2-m removal and, therefore, exert an influence on the high plasma concentrations typical in ESRD. As shown in chapter 5, the intradialytic removal of ß2-m is negligible for low-flux dialysers due to its molecular weight of 11,818 (see **figure 5.15**) and differs for the various high-flux dialysers (see **figures 5.16-5.19**). This is due to the primary, membrane-specific mechanism of ß2-m removal for the particular high-flux dialyser, i.e. adsorption (e.g. PMMA), diffusion (e.g. some cellulose triacetate membranes, particularly at high blood flow) or convection (e.g. high-flux polysulfone) (see chapter 5). The removal of ß2-m has additionally been improved by new developments in membrane structure: these enhanced ß2-m removal without loss of albumin retention capacity (e.g. the Helixone® membrane from Fresenius Medical Care) (see chapter 6.3 and **figure 6.16**). It is, therefore, not surprising that high-flux dialysis significantly reduces the predialysis ß2-m levels. This was shown in several clinical trials comparing high-flux and low-flux haemodialysis: e.g. high-flux polysulfone vs. regenerated cellulose [245] or high-flux polysulfone vs. low-flux polysulfone [245, 264, 386]; regenerated cellulose versus high-flux polysulfone [385, 386] or polyacrylonitrile [385]; and regenerated cellulose versus polyacrylonitrile (AN69®)[382]. Speaking quantitatively, reductions in predialysis ß2-m levels between 13 and 70% were reported with high-flux dialysers (see chapter 5.3.2 for details).

Several clinical studies reported an influence of high-flux membranes on clinical signs of ß2-m amyloidosis. In two studies, the severity of bone lesions correlated positively with the duration of dialysis using regenerated cellulose (Cuprophan®) membranes and negatively with the duration of dialysis using polyacrylonitrile membranes (AN69®, Hospal) [375, 382]. Survival without bone amyloidosis was also found to be better with polyacrylonitrile (AN69®, Hospal) than with regenerated cellulose (Cuprophan®) [375] (see **figure 10.17**). Two other studies failed to see such statistically significant associations [377, 387], however neither of these used strict criteria for the identification of amyloid bone cysts. Furthermore, patients were not treated consistently with only one membrane in one of these studies [387]. A lower risk of carpal tunnel surgery, another common aftermath of ß2-m amyloidosis, was reported by Chanard et al. for patients treated with the high-flux membrane AN69® compared to patients dialysed with cellulosic membranes ($p < 0.012$, follow-up period of over 5 years, $n = 85$) [388]. In another clinical study, high-flux dialysis with polysulfone (F60, Fresenius Medical Care) inhibited the development of a carpal tunnel syndrome (CTS) in 10 patients, whereas 8 of

10 patients treated with regenerated cellulose (Cuprophan®) developed CTS during the 72 months of observation [389]. Koda et al. successively switched patients from low-flux, cellulosic membranes (77.4% regenerated cellulose, 19.9% cellulose acetate, 2.7% others) to high-flux dialysis (polymethylmethacrylate: 32.4%, cellulose triacetate 28.6%, polyacrylonitrile 17.2%, polysulfone 16.7%, PEPA® 4.4% and others 2.7%) and found a significantly decreased relative risk of CTS in the high-flux group versus the conventional one (0.53 versus 1.0, $p = 0.05$) [297]. Finally, Schiffl et al., attempting to evaluate the effects of dialyser biocompatibility and flux in three different patient groups (group I: treated with regenerated cellulose; group II: treated with low-flux polysulfone or polymethylmethacrylate; and group III: treated with high-flux polysulfone or polyacrylonitrile), made the following retrospective observation (mean time on dialysis approximately 135 months per group): signs of ß2-m amyloidosis, such as carpal tunnel syndrome, arthropathy and bone cysts, were significantly higher in group I compared to group III [385] (see **table 10.11**). Although improved dialyser biocompatibility had a significant positive effect on predialysis ß2-m levels in this study, only increased dialyser flux positively influenced clinical signs of amyloidosis to a statistically significant extent.

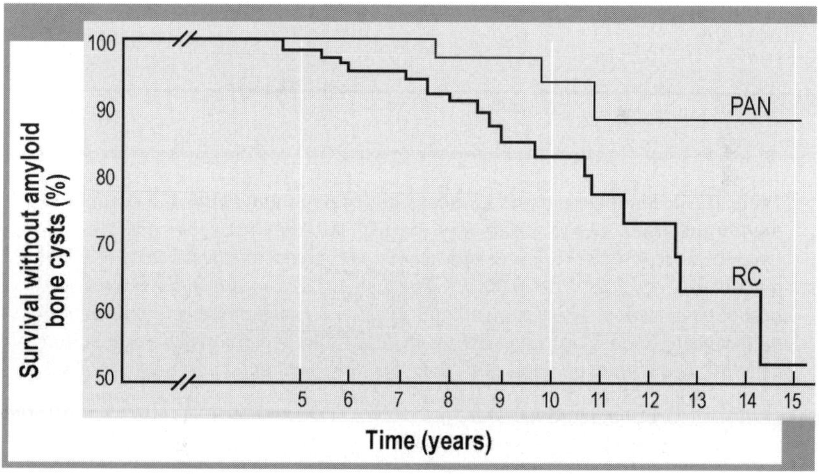

Figure 10.17: Kaplan Meier survival curves without amyloid bone cysts in patients treated exclusively with either polyacrylonitrile PAN (AN69®, Hospal) or regenerated cellulose (RC) (Cuprophan®). *Survival without amyloid bone cysts is significantly better for AN69® than for Cuprophan® ($p = 0.003$ for log rank, $p = 0.13$ for Gehan test) (adapted from [375]).*

Biochemical/ clinical data	Group I: low-flux regenerated cellulose (n = 29)	Group II: low-flux polysulfone/ polymethyl-methacrylate (n = 34)	Group III: high-flux polysulfone/ polyacrylonitrile (n = 26)
Predialysis ß2-m (mg/dl)	56 ± 10	45 ± 9*	30 ± 9*
Serum aluminium (µg/l)	43 ± 15	48 ± 12	45 ± 17
PTH (pg/ml)	60 ± 30	48 ± 32	55 ± 25
CRP (mg/dl)	0.8 ± 0.4	0.6 ± 0.3	0.9 ± 0.3
CTS	21 (72%)	14 (41%)	7 (27%)**
Arthropathy	19 (66%)	10 (29%)	6 (23%)**
Bone cysts	20 (69%)	13 (38%)	7 (27%)**

Table 10.11: Biochemical and clinical signs of ß2-m amyloidosis according to membrane used. *Dialysis with low- or high-flux biocompatible dialysers decreased predialysis ß2-m levels significantly compared to dialysis with low-flux regenerated cellulose (*p < 0.005). Clinical signs of ß2-m amyloidosis were less pronounced when low-flux synthetic dialysers (polysulfone or polymethylmethacrylate (details not specified)) were used than when low-flux regenerated cellulose was employed. However, only high-flux, synthetic membranes (polysulfone or polyacrylonitrile, (**p < 0.005)) yielded significant decreases compared to regenerated cellulose (adapted from [385]).*

Haemodiafiltration/haemofiltration versus haemodialysis

Increased convective solute removal by renal replacement modes with high filtrate flows, i.e. haemodiafiltration (HDF) and haemofiltration (HF) (see **figures 5.13** and **5.14**), has been discussed as one approach towards optimising ß2-m removal [21-24, 245, 390, 391]. A pre- to postdialysis reduction of up to 70% has been reported (see chapter 5.3.2). This may have led to the HDF/HF reductions in predialysis levels of about 30% to 18 mg/l after 18 months observed in one study [22]. Canaud et al. recorded the progress of clinical symptoms in 21 ESRD patients treated with HDF for 5 years using high-flux polysulfone membranes (HF80, Fresenius Medical Care): HDF was the first and only renal replacement mode employed in 10 of these patients, and none of them developed any clinical symptoms of ß2-m related amyloidosis [24]. Furthermore, no radiological signs of amyloidosis were detected [24]. However, first radiological and clinical signs of ß2-m related amyloidosis in HD patients treated with biocompatible membranes are not expected to develop before at least 7 and 8 years of dialysis treatment, respectively [375]. In the Canaud study, symptomatology was not improved (with the exception of pain relief) in 9 patients in whom ß2-amyloidosis was present before start of HDF 3-6 months after switching to HDF [32]. In another study comparing

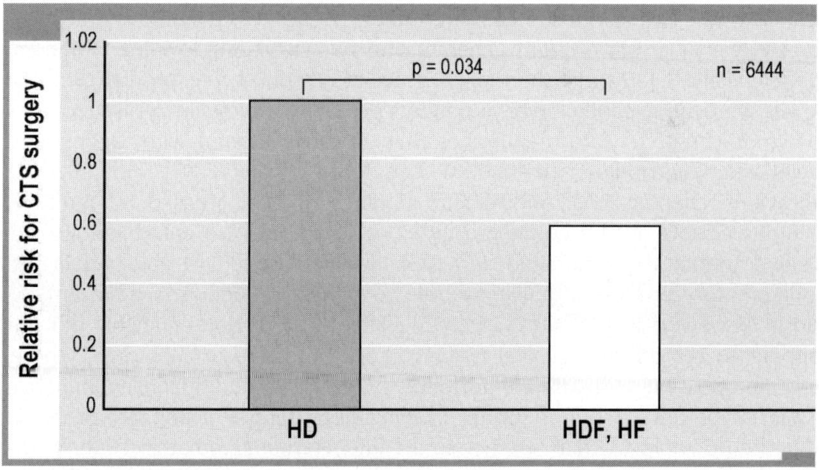

Figure 10.18: Relative risk of undergoing carpal tunnel surgery in patients treated with HDF/HF and HD. *The relative risk of having carpal tunnel surgery was 41% lower in patients on convective therapies compared to HD (RR = 0.59, 95% CI 0.36 - 0.96, p = 0.034) adapted from data from [392]).*

standard haemodialysis with haemodiafiltration or haemofiltration, the relative risk of carpal tunnel syndrome requiring surgical therapy was 42% lower for HDF/HF patients [392] (see **figure 10.18**). In a multicentre evaluation by the Japanese Society for Dialysis Therapy of 1196 patients who were on haemopurification therapy as of the end of 1998 and developed dialysis-related amyloidosis during 1999, the use of off-line, on-line or push/pull haemodiafiltration reduced the risk of developing amyloidosis compared to low-flux and high-flux dialysis; risks were 0.117, 0.013 and 0.017 vs. 1.0 for low-flux dialysis and 0.489 for high-flux dialysis, respectively) [393].

Dialyser biocompatibility

Mainly dialyser biocompatibility characteristics that influence the inflammatory state, oxidative and carbonyl stress are thought to contribute to ß2-m amyloidosis [334]. When ß2-m levels were compared in patients treated with low-flux biocompatible and low-flux bioincompatible membranes, varying results were obtained. Whereas Locatelli et al. did not find any difference in predialysis ß2-m levels comparing regenerated cellulose membranes (Cuprophan®) with low-flux polysulfone [245], Hakim et al. reported that the use of the low-flux, biocompatible polymethylmethacrylate membrane prevented an increase in ß2-m levels compared to regenerated cellulose (ß2-m levels were 6.2 mg/l versus 11.8 mg/l after 18 months, $p < 0.001$) and interpreted this as a sign of ß2-m generation or release during low-flux bioincompatible dialysis [394]. Furthermore, Schiffl et al. found that predialysis ß2-m levels were significantly lower in patients treated with low-flux polysulfone or polymethylmethacrylate membranes than in those treated with regenerated cellulose (Cuprophan®) ($p < 0.005$) (see **table 10.11**) [385]. However, as shown in chapter 7.3.4, the *in vitro* findings of an increased ß2-m mRNA synthesis could not be confirmed by *in vivo* data. *In vitro* data have also revealed that both unmodified and AGE-modified ß2-m are involved in the inflammatory processes that contribute to bone destruction in ß2-m amyloidosis (reviewed in [47, 48, 374, 395]). However, diabetes mellitus did not appear to constitute a clinical risk factor for amyloidosis [376, 396]. Therefore, the possibility that different aspects of dialyser biocompatibility influence ß2-m amyloidosis requires further investigation, even if it appears probable that the documented dialyser membrane effects on inflammatory state, oxidative and carbonyl stress are involved in ß2-m pathogenesis (see **table 10.10**).

Additional bacterial contamination of the dialysis fluid

Dialysis fluid impurity is another factor that can contribute to ß2-m amyloidosis [379-381]. The well known studies of Baz et al. and Kleophas et al. revealed a lower incidence of carpal tunnel syndrome in patients dialysed partially with low-flux cellulosic dialysers and ultrapure dialysis fluid (CFU < 1/ml) compared to standard dialysis fluid [379, 381]. Schiffl et al., who primarily found an increase in clinical signs of ß2-m amyloidosis in patients treated with regenerated cellulose compared to those on biocompatible high-flux dialysis (polysulfone, polyacrylonitrile), identified bacterial contamination of the dialysis fluid (CFU > 200/ml) as an additional independent risk factor [385]. Finally, Schwalbe et al. reviewed the prevalence of carpal tunnel syndrome or radiological signs of ß2-m amyloidosis in 1996 compared to 1988 and found a decrease of symptoms of approximately 80%, even if the relative overall contribution of high-flux treatment time to the total haemodialysis treatment time only increased from 6% in 1988 to 13% in 1996. The authors speculate that factors other than improved removal may be involved, for example dialysis fluid composition and purity [380].

Does increased treatment frequency affect the development of ß2-m amyloidosis?

ß2-m removal may be enhanced by increasing the frequency of dialysis treatment; however, also in frequent treatment modes, the choice of dialysis membrane and whether or not it is reused remain major factors of influence (reviewed in [397, 398]). ß2-m-removal is reported to be four times higher in nocturnal home haemodialysis than in conventional modes [399]. A comparison of nocturnal haemodialysis (NHD) (6 nights per week, 8 hours treatment time, high-flux polysulfone (F40, Fresenius Medical Care)) with conventional high-flux dialysis (3 times weekly, 4 hours, F80, Fresenius Medical Care) revealed that predialysis ß2-m levels progressively declined from 27.2 ± 11.7 mg/dl at initiation of NHD to 13.7 ± 4.4 mg/dl over 9 months and remained stable thereafter while continuating therapy [400]. When patients on standard on-line haemodiafiltration (HF 80, Fresenius Medical Care, trice weekly 4 hours treatment, no reuse) were changed to short daily haemodiafiltration (2 - 2.5 hours treatments, six times per week) without changing the dialyser or prescriptions such as blood, dialysis fluid flow or infusion flow, ß2-m removal increased by 67% [401]. To date, no long-term studies have been performed that investigate a possible association between increased frequencies of treatments and a delayed development of clinical signs of ß2-m amyloidosis.

Does high-flux dialysis combined with specific ß2-m adsorption columns have an effect on ß2-m related amyloidosis?

The adsorption column Lixelle™ (Kaneka Co, Osaka) for direct haemoperfusion has been commercially available in Japan since 1996 and has been shown to remove ß2-m efficiently [402-404]. It contains 350 ml of porous cellulose adsorbent beads with a diameter of about 460 µm, in which a hexadecyl group with high hydrophobicity is used as ligand. Hydrophobic peptides and proteins with a molecular weight of 4000 to 20,000 are eliminated by the molecule sieving effect of the surface pores of the beads. For example, ß2-m, as hydrophobic protein, is bound by the hydrophobic hexadecyl hydrocarbonate group [reviewed in 404]. The column is used in combination with high-flux dialysis, being included in the blood circuit during the haemodialysis treatment. A recent study investigated the effect of combined ß2-m adsorption by column and high-flux dialysis on ß2-m levels and symptoms of dialysis related amyloidosis in 17 long-term haemodialysis patients (mean time on dialysis: 20.2 ± 4.5 years; membranes: polysulfone, polyarylethersulfone, cellulose triacetate, modified regenerated cellulose) [404]. ß2-m serum levels and clinical parameters (such as pinch strength, motor terminal latency, degree of joint pain), and features such as frequency of nocturnal awakenig by pain and activities of daily life were all stable during the 12 month observation period preceeding the combined treatment (note: all patients were on high-flux dialysis). After 12 months treatment with the combined adsorber-dialysis system, ß2-m levels dropped significantly (from 34.6 ± 9.3 to 28.8 ± 7.3 mg/l ($p < 0.05$)) and the following clinical parameters improved: pinch strength ($p < 0.001$); median motor terminal latency ($p < 0.05$); frequency of nocturnal awakening due to pain ($p < 0.01$); and subjective evaluation of activities related to the upper extremities ($p < 0.005$). An aggravation of dialysis-related hypotension and anaemia was reported as side-effects in a previous study [405]; this was counteracted by extra saline and early initiation of erythropoietin therapy in another study [404].

Summary

Reviewing studies addressing the influence of dialyser characteristics on ß2-m amyloidosis, one finds that predialysis plasma ß2-m levels decreased significantly during months of observation in patients treated by standard high-flux dialysis, daily high-flux dialysis, haemodiafiltration and haemofiltration, but that they still remain much higher than in healthy people. This is because weekly removal rates by all forms of renal replacement therapy are much lower than the production. The dual question remains unanswered: what level of ß2-m removal by renal replacement therapy targeting which predialysis ß2-m threshold level is sufficient to postpone or inhibit the development of ß2-m amyloidosis? Clinical studies reveal that especially high-flux dialysis with synthetic membranes and haemodialfiltration/haemofiltration seem to reduce not only predialysis ß2-m levels but also may postpone or inhibit clinical symptoms, such as bone cysts and carpal tunnel syndrome. The combined high-flux dialysis - adsorption system available up to now only in Japan reduces ß2-m levels and associated symptoms in a small number of patients suffering from amyloidosis. However the treatment approach is so new that possible long-term side-effects cannot yet be assessed. The contribution of dialyser biocompatibility to ß2-m related amyloidosis has to be studied further in the future. The addition of dialysis fluid impurity appears to aggravate symptoms. Recently published European Best Practice Guidelines recommend the use of synthetic, high-flux membranes and additional strategies, such as the addition of a convective component to the treatment or increasing haemodialysis time and frequency, to maximise ß2-m removal (guideline II.2.2 [20]).

10.8 Pruritus

Chronic pruritus is common in end-stage renal disease (ESRD): 20 - 90% of the patients suffer from this problem [406-411], with prevalence declining from approximately 90% in the early seventies to 20% in the late nineties (reviewed in [411]) The exact pathophysiology of pruritus in ESRD remains elusive, mainly because of its subjective nature and the strong influence of psychological factors [406, 408]. Xerosis ("dry skin") [407], peripheral neuropathy, elevated concentrations of calcium, magnesium, phosphate, presence as well as degree of hyperparathyroidism, higher levels of serum bile acids [412], lower serum transferrin and albumin levels together with higher ferritin levels in the context of chronic inflammation [413] and, finally, activation of th1 lymphocytes by the presence of an inflammatory state [411, 414] may all contribute to pruritus [408]. However, not all patients suffering from pruritus have any of these conditions [407, 412, 415, 416], and the conditions are also not found to correlate with symptom severity [416]. Adequate nutrition and dialysis dose were associated with a reduction in pruritus [407, 415] in some studies, but not in all [412, 416].

In ESRD patients, pruritus may additionally be aggravated by the haemodialysis treatment itself [408, 417]. Histamine, mainly released by skin mast cells, is known to trigger itching in allergic skin affections. Such a sensitisation may be elicited during dialysis by residuals of ethylene oxide (EtO) or formaldehyde in new or reused dialysers, respectively [408]. Furthermore, products of complement activation, such as C3a, C4a and C5a, develop during dialysis; these may induce histamine release from mast cells and basophils (reviewed in [408]) and contribute to augmented pruritus during the treatment.

The severity of pruritus was found to be lower with the use of synthetic membranes, such as high-flux polysulfone (PSu) [410, 416], polyacrylonitrile (PAN) [418] and polymethylmethacrylate (PMMA) [410], than when regenerated cellulose [410, 416, 418] or cellulose triacetate [410] membranes were used. Whether this results are due to a better biocompatibility of synthetic membranes (see chapters 7 and 8) or an increased removal of middle molecular weight substances that possibly contribute to uraemic pruritus [418] (and see chapter 5), or from a combination of both, remains unclear.

10.9 Peripheral nerve function

Uraemic neuropathy is a well-known and frequent complication of ESRD whose exact cause is unknown [419]. However, dialysis adequacy, dialyser biocompatibility, the retention of middle and high molecular uraemic toxins and a depletion of members of the vitamin B_6 complex are discussed as possible causes [420-423]. High patient age and the presence of diabetes mellitus are also contributing factors [421].

Does the choice of dialyser or the use of haemofilters influence neuropathic impairment in ESRD patients?

In particular, the removal ability of a dialyser or haemofilter for middle and high molecular weight proteins was thought to influence neuropathic impairment. Some studies demonstrate a slight positive influence of high-flux, synthetic membranes compared to the low-flux cellulosic ones [419, 420, 424], but this was not found in one other study [421]. Robles et al. measured sensory and motor nerve conduction velocities one year after having switched eleven patients from regenerated cellulose membranes (Cuprophan®) to high-flux polysulfone (HF-80, Fresenius Medical Care), and found a significant increase of the postdialysis sensory nerve conduction (SNC) values after having used polysulfone for 12 months. However, the membranes tested did not differ regarding postdialysis improvements in motor conduction velocities (MNC), predialysis SNC and predialysis MNC values [419]. In another study, haemodialysis with polyacrylonitrile (AN69®) compared to regenerated cellulose membranes (Cuprophan®) also acutely improved SNC and even MNC; however, no long-term follow-up of predialysis values was carried out [424]. No difference was found in one study comparing neuropathic impairment in patients dialysed with low-flux dialysers (regenerated cellulose (Cuprophan®)) and high-flux dialysers (polyacrylonitrile (AN69®) [421].

A comparison of haemodialysis using regenerated cellulose (Cuprophan®) with haemodiafiltration using high-flux polysulfone (BL 627, Bellco) revealed that SNC and MNC parameters were stable in the haemodiafiltration group during the observation period of one year, but declined in the haemodialysis group [420].

In conclusion, there are some indications that a better removal of uraemic toxins by high-flux, synthetic membranes - especially when used in haemodiafiltration - may positively influence peripheral neuropathy in ESRD. However, more controlled studies with longer follow-up periods are necessary to confirm this.

References

1. Lowrie EG, Laird NM, Parker TF, Sargent JA: Effect of the haemodialysis prescription on patient morbidity: report from the National Cooperative Dialysis Study. N Engl J Med 305(20): 1176-1181, 1981

2. Charra B, Calemard E, Ruffet M, Chazot C, Terrat JC, Vanel T, Laurent G: Survival as an index of adequacy of dialysis. Kidney Int 41: 1286-1291, 1992

3. Owen WF jr, Lew NL, Liu Y, Lowrie EG, Lazarus JM: The urea reduction ratio and serum albumin concentration as predictors of mortality in patients undergoing hemodialysis. N Engl J Med 329(14): 1001-1006, 1993

4. Kopple JD, Hakim RM, Held PJ, Keane WF, King K, Lazarus JM, Parker III TF, Teehan BP: Recommendations for reducing the high morbidity and mortality of United States maintenance dialysis patients. Am J Kidney Dis 24(6): 968-973, 1994

5. Held PJ, Carrol CE, Liska DW, Turenne MN, Port FK: Hemodialysis therapy in the United States: what is the dose and what does it matter? Am J Kidney Dis 24(6): 974-980, 1994

6. Parker III TF: Role of dialysis dose on morbidity and mortality in maintenance hemodialysis patients. Am J Kidney Dis 24(6): 981-989, 1994

7. Consensus conference on morbidity and mortality of renal disease: a NIH consensus conference panel. Ann Intern Med 121: 62-70, 1994

8. Held PJ, Port FK, Wolfe RA, Stannard DC, Caroll CE, Daugirdas JT, Bloembergen WE, Greer JW, Hakim RM: The dose of haemodialysis and patient mortality. Kidney Int 50(2): 550-556, 1996

9. Shinzato T, Nakai S, Akiba T, Vamazaki C, Sasaki R, Kitaoka T, Kubo K, Shinoda T, Kurokawa K, Marumo F, Sato T, Maeda K: Survival in long-term haemodialysis patients: results from the annual survey of the Japanese Society for Dialysis Therapy. Nephrol Dial Transplant 12: 884-888, 1997

10. Port FK, Orzol SM, Held PJ, Wolfe RA: Trends in treatment and survival for hemodialysis patients in the United States. Am J Kidney Dis 32(6, Suppl 4): S34-S38, 1998

11. Lowrie EG, Chertow GM, Lew NL, Lazarus JM, Owen WF: The urea (clearance x dialysis time) product (Kt) as an outcome-based measure of haemodialysis dose. Kidney Int 56: 729-737, 1999

12. Okechukwu CN, Lopes AA, Stack AG, Feng S, Wolfe RA, Port FK: Impact of years of dialysis therapy on mortality risk and the characteristics of longer term dialysis survivors. Am J Kidney Disease 39(3): 533-538, 2002

13. The United States data report on chronic renal disease (URSDS), chapter 9: p152-164, 2002

14. Port FK, Ashby VB, Dhingra RK, Roys EC, Wolfe RA: Dialysis dose and body mass index are strongly associated with survival in hemodialysis patients. J Am Soc Nephrol 13: 1061-1066, 2002

15. Wolfe RA, Held PJ, Hulbert Shearon TE, Ashby VB, Port FK: URR > 75% is associated with lower mortality among females but not among males. (Abstract) J Am Soc Nephrol 13(9): 20A, 2002

16. Bosch JA, Nabut J, Hegbrant J, Alquist M, Walters BA: Increased survival for hemodialysis patients with a dialysis dose above the KDOQI guidelines. (Abstract) J Am Soc Nephrol 13(9): 21A, 2002

17. Haemodialysis adequacy workgroup: National Kidney Foundation DOQI™: Clinical practice guidelines for hemodialysis adequacy, 2000 update. Am J Kidney Dis 37(Suppl 1): S7-S64, 2001

18. The Renal Association. Recommended standards for haemodialysis. Royal college of physicians London. Treatment of adult patients with renal failure. Recommended standards and audit measure: 17-29, 1997

19. The Canadian Society of Nephrology: clinical practice guidelines for the delivery of haemodialysis. J Am Soc Nephrol 10: S306-S319, 1999

20. Kessler M, Canaud B, Pedrini LA, Tattersall J, ter Wee PM, Vanholder R, Wanner C: European Best Practice Guidelines for haemodialysis (part 1). Nephrol Dial Transplant 17(Suppl 7): 1-107, 2002

21. Maduell F, del Pozo C, Garcia H, Sanchez L, Hdez-Jaras J, Albero MD, Calvo C, Torregrosa I, Navarro V: Change from conventional haemodiafiltration to on-line haemodiafiltration. Nephrol Dial Transplant 14(5): 1202-1207, 1999

22. Wizemann V, Lotz C, Techert F, Uthoff S: On-line haemofiltration versus low-flux haemodialysis. A prospective randomized study. Nephrol Dial Transplant 15(Suppl 1): 43-48, 2000

23. Lornoy W, Becaus I, Billiouw JM, Sierens L, Van Malderen P, D'Haenens P: On-line haemodiafiltration. Remarkable removal of ß2-microglobulin. Long-term clinical observations. Nephrol Dial Transplant 15(Suppl 1): 49-54, 2000

24. Canaud B, Bosc JY, Leray-Moragues H, Stec F, Argiles A, Leblanc M, Mion C: On-line haemofiltration. Safety and efficacy in long-term clinical practice. Nephrol Dial Transplant 15(Suppl 1): 60-67, 2000

25. Lonnemann G, Koch KM, Shaldon S, Dinarello CA: Studies on the ability of hemodialysis membranes to induce, bind, and clear human interleukin. J Lab Clin Med 112(1): 76-86, 1988

26. Laude-Sharp M, Caroff M, Simard L, Pusineri C, Kazatchkine MD, Haeffner-Cavaillon N: Induction of IL-1 during hemodialysis: transmembrane passage of intact endotoxins (LPS). Kidney Int 38: 1089-1094, 1990

27. Ureña P, Herbelin A, Zingraff J, Lair M, Man NK, Descamps-Latscha B, Drüeke T: Permeability of cellulosic and non-cellulosic membranes to endotoxin subunits and cytokine production during in-vitro haemodialysis. Nephrol Dial Transplant 7: 16-28, 1992

28. Bommer J, Becker KP, Urbaschek R: Potential transfer of endotoxin across high-flux polysulfone membranes. J Am Soc Nephrol 7: 883-888, 1996

29. Schindler R, Krautzig S, Lufft V, Lonnemann G, Mahiout A, Marra MN, Shaldon S, Koch KM: Induction of interleukin-1 and interleukin1-receptor antagonist during contaminated in vitro dialysis with whole blood. Nephrol Dial Transplant 11(1): 101-108, 1996

30. Weber C, Linsberger I, Rafiee-Tehrani M, Falkenhagen D: Permeability and adsorption capacity of dialysis membranes to lipid A. Int J Artif Organs 20: 144-152, 1997

31. Bonnie-Schorn E, Grassmann A, Uhlenbusch-Körwer I, Weber C, Vienken J: Transfer of contaminants across dialysis membranes in *Water quality in hemodialysis*, edited by Vienken J, Pabst Science Publishers, Lengerich: 35-49, 1998

32. Lonnemann G: The quality of dialysate: an integrated approach. Kidney Int 58(Suppl 76): S112-119, 2000

33. Niwa T, Asada H, Tsutsui S, Miyazaki T: Efficient removal of albumin-bound furancarboxylic acid by protein-leaking hemodialysis. Am J Nephrol 15(6): 463-467, 1995

34. Yamada S, Kataoka H, Kobayashi H, Ono T, Minakuchi J, Kawano Y: Identification of an erythropoietic inhibitor from the dialysate collected in the hemodialysis with PMMA membrane (BK-F). Contrib Nephrol 125: 159-172, 1999

35. Seres DS, Strain GW, Hashim SA, Goldberg IJ, Levin NW: Improvement of plasma lipoprotein during high-flux dialysis. J Am Soc Nephrol 3(7): 1409-1415, 1993

36. de Precigout V, Higueret D, Larroumet N, Combe C, Iron A, Blanchetier V, Potaux L, Aparicio M: Improvement in lipid profiles and triglyceride removal in patients on polyamide membrane hemodialysis. Blood Purif 14(2): 170-176, 1996

37. Cheung Ak, Parker CJ, Ren K, Iverius PH: Increased lipase inhibition in uremia: identification of pre-ß HDL as a major inhibitor in normal and uraemic plasma. Kidney Int 49(5): 1360-1371, 1996

38. Wanner C, Bahner U, Mattern R, Lang D, Passlick-Deetjen J: Influence of a new high-flux membrane on apolipoprotein -& lipid profile of ESRD patients. (Abstract) J Am Soc Nephrol 13(9): 600A, 2002

39. Henning BF, Riezler R, Tepel M, Langer K, Raidt H, Graefe U, Zidek W: Evidence of altered homocysteine metabolism in chronic renal failure. Nephron 83(4): 314-322, 1999

40. Mueller A, Klemm A, Stein G, Hein GE, Busch M: Influence of hemodialysis therapy on serum levels of homocysteine, methionine, dimethylglycine and cysthationine. (Abstract) J Am Soc Nephrol 13(9): 416A, 2002

41. Haag Weber M, Hörl WH: Effect of biocompatible membranes on neutrophil function and metabolism. Clin Nephrol 42(Suppl 1): S31-S36, 1994

42. Cappelli A, DiFelice A, Perrone S, Ballestri M, Bonucchi D, Savazzi AM, Ciuffreda A, Lusvarghi E: Which level of cytokine production is critical in haemodialysis? Nephrol Dial Transplant 13(Suppl 7): 55-66, 1998

43. Gesualdo L, Pertosa G, Grandaliano G, Schena FP: Cytokines and biocompatibility. Nephrol Dial Transplant 13: 1622-1626, 1998

44. Clark WR, Hamburger RJ, Lysaght MJ: Effect of membrane composition and structure on solute removal and biocompatibility in hemodialysis. Kidney Int 56: 2005-2015, 1999

45. Riella MC: Malnutrition in dialysis: malnourishment or uremic inflammatory response? Kidney Int 57(3): 1211-32, 2000

46. Deppisch RM, Beck W, Goehl H, Ritz E: Complement components as uremic toxins and their potential role as mediators of microinflammation. Kidney Int 59(Suppl 78): S271-277, 2001

47. Hörl WH: Hemodialysis membranes: interleukins, biocompatibility, and middle molecules. J Am Soc Nephrol 13: S62-S71, 2002

48. Lonnemann G, Koch KM: β2-microglobulin amyloidosis: effects of ultrapure dialysate and type of dialyser membrane. J Am Soc Nephrol 13: S72-S77, 2002

49. McIntyre C, Harper I, Macdougall IC, Raine AE, Williams A, Baker LR: Serum C-reactive protein as a marker for infection and inflammation in regular dialysis patients. Clin Nephrol 48(6): 371-374, 1997

50. Kimmel PL, Phillips TM, Simmens SJ, Peterson RA, Weihs KL, Alleyne S, Cruz I, Yanovski JA, Veis JH: Immunologic function and survival in hemodialysis patients. Kidney Int 54: 236-244, 1998

51. Zimmermann J, Herrlinger S, Pruy A, Metzger T, Wanner C: Inflammation enhances cardiovascular risk and mortality in hemodialysis patients. Kidney Int 55(2): 648-658, 1999

52. Schindler R, Boenisch O, Fischer C, Frei U: Effect of the hemodialysis membrane on the inflammatory reaction in vivo. Clin Nephrol 53(6): 452-459, 2000

53. Panichi V, Migliori M, De Pietro S, Metelli MR, Taccola D, Perez R, Palla R, Rindi P, Cristofani R, Tetta C: Plasma C-reactive protein in hemodialysis patients: a cross-sectional, longitudinal clinical survey. Blood Purif 18(1): 30-36, 2000

54. Galli F, Canestrari F, Bellomo G: Pathophysoiology of the oxidative stress and its implication in uremia and dialysis. Contrib Nephrol 127: 1-31, 1999

55. Miyata T, Kurokawa K, Van Ypersele de Strihou C: Relevance of oxidative and carbonyl stress to long-term uremic complications. Kidney Int 58(Suppl 76): S120-125, 2000

56. Haverkate F, Thompson SG, Pype SDM, Gallimore JR, Pepys MB: Production of C-reactive protein and risk of coronary events in stable and unstable angina. Lancet 349: 462-466, 1997

57. Vallance P, Collier J, Bhagat K: Infection, inflammation, and infarction: does acute endothelian dysfunction provide a link? Lancet 349: 1391-1392, 1997

58. Ridker PM, Cushman M, Stampfer MJ, Russell PT, Hennekens CH: Inflammation, aspirin, and the risk of cardiovascular disease in apparently healthy men. N Engl J Med 336: 973-979, 1997

59. Ross R: Atherosclerosis- an inflammatory disease. N Engl J Med 340: 115-126, 1999.

60. Lowrie EG, Lew NL: Death risk in hemodialysis patients: the predictive value of commonly measured variables and an evaluation of death rate differences between facilities. Am J Kidney Dis 15(5): 458-482, 1990

61. Bergström J, Heimbürger O, Lindholm B, Qureshi AR: Elevated C-reactive protein is a strong predictor of increased mortality and low serum albumin in hemodialysis (HD) patients. (Abstract) J Am Soc Nephrol 6: 573, 1995

62. Bologa RM, Levine DM, Parker TS, Cheigh JS, Serur D, Stenzel KH, Rubin AL: Interleukin-6 predicts hypoalbuminemia, hypocholesterolemia, and mortality in hemodialysis patients. Am J Kidney Dis 32(1): 107-114, 1998

63. Yeun JY, Levine RA, Mantadilok V, Kaysen GA: C-reactive protein predicts all-cause and cardiovascular mortality in hemodialysis patients. Am J Kidney Dis 35(3): 469-476, 2000

64. Qureshi AR, Alvestrand A, Divino-Filho JC, Gutierrez A, Heimbürger O, Lindholm B, Bergström: Inflammation, malnutrition, and cardiac disease as predictors of mortality in hemodialysis patients. J Am Soc Nephrol 13: S28-S36, 2002

65. Santoro A, Mancini E: Cardiac effects of chronic inflammation in dialysis patients. Nephrol Dial Transplant 17(Suppl 8): 10-15, 2002

66. Zoccali C, Mallamaci M, Tripepi G: Atherosclerosis in dialysis patients: does chlamydia pneumoniae infection contribute to cardiovascular damage? Nephrol Dial Transplant 17(Suppl 8): 25-28, 2002

67. Coresh J, Longenecker JC, Eustace J, Liu Y, Fink N, Levin N, Tracy RP, Powe NR, Klag MJ: C-reactive protein and mortality among incident dialysis patients the CHOICE study. (Abstract) J Am Soc Nephrol 13(9): 423A, 2002

68. Bayés B, Pastor MC, Bonal J, Juncà J, Hernandez JM, Riutort N, Foraster A, Romero R: Homocysteine, C-reactive protein, lipid peroxidation and mortality in haemodialysis patients. Nephrol Dial Transplant 18: 106-112, 2003

69. Papagianni A, Kalovoulos M, Kirmizis D, Vainas A, Belechri AM, Alexopoulos E, Memmos D: Carotid atherosclerosis is associated with inflammation and endothelial cell adhesion molecules in chronic haemodialysis patients. Nephrol Dial Transplant 18: 113-119, 2003

70. Ikizler TA, Wingard RL, Harvell J, Shyr Y, Hakim RM: Association of morbidity with markers of nutrition and inflammation in chronic hemodialysis patients: a prospective study. Kidney Int 55(5): 1945-1951, 1999

71. Stenvinkel P, Heimbürger O, Paultre F, Diczfalusy U, Wang T, Berglund L, Jogestrand T: Strong association between malnutrition, inflammation, and atherosclerosis in chronic renal failure. Kidney Int 55(5): 1899-1991, 1999

72. Ikizler TA: Epidemiology of vascular disease in renal failure. Blood Purif 20: 6-10, 2002

73. Stenvinkel P, Heimbürger O, Jogestrand T: Elevated Interleukin-6 predicts progressive carotid artery atherosclerosis in dialysis patients: association with chlamydia pneumoniae seropositivity. Am J Kidney Dis 39(2): 274-282, 2002

74. Zoccali C, Benedetto FA, Maas R, Mallamaci F, Tripepi G, Malatino L, Böger R: Asymmetric dimethylarginine, c-reactive protein, and carotid intima-media thickness in end-stage renal disease. J Am Soc Nephrol 13: 490-496, 2002

75. Kato A, Odamaki M, Takita T, Maruyama Y, Kumagai H, Hishida A: Association between interleukin-6 and carotid atherosclerosis in hemodialysis patients. Kidney Int 61: 1143-1152, 2002

76. Kaizu Y, Kimura M, Yoneyama T, Miyaji K, Hibi I, Kumagai H: Interleukin-6 may mediate malnutrition in chronic hemodialysis patients. Am J Kidney Dis 31(1): 93-100, 1998

77. Stenvinkel P, Heimbürger O, Lindholm B, Kaysen GA, Bergström J: Are there two types of malnutrition? Evidence for relationships between malnutrition, inflammation and atherosclerosis (MIA syndrome). Nephrol Dial Transplant 15: 953-960, 2000

78. Kaysen GA, Dubin JA, Muller HG, Mitch WE, Rosales LM, Levin NW: Relationships among inflammation nutrition and physiologic mechanisms establishing albumin levels in hemodialysis patients. Kidney Int 61(6): 2240-2249, 2002

79. Stenvinkel P, Barany P, Chung SH, Lindholm B, Heimbürger: A comparative analysis of nutritional parameters as predictors of outcome in male and female ESRD patients. Nephrol Dial Transplant 17: 1266-1274, 2002

80. Stenvinkel P, Barany P, Heimbürger O, Pecoits-Filho R, Lindholm B: Mortality, malnutrition, and atherosclerosis in ESRD: what is the role of interleukin-6? Kidney Int 61(Suppl 80): S103-S108, 2002

81. Barany P, Divino JC, Bergström J: High C-reactive protein is a strong predictor of resistance to erythropoietin in hemodialysis patients. Am J Kidney Dis 29: 565-568, 1997

82. Goicoechea M, Martin J, de Sequera P, Quiroga JA, Ortiz A, Carreño V, Caramelo C: Role of cytokines in the response to erythropoietin in hemodialysis patients. Kidney Int 54(4): 1337-1343, 1998

83. Gunnell J, Yeun JY, Depner CA, Kaysen GA: Acute phase response predicts erythropoietin resistance in hemodialysis and peritoneal dialysis patients. Am J Kidney Dis 33: 63-72, 1999

84. Sitter T, Bergner A, Schiffl H: Dialysate related cytokine induction and response to recombinant human erythropoietin in haemodialysis patients. Nephrol Dial Transplant 15(8): 1207-1211, 2000

85. Stenvinkel P: The role of inflammation in the anaemia of end-stage renal disease. Nephrol Dial Transplant 16(Suppl 7): 36-40, 2001

86. Ridker PM, Buring JE, Sgih J, Matias M, Hennekens CH: Prospective study of C-reactive protein and the risk of future cardiovascular events in healthy women. Circulation 98: 731-733, 1998

87. Stenvinkel P: Inflammatory and atherosclerotic interactions in the depleted uremic patient. Blood Purif 19: 53-61, 2001

88. Kaysen GA, Dubin JA, Müller HG, Rosales LM, Levin NW, and the HEMO Group: The acute-phase response varies with time and predicts serum albumin levels in hemodialysis patients. Kidney Int 58(1): 346-352, 2000

89. Ayus JC, Sheikh Hamad D: Silent infection in clotted hemodialysis grafts. J Am Soc Nephrol 9: 1314-1321, 1998

90. Nassar GM, Fishbane S, Ayus JC: Occult infection of old nonfunctioning arteriovenous grafts: a novel cause of erythropoietin resistance and chronic inflammation in hemodialysis patients. Kidney Int (Suppl 80): 49-54, 2002

91. Tetta S, Biasioli S Schiavon R, Inguaggiato P, David S, Panichi V, Wratten ML: An overview of haemodialysis and oxidative stress. Blood Purif 17: 118-126, 1999

92. Miyata T, van Ypersele de Strihou C, Kurokawa K, Baynes JW: Alterations in nonenzymatic biochemistry in uremia: origin and significance of "carbonyl stress" in long-term uremic complications. Kidney Int 55: 389-399, 1999

93. Nguyen-Khoa T, Massy ZA, De Bandt JP, Kebede M, Salama L, Lambrey G, Witko-Sarsat V, Drüeke TB, Lacour B, Thévenin M: Oxidative stress and haemodialysis: role of inflammation and duration of dialysis treatment. Nephrol Dial Transplant 16(2): 335-340, 2001

94. Galle J: Oxidative stress in chronic renal failure: Nephrol Dial Transplant 16: 2135-2137, 2001.

95. Spittle MA, Hoenich NA, Handelman GJ, Adhikarla R, Homel P, Levin NW: Oxidative stress and inflammation in hemodialysis patients. Am J Kidney Dis 38(6): 1408-1413, 2001

96. Descamps-Latscha B, Drueke T, Witko-Sarsat V: Dialysis-induced oxidative stress: biological aspects, clinical consequences, and therapy. Semin Dial 14(3): 193-199, 2001

97. Miyata T, Sugiyama S, Saito A, Kurokawa K: Reactive carbonyl compounds related uremic toxicity ("carbonyl stress"). Kidney Int 59(Suppl 78): S25-31, 2001

98. Schwedler S, Schinzel R, Vaith P, Wanner C: Inflammation and advanced glycation end products in uremia: simple coexistance, potentiation or causal relationship? Kidney Int 58(Suppl 78): S32-36, 2001

99. Blackburn GL: Pasteur's quadrant and malnutrition. Nature 409: 397- 401, 2001

100. Kaysen GA: Role of inflammation and its treatment in ESRD patients. Blood Purif 20: 70-80, 2002

101. Guth HJ, Gruska S, Kraatz G: The measurement of cytokine production capacity during dialysis-a new dynamic method for the evaluation of biocompatibility? Int J Artif Organs 23(10): 675-679, 2000

102. Kaysen GA: The microinflammatory state in uremia: causes and potential consequences. J Am Soc Nephrol 12: 1549-1557, 2001

103. Lonnemann G, Behme TC, Lenzner B, Floege J, Schulze M, Colton CK, Koch KM, Shaldon S: Permeability of dialyzer membranes to TNF alpha-inducing substances derived from water bacteria. Kidney Int 42(1): 61-68, 1992

104. Lonnemann G, Schindler R, Lufft V, Mahiout A, Shaldon S, Koch KM: The role of plasma coating on the permeation of cytokine-inducing substances through dialyser membranes. Nephrol Dial Transplant 10: 207-211, 1995

105. Jaber BL, Gonski JA, Cendoroglo M, Balakrishnan VS, Razeghi P, Dinarello CA, Pereira BJ: New polyether sulfone dialyzers attenuate passage of cytokine-inducing substances from pseudomonas aeruginosa contaminated dialysate. Blood Purif 16(4): 210-219, 1998

106. Lonnemann G, Sereni L, Lemke HD, Tetta C: Pyrogen retention by highly permeable synthetic membranes during in vitro dialysis. Artif Organs 25(12): 951-960, 2001

107. Schindler R, Christ-Kohlrausch F, Frei U, Shaldon S: Differences in the permeability of high-flux dialyzer membranes for bacterial products. Clin Nephrol 59(6): 447-454, 2003

108. Weber V, Linsberger I, Rossmanith E, Weber C, Falkenhagen D: Pyrogen transfer across high and low-flux hemodialysis membranes. Artif Org: accepted for publication in Feb. 2004

109. Linnenweber S, Lonnemann G: Pyrogen retention by the Asahi APS-650 polysulfone dialyzer during in vitro dialysis with whole human donor blood. ASAIO J 46(4): 444-447, 2000

110. Schindler R, Lonnemann G, Schäffer J, Shaldon S, Koch KM, Krautzig S: The effect of ultrafiltered dialysate on the cellular content of interleukin-1 receptor antagonist in patients on chronic hemodialysis. Nephron 68: 229-233, 1994

111. Panichi V, De Pietro S, Andreini B, Migliori M, Tesore V, Taccola D, Rindi P, Palla R, Tetta C: Cytokine production in haemodiafiltration: a multicentre study. Nephrol Dial Transplant 13: 1737-1744, 1998

112. Panichi V, Migliori M, De Pietro S, Taccola D, Andreini B, Metelli MR, Giovanni L, Palla R: The link of biocompatibility to cytokine production. Kidney Int 58(Suppl 76): S96-103, 2000

113. Honkanen E, Grönhagen-Riska C, Teppo AM, Maury CPJ, Meri S: Acute-phase proteins during hemodialysis: correlations with serum interleukin-1 beta levels and different dialysis membranes. Nephron 57(3): 283-287, 1991

114. Qian Z, Yu Z, Dai H, Zhang Q, Chen S: Influence of hemodialysis membrane on gene expression and plasma levels of interleukin-1ß. Artif Organs 19(8): 842-846, 1995

115. Memoli B, Postiglione L, Cianciaruso B, Bisesti V, Cimmaruta C, Marzano L, Minutolo R, Cuomo V, Guida B, Andreucci M, Rossi G: Role of different dialysis membranes in the release of interleukin-6-soluble receptor in uremic patients. Kidney Int 58(1): 417-424, 2000

116. Bingel M, Lonnemann G, Koch KM, Dinarello CA, Shaldon S: Plasma interleukin-1 activity during hemodialysis: the influence of dialysis membranes. Nephron 50: 273-276, 1988

117. Haeffner-Cavaillon N, Cavaillon JM, Ciancioni CH, Bacle F, Delons S, Kazatchkine MD: In vivo induction of interleukin-1 during hemodialysis. Kidney Int 35: 1212-1218, 1989

118. Rosenkrantz AR, Körmöczi GF, Thalhammer F, Menzel EJ, Hörl WH, Mayer G, Zlabinger G: Novel C5-dependant neutrophil stimulation by bioincompatible dialyser membranes. Nephrol Dial Transplant 10: 128-135, 1999

119. Rousseau Y, Carreno MP, Poignet JL, Kazatchkine MD, Haeffner-Cavaillon N: Dissociation between complement activation, intergrin expression and neutropenia during hemodialysis. Biomaterials 20(20): 1959-1967, 1999

120. Schouten WE, Grooteman MP, van Houte AJ, Schoorl M, van Limbeek J, Nubé MJ: Effects of dialyser and dialysate on the acute phase reaction in clinical bicarbonate dialysis. Nephrol Dial Transplant 15(3): 379-384, 2000

121. Linnenweber S, Lonnemann G: Effects of dialyzer membrane on interleukin-1ß (IL-1ß) and IL-1ß-converting enzyme in mononuclear cells. Kidney Int 59(Suppl 78): S282-S285, 2001

122. Combe C, Pourtein M, de Précigout V, Baquey A, Morel D, Potaux L, Vincendeau P, Bézian JH, Aparicio M: Granulocyte activation and adhesion molecules during hemodialysis with cuprophane and a high-flux biocompatible membrane. Am J Kidney Dis 24(3): 437-442, 1994

123. Memoli B, Minutolo R, Bisesti V, Postiglione L, Conti A, Marzano L, Capuano A, Andreucci M, Baletta MM, Guida B, Tetta C: Changes of serum albumin and C-reactive protein are related to changes of interleukin-6 release by peripheral blood mononuclear cells in hemodialysis patients treated with different membranes. Am J Kidney Dis 39(2): 266-273, 2002

124. Schindler R, Lonnemann G, Shaldon S, Koch KM, Dinarello CA: Transcription, not synthesis of interleukin-1 and tumor necrosis factor by complement. Kidney Int 37: 85-93, 1990

125. Gu Y, Ding F, Qin H, Zhao H, Lin S: Synergetic effect of dialyzer membrane and lipopolysaccharide on peripheral blood mononuclear cell cytokine production in uremic patients. Chin Med J 113(4): 315-319, 2000

126. Schindler R, Eichert F, Lepenies J, Frei U: Blood components influence cytokine induction by bacterial substances. Blood Purif 19(4): 380-387, 2001

127. Ward RA, McLeish KR: Oxidant stress in hemodialysis patients: what are the determining factors? Artif Organs: 27(3): 230-236, 2003

128. Handelmann GJ: Current studies on oxidant stress in dialysis. Blood Purif 21: 45-50, 2003

129. Locatelli F, Canaud B, Eckardt KU, Stenvinkel P, Wanner C, Zoccali C: Oxidative stress in end-stage renal disease: An emerging threat to patient outcome. Nephrol Dial Transplant 18: 1272-1280, 2003

130. Vanholder R, De Smet R, Glorieux G, Argiles A, Baurmeister U, Brunet P, Clark W, Cohen G, De Deyn PP, Deppisch R, Descamps-Latscha B, Henle T, Jorres A, Lemke HD, Massy ZA, Passlick-Deetjen J, Rodriguez M, Stegmayr B, Stenvinkel P, Tetta C, Wanner C, Zidek W; European Uremic Toxin Work Group (EUTox): Review on uremic toxins: classification, concentration, and interindividual variability. Kidney Int 63(5): 1934-1943, 2003

131. Samouilidou E, Grapsa E: Effect of dialysis on plasma total antioxidant capacity and lipid-peroxidation products in patients with end-stage renal disease. Blood Purif 21: 209-212, 2003

132. Himmelfarb J, McMonagle E: Albumin is the major plasma protein target of oxidant stress in uremia. Kidney Int 60(1): 358-363, 2001

133. Vanholder R, Glorieux G, Lameire N for the European Uremic Toxic Work Group (EUTox): Uraemic toxins and cardiovascular disease. Nephrol Dial Transplant 18(3): 463-466, 2003

134. Kosch M, Levers A, Fobker M, Barenbrock M, Schaefer RM, Ran KH, Hausberg M: Dialysis filter type determines acute effect of haemodialysis on endothelian function and oxidative stress. Nephrol Dial Transplant 18: 1370-1375, 2003

135. Wratten ML, Tetta C, Ursini F, Sevanian A: Oxidant stress in hemodialysis: prevention and treatment strategies. Kidney Int 58 (Suppl 76): S126-132, 2000

136. Amore A, Coppo R: Immunological basis of inflammation in dialysis. Nephrol Dial Transplant 17(Suppl 8): 16-24, 2002

137. Wanner C, Metzger T: C-reactive protein a marker for all-cause and cardiovascular mortality in haemodialysis patients. Nephrol Dial Transplant 17(Suppl 8): 29-32, 2002

138. Zoccali C, Mallamaci F, Tripepi G: Inflammation and atherosclerosis in end-stage renal disease. Blood Purif 21: 29-36, 2003

139. Inal M, Kanbak G, Sen S, Akyuz F, Sunal E: Antioxidant status and lipid peroxidation in hemodialysis patients undergoing erythropoietin and erythropoietin-vitamin E combined therapy. Free Radic Res 31(3): 211-216, 1999

140. Bonnefont-Rousselot D, Lehmann E, Jaudon MC, Delattre J, Perrone B, Rechke JP: Blood oxidative stress and lipoprotein oxidizability in haemodialysis patients: effect of the use of a vitamin E-coated dialysis membrane. Nephrol Dial Transplant 15(12): 2020-2028, 2000

141. Galli F, Varga Z, Balla J, Ferraro B, Canestrari F, Floridi A, Kakuk G, Buoncristiani U: Vitamin E, lipid profile, and peroxidation in hemodialysis patients. Kidney Int (Suppl. 78): S148-154, 2001

142. Morena M, Cristol JP, Canaud B: Why hemodialysis patients are in a pro-oxidant state? What could be done to correct the pro/antioxidant imbalance. Blood Purif 18(3): 191-199, 2000

143. Himmelfarb J, McMonagle E: Manifestations of oxidant stress in uremia. Blood Purif 19: 200-205, 2001

144. Biasioli S, Schiavon R, Petrosino L, Cavallini L, Cavalcanti G, De Fanti E: Dialysis kinetics of homocysteine and reactive oxygen species. ASAIO J 44(5): M423-432, 1998

145. Tepel M, van der Giet M, Jankowski J, Zidek W: The antioxidant acetylcysteine reduces cardiovascular events in patients with end-stage renal failure: a randomized, controlled trial. Circulation 107(7): 992-995, 2003

146. Taccone-Galucci M, Lubrano R, Meloni C: Vitamin E as an antioxidant agent in *Vitamin E bounded membrane. A further step in dialysis optimization,* edited by Ronco C, La Greca G. Contrib Nephrol, Karger, Basel, 127: 32-43, 1999

147. Hultqvist M, Hegbrandt J, Nilsson-Thorell C, Lindholm T, Nilsson P, Lindén T, Hultqvist-Bengtsson U: Plasma concentrations of vitamin C, Vitamin E and/or malondialdehyde as markers of oxygen free radical production during hemodialysis. Clin Nephrol 47(1): 37-46, 1997

148. Morena M, Cristo JP, Descombs B, Canaud B. Does vitamin E bound on dialysis membrane improve the LDL susceptibility to oxidation? Lessons from an in vitro model in *Vitamin E bounded membrane. A further step in dialysis optimization,* edited by Ronco C, La Greca G. Contrib Nephrol Karger, Basel, 127: 128-138, 1999

149. Galli F, Rovidati S, Benedetti S, Canestrari F, Ferraro B, Floridi A, Buoncristiani U: Lipid peroxodation, leukocyte function and apoptosis in hemodialysis patients treated with vitamin E modified filters in *Vitamin E bounded membrane. A further step in dialysis optimization,* edited by Ronco C, La Greca G. Contrib Nephrol, Karger, Basel, 127: 156-171, 1999

150. Mune M, Yukawa S, Kishino M, Otani H, Kimura K, Nishikawa O, Takahashi T, Kodama N, Saika Y, Yamada Y: Effect of vitamin E on lipid metabolism and atherosclerosis in ESRD patients. Kidney Int (Suppl.71): S126-129, 1999

151. Clermont G, Lecour S, Cabanne JF, Motte G, Guilland JC, Chevet D, Rochette L: Vitamin E-coated dialyzer reduces oxidative stress in hemodialysis patients. Free Radic Biol Med 31(2): 233-241, 2001

152. Galli F, Rovidati S, Chiarantini L, Campus G, Canestrari F, Buoncristiani U: Bioreactivity and biocompatibility of a vitamin E-modified multi-layer hemodialysis filter. Kidney Int 54(2): 580-589, 1998

153. Stephens NG, Parsons A, Schofield PM, Kelly F, Cheeseman K, Mitchinson MJ: Randomised controlled trial of vitamin E in patients with coronary disease: Cambridge Heart Antioxidant Study (CHAOS). Lancet 347(9004): 781-786, 1996

154. GISSI-Prevenzione Investigators (Gruppo Italiano per lo Studio della Sopravivenza nell'Infarto miocardico): Dietary supplementation with n-3 polyunsaturated fatty acids and vitamin E after myocardial infarction: results of the GISSI-Prevenzione trial. Lancet 354: 447-455, 1999

155. Yusuf S, Dagenais G, Pogue J, Bosch J, Sleight P: Vitamin E supplementation and cardiovascular events in high-risk patients. The Heart Outcomes Prevention Evaluation Study Investigators. N Engl J Med 342(3): 154-160, 2000

156. Lonn E: Modifying the natural history of atherosclerosis: the SECURE trial. Int J Pract 117(Suppl Jan): 13-18, 2001

157. Lonn E, Yusuf S, DsarvikV et al: Effects of ramipril and vitamin E on atherosclerosis : the study to evaluate carotid ultrasound changes in patients treated with ramipril and Vitamin E (SECURE). Circulation 103: 919-925, 2001

158. Mancini GB, Stewart DJ: Why were the results of the Heart Outcome Prevention Evaluation (HOPE) trial so astounding? Can J Cardiol 17(Suppl A): 15A-17A, 2001

159. Brown BG, Zhao XQ, Chait A, Fisher LD, Cheung MC, Morse JS, Dowdy AA, Marino EK, Bolson EL, Alaupovic P, Frohlich J, Albers JJ: Simvastatin and niacin, antioxidant vitamins, or the combination for the prevention of coronary disease. N Engl J Med 345(22): 1583-159, 2001

160. MRC/BHF/MRC/BHF Heart Protection Study on anti-oxidant vitamin supplementation in 20,536 high-risk individuals: a randomised placebo controlled trial. Lancet 360: 23-33, 2002

161. Boaz M, Smetana S, Weinstein T, Matas Z, Gafter U, Iaina A, Knecht A, Weissgarten Y, Brunner D, Fainaru M, Green MS: Secondary prevention with antioxidants of cardiovascular disease in endstage renal disease (SPACE): randomised placebo-controlled trial. Lancet 356(9237): 1213-1218, 2000

162. Schieke G, Gwinner W, Radermacher J, Bahlmann J, Lonnemann G: Long-term effects of vitamin E bonded membrane on mononuclear cell activation, malondialdehyde generation and endothelian function in ESRD patients in *Vitamin E bonded membrane. A further step in dialysis optimization*, edited by Ronco C, La Greca G, Basel, Karger. Contrib Nephrol 127: 243-250, 1999

163. Khajehdehi P: Effect of vitamins on the lipid profile of patients on regular hemodialysis. Scand J Urol Nephrol 34(1): 62-66, 2000

164. Miyazaki H, Matsuoka H, Itabe H, Usui M, Ueda S, Okuda S, Imaizumi T: Hemodialysis impairs endothelial function via oxidative stress: effects of vitamin E-coated dialyzer. Circulation 101(9): 1002-1006, 2000

165. Kobayashi S, Moriya H, Ohtake T: Vitamin E-bonded hemodialyzer improves atherosclerosis associated with a rheological improvement of circulating red blood cells. Kidney Int 63: 1881-1887, 2003

166. Cristol JP, Bosc JY, Badiou S, Leblanc M, Lorrho R, Descombs B, Canaud B: Erythropoietin and oxidative stress in hemodialysis: beneficial effects of vitamin E supplementation. Nephrol Dial Transplant 12: 2312-2317, 1997

167. Túri S, Németh I, Varga I, Matkovics B: Erythropoietin and oxidative stress in haemodialysis: beneficial effects of vitamin E supplementation. (Letter) Nephrol Dial Transplant 14(1): 252-253, 1999

168. Usberti M, Bufano G, Lima G, Gazotti RM, Tira P, Gerardi G, Di Lorenzo D: Increased red blood cell survival reduces the need of erythropoietin in hemodialyzed patients treated with exogenous gluthathione and vitamin E-modified membrane in *Vitamin E bonded membrane. A further step in dialysis optimization*, edited by Ronco C, La Greca G, Karger, Basel. Contrib Nephrol 127: 208-214, 1999

169. Satoh M, Yamasaki Y, Nagake Y, Kasahara J, Hashimoto M, Nakanishi N, Makino H: Oxidative stress is reduced by the long-term use of vitamin E-coated dialysis filters. Kidney Int 59(5): 1943-1950, 2001

170. Richardson D, Lindley EJ, Bartlett C, Will EJ: A randomized, controlled study of the consequences of hemodialysis membrane composition on erythropoietic response. Am J Kidney Dis 42(3): 551-560, 2003

171. Eiselt J, Racek J, Trefil L, Opatrný K Jr: Effects of a vitamin E-modified dialysis membrane and vitamin C infusion on oxidative stress in hemodialysis patients. Artif Organs 25(6): 430-436, 2001

172. Huraib S, Tanimu D, Shaheen F, Hejaili F, Giles C, Pagayon V: Effect of vitamin-E-modified dialysers on dialyser clotting, erythropoietin and heparin dosage comparative crossover study. Am J Nephrol 20(5): 364-368, 2000

173. Cianciolo G, Donati G, Manna C, Grammatico F, Mosconi G, Raimondi C, Coli L, Stefoni S: Platelet and coagulative activation, lipid profile during hemodialysis: standard versus low molecular weight heparin. (Abstract) Nephrol Dial Transplant 15(9): A147, 2000

174. Woods HF: Does choice of membrane or modality impact oxidant stress in hemodialysis therapy? Kidney Int 60(4): 1611, 2001

175. Tsuruoka S, Kawaguchi A, Nishiki K, Hayasaka T, Fukushima C, Sugimoto K, Saito T, Fujimura A: Vitamin E-bonded hemodialyzer improves neutrophil function and oxidative stress in patients end-stage renal failure. Am J Kidney Dis 39(1): 127-133, 2002

176. Girndt M, Lengler S, Kaul H, Sester U, Sester M, Kohler H: Prospective crossover trial of the influence of vitamin E-coated dialyzer membranes on T-cell activation and cytokine induction. Am J Kidney Dis 35(1): 95-104, 2000

177. Dhondt A, Vanholder R, Glorieux G, Waterloos MA, De Smet R, Lesaffer G, Lameire N: Vitamin E-bonded cellulose membrane and hemodialysis bioincompatibility: absence of an acute benefit on expression of leukocyte surface molecules. Am J Kidney Dis 36(6): 1140-1146, 2001

178. Yoshida K, Kitauchi T, Kimura S, Yoneda T, Uemura H, Ozono S, Hirao Y: Serum neopterin monitoring and vitamin E-modified, regenerated hemodialyzer membrane influence on biocompatibility. Artif Organs 26(1): 54-57, 2002

179. Shimazu T, Kondo S, Toyama K, Komurai M, Ohminato M, Yasuda T, Sato T, Maeba T, Maruyama H, Owada S, Ishida M: Effect of vitamin E modified regenerative cellulosic membrane on neutrophil superoxide anion radical production and lipid peroxidation in *Vitamin E bonded membrane. A further step in dialysis optimization*, edited by Ronco C, La Greca G, Karger, Basel. Contrib Nephrol 127: 251-260, 1999

180. Biasioli S, Schiavon R, Petrosino L, Cavallini L, Cavalcanti G, De Fanti E, Zambello A, Borin D: Effect of several cellulosic dialytic membranes on hyperhomocysteinemia and on the oxidative stress in dialysis patients: any role for Curay + vitamin E? Contrib Nephrol 127: 96-112, 1999

181. Biasioli S, Schiavon R, Petrosino L, Cavallini L, Cavalcanti G, De Fanti E, Zambello A, Borin D: Role of cellulosic and noncellulosic membranes in hyperhomocysteinemia and oxidative stress. ASAIO J 46(5): 625-634, 2000

182. Walker RJ, Sutherland WHF, deJong S: Long-term effects of changing from cellulose acetate to polysulfone dialysis membranes on markers of protein oxidation and inflammation. (Abstract) J Am Soc Nephrol 13(9): 603A, 2002

183. Lucchi L, Bergamini S, Botti B, Rapanà R, Ciuffreda A, Ruggiero P, Ballestri M, Tomasi A, Albertazzi A: Influence of different hemodialysis membranes on red blood cell susceptibility to oxidative stress. Artif Organs 24(1): 1-6, 2000.

184. Ghezi PM, Ronco C: Excebrane: hemocompatibility studies by the intradialytic monitoring of oxygen saturation in *Vitamin E-bounded membrane. A further step in dialysis optimization*, edited by Ronco C, La Greca D, Karger, Basel. Contrib Nephrol 127: 177-191, 1999

185. Sanaka T, Omata M, Nishimura H, Shinobe M, Higushi C: Suppressive effect of vitamin E-coated dialysis membrane on hemodialysis induced cell activation in *Vitamin E-bounded membrane. A further step in dialysis optimization*, edited by Ronco C, La Greca D, Karger, Basel. Contrib Nephrol 127: 261-268, 1999

186. Galle J, Seibold S: Has time come to use antioxidant therapy in uraemic patients? Nephrol Dial Transplant 18: 1452-1455, 2003

187. Brown BG, Cheung MC, Lee AC, Zhao XQ, Chait A: Antioxidant vitamins and lipid therapy: end of a long romance? Arterioscler Thromb Vasc Biol 22: 1535-1546, 2002

188. Pru C, Eaton J, Kjellstrand C: Vitamin C intoxication and hyperoxalemia in chronic hemodialysis patients. Nephron 39: 112-116, 1985

189. Van Ypersele de Strihou C: Advanced glycation in uraemic toxicity. EDTNA ERCA J 29(3): 148-150, 2003

190. Miyata T, Ueda Y, Shinzato T, Iida Y, Tanaka S, Kurokawa K, van Ypersele de Strihou C, Maeda K: Accumulation of albumin-linked and free-form pentosidine in the circulation of uremic patients with end-stage renal failure: renal implications in the pathophysiology of pentosidine. J Am Soc Nephrol 7(8): 1198-1206, 1996

191. Schwedler SB, Metzger T, Schinzel R, Wanner C: Advanced glycation end products and mortality in hemodialysis patients. Kidney Int 62: 301-310, 2002

192. Uchimura T, Mortomiya Y, Hashagushi T, Iwamoto H, Maruyama I: Advanced glycation end-products was a risk factor of progression of atherosclerosis in the maintenance haemodialysis patients. Abstract (F-PO753), ASN, 2003

193. Hou FF, Jiang JP, Guo JQ, Wang GB, Zhang X, Stern DM, Schmidt AM, Owen WFjr: Receptor for advanced glycation end products on human synovial fibroblasts: role of the pathogenesis of dialysis-related amyloidosis. J Am Soc Nephrol 13: 1296-1306, 2002

194. Shimoike T, Inoguchi T, Umeda F, Nawata H, Kawano K, Ochi H: The meaning of serum levels of advanced glycolisation end products in diabetic nephropathy. Metabolism 49(8): 1030-1035, 2000

195. Henle T, Deppisch R, Beck W, Hergesell O, Hänsch GM, Ritz E: Advanced glycated end-products (AGE) during haemodialysis treatment: discrepant results with different methodologies reflecting the heterogeneity of AGE compounds. Nephrol Dial Transplant 14: 1968-1975, 1999

196. Odetti P, Cosso L, Prozanto MA, Dapino D, Gurreri G: Plasma advanced glycosylation end-products in maintenance haemodialysis patients. Nephrol Dial Transplant 10: 2110-2113, 1995

197. Miyata T, Ueda Y, Yoshida A, Sugiyama S, Iida Y, Jadoul M, Maeda K, Kurokawa K, Van Ypersele de Strihou C: Clearance of pentosisine, an advanced glycation end product, by different modalities of renal replacement therapy. Kidney Int 51: 880-887, 1997

198. Jadoul M, Ueda Y, Yasuda Y, Saito A, Robert A, Ishida N, Kurokawa K, Van Ypersele de Strihou C, Miyata T: Influence of hemodialysis membrane on pentosidine plasma level, a marker of "carbonyl stress". Kindey Int 55: 2487-2492, 1999

199. Izuhara Y, Miyata T, Saito K, Saito A, Nangaku M, Kurokawa K, van Ypersele de Strihou C: Ultrapure dialysate decreases plasma pentosidine, a marker of "carbonyl stress". Abstract (SU-PO871), ASN, 2003

200. Bergström J: Nutrition and mortality in hemodialysis. J Am Soc Nephrol 6(5): 1329-1341, 1995

201. Kopple JD: Nutritional status as a predictor of mortality in maintenance dialysis patients. ASAIO Journal: 246-250, 1997

202. Foley RN, Parfrey PS, Harnett JD, Kent GM, Murray DC, Barre PF: Hypalbuminemia, cardiac morbidity, and mortality in end-stage renal disease. J Am Soc Nephrol 7: 728-736, 1998

203. Herselman M, Moosa MR, Kotze TJ, Kritzinger M, Wuister S, Mostert D: Protein-energy malnutrition as a risk factor for increased morbidity in long-term hemodialysis patients. J Ren Nutr 10(1): 7-15, 2000

204. The United States data report on chronic renal disease (URSDS), chapter 6: 106-120, 2002

205. Pifer TB, McCullough KP, Port FK, Goodkin DA, Maroni BJ, Held PJ, Young EW: Mortality risk in hemodialysis patients and changes in nutritional indicators: DOPPS. Kidney Int 62(6): 2238-2245, 2002

206. Eknoyan G, Beck GJ, Cheung AK, Daugirdas JT, Greene T, Kusek JW, Allon M, Bailey J, Delmez JA, Depner TA, Dwyer JT, Levey AS, Levin NW, Milford E, Ornt DB, Rocco MV, Schulman G, Schwab SJ, Teehan BP, Toto R for the Hemodialysis (HEMO) Study Group: Effect of dialysis dose and membrane flux in maintenance hemodialysis. N Engl J Med 347(25): 2010-2019, 2002

207. Lindholm B, Wang T, Heimbürger O, Bergström J: Influence of different treatments and schedules on the factors conditioning the nutritional status in dialysis patients. Nephrol Dial Transplant 13(Suppl 6): 66-73, 1998

208. Qureshi AR; Alvestrand A, Danielsson A, Divino-Filho JC, Gutierrez A, Lindholm B, Bergström J: Factors predicting malnutrition in hemodialysis patients: a cross sectional study. Kidney Int (53): 773-782, 1998

209. Frankenfield DI, McClellan WM, Helgerson SD, Lowrie EG, Rocco MV, Owen WF Jr: Relationship between urea reduction ratio, demographic characteristics, and body weight for patients in the 1996 National ESRD Core Indicator Project. Am J Kidney Dis 33(3): 584-591, 1999

210. Tayeb JS, Provenzano R, El-Ghoroury M, Bellovich K, Khairullah Q, Pieper D, Morrison L, Calleja Y: Effect of biocompatibility of hemodialysis membranes on serum albumin levels. Am J Kidney Dis 35(4): 606-610, 2000

211. Rocco MV, Paranandi L, Burrowes JD, Cockram DB, Dwyer JT, Kusek JW, Leung J, Makoff R, Maroni B, Poole D, for the HEMO study group: Nutritional status in the HEMO study cohort at baseline. Am J Kidney Dis 39(2): 245-256, 2002

212. Steiber AL, Handu DJ, Cataline DR, Deighton TR, Weatherspoon LJ: The impact of nutrition intervention on a reliable morbidity and mortality indicator: the hemodialysis-prognostic nutrition index. J Ren Nutr 13(3): 186-190, 2003

213. Greene T, Beck GJ, Gassman JJ, Gotch FA, Kusek JW, Levey AS, Levin NW, Schulman G, Eknoyan G: Design and statistical issues of the hemodialysis (HEMO) study. Control Clin Trials 21(5): 502-525, 2000

214. Gutierrez A: Protein catabolism in maintenance haemodialysis: the influence of the dialysis membrane. Nephrol Dial Transplant 11(Suppl 2): 108-111, 1996

215. Norton PA: Affect of serum leptin on nutritional status in renal disease. J Am Diet Assoc 102(8): 1119-1125, 2002

216. Kaysen GA, Don BR: Factors that affect albumin concentration in dialysis patients and their relationship to vascular disease. Kidney Int 63 (Suppl 84): S94-S97, 2003

217. Lofberg E, Essen P, McNurlan M, Wernerman J, Garlick P, Anderstam B, Bergström J, Alvestrand A: Effect of hemodialysis on protein synthesis. Clin Nephrol 54(4): 284-294, 2000

218. Ikizler TA, Pupim LB, Brouillette JR, Levenhagen DK, Farmer K, Hakim RM, Flakoll PJ: Hemodialysis stimulates muscle and whole body protein loss and alters substrate oxidation. Am J Physiol Endocrinol Metab 282(1): E107-116, 2002

219. Sanaka T: Nutritional effect of dialysis therapy. Artif Organs 27(3): 224-226, 2003

220. Kopple JD: Effect of nutrition on morbidity and mortality in maintenance dialysis patients. Am Jm Kidney Dis 24(6): 1002-1009, 1994

221. Navarro JF, Marcén R, Teruel JE, Martin del Río R, Gámez C, Mora C, Ortuño J: Effect of different dialysis membranes on amino-acid losses during haemodialysis. Nephrol Dial Transplant 13: 113-117, 1998

222. Navarro JF, Mora C, León C, Martín-Del Rio R, Macía ML, Gallego E, Chahin J, Méndez ML, Rivero A, García J: Amino acid losses during hemodialysis with polyacrylonitrile membranes: effect of intradialytic amino acid supplementation on plasma amino acid concentrations and nutritional variables in nondiabetic patients. Am J Clin Nutr (3): 765-773, 2000

223. Gutierrez A, Alvestrand A, Wahren J, Bergström J: Effect of in vivo contact between blood and dialysis membranes on protein catabolism in humans. Kidney Int 38(3): 487-494, 1990

224. Veenemann JM, Kingma HA, Stellaard F, De Jong PE, Reijngoud DJ, Huisman RM: Dialysis membrane biocompatibility does not influence whole body protein metabolism. (Abstract) J Am Soc Nephrol 13(9): 602A, 2002

225. Mujais SK: Protein permeability in dialysis. Nephrol Dial Transplant 15: 10-14, 2000

226. Ikizler TA, Flakoll PJ, Parker RA, Hakim RM: Amino acid and albumin losses during haemodialysis. Kidney Int 46(3): 830-837, 1994

227. Sombolos K, Tsitamidou Z, Kyriazis G, Karagianni A, Kantaropoulou M, Progia E: Clinical evaluation of four high-flux hemodialyzers under conventional conditions in vivo. Am J Nephrol 17: 406-412, 1997

228. Rocco M, Dwyer J, for the HEMO study group: Effects of dose and flux interventions on nutritional parameters. Results from the Hemodialysis study. (Abstract) J Am Soc Nephrol 13(9): 421A, 2002

229. Ledebo I: Does convective dialysis therapy applied daily approach renal blood purification? Kidney Int 59(Suppl 78): S286-291, 2001

230. Clark WR, Gao D: Low-molecular weight proteins in end-stage renal disease: potential toxicity an dialytic removal mechanisms. J Am Soc Nephrol 13: S41-S47, 2002

231. Samtleben W, Dengler C, Reinhardt B, Nothdurft A, Lemke HD: Comparison of the new polyethersulfone high-flux membrane DIAPES® HF800 with conventional high-flux membranes during on-line haemodiafiltration. Nephrol Dial Transplant 18: 2382-2386, 2003

232. Krieter DH, Canaud B: High permeability of dialysis membranes: what is the limit of albumin loss? Nephrol Dial Transplant 18: 651-654, 2003

233. Nensel U, Rockel A, Hillenbrand T, Bartel J: Dialyzer permeability for low-molecular-weight proteins. Comparison between polysulfone, polyamide and cuprammonium-rayon dialyzers. Blood Purif 12(2): 128-34,1994

234. Combarnous F, Tetta C, Cellier CC, Wratten ML, Custaud, De Catheu T, Fouque D, David S, Carraro G, Laville M: Albumin loss in on-line hemodiafiltration. Int J Artif Organs 25(3): 203-209, 2002

235. Beck W, Deppisch R, Göhl H: May albumin loss through dialyzer membranes contribute to low serum albumin levels in hemodialysis patients? (Abstract) Blood Purif 16: 231, 1998

236. Ahrenholz P, Tiess M, Ramlow W, Winkler RE: Characteristics of high-flux dialysers in pre- and post-dilution hemofiltration (HDF). (Abstract) J Am Soc Nephrol 13(9): 239A-240A, 2002

237. Miwa M, Shinzato T: Push/pull hemodiafiltration: technical aspects and clinical effectiveness. Artif Organs 23(12): 1123-1126, 1999

238. Ahrenholz PG, Winkler RE, Mechelsen A, Lang DA, Bowry SK: Dialysis membrane-dependent removal of middle molecule during haemodiafiltration; the ß2-microglobulin/albumin relationship. Clin Nephrol, submitted for publication in 2004

239. Kim ST, Yamamoto C, Taoka M, Takasugi M: Programmed filtration, a new method for removing large molecules and regulating albumin leakage during hemodiafiltration treatment. Am J Kidney Dis 38(Suppl 1): S220-223, 2001

240. Bolasco P, Altieri P, Andrulli S, Basile C, Di Filippo S, Feriani M, Pedrini L, Santoro A, Zoccali S, Sau G, Locatelli F: Convection versus diffusion in dialysis: an Italian prospective multicentre study. Nephrol Dial Transplant 18(Suppl 7): vii50-vii54, 2003

241. Gutierrez A, Bergström J, Alvestrand A: Protein catabolism in sham-hemodialysis: the effect of different membranes. Clin Nephrol 38(1): 20-29, 1992

242. King AJ, Kehayias JJ, Roubenoff R, Schmid CH, Pereira BJ: Cytokine production and nutritional status in hemodialysis patients. Int J Artif Organs 21(1): 4-11, 1998

243. Ducci D, Bilancioni R, Pistocchi E, Baldrati L, Capponcini C, Delvecchio C, Feletti C: Evolution of serum prealbumin following hemodialysis: effect of different dialysis membranes. Nephron 62(2): 145-149, 1992

244. Parker III TF, Wingard RL, Husni L, Ikizler TA, Parker RA, Hakim RM: Effect of membrane biocompatibility on nutritional parameters in chronic hemodialysis patients. Kidney Int 49: 551-556, 1996

245. Locatelli F, Mastrangelo F, Redaelli B, Ronco C, Marcelli D, La Greca G, Orlandini G: Effects of different membranes and dialysis technologies on patient treatment tolerance and nutritional parameters. Kidney Int 50: 1293-1302, 1996

246. Locatelli F for the Italian Cooperative Dialysis Study Group: Effect of hemodialysis membranes on serum albumin. (Letter) Am J Kidney Dis 37(2): 455-456, 2001

247. Young EW: Dialysis dose, membrane type, and anemia control. Am J Kidney Dis 6(Suppl 4): S157-S160, 1998

248. Xia H, Ebben J, Ma JZ, Collins AL: Hematocrit levels and hospitalization risks in hemodialysis patients J Am Soc Nephrol 10: 1309-1316, 1999

249. Ma JZ, Ebben J, Xia H, Collins AL: Hemoatocrit level and associated mortality in hemodialysis patients. J Am Soc Nephrol 10: 610-619, 1999

250. Hegarty J, Foley RN: Anaemia, renal insufficiency and cardiovascular outcome. Nephrol Dial Transplant 16(Suppl 1): 102-104, 2001

251. Rocco MV, Bedinger MR, Milam R, Greer JW, McClellan WM, Frankenfield DL: Duration of dialysis and its relationship to dialysis adequacy, anemia management, and serum albumin level. Am J Kidney Dis 38(4): 813-823, 2001

252. Valderrábano F: Anaemia management in chronic kidney disease patients: an overview of current clinical practice. Nephrol Dial Transplant 17(Suppl 1): 13-18, 2002

253. Ofsthun N, LaBreque J, Lacson E, Keen M, Lazarus JM: The effects of higher hemoglobin levels on mortality and hospitalization in hemodialysis patients. Kidney Int 63: 1908-1914, 2003

254. Lacson E Jr, Ofsthun N, Lazarus JM: Effect of variability in anemia management on hemoglobin outcomes in ESRD. Am J Kidney Dis 41(1): 111-124, 2003

255. Ifudu O, Feldman J, Friedman EA: The intensity of hemodialysis and the response to erythropoeitin in patients with end-stage renal disease. N Engl Med 334: 420-425, 1996

256. Frankenfield D, Johnson CA, Wish JB, Rocco MV, Madore F, Owen WF jr: Anemia management of adult hemodialysis patients in the US results: from the 1997 ESRD Core Indicators Project. Kidney Int 57(2): 578-589, 2000

257. Ifudu O, Uribarri J, Rajwani I, Vlacich V, Reydel K, Delosreyes G, Friedman EA: Adequacy of dialysis and differences in hematocrit among dialysis facilities. Am J Kidney Dis 36(6): 1166-1174, 2000

258. NKF-K/DOQI clinical practice guidelines for anaemia, update 2000, www.kidney.org/professionals/kdoqi/index/cfm

259. European Best Practice Guidelines for the management of anaemia in patients with chronic renal failure. Nephrol Dial Transplant 14(Suppl 5): 1-50, 1999

260. Villaverde M, Pérez-Garcia R, Verde E, López-Gómez M, Jofré R, Junco E, Luño J: La polisulfona de alta permeabilidad mejora la repuestza de la anemia a la eritropoyetina en hemodialisis. Nefrologia 19(2): 161-167, 1999

261. Locatelli F, Andrulli S, Pecchini F, Pedrini L, Agliata S, Lucchi L, Farina M, La Milia V, Grassi C, Borghi M, Redaelli B, Conte F, Ratto G, Cabiddu G, Grossi C, Modenese R: Effect of high-flux dialysis on the anaemia of haemodialysis patients. Nephrol Dial Transplant 15: 1399-1409, 2000

262. Cortes G, Sanchez Perales S, Liebana A, Gil GM, Borrego FJ, Borrego J, Perez del Barrio P, Serrano P, Perez Banasco V: Beneficial effect of AN69 membrane on anemia in hemodialyzed patients. Nefrologia 21(4): 370-375, 2001

263. Opatrný K Jr, Reischig T, Vienken J, Eiselt J, Vít L, Opatrna S, Šefrna F, Racek J, Brown GS: Does treatment modality have an impact on anemia in patients with chronic renal failure? Effect of low- and high-flux biocompatible dialysis. Artif Organs 26(2): 181-188, 2002

264. Godino JIM, Rentero R, Orlandini G, Marcelli D, Ronco C: Results from the EuCliD® (European Clinical Dialysis Database): impact of shifting treatment modality. Int J Artif Org 25(11): 1049-1060, 2002

265. Schrander-v.d. Meer AM, ter Wee PM, Donker AJM, van Dorp WT: Dialysis efficacy during acetate-free biofiltration. Nephrol Dial Transplant 13(2): 370-274, 1998

266. Ward RA, Schmidt B, Hullin J, Hillebrand G, Samtleben W: A comparison of on-line hemodialfiltration and high-flux hemodialysis: A prospective clinical study. J Am Soc Nephrol 11: 2344-2350, 2000

267. Eiselt J, Racek J, Opatrný K Jr: The effect of hemodialysis and acetate-free biofiltration on anemia. Int J Artif Organs 23(3): 173-180, 2000

268. Basile C, Giordano R, Montanaro A, De Maio P, De Padova F, Marangi AL, Semeraro A: Effect of acetate free biofiltration on the anaemia of haemodialysis patients: a prospective cross-over study. Nephrol Dial Transplant 16: 1914-1919, 2001

269. Eckardt KU: Anaemia correction-does the mode of dialysis matter? Nephrol Dial Transplant 15: 1278-1280, 2000

270. Movilli E, Cancarini GC, Zani R, Camerini C, Sandrini M, Maiorca R: Adequacy of dialysis reduces the doses of recombinant erythropoietin independently from the use of biocompatible membranes in haemodialysis patients. Nephrol Dial Transplant 16(1): 111-114, 2001

271. Coladonato JA, Frankenfield DL, Reddan DN, Klassen PS, Szczech LA, Johnson CA, Owen WFJr: Trends in anemia management among US hemodialysis patients. J Am Soc Nephrol 13(5): 1288-1295, 2002

272. Moist LM, Port FK, Orzol SM, Young EW, Ostbye T, Wolfe RA, Hulbert-Shearon T, Jones CA, Bloembergen WE: Predictors of loss of residual renal function among new dialysis patients. J Am Soc Nephrol 11(3): 556-564, 2000

273. Ravid M, Lang R, Rolson M: The importance of daily urine volume and residual renal function in patients treated with hemodialysis. Dial Transplant 9: 763-765, 1985.

274. Suda T, Hiroshige K, Ohta T, Watanabe Y, Iwamoto M, Kanegae K, Ohtani A, Nakashima Y: The contribution of residual renal function to overall nutritional status in chronic haemodialysis patients. Nephrol Dial Transplant 15(3): 396-401, 2000

275. Adequacy of dialysis and nutrition in continuous peritoneal dialysis: association with clinical outcomes. Canada-USA (CANUSA) Peritoneal Dialysis Study. J Am Soc Nephrol 7(2): 198-207, 1996

276. Bargman J, Thorpe K, Churchil D: The importance of residual renal function for survival in patients on peritoneal dialysis. (Abstract) J Am Soc Nephrol 8(9): 185A, 1997

277. Iest CG, Vanholder RC, Ringoir SM: Loss of residual renal function in patients on regular hemodialysis. Int J Artif Organs12(3): 159-164, 1989

278. Hakim RA, Wingard RL, Parker RA: Effects of dialysis membrane in the treatment of patients with acute renal failure. New Engl J Med 331(20): 1338-1342, 1995

279. Schiffl H, Lang SM, Fischer R: Ultrapure dialysis fluid slows loss of residual renal function in new dialysis patients. Nephrol Dial Transplant 17(10): 1814-1818, 2002

280. Hartmann J, Fricke H, Schiffl H: Biocompatible membranes preserve residual renal function in patients undergoing regular hemodialysis. Am J Kidney Dis 30(3): 366-373, 1997

281. McCarthy JT: The use of polysulfone (PS) dialyzers slows the rate of intrinsic renal function loss in chronic hemodialysis patients. (Abstract) J Am Soc Nephrol 4: 367, 1993

282. Mc Kane WS, Tattersall JE, Farrigton K: Preservation of residual renal function in high flux dialysis. (Abstract) Nephrol Dial Transplant 9: 1994

283. Van Stone JC: The effect of dialyzer membrane and etiology of kidney disease on the preservation of residual renal function in chronic hemodialysis patients. ASAIO J 41(3): M713-716, 1995

284. Caramelo C, Alcazar R, Gallar P, Teruel JL, Velo M, Ortega O, Galera A, Da Silva M: Choice of dialysis membrane does not influence the outcome of residual renal function in haemodialysis patients. Nephrol Dial Transplant 9(6): 675-677, 1994

285. McCarthy JT, Jenson BM, Squillace DP, Williams AW: Improved preservation of residual renal function in chronic hemodialysis patients using poysulfone dialyzers. Am J Kidney Diseases 29(4): 576-583, 1997

286. McKane W, Chandna SM, Tattersell JE, Greenwood RN, Farrington K: Identical decline of residual renal function in high-flux biocompatible hemodialysis and CAPD. Kidney Int 61: 256-265, 2002

287. Locatelli F, Hannedouche T, Jacobson S, La Greca G, Loureiro A, Martin-Malo A, Papadimitriou M, Vanholder R: The effect of membrane permeability on ESRD: design of a prospective randomised multicentre trial. J Nephrol 12(2): 85-88, 1999

288. The United States data report on chronic renal disease (URSDS), chapter 10, cardiovascular special studies: 166-176, 2002

289. Foley RN, Parfrey PS, Sarnak: Clinical epidemiology of cardiovascular disease in chronic renal disease. Am J Kidney Dis 32(5, Suppl 3): S112-119, 1998

290. Joki N, Hase H, Nakamura R, Yamaguchi T: Onset of coronary artery disease prior to initiation of haemodialysis in patients with end-stage renal disease. Nephrol Dial Transplant 12: 718-723, 1997

291. Drüeke TB: Aspects of cardiovascular burden in pre-dialysis patients. Nephron 85(Suppl 1): 1-9, 2000

292. Shoji T, Emoto M, Tabata T, Kimoto E, Shinohara K, Maekawa K, Kawagishi T, Tahara H, Ishimura E, Nishizawa Y: Advanced atherosclerosis in predialysis patients with chronic renal failure. Kidney Int 61: 2187-2192, 2002

293. Goodman WG, Godin J, Kuizon BD, Yoon C, Gales B, Sider D: Coronary artery calcifications in young adults with end-stage renal disease who are undergoing dialysis. New Engl J Med 342: 1478-1483, 2000

294. Nishizawa Y, Shoji T, Kawagishi T, Morii H: Atherosclerosis in uremia: Possible role of hyperparathyroidism on intermediate density lipoprotein accumulation. Kidney Int 52(Suppl 62): S90-S92, 1997

295. O'Hare A, Hsu CY, Bacchetti P, Johansen KL: Peripheral vascular disease risk factors among patients undergoing hemodialysis. J Am Soc Nephrol 13: 497-503, 2002

296. Hakim RM, Held PJ, Stannard DC, Wolfe RA, Port FK, Daugirdas JT, Agodoa L: Effect of the dialysis membrane on mortality of chronic hemodialysis patients. Kidney Int 50: 566-570, 1996

297. Koda Y, Nishi S, Miyazaki S, Haginoshita S, Sakurabayashi T, Suzuki M, Sakai S, Yuasa Y, Hirasawa Y, Nishi T: Switch from conventional to high-flux membrane reduces the risk of carpal tunnel syndrome and mortality of hemodialysis patients. Kidney Int 52(4): 1096-1101, 1997

298. Bloembergen WE, Hakim RM, Stannard DC, Held PJ, Wolfe RA, Agodoa Port FK: Relationship of dialysis membrane and cause-specific mortality. Am J Kidney Dis 33(1): 1-10, 1999

299. Woods HF, Nandakumar M: Improved outcome for haemodialysis patients treated with high-flux membranes. Nephrol Dial Transplant 15(Suppl 1): 36-42, 2000

300. Hakim RM: Influence of high-flux biocompatible membrane on carpal tunnel syndrome and mortality. Am J Kidney Dis 32(2): 338-40; discussion 340-43, 1998

301. Himmelfarb JT: Success and challenge in dialysis therapy. N Engl J Med 247(25): 2068-2070, 2002

302. Scribner BH, Blagg CR: Effect of dialysis dose and membrane flux in maintenance hemodialysis. (Letter) N Engl J Med 348(15): 1491-1492, 2003

303. Friedman EA: Effect of dialysis dose and membrane flux in maintenance hemodialysis. (Letter) N Engl J Med 348(15): 1492, 2003

304. Hoenich NA: Effect of dialysis dose and membrane flux in maintenance hemodialysis. (Letter) N Engl J Med 348(15): 1492, 2003

305. Locatelli F: Effect of dialysis dose and membrane flux in maintenance hemodialysis. N (Letter) Engl J Med 348(15): 1492-1493, 2003

306. Levin N, Greenwood R: Reflections on the HEMO study: the American viewpoint. Nephrol Dial Transplant 18(6):1059-1060, 2003

307. Locatelli F: Dose of dialysis, convection and haemodialysis patients outcome–what the HEMO study doesn't tell us: the European viewpoint: Nephrol Dial Transplant 18(6):1061-1065, 2003

308. Prichard S: ADEMEX and HEMO trials: Where are we going? Blood Purif 21: 42-45, 2003

309. Wanner C: Fettstoffwechselstörungen in *Blutreinigungsverfahren*, edited by Franz E, Hörl WH, 5th edition, Thieme Verlag Stuttgart, New York: 175-181, 1997

310. Wheeler DC: Should hyperlipidaemia in dialysis patients be treated? Nephrol Dial Transplant 12: 19-21, 1997

311. Wanner C: Importance of hyperlipidaemia and therapy in renal patients. Nephrol Dial Transplant 15(Suppl 5): 92-96, 2000

312. De Gomez Dumm NT, Giammona AM, Touceda LA, Raimondi C: Lipid abnormalities in chronic renal failure patients undergoing hemodialysis. Medicina (B Aires) 61(2): 142-146, 2001

313. Fleischmann EH, Bower JD, Salahudeen A: Are conventional cardiovascular risk factors predictive of two-year mortality in hemodialysis patients? Clin Nephrol 56(3): 221-230, 2001

314. Fleischmann EH, Bower JD, Salahudeen AK: Risk factor paradox in hemodialysis: better nutrition as a partial explanation. ASAIO J 47(1): 74-81, 2001

315. Longenecker JC, Liu Y, Klag MJ, Marcovina M, Powe NR, Levey AS, Fink NE, Giaculli F, Coresh J: High lipoprotein (a) level and small apolipoprotein(a) size prospectively predict cardiovascular disease events in end-stage renal disease: the CHOICE study. (Abstract) J Am Soc Nephrol 13(9): 423A, 2002

316. Blankestijn PJ, Vos PF, Rabelink TJ, van Rijn HJ, Jansen H, Koomans HA: High-flux dialysis membranes improve lipid profile in chronic hemodialysis patients. J Am Soc Nephrol 5(9): 1703-1798, 1995

317. Goldberg IJ, Kaufmann AM, Lavarias VA, Vanni-Reyes T, Levin NW: High flux dialsis membranes improve plasma lipoprotein profiles in patients with end-stage renal disease. Nephrol Dial Transplant 11(Suppl 2): 104-107, 1996

318. Ingram AJ, Parbtani A, Churchill DN: Effects of two low-flux cellulose acetate dialysers on plasma lipids and lipoproteins- a cross over trial. Nephrol Dial Transplant 13: 1452-1457, 1998

319. House AA, Wells GA, Donnelly JG, Nadler SP, Hebert PC: Randomized trial of high-flux vs low-flux haemodialysis: effects on homocysteine and lipids. Nephrol Dial Transplant 15(7): 1029-1034, 2000

320. Cressmann MD, Heyka RJ, Paganini EP, O'Neil J, Skibinski CI, Hoff HF: Lipoprotein(a) is an independent risk factor for cardiovascular disease in hemodialysis patients. Circulation 86: 475-482, 1992

321. Jaar BJ, Astor B, Longenecker JC, Fink N, Klag MJ, Powe NR, Selhub J, Tracy RP, Marcovina S, Coresh J: Lipoprotein (a) and C-reactive protein are predictors of peripheral vascular disease among incident dialysis patients: the CHOICE study. (Abstract) J Am Soc Nephrol 13(9): 424A, 2002

322. Koch M, Kutkuhn B, Trenkalder E, Back D, Grabensee B, Dieplinger H, Kronengerg F: Apolipoprotein B, Fibrinogen, HDL, Cholesterol and apoliporotein (a) phenotypes predict coronary heart disease in hemodialysis aptients. J Am Soc Nephrol 8: 1889-1989, 1997

323. Zoccali C: Cardiovascular risk in uraemic patients - is it fully explained by classical risk factors? Nephrol Dial Transplant 15: 454-457, 2000

324. Pignone M, Phillips C, Mulrow C: Use of lipid lowering drugs for primary prevention of coronary heart disease: meta-analysis of randomised trials. BMJ 321(7267): 983-986, 2000

325. Ritz E, Bianchi G, London GM, Marcelli D, Massy ZA, Parfrey PS, Passlick-Deetjen J, Rabelink TJ, Wanner Chr: Clinical algorithms on cardiovascular risk factors in renal patients. Nephrol Dial Transplant 15(Suppl. 5): 125-154, 2000

326. Seliger SL, Weiss NS, Daniel L, Gillen DL, Kestenbaum B, Ball A, Sherrard DJ, Stehman-Breen CO: HMG-CoA reductase inhibitors are associated with reduced mortality in ESRD patients. Kidney Int 61(1): 297-304, 2002

327. Saltissi D, Morgan C, Rigby RJ, Westhuyzen J: Safety and efficacy of simvastatin in hypercholestrolemic patients undergoing chronic renal dialysis. Am J Kidney Dis 39(2): 283-290, 2002

328. Josephson MA, Fellner SK, Dasgupta A: Improved lipid profiles in patients undergoing high-flux dialysis. Am J Kidney Dis 20(4): 361-366, 1992

329. Docci D, Capponcini C, Mengozzi S, Baldrati L, Neri L, Feletti C: Effects of different dialysis membranes on lipid and lipoprotein serum profiles in hemodialysis patients. Nephron 69(3): 323-326, 1995

330. Tanaka H, Omachi T, Nishikawa O, Yukawa S, Yoshimoto M, Nishide T: Can dialysis membrane improve serum lipid profile in maintenance hemodialysis patients? (Abstract) EDTA Congress, Genf, 1997

331. Kimak E, Solski J, Janicka L, Wojtysiak B, Zagojska M: Effect of dialysis membranes on lipoprotein profile of serum in haemodialysed patients. Int Urol Nephrol 30(6): 789-798, 1998

332. Ottosson P, Attman PO, Knight C, Samuelsson O, Weiss L, Alaupovic P: Do high-flux dialysis membranes affect renal dyslipidemia? ASAIO J 47(3): 229-23, 2001

333. Sperschneider H, Deppisch R, Beck W, Wolf H, Stein G: Impact on membrane choice and blood flow pattern on coagulation and heparin requirement-potential consequences on blood lipid concentrations. Nephrol Dial Transplant 12: 2638-2646, 1997

334. Stampfer MJ, Malinow MR, Willett WC, Newcomer LM, Upson B, Ullmann D, Tishler PV, Hennekens CH: A prospective study of plasma homocysteine and risk of myokardial infarction in US physicians. JAMA 268(7): 877-881, 1992

335. Boushey CJ, Beresford SA, Omenn GS, Motulsky AG: A quantitative assesssment of plasma homocyteine as a risk factor for vascular disease. Probable benefits of increasing folic acid intakes. JAMA 274(13): 1049-1057, 1995

336. Perry IJ, Refsum H, Morris RW, Ebrahim SB, Ueland PM, Shaper AG: Prospective study of serum total homocysteine concentration and risk of stroke in middle-aged British men. Lancet 346(8987): 1395-1398, 1995

337. Anderson JL, Muhlestein JB, Horne BD, Carlquist JF, Bair TL, Madsen TE, Pearson RB: Plasma homcysteine predicts mortality independently of traditional risk factors and c-reactive protein in patients with angiographically defined coronary artery disease. Circulation 102(11): 1227- 1236, 2000

338. Bachmann J, Tepel M, Raidt H, Riezler R, Graefe U, Langer K, Zidek W: Hyperhomocysteinemia and the risk for vascular disease in hemodialysis patients. J Am Soc Nephrol 6(1): 121-125, 1995

339. Bostom AG, Shenim D, Lapane KL, Miller JW, Sutherland P, Nadeau M, Seyoum E, Hartman W, Prior R, Wilson PW: Hyperhomocysteinemia and traditional disease risk factors in end-stage renal disease patients on dialysis: a case control study. Atherosclerosis 114(1): 93-103, 1995

340. Robinson K, Gupta A, Dennis V, Arheart K, Chaudhary D, Green R, Vigo P, Mayer EL, Selhub J, Kutner M, Jacobsen DW: Hyperhomocysteinemia confers an independent increased risk of atherosclerosis in end-stage renal disease and is closely linked to plasma folate and pyridoxine concentrations. Circulation 94(11): 2743-2748, 1996

341. Moustapha A, Naso A, Nahlawi M, Gupta A, Arheart KL, Jacobsen DW, Robinson K, Dennis VW: Prospective study of hyperhomocysteinemia as an adverse cardiovascular risk factor in end-stage renal disease. Circulation 97(2): 138-141, 1998

342. Mallamaci F, Zoccali C, Tripepi G, Fermo I, Benedetto FA, Cataliotti A, Bellanuova I, Malatino LS, Soldarini A: Hyperhomocysteinemia predicts cardiovascular outcomes in hemodialysis patients. Kidney Int 61(2): 609-614, 2002

343. Descombes E, Boular O, Perriard F: Water-soluble vitamin levels in patients undergoing high-flux hemodialysis and receiving long-term oral postdialysis vitamin supplementation. Artif Organs 24(10): 773-778, 2000

344. Henning BF, Tepel M, Graefe U, Zidek W: Homocysteine and its metabolites in chronic renal insufficiency and the effect of a vitamin replacement. Med Klin 95(9): 477-481, 2000

345. Leblanc M, Pichette V, Geadah D, Ouimet D: Folic acid and pyridoxal-5'-phosphate losses during high-efficiency hemodialysis in patients without hydrosoluble vitamin supplementation. J Ren Nutr 10(4): 1196-201, 2000

346. Oishi K, Nagake Y, Yamasaki H, Fukuda S, Ichikawa H, Ota K, Makino H: The significance of serum homocysteine levels in diabetic patients on haemodialysis. Nephrol Dial Transplant 15(6): 851-855, 2000

347. Tremblay R, Bonnardeaux A, Geadah D, Busque L, Lebrun M, Ouimet D, Leblanc M: Hyperhomocysteinemia in hemodialysis patients: effects of 12-month supplementation with hydrosoluble vitamins. Kidney Int 58(2): 851-858, 2000

348. Bayés B, Pastor MC, Bonal J, Juncà J, Romero R: Homocysteine and lipid peroxidation in haemodialysis: role of folinic acid and vitamin E. Nephrol Dial Transplant 16(11): 2172-2175, 2001

349. Buccianti G, Bamonti Catena F, Patrosso C, Corghi E, Novembrino C, Baragetti I, Lando G, De Franceschi M, Maiolo AT: Reduction of the homocysteine plasma concentration by intravenously administered folinic acid and vitamin B(12) in uraemic patients on maintenance haemodialysis. Am J Nephrol 21(4): 294-299, 2001

350. Lasseur C, Parrot F, Delmas Y, Level C, Ged C, Redonnet-Vernhet I, Montaudon D, Combe C, Chauveau P: Impact of high-flux/high-efficiency dialysis on folate and homocysteine metabolism. J Nephrol 14(1): 32-35, 2001

351. Van Tellingen A, Muriël PC, Grooteman MP, Bartels PC, Van Limbeek J, Van Guldener C, Wee PM, Nubé MJ: Long-term reduction of plasma homocysteine levels by super-flux dialyzers in hemodialysis patients. Kidney Int 59(1): 342-347, 2001

352. Lindner A, Banksson DD, Stehman-Breen C, Mahuren JD, Coburn SP: Vitamin B6 metabolism and homocysteine in end-stage renal disease and chronic renal insufficiency. Am J Kidney Dis 39(1): 134-145, 2002

353. Friedman AN, Bostom AG, Levey AS, Rosenberg IH, Selhub J, Pierratos A: Plasma total homocysteine levels among patients undergoing nocturnal versus standard hemodialysis. J Am Soc Nephrol 13(1): 265-268, 2002

354. De Vriese AS, Verbeke F, Schrijvers BK, Lameire NH: Is folate a promising agent in the prevention and treatment of cardiovascular disease in patients with renal failure? Kidney Int 61: 1199-1209, 2002

355. Guttormsen AB, Ueland PM, Svarstad E, Refsum H: Kinetic basis of hyperhomocysteinemia in patients with chronic renal failure. Kidney Int 52(2): 495-502, 1997

356. Bostom AG, Lathorp L: Hyperhomocysteinemia in end-stage renal disease: prevalence, etiology, and potential relationship to arteriosclerotic outcomes. Kidney Int 52(1): 10-20, 1997

357. Van Guldener C, Donker AJ, Jakobs C, Teerlink T, de Meer K, Stehouwer CD: No net renal extraction of homocysteine in fasting humans. Kidney Int 54(1): 166-169, 1998

358. Huang JW, Yen CJ, Pai MF, Wu KD, Tsai TJ, Hsieh BS: Association between serum aspartate transaminase and homocysteine levels in hemodialysis patients. Am J Kidney Dis 40(6): 1195-1201, 2002

359. Arnadottir M, Berg AL, Hegbrant J, Hultberg B: Influence of haemodialysis on plasma total homocysteine concentration. Nephrol Dial Transplant 14(1): 142-146, 1999

360. Bloembergen WE, Port FK: Epidemiological perspective on infections in chronic dialysis patients. Adv Ren Replace Ther 3(3): 201-207, 1996

361. Vanholder R, Van Biesen W: Incidence and infectious morbidity and mortality in dialysis patients. Blood Purif 20(5): 477-489, 2002

362. Himmelfarb J, Hakim RM: Biocompatibility and the risk of infection in haemodialysis patients. Nephrol Dial Transplant 9(Suppl 2): 138-144, 1994

363. Bonomini V, Coli L, Scolari MP, Stefoni S: Structure of dialysis membranes and long-term clinical outcome. Am J Nephrol 15(6): 455-462, 1995

364. Churchill DN: Clinical impact of biocompatible dialysis membranes on patient morbidity and mortality an appraisal of the evidence. Nephrol Dial Transplant 10(Suppl 10): 52-56, 1995

365. Pertosa G, Grandaliano G, Gesualdo L, Schena FP: Clinical relevance of cytokine production in hemodialysis. Kidney Int 58(Suppl 76): S104-S111, 2000

366. Cohen G: Immune dysfunction in uremia. Int J Artif Org 25(7): 610-611, 2002

367. Vanholder R, Ringoir S, Dhondt A: Phagocytosis in uremic and hemodialysis patients: a prospective and cross sectional study. Kidney Int 39(2): 320-327, 1991

368. Lonnemann G, Novick D, Rubinstein M, Passlick-Deetjen J, Lang D, Dinarello CA: A switch to high-flux Helixone membranes reverses suppressed interferon-γ production in patients on low-flux dialysis. Blood Purif 21: 225-231, 2003

369. Hoen B, Paul-Dauphin A, Hestin D, Kessler M: EPIBACDIAL: a multicenter prospective study of risk factors for bacteremia in chronic hemodialysis patients. J Am Soc Nephrol 9(5): 869-876, 1998

370. Hornberger JC, Chernew M, Petersen J, Garber AM: A multivariate analysis of mortality and hospital admissions with high-flux dialysis. J Am Soc Nephrol 3(6):1227-1237, 1992

371. Allon M, Depner TA, Radeva M, Bailey J, Beddhu S, Butterly D, Coyne DW, Gassman JJ, Kaufman AM, Kaysen GA, Lewis JA, Schwab SJ; HEMO Study Group: Impact of dialysis dose and membrane on infection-related hospitalization and death: results of the HEMO Study. J Am Soc Nephrol 14(7): 1863-1870, 2003

372. Locatelli F: How will the results of the HEMO study impact dialysis practice? Sem Dial 16(1): 20-21, 2003

373. Jadoul M: Dialysis-related amyloidosis: importance of biocompatibility and age. Nephrol Dial Transplant 13(Suppl7): 61-64, 1998

374. Drüeke TB: ß2-microglobulin and amyloidosis. Nephrol Dial Transplant 15(Suppl 1) 17-24, 2000

375. Van Ypersele de Strihou C, Jadoul M, Malghem J, Maldague J, Jamart J and the working party on dialysis amyloidosis: Effect of dialysis membrane and patient's age on signs of dialysis-related amyloidosis. Kidney Int 39(5): 1012-1019, 1991

376. Jadoul M, Garbar C, Noel H, Sennesael J, Vanholder R, Bernaert P, Rorive G, Hanique G, van Ypersele de Strihou C: Histological prevalence of beta 2-microglobulin amyloidosis in hemodialysis: a prospective post-mortem study. Kidney Int 51(6): 1928-1932, 1997

377. Kessler M, Netter P, Azoulay E, Mayeux D, Pere P, Gaucher A: Dialysis-associated arthropathy: a multicentre survey of 171 patients receiving haemodialysis for over 10 years. The Co-operative Group on Dialysis-associated Arthropathy. Br J Rheumatol 31(3): 57-162, 1992

378. Harris SAC, Brown EA: Patients surviving more than 10 years on haemodialysis. The natural history of the complications of treatment. Nephrol Dial Transplant 13(5): 1226-1233, 1998

379. Baz M, Durand C, Ragon A, Jaber K, Andrieu D, Merzouk T, Purgus R, Olmer M, Reynier JP, Berland Y: Using ultrapure water in hemodialysis delays carpal tunnel syndrome. Int J Artif Organs 14(11): 681-685, 1991

380. Schwalbe S, Holzhauer M, Schaeffer J, Galanski M, Koch KM, Floege J: ß2-microglobulin associated amyloidosis: a vanishing complication of long-term hemodialysis. Kidney Int 52: 1077-1083, 1997

381. Kleophas W, Haastert B, Backus G, Hilgers P, Westhoff A, van Endert G: Long-term experience with an ultrapure individual dialysis fluid with a batch type machine. Nephrol Dial Transplant 13: 3118-3125, 1998

382. Miura Y, Ishiyama T, Inomata A, Takeda T; Senma S, Okuyama K, Susuki Y: Radionlucent bone cysts and the type of dialysis membrane used in patients undergoing long-term hemodialysis. Nephron 60: 268-273, 1992

383. Van Ypersele de Strihou C, Floege J, Jadoul M, Koch KM: Amyloidosis and its relationship to different dialysers. Nephrol Dial Transplant 9(Suppl 2): 156-161, 1994

384. Van Ypersele de Strihou C: Are biocompatible membranes superior for hemodialysis therapy? Kidney Int 52(Suppl 62): S101-S104, 1997

385. Schiffl H, Fischer R, Lang SM, Mangel E: Clinical manifestations of AB-amyloidosis: effects of biocompatibility and flux. Nephrol Dial Transplant 15: 840-845, 2000

386. Pickett TM, Cruickshank A, Greenwood RN, Taube D, Davenport A, Farrington K: Membrane flux not biocompatibility determines beta-2-microglobulin levels in hemodialysis patients. Blood Purif 20(2): 161-166, 2002

387. Brunner FP, Brynger H, Ehrich JHH, Fassbinder W, Geerlings W, Rizzono G, Selwood NH, Tufveson G, Wing AJ: Case contol study on dialysis arthropathy: the influence of two different dialysis membranes: data from the EDTA registry. Nephrol Dial Transplant 5: 432-436, 1990

388. Chanard J, Bindi P, Lavaud S, Toupnce O, Maheut H, Lacour F: Carpal tunnel syndrome and type of dialysis membrane. BMJ 298: 867-868, 1989

389. Küchle C, Fricke H, Held E, Schiffl H: High-flux hemodialysis postpones clinical manifestation of dialysis related amyloidosis. Am J Nephrol 16(6): 484-488, 1996

390. Takenaka T, Itaya Y, Tsichiya Y, Kobayashi K, Suszuki H: Fitness of biocompatible high-flux hemofiltration for dialysis-related amyloidosis. Blood Purif 19(1): 10-14, 2001

391. Lin CL, Yang CW, Chiang CC, Chang CT, Huang CC: Long-term on-line hemodiafiltration reduces predialysis beta-2-microglobulin levels in chronic hemodialysis patients. Blood Purif 19(3): 301-307, 2001

392. Locatelli F, Marcelli D, Conte F, Limido A, Malberti F, Spotti D: Comparison of mortality in ESRD patients on convective and diffusive extracorporeal treatments. The registro Lombardo Dialyisi E Trapianto. Kidney Int 55(1): 286-293, 1999.

393. Nakai S, Iseki K, Tabei K, Kubo K, Masakane I, Fushimi K, Kikuchi K, Shinzato T, Sanaka T, Akiba T: Outcomes of hemodiafiltration based on Japanese dialysis patient registry. Am J Kidney Dis 38(4, Suppl 1): S212-216, 2001

394. Hakim RM, Wingerd RL, Husni L, Parker RA, Parker III TF: The effect of membrane biocompatibility on plasma ß2-microglobulin levels in chronic hemodialysis patients. J Am Soc Nephrol 7(3): 472-478, 1996

395. Campistol JM, Bernard D, Papastoitsis G, Sole M, Kasirsky J, Skinner M: Polymerization of normal and intact ß2-microglobulin as amyloidogenic protein in dialysis-amyloidosis. Kidney Int 50: 1262-1257, 1996

396. Lehnert H, Jakob C, Marzoll I , Schmidt-Gayk H, Stein G, Ritz E: Prevalence of dialysis related amyloidosis in diabetic patients. Nephrol Dial Transplant 11(19): 2004-2007, 1996

397. Goldfarb-Rumyantzev AS, Cheung AK, Leypold JK: Computer simulation of small-solute and middle-molecule removal during short daily and long thrice-weekly hemodialysis. Am J Kidney Dis 40(6): 1211-1218, 2002

398. Gotch FA, Levin NW: Daily dialysis: the long and the short of it. Blood Purif 21: 271-281, 2003

399. Pierratos A: Nocturnal haemodialysis: an update on a 5-years experiance. Nephrol Dial Transplant 14: 2835-2840, 1999

400. Raj DSC, Ouwendyk M, Francoeur R, Pierratos A: ß2-microglobulin kinetics in nocturnal haemodialysis. Nephrol Dial Transplant 15: 58-64, 2000

401. Maduell F, Navarro V, Torregrosa E, Rius A, Dicenta F, Cruz MC, Ferrero JA: Change from three times a week on-line hemodiafiltration to short daily on-line hemodiafiltration. Kidney Int 64: 305-313, 2003

402. Hiyama E, Hyodo T, Kondo M, Otsuka K, Honma T, Taira T, Yoshida K, Uchida T, Endo T, Sakai T, Baba S, Hidai H: Performance of the newer type (Lixelle Type S-15) on direct hemoperfusion beta-2-microglobulin adsorption column for dialysis-related amyloidosis. Nephron 92(2): 501-502, 2002

403. Suzuki K, Shimazaki M, Kutsuki H: Beta2-microglobulin-selective adsorbent column (Lixelle) for the treatment of dialysis-related amyloidosis. Therap Apher Dial 7(1): 104-107, 2003

404. Abe T, Uchita K, Orita H, Kamimura M, Oda M, Hasegawa H, Kobata H, Fukunishi M, Shimazaki M, Abe T, Akizawa T, Ahmad S: Effect of beta(2)-microglobulin adsorption column on dialysis-related amyloidosis. Kidney Int 64(4): 1522-1528, 2003

405. Kazama JJ, Maruyama H, Gejyo F: Reduction of circulating ß2-microglobulin level for the treatment of dialysis-relates amyloidosis. Nephrol Dial Transplant 16(Suppl 4): 31-35, 2001

406. Virga G, Mastrosimone S, Amici G, Munaretto G, Gastaldon F, Bonadonna A: Symptoms in hemodialysis patients and their relationship with biochemical and demographic parameters. Int J Artif Organs 21(12): 788-93, 1998

407. Goicoechea M, de Sequera P, Ochando A, Andrea C, Caramelo C: Uremic pruritus: an unresolved problem in hemodialysis patients. Nephron 82(1): 73-74, 1999

408. Schwartz IF, Iaina A: Uraemic pruritus. Nephrol Dial Transplant 14: 834-839, 1999

409. Merkus MP, Jager KJ, Dekker FW, de Haan RJ, Boeschoten EW, Krediet RT: Physical symptoms and quality of life in patients on chronic dialysis: results of The Netherlands Cooperative Study on Adequacy of Dialysis (NECOSAD). Nephrol Dial Transplant 14(5): 1163-1170, 1999

410. Kato A, Takita T, Furuhashi M, Takahashi T, Watanabe T, Maruyama Y, Hishida A: Polymethylmethacrylate efficacy in reduction of renal itching in hemodialysis patients: crossover study and role of tumor necrosis factor-α. Artif Organs 25(6): 441-447, 2001

411. Mettang T, Pauli-Magnus C, Alscher DM: Uraemic pruritus- new perspectives and insights from recent trials. Nephrol Dial Transplant 17: 1558-1563, 2002

412. Mamianetti A, Tripodi V, Vescina C, Garrido D, Viziolo N, Carducci C, Carreño AC: Serum bile acids and pruritus in hemodialysis patients. Clin Nephrol 53(3): 194-198, 2000

413. Virga G, Visentin I, La Milia V, Bonadonna A: Inflammation and pruritus in haemodialysis patients. Nephrol Dial Transplant 17: 2164-2169, 2002

414. Kimmel M, Alscher D, Dunst R, Kuhlmann U, MettangT: The role of inflammation in uraemic pruritus. (Abstract) Nephrol Dial Transpl 18(Suppl 4): 206-207, 2003

415. Hiroshige K, Kabashima N, Tagasugi M, Kuroiwa A: Optimal dialysis improves uremic pruritus. Am J Kidney Dis 25: 413-419, 1995

416. Kato A, Hamada M, Maryama T, Matyama Y, Hishida A: Pruritus and hydration state of stratum corneum in hemodialysis patients. Am J Nephrol 20: 437-442, 2000

417. Ståhle-Backdahl M, Wahlgren CF, Hägermark O: Computerized recording of itch in patients on maintenance hemodialysis. Acta Derm Venereol 69(5): 410-414, 1989

418. Dimkovic N, Djukanovic L, Radmilovic A, Bojic P, Juloski T: Uremic pruritus and cell mast cells. Nephron (61): 5-9, 1992

419. Robles NR, Murga L, Galvan S, Esparrago JF, Sanchez-Casado E: Hemodialysis with cuprophane or polysulfone: effects on uremic polyneuropathy. Am J Kidney Dis 21(3): 282-287, 1993

420. Malberti F, Surian M, Farina M, Vitelli E, Mandolfo S, Guri L, De Petri GC, Castellani A: Effect of hemodialysis and hemodiafiltration on uremic polyneuropathy. Blood Purif 9(5-6): 285-295, 1991

421. Robles NR, Solis M, Albarran L, Esperrago JF, Roncero F, Sanchez-Casado E: Sympathetic skin response in hemodialysis patients: correlation with nerve conduction studies and adequacy in dialysis. Nephron 82(1): 12-6, 1999

422. Laaksonen S, Voipio-Pulkki, Erkinjuntti M, Asola M, Falck B: Does dialysis therapy improve autonomic and peripheral nervous system abnormailties in chronic uraemia? J Intern Med 248(1): 21-28, 2000

423. Okada H, Moriwaki K, Kanno Y, Sugahara S, Nakamoto H, Yoshizawa M, Suzuki H: Vitamin B6 supplementation can improve peripheral polyneuropathy in patients with chronic renal failure on high-flux haemodialysis and human recombinant erythropoietin. Nephrol Dial Transpl 15: 1410-1413, 2000

424. Robles NR, Cancho B, Pizarro J, Solis M, Alvarez Mato C, Sanchez-Casado E: Acute effect of hemodialysis with polyacrylonitrile membrane on nerve conduction velocities. Ren Fail 23(2): 251-257, 2000

11. Cumulative effects of patient, treatment and device factors on mortality

Although mortality in end stage renal disease (ESRD) has decreased over the past few decades, it is still substantially higher than in the general, non-dialysis population. For example, recently, all-cause death rates in the U.S. were shown to be almost four times higher in dialysis patients aged 65 or older than in the general Medicare population, irrespective of gender, race or diabetic status; the expected remaining life-span in the dialysis patient group was estimated to be less than one quarter to one fifth of that of the general population [1]. This reflects that, in addition to the generally recognised mortality risk factors, ESRD involves further specific uraemia-associated risk factors. Some of these are already present at the chronic kidney disease stage, meaning that the mortality risk in chronic renal failure is already increased compared to the general population, and that this risk reaches its maximum in end-stage renal disease (see **figure 11.1**). The specific uraemia-associated mortality risk factors will be described in detail below (chapter 11.1).

As was shown in sections B and C and in chapter 10, dialyser and haemofilter characteristics essentially determine dialysis adequacy and biocompatibility and, thus, may directly or indirectly contribute to major clinical problems in ESRD. These problems comprise both disturbed pathophysiological pathways (e.g. chronic inflammatory state, oxidative and carbonyl stress) and defined illnesses, such as malnutrition, renal anaemia, loss of residual renal function, atherosclerosis, susceptibility to infection, amyloidosis, pruritus and peripheral nerve dysfunction (see **figure 10.1**). In this chapter, many of these diseases are identified as risk factors for mortality in ESRD. The possible association between dialyser and haemofilter choice and mortality in ESRD will be addressed in chapter 11.2.

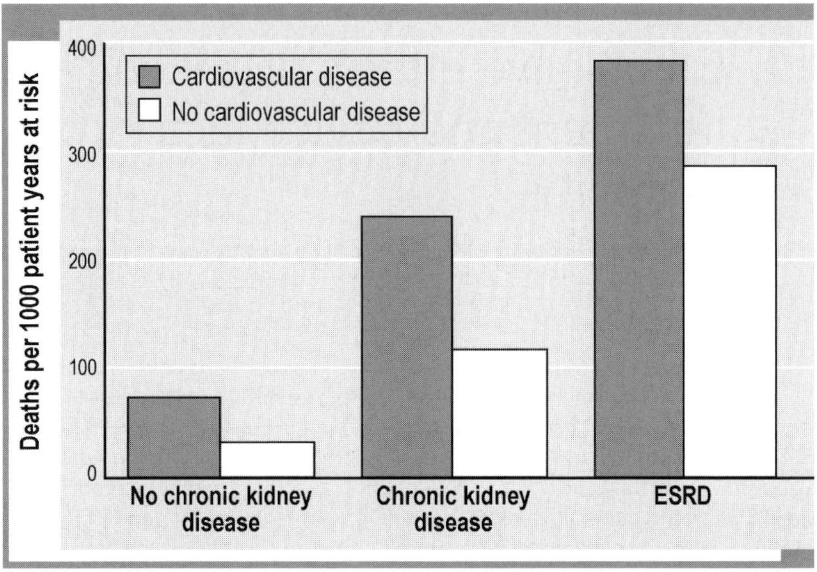

Figure 11.1: Cardiovascular and non-cardiovascular mortality in the dialysis population, patients with chronic kidney disease and the general Medicare population in patients aged 65 and older. *Mortality rates, irrespective of cardiovascular disease, are already elevated in chronic kidney disease and reach a maximum in ESRD (adapted from [1]).*

11.1 Specific ESRD-associated mortality factors

In addition to the generally recognised risk factors contributing to mortality, such as age, gender, race, hypertension, smoking, dyslipidaemia and hyperglycaemia, dialysis patients are subject to additional uraemia-associated risk factors. Increasing insight into these has been gained over the past decades of dialysis therapy development, and ongoing research and/or large observational mortality statistics in ESRD patients provide us with even more details. Evidence-based therapeutic recommendations for risk prevention have already been developed for some well-known uraemia-associated risk factors. Examples are dialysis adequacy (e.g. [2-5]), anaemia (e.g. [6, 7]), malnutrition (e.g. [8]), cardiovascular (atherosclerotic) risk factors (e.g. [5, 9, 10, 11]), dialysis-associated infections and chronic inflammation (e.g. [5]), hyperphosphat-

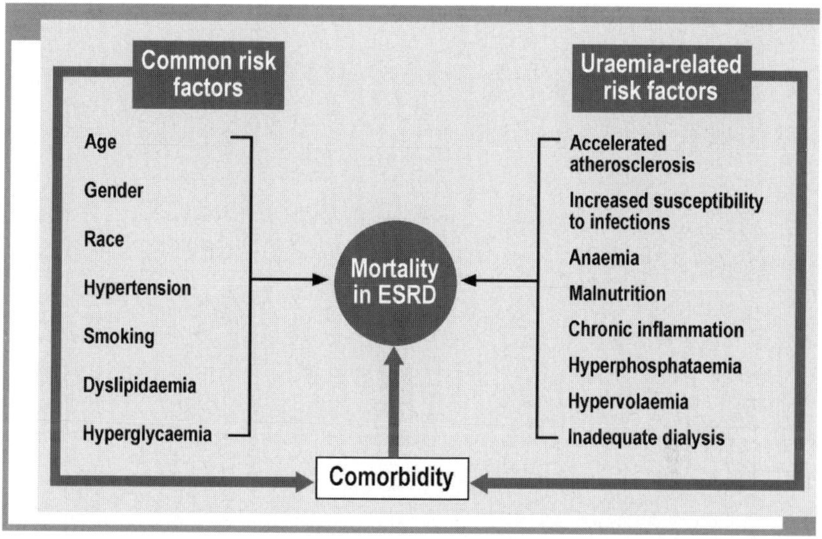

Figure 11.2: Common and uraemia-related risk factors that influence mortality of ESRD patients.

aemia (e.g. [5, 12]) and interdialysis hypervolaemia (e.g. [5]). The impact of these risk factors on mortality in ESRD is summarised in **table 11.1**; the table also includes some official guidelines for prevention and therapy, as well as possible influences of dialysis adequacy and dialyser characteristics on these factors. The possible contribution of dialyser characteristics to mortality will be discussed in chapter 11.2 in more detail. Finally, the common presence of comorbid conditions amplifies the problem in ESRD, as shown in **figure 11.2** (see also [14, 21, 24, 32, 34, 61-64]).

Mortality risk factor in ESRD	Parameters studied	Impact on mortality in ESRD	Official therapy or prevention guidelines	Influence of dialysis adequacy	Possible influence of dialyser characteristics
Accelerated atherosclerosis	Deaths due to cardio-, cerebro- and peripheral vascular diseases	One report of a 3 - 7 times increased cardiovascular mortality compared to the general population (depending on patients age) [1] (see **fig. 11.3**). Association between atherosclerosis and mortality (e.g. [13,14])	DOQI™ guidelines for managing dyslipidaemia in CKD: regular assessment of lipid status, treatment of dyslipidaemia [9] EBP guidelines VII.1-2: regular assessment of cardiovascular risk factors (smoking, hyperglycaemia, dyslipidaemia, hypertension) and treatment thereof [5]	?	Probable (see chapter 10.5)
Increased susceptibility to infections	Deaths due to infection	Constitutes 7 - 12% (e.g. [1, 15, 16]) up to 23% [17] of the deaths in ESRD. Sepsis-associated mortality in ESRD is 30 - 50 times higher than in the general population [18, 19]	EBP guideline VI.I: guaranteed dialysis adequacy, prevention of malnutrition, satisfactory haemoglobin level, avoidance of iron overload, use of biocompatible membranes [5]	Yes	Possible (see chapters 8 and 10.6)

Anaemia	Hb, Hct	Association between degree of anaemia and mortality (e.g. [1, 20-22])	DOQI™: Hb 11-12 g/dl (Hct 33 - 36%) [7] EBP-guideline 5: Hb > 11 g/dl (Hct > 33%) [6]	Yes	Possible (see chapter 10.3)
Malnutrition	Plasma albumin, weight, BMI, PNA anthropometry, subj. glob. nutr. ass., hand grip strength and others	Association between malnutrition and mortality (e.g. [1, 13, 14, 23-38])	DOQI™: stipulates levels of several clinical and laboratory parameters, e.g. serum albumin > 4 g/dl [8]	Yes	Probable (see chapter 10.5)
Chronic inflammation	CRP, IL-6 and others	Association between mortality and higher levels of acute phase proteins and/or pro-inflammatory cytokines (e.g. [14, 33, 37, 39-45])	EBP guidelines VII 5.1-2: 3-monthly CRP testing; if CRP levels > 8 mg/l then screening for silent infection of haemodialysis access grafts, paradontitis or other low-grade infections, also checking of membrane biocompatibility and dialysis fluid purity [5]	?	Probable (see chapter 10.1.1)

Mortality risk factor in ESRD	Parameters studied	Impact on mortality in ESRD	Official therapy or prevention guidelines	Influence of dialysis adequacy	Possible influence of dialyser characteristics
Hyper-phosphataemia	Phosphate level, calcium-phosphate product	Association between mortality and phosphate and/or calcium-phosphate product levels (e.g. [21, 46, 47])	DOQI™ guidelines for bone metabolism and disease in CKD: target ranges: 1.13-1.78 mmol/l (i.e.3.5 - 5.5 mg/dl) for serum phosphate; 150 - 300 pg/ml for PTH; < 55 mg^2/dl^2 for normal calcium-phosphate product level [12] EBP guideline VII.3: target ranges: 0.8 - 1.8 mmol/l (i.e. 2.5 - 5.5 mg/dl) for serum phosphate; < 55 mg^2/dl^2 for normal calcium-phosphate product level [5]	Yes (?)	Probably (see chapter 5.2)
Dialysis prescription: *time*	Interdialytic hypertension, ultrafiltration volume	Association between haemodialysis time and mortality (e.g. [23, 28, 48])	EBP guideline II.5.1: weekly treatment times of $\geq 3 \times 4$ h [5]	-	-
Dialysis prescription: *adequacy*	Kt/V, URR	Association between dialysis adequacy and mortality (e.g. [1, 21, 24, 28, 34, 49-60])	DOQI™/ The Ren. Assoc. (UK) / Can. Soc. Nephrol.: minimum e-Kt/V ≥ 1.0 (sp-Kt/V ≥ 1.2), URR ≥ 65% [2-4] EBP-guideline II.1.3: e-Kt/V ≥ 1.2 (sp-Kt/V ≥ 1.4) [5]	-	Yes

Table 11.1: Specific uraemia-associated risk factors that influence mortality in ESRD. *The impact of various mortality risk factors, some official guidelines for prevention and therapy, and possible influences of dialysis adequacy and dialyser characteristics are shown. BMI: body mass index; PNA: protein nitrogen appearance; PTH: parathyroidhormone; e: equilibrated; sp: single-pool; Hb: haemoglobin; Hct: haematocrit; CKD: chronic kidney disease; EBP: European Best Practice Guidelines; DOQI™: Kidney Disease Outcomes Quality Initiative from the US National Kidney Foundation; URR: urea reduction ratio; subj. glob. nutr. ass.: subjective, global nutritional assessment.*

The actual impact of the aforementioned risk factors on mortality in ESRD can best be explained using key figures from selected studies. **Figures 11.1, 11.3** and **11.4** show the high incidence of cardiovascular mortality in ESRD compared to the general population (a consequence of the accelerated atherosclerosis commonly present dialysis patients (see **figure 10.14**)); the difference is greatest at younger ages (**figure 11.3**) [16, 65]. **Figure 11.4** also demonstrates that not only cardiac problems, but also infections contribute significantly to death in ESRD. It further illustrates that the primary cause of end-stage renal failure plays a similar role in both all-cause and cardiac mortality in ESRD. **Figure 11.5** depicts the association between haemoglobin level and death risk, showing an increased risk of death at haemoglobin values below 10 -11 g/dl [1]. **Figure 11.6** demonstrates the relationship between malnutrition and survival in ESRD [14]. **Figures 11.7** and **11.8** show the association between mortality in ESRD and levels of C-reactive protein and interleukin-6, respectively; both these markers are indicators of chronic inflammation which, in turn, contributes to the three main diseases atherosclerosis, anaemia and malnutrition [40, 43].

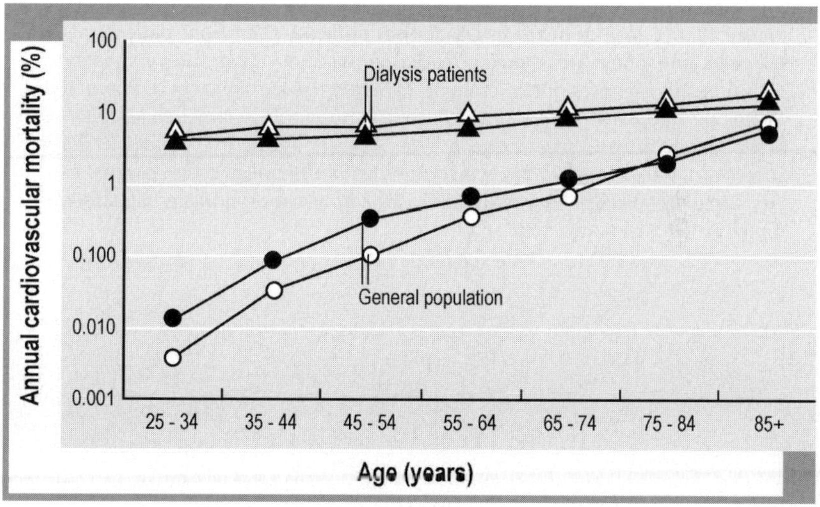

Figure 11.3: Cardiovascular mortality by age and race in the general population and in dialysis patients. *Filled and open symbols represent the black and the white population, respectively (adapted from [65]).*

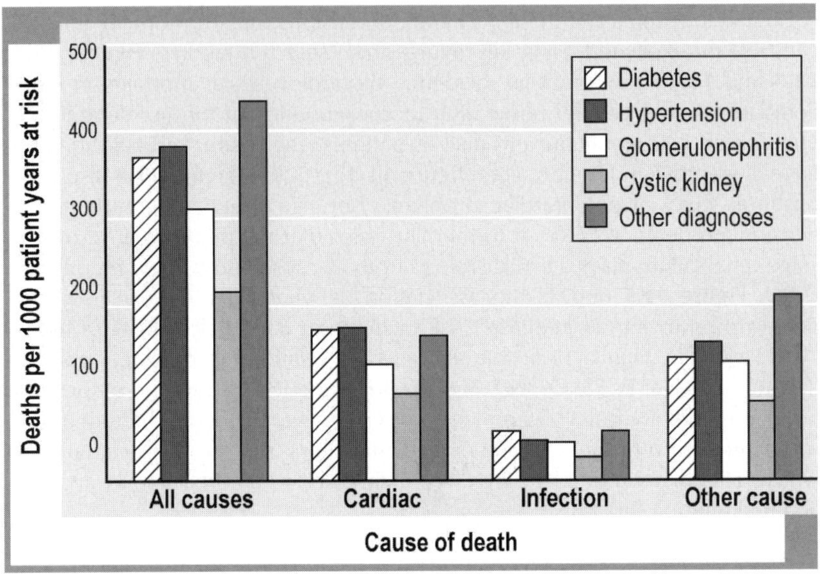

Figure 11.4: Cause of death in US dialysis patients. Data from patients aged 65 years and older are shown. *Unadjusted all-cause death rates for patients with primary diagnoses of diabetes and hypertension are similar at 370 and 382 deaths per thousand patient years. Patients with chronic glomerulonephritis or cystic kidney disease have mortality rates lower than these (311 and 215, respectively) and lower than those associated with other diagnoses (i.e. renal cancer, vasculitis, AIDS nephropathy). Cardiac and all-cause mortality rates follow similar patterns (adapted from [1]).*

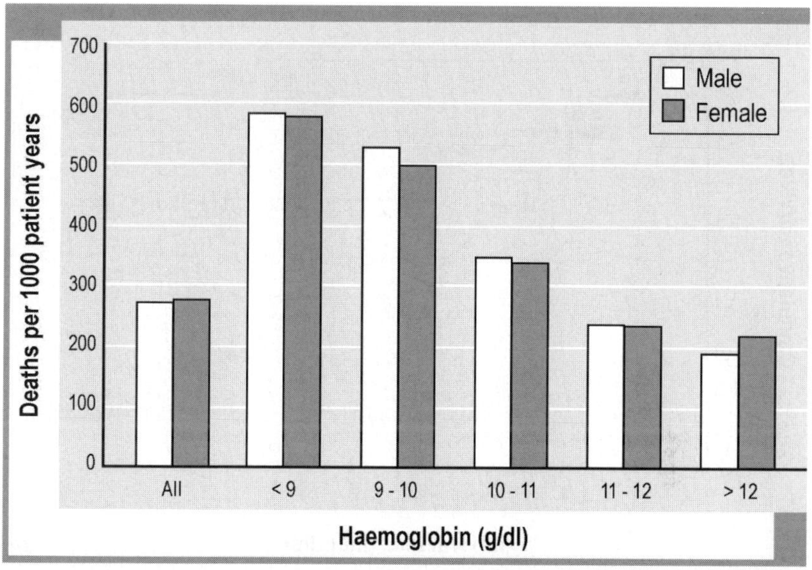

Figure 11.5: Haemoglobin level and survival in ESRD. *One-year mortality rates are adjusted for urea reduction rate (from the USRDS data report 2002 [1]).*

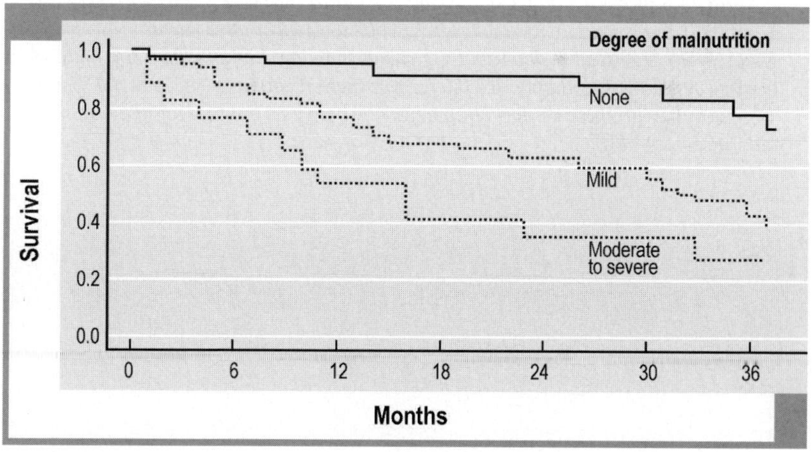

Figure 11.6: Malnutrition and survival in haemodialysis patients. *Kaplan-Meier survival curves for patients with normal nutritional status (n = 46), mild malnutrition (n = 65) and moderate to severe malnutrition (n = 17) based on subjective global nutritional assessment (adapted from [14]).*

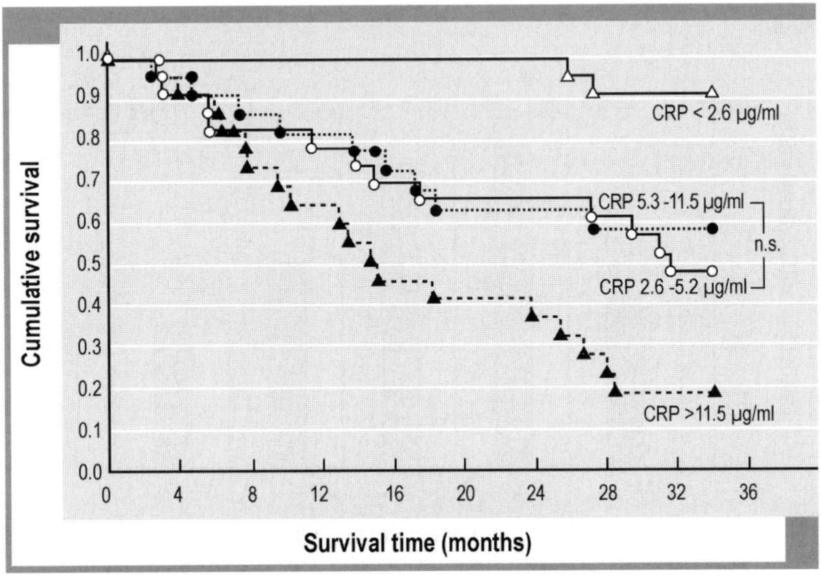

Figure 11.7: CRP levels and survival in haemodialysis patients. *Kaplan–Meier estimates of survival in 91 haemodialysis patients. Serum C-reactive protein (CRP, µg/ml) quartiles were CRP > 11.5 µg/ml (highest quartile), CRP between 5.3 and 11.5 µg/l, CRP between 2.6 and 5.2 µg/ml, and CRP < 2.6 µg/ml (lowest quartile). Lower serum CRP values are associated with better survival. All differences were statistically significant (p values ranging from 0.0001 for highest quartile vs. lowest quartile to 0.012 for highest quartile vs. quartile 5.3 - 11.5 µg/ml), with the exception of differences between the two middle quartiles (adapted from [43]).*

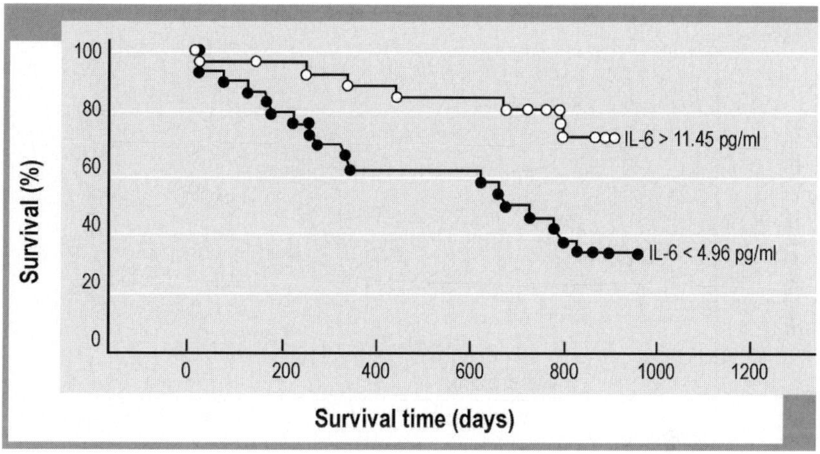

Figure 11.8: Interleukin-6 levels and survival in haemodialysis patients. *Kaplan-Meier survival plots adjusted for age, albumin level and body mass index in 89 patients stratified by interleukin-6 values (IL-6). Data for patients with IL-6 levels in the highest and lowest tertiales are shown, i.e. IL-6 values > 11.45 pg/ml and < 4.96 pg/ml, respectively. The adjusted mortality rate for patients with the lower IL-6 values was 33%; this was significantly higher (58%, p < 0.001) for those patients with higher IL-6 values (adapted from [40]).*

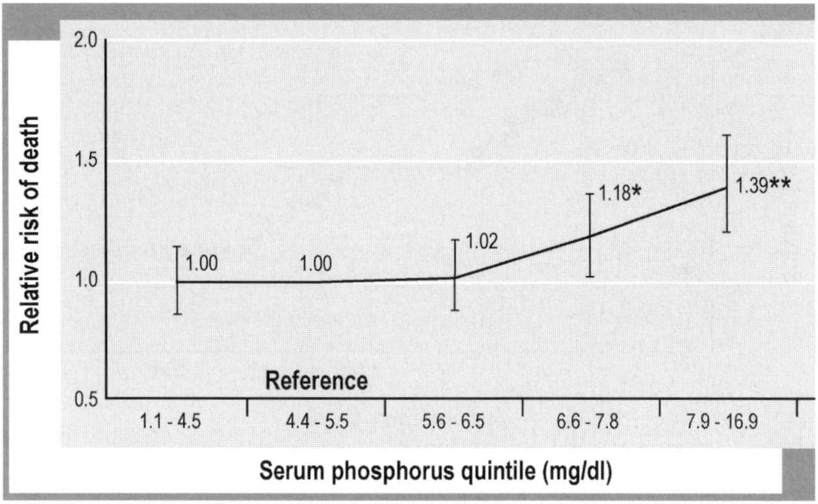

Figure 11.9: Phosphorus levels and mortality. *The relative risks of death (RR) for quintiles of serum phosphorus levels in 6407 dialysis patients are shown. Vertical bars indicate the 5% to 95% confidence intervals. RR increases with serum phosphorus level > 6.5 mg/dl. *p < 0.03, **p < 0.0001 vs. reference (adapted from [46]).*

Figure 11.9 illustrates an increased relative risk of death in patients with phosphorus levels above 6.5 mg/dl, probably due to the augmented risk of hyperparathyroidism, extraskeletal calcification and vascular sclerosis [46]. A study on the association between adherence to the proposed NKF-K/DOQI™ bone metabolism and disease guidelines (see **table 11.1**) and mortality was recently published and involved several thousand US patients. Patients within both serum parathyroid hormone and calcium phosphate product guideline ranges demonstrated a significantly lower risk of mortality ($p < 0.001$) than those with one of these parameters outside the recommended range. In addition, patients with calcium phosphate product values within the recommended range had a lower mortality than those with values above the range ($p < 0.001$) [47]. In **figures 11.10** and **11.11**, the influence of the two dialysis treatment parameters "time spent per treatment" and "dialysis dose delivered" on the relative risk of death are presented. Dialysis adequacy has long been recognised as a mortality risk (e.g. [1, 21, 24, 28, 34, 49-59]). Consequently, most guidelines define the minimum threshold value for dialysis dose to be between 1.0 and 1.2 eKt/V (see **table 11.1**). However, in the study

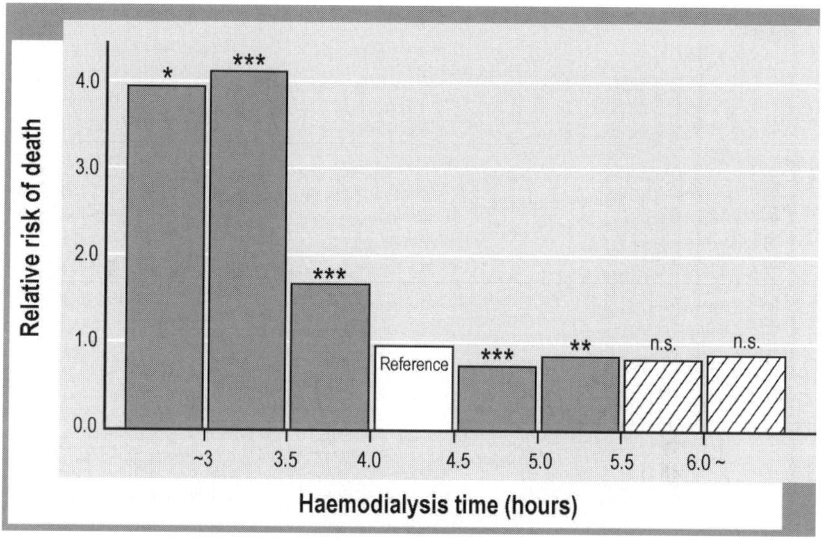

Figure 11.10: Haemodialysis time and death risk. *The relative risk of death increases sharply at dialysis treatment times of less than four hours, and is lowest at treatment times of 4.5 to 5 hours. The slight reincrease in relative risk of death for dialysis times above five hours might be due to other risk factors in the patient group that demand such long treatment times, e.g. cardiovascular instability or excessive interdialysis weight gain. *p < 0.05, **p < 0.01, ***p < 0.0001 vs. reference (adapted from [28]).*

presented in **figure 11.11**, increasing Kt/V values even up to 1.8 decreased the death risk in a selected Asian patient population (small body size) [28]. These results were supported by another large observational survey of 33,608 US patients: percentage survival time increased by up to 146% when spKt/V was increased from 1.2 to 1.6 ($p < 0.001$) [59]. Recently published results of the HEMO study did not show this dose effect on all-cause mortality in 1846 patients when an eKt/V of 1.16 ± 0.08 was compared with an eKt/V of 1.53 ± 0.09 [36]. Analysis of subgroups showed possible interactions between dialysis dose and sex: a higher dialysis dose decreased mortality in females, but not in males ($p = 0.01$) ([36], reviewed in [60]). This positive effect of dialysis dose on mortality in females was also found in another study, which compared urea reduction rates of >70% with those of 65-70% [58]. These results exemplify the ongoing research and debate in evaluating patient mortality in relation to dialysis adequacy. Whereas some authors state that the results of

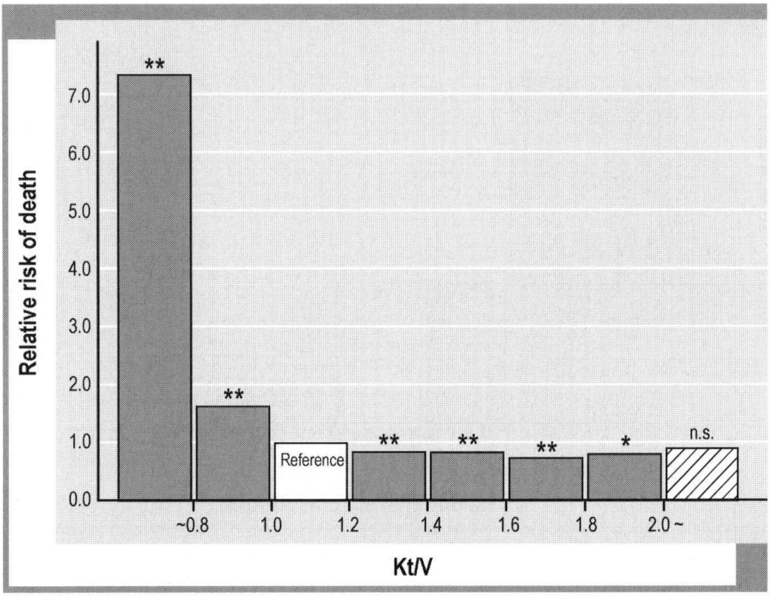

Figure 11.11: Haemodialysis adequacy and death risk. *The relative risk of death in 53,867 Japanese patients was determined for varying values of Kt/V. The relative risk of death decreased with an increasing Kt/V up to 1.8. *p < 0.005, **p < 0.0001 vs. reference (adapted from [28]).*

the HEMO study support the theory that a dialysis dose of 1.3 spKt/V (corresponding to an URR of 65%) is fully adequate [66, 67], others do not completely agree and urge further exploration of the subject [68-72]. Reasons for disagreement are, for example, the wide treatment time window (2.5 - 4.5 hours), the use of dialysers that were reused up to 20 times, the exclusion of patients with large body sizes (> 90 kg) by the randomisation mode [68], and the high percentage (60%) of patients on high-flux dialysis with a mean spKt/V of 1.6 at initiation of the study. The last point possibly resulted in actual dose reduction after enrolment in the standard dialysis group, with an ensuing carryover effect [70]. Further insight into the effects of increasing dialysis dose on mortality will, hopefully, become available after publication of other studies now in progress (e.g. [73]) and/or after complete analysis of the subgroups and statistics in the HEMO study [36, 74-76]. Treatment time is a major determinant of dialysis dose, being the "t" in Kt/V: treatment times below 4 hours were also associated with increased mortality, as shown in **figure 11.10**.

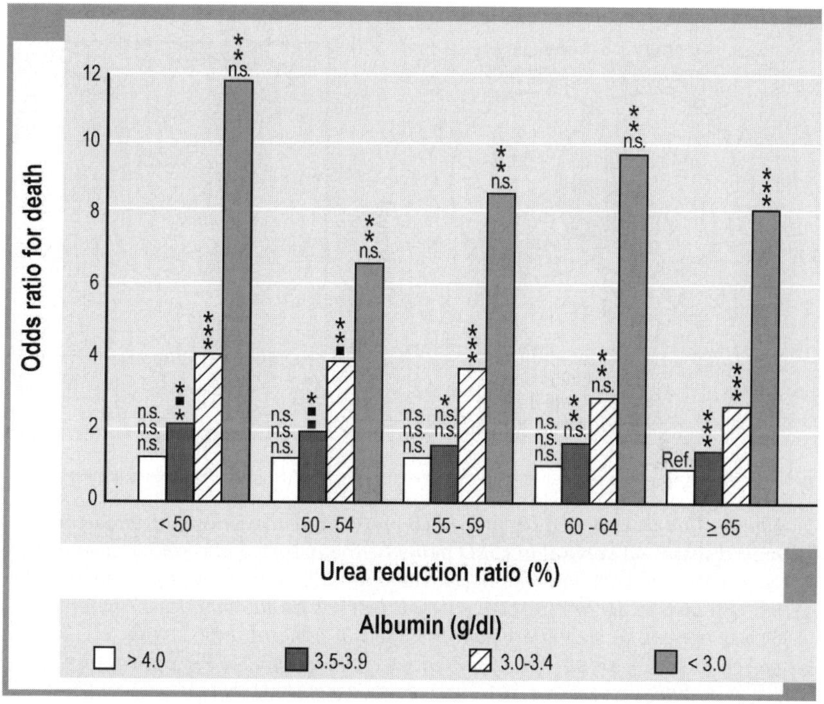

Figure 11.12: Impact of serum albumin and urea reduction rate on mortality. *Odds ratios for death were calculated for 13,473 haemodialysis patients with various serum albumin concentrations and urea reduction ratios. Low urea reduction rates were associated with increased odds ratio for death. These risks are enhanced by inadequate nutrition. An odds ratio of 1.0 was assigned to the reference group (Ref.) with an urea reduction ratio (URR) of ≥ 65% and a serum albumin concentration of ≥ 4.0 g/dl. The top symbols on the bars indicate the statistical significance compared to the reference group; the middle symbols indicate p values for comparisons with a serum albumin level of ≥ 4.0 g/dl; and the bottom symbols indicate p values for comparisons with an URR of ≥ 65%. n.s: not significant (p > 0.05); ▪ p = 0.05 to> 0.01, * p ≤ 0.01 (adapted from [24])*

Finally, the common presence of comorbid conditions amplifies the risk of death in ESRD. Even almost ten years ago, the cumulative effect of low albumin values (a measure for malnutrition) and low urea reduction rates (a measure for low dialysis dose) on patient mortality was described (**figure 11.12**) [24]. The amplified influence of the presence of cardiovascular dis-

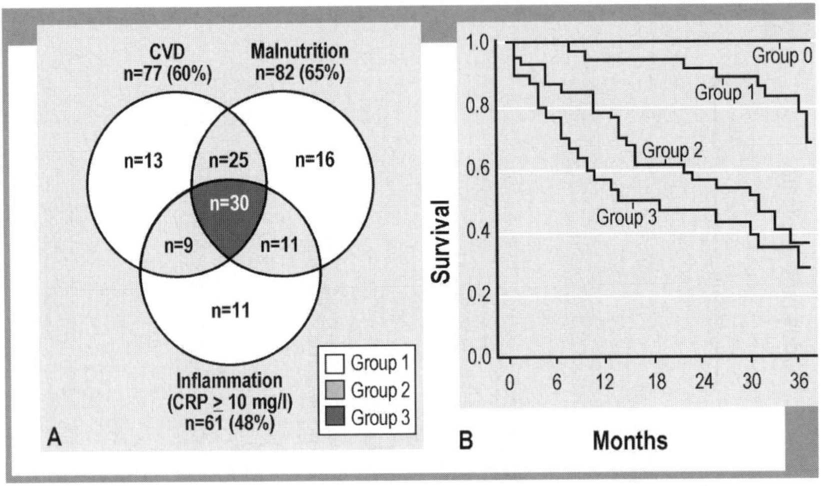

Figures 11.13A and 11.13B: Individual and cumulative effects of three common diseases on survival in ESRD patients. *The presence of cardiovascular disease (CVD), malnutrition and inflammation in 128 haemodialysis patients studied is shown in figure A. Patient survival depends on the number of these risk factors present, as shown in figure B. Group 0: none of these risk factors (RF) present (n = 13); group 1: 1 RF present (n = 39); group 2: 2 RFs present (n = 4; group 3: 3 RFs present (n = 30). Survival was significantly different (log-rank test) between groups 0 and 2 (p = 0.007), 0 and 3 (p = 0.003), 1 and 2 (p = 0.0002), and 1 and 3 (p = 0.0001), but not between groups 0 and 1 (p = 0.17) and 2 and 3 (p = 0.29) (adapted from [14]).*

ease, malnutrition (defined by subjective global nutritional assessment) and inflammation (serum CRP ≥ 10 mg/dl) on mortality in ESRD was recently studied in 128 haemodialysis patients. The distribution of these three common diseases, each an independent risk factor for mortality, among the patients studied is shown in **figure 11.13A**. The cumulative effect of the presence of multiple risk factors on mortality is shown in **figure 11.13B**: after 36 months of observation, mortality was 0% when none of these complications were present, but was 75% in those patients having all three risk factors at baseline [14].

11.2 Influence of dialyser and haemofilter characteristics on mortality

In chapter 10, the possible influence of dialyser characteristics on those diseases and treatment aspects classified above as "uraemia-associated risk factors for mortality" was discussed in some detail; a short summary has been presented in **table 11.1**. Because dialyser characteristics contribute to most of these factors, one could expect that dialyser choice would influence mortality in ESRD. However, the clinical risk factors have multifactorial origins (with the exception of "dialysis prescription dose" and "dialysis prescription time"). Consequently, the dialyser is probably only one - major or minor - puzzle piece in the complicated aetiology of the complete disease. Interpretation of studies on the influence of dialyser characteristics on patient mortality is further complicated by the effects of comorbidity (which is common in ESRD patients), the variety of dialysers available (e.g. low-flux, high-flux, bioincompatible and biocompatible) and their application in different dialysis treatment modalities (i.e. the predominantly diffusive mode of haemodialysis or more convective haemodiafiltration and haemofiltration modes). Furthermore, technical details of the treatment procedure, such as the use of machines with ultrafiltration control, the degree of dialysis fluid purity and the practice of dialyser reprocessing, may also exert an additional influence on patient mortality rates. The key studies examining the effects of dialyser characteristics on mortality in ESRD are summarised in **table 11.2**. Unfortunately, almost all studies published to date are either retrospective or so-called "historical prospective" in nature and their design does often not allow a clear distinction between the effects of dialyser biocompatibility and flux on mortality. Therefore, the following studies will be analysed irrespective of these eventual overlapping influences, and the focus of attention will be placed on, three major points of interest: (1) studies comparing regenerated cellulose membranes with other membranes; (2) studies comparing modified cellulose membranes and synthetic membranes; and (3) studies comparing low-flux and high-flux dialysers.

Author/ year/ study design	Number of patients	Follow-up period	Membranes tested	Study characteristics	Effect on mortality
Levin et al. 1991 [77] Retrospective	986	5 years	RC (n = 438) Hf-PSu (n = 548)	No information on comorbidity or Kt/V	Relative risk of death was 1.0 for RC and 0.19 for Hf-PSu
Hornberger et al. 1992 [78] Retrospective, cross-over	253	1987-1991	RC (n = 146) Hf-PSu (n = 107)	Data adjusted for comorbidity but not for Kt/V: Kt/V Hf-PSu > RC (1.14 vs. 1.04)	80 deaths occurred (RC: 69; Hf-PSu: 11); annual mortality for Hf-PSu was 7% compared to 20% with RC ($p < 0.001$)
Chandran et al. 1993 [79] Retrospective	352	1981-1991	All pat. treated with PAN (AN69®), data compared to USRDS data of pat. treated with RC membranes	Pat. in the PAN group were younger (5 years), had higher PCR and serum alb. values, but lower Kt/V (0.93 vs. 1.46)	According to USRDS, 203 deaths would have been expected - only 132 deaths were recorded in the PAN group ($p < 0.001$)
Hakim et al. 1994 [80] Prospective	2325	?	RC (n = 1407) CDA / HE (n = 388) Hf-PSu / PAN (n = 530)	Kt/V and comorbidity controlled	Relative risk of death was 1.33 for RC, 1.03 for CDA / HE and 1.0 for Hf-PSu / PAN
Bonomini et al. 1995 [81] Retrospective	122	1963-1993	Cellul. (n = 64) (RC predominant at start of observation, 51% at end, CA 40% after 10 years) Synth. (n = 58) (PAN, PSu, PMMA)	Kt/V and albumin not different among the groups; no adjustment for comorbidity	No difference in survival between the groups

Hakim et al. 1996 [82] Hist. prospective	2410	1990-1991	RC (65%) Mod. C (16.1%): CA, CDA, CTA, HE Synth. (18.1%): PSu, PMMA, PAN, PA	Adjustment for comorbidity, Kt/V and patient demographics	Relative risk of death was 1.0 for RC, 0.74 for mod. C and 0.75 for synth. ($p < 0.002$)
Koda et al. 1997 [83] Retrospective	819	1968-1994	Lf: RC (77.4%), CA (19.9%), others (2.7%) Hf: PMMA (32.4%), CTA (28.6%), PAN (17.2%), PSu (16.7%), PEPA (3.4%), others (2.7%)	Kt/V only partially controlled, dialysis technology changed during the long observation period	Relative risk of death was 1.0 for Lf and 0.63 for Hf treatment ($p < 0.05$)
Port et al. 1998 [56] Retrospective	3563 (CMS study) 6585 (CMA study) 4619 (DMMS w1) 2037 (DMMS w2)	1986-1997	RC (70% in 1986, 22% in 1996) Mod. C (17% in 1986, 20% in 1996) Synth. (9% in 1986, 55% in 1996)	Kt/V increased by 0.2 during observation period	Extrapolation of a 5% reduction in mortality risk when synth. or mod. C are used compared to RC
Bloembergen et al. 1999 [84] Hist. prospective	6714 (Data from CMA study)	1990-1991	RC (62%) Mod. C (38%): CA, CDA, CTA, HE Synth. (19%): PSu, PMMA, PAN, PA	Data adjusted for comorbidity and Kt/V	Reduction of relative risk of death to 0.82 with mod. C / synth. vs. RC (1.0) ($p < 0.002$); no difference between mod.C and synth.

Author/ year/ study design	Number of patients	Follow-up period	Membranes tested	Study characteristics	Effect on mortality
Leypold et al. 1999 [85] Hist. prospective	1771 (Data from CMA study)	1990-1991	Membranes grouped according to middle molecule removal ability (total removal of vit. B_{12})	Data adjusted for Kt/V	A 10% increase in vit B_{12} Kt/V resulted in an approximately 5% reduction of mortality risk (RR = 0.952, $p < 0.0001$ vs. 1.0)
Locatelli et al. 1999 [86] Retrospective	6444	1983-1995	HD HDF/HF, membranes not specified	Data adjusted for comorbidity and Kt/V	No difference in adjusted death rate between HD and HDF/HF
Woods et al. 2000 [87] Retrospective	715	1991-1996	Lf-PSu (n = 252) Hf-PSu (n = 463)	Data partially adjusted for comorbidity; Kt/V higher in Hf-PSu than in Lf-PSu group (1.56 vs. 1.52, $p < 0.001$)	30% better survival with Hf-PSu than with Lf-PSu for non-diabetic patients ($p = 0.029$)
Port et al. 2001 [88] Retrospective	12,791	Start 1993	RC: 40%, Mod. C: 23% Synth. Hf: 26% Synth. Lf: 11%	Data adjusted for comorbidity and Kt/V	After adjustment for reuse agent and dialysis facility: lower risk of death for synth-Hf compared to all other types of membranes combined (RR: 0.82, $p = 0.0002$)

Eknoyan et al. for the HEMO study group, 2002 [36] Prospective	1846	1995-2001	Lf-membranes (ß2-m clear. < 10 ml/min (mean 3 ± 7 ml/min)) vs. Hf-membranes (ß-2m clear. > 20 ml/min (mean 34 ± 11 ml/min). Most common Lf dialysers: Lf-PSu (46%), CA (43%) (RC not allowed). Most common Hf dialysers: Hf-Psu (43%), CTA (48%)	*Targeted:* "Standard" HD dose (eKt/V of 1.04) vs. "high" HD dose (eKt/V of 1.45) *Mean values attained*: "standard" HD dose: eKt/V 1.16 ± 0.08 vs. "high" dose: eKt/V1.53 ± 0.09	No differences in all-cause mortality between Lf- and Hf-dialysis and between "standard" and "high" HD dose. Analysis of subgroups: Positive effect of dialysis dose on mortality in females ($p < 0.01$) Positive effects of Hf dialysis on cardiac deaths ($p < 0.05$) and on survival in patients dialysed > 3.7 years before study start ($p = 0.0071$)

Table 11.2: Effect of dialyser characteristics on patient mortality. *Data from selected studies are shown. Hf: high-flux; Lf: low-flux; RC: regenerated cellulose; mod. C: modified cellulose; CA: cellulose acetate; CDA: cellulose diacetate; CTA: cellulose triacetate, HE: Hemophan®; hist.: historical; cellul.: cellulosic; synth.: synthetic; PSu: polysulfone; PAN: polyacrylonitrile; PMMA: polymethylmethacrylate; PA: polyamide; Pat.: patients; clear.: clearance; CMS: case mix study; CMA: case mix adequacy study; DMMS: dialysis morbidity and mortality study; w1: wave 1; w2: wave2; HEMO study: haemodialysis membrane outcome study; RR: relative risk; vit.: vitamin; alb.: albumin.*

Regenerated cellulose membranes versus membranes made from other materials

Several studies report a negative influence of the use of membranes made from regenerated cellulose [77-80, 82, 84] or predominantly regenerated cellulose [56, 83] on patient mortality compared to the use of synthetic membranes [77-79] or a mixed group of modified cellulosic and synthetic membranes [56, 80, 82-84]. These studies often involved large patient populations of several thousand individuals [56, 80, 82, 84], but data were sometimes not adjusted for comorbidity [77, 79, 81] or Kt/V [77, 78, 83, 87], both of which are known to influence mortality in ESRD. In addition, regenerated cellulose dialysers are sometimes compared with dialysers of varying biocompatibility *and* performance characteristics. For example, modified cellulosic and synthetic membranes are often grouped together, although the modified cellulose membranes are predominantly low-flux while the synthetic membranes can be either low-flux or high-flux. This makes it virtually impossible to differentiate between effects due biocompatibility and effects due performance [56, 81]. Only in two of the studies in which membranes made from regenerated cellulose were used predominantly and during most of the observation period, no influence of dialyser choice on mortality was found [81, 86]. Up to now, no proof has been presented for superior survival with low-flux biocompatible dialysers compared to their low-flux bioincompatible counterparts [5].

Modified cellulosic membranes versus synthetic membranes

Patient mortality using modified cellulosic membranes did not differ from that using synthetic membranes in two studies. One of these studies compared cellulose diacetate or Hemophan® with high-flux polysulfone or polyacrylonitrile [80], and the other compared cellulose acetate, cellulose diacetate, cellulose triacetate or Hemophan® with polysulfone, polymethylmethacrylate, polyacrylonitrile or polyamide [82]. Another study involving 12,791 patients found a reduced relative risk of death ($RR = 0.82$, $p = 000.2$), in patients treated with synthetic high-flux membranes (26% of all patients) compared to patients treated with all other types of membranes combined (regenerated cellulose (40%), modified cellulose (23%), synthetic low-flux (11%)) [88].

Low-flux versus high-flux membranes

A number of studies compared mortality rates with low-flux and high-flux dialysers; the low-flux membranes investigated were regenerated cellulose [81, 83], cellulose acetate [81, 83], cellulose diacetate [80] and Hemophan® [80], and the high-flux membranes were cellulose triacetate [83], polymethyl-methacrylate [81, 83], polyacrylonitrile [81, 83], polysulfone [81, 83] and PEPA® [81]. In one study [83], the relative risk of death was found to be lower in the high-flux group than the low-flux group (0.63 versus 1.0; $p < 0.05$). However, the other studies found no difference between the groups [80, 81]. Regardless of biocompatibility considerations, the removal of larger molecules had a positive influence on mortality in three other studies [85, 87, 88], although Kt/V was higher in the high-flux group than the low-flux group in one of these studies [87]. According to recent results of the HEMO study, high-flux dialysis did not reduce all-cause mortality when compared to low-flux dialysis. However, analysis of subgroups showed that all-cause mortality was reduced by 32% with high-flux compared to low-flux dialysis for patients who were on dialysis for a prolonged period of time before entering the study (> 3.7 years) ($p = 0.005$) [36]. In addition, high-flux dialysis may improve cardiac outcome by reducing the risk of cardiac death: the relative risk of death was reported to be 0.78 with high-flux dialysis compared to 1.0 with low-flux dialysis ($p < 0.05$) [36]. These different subgroup analyses of the HEMO study must be interpreted with caution because they bear the risk for creating false positive results. It is also of note that the design of the HEMO study favoured a selection of patients which were already relatively long on dialysis before entering the study, and excluded patients with advanced age, with severe comorbidities and with serious access problems – all conditions that are more common in the average dialysis population. Therefore, it cannot be ruled out that in particular these patient groups could have benefited from high-flux dialysis [72, 89-93]. In addition, the practice of dialyser reuse, which was permitted in the HEMO study, might have interfered with dialyser performance characteristics (see chapter 12) and, thus, masked potential differences in outcome. Very recently, data from the French Study Group of Nutrition in Dialysis showed a better survival when high-flux membranes were used, especially in patients who were on dialysis for over three years (as also found in the HEMO study). The authors speculate that short-term survival might predominately result from comorbidity, whereas haemodialysis technique may influence long-term survival [94].

Taken together, the results of the above-mentioned studies indicate that membrane flux, rather than biocompatibility, may influence mortality in dialysis patients. This subject is also the main concern of the ongoing European Membrane Permeability (MPO) study [73] which, in contrast to the HEMO study, allocates patients who are no longer than 2 months on dialysis to either high-flux or low-flux dialysis with new dialysers for an observation period of 3-6 years.

In conclusion, some studies support the theory that mortality is higher in ESRD patients treated with regenerated cellulose membranes, and some data indicate an increased survival with the use of membranes allowing the removal of larger molecules (especially high-flux synthetic membranes). However, almost all these studies are retrospective in nature and very different in their designs. Furthermore, the results are often not, or only partially, adjusted for other parameters that influence survival in ESRD, such as dialysis adequacy and comorbidity. Clinical data from single, experienced centres have shown very good survival rates even for patients formerly dialysed predominantly with regenerated cellulose, but with excellent control of hydration status, hypertension and dialysis fluid purity [48, 50, 95, 96]. Patient compliance, psychosocial situation and quality of care are factors that also contribute to patient mortality in ESRD [4-8, 23, 28, 56, 97-101]. Perhaps large, prospective ongoing studies, such as the Membrane Permeability and ESRD Outcome study (MPO) in Europe [73], or further subanalysis of the HEMO study in the USA [36, 74] will provide more insight. Nevertheless, the recently published European Best Practice Guidelines for Haemodialysis already recommend the use of "large pore/high-flux biocompatible dialysers to improve clinical outcome regarding morbidity/mortality" (EBP guideline III.2 [5]).

References

1. The United States data report on chronic renal disease (USRDS), Chapter 9, p152-164, 2002

2. The Renal Association. Recommended standards for Haemodialysis. Royal college of physicians London. Treatment of adult patients with renal failure. Recommended standards and audit measure: 17-29, 1997

3. The Canadian Society of Nephrology. Clinical practice guidelines for the delivery of haemodialysis. J Am Soc Nephrol 10: S306-S319, 1999

4. Haemodialysis adequacy workgroup: National Kidney Foundation DOQI™: clinical practice guidelines for hemodialysis adequacy, 2000 update. Am J Kidney Dis 37(Suppl 1): S7-S64, 2001

5. Kessler M, Canaud B, Pedrini LA, Tattersall J, ter Wee PM, Vanholder R, Wanner C: European Best Practice Guidelines for Haemodialysis (Part 1). Nephrol Dial Transplant 17(Suppl 7): 1-107, 2002

6. European Best Practice Guidelines for the management of anemia in patients with chronic renal failure. Nephrol Dial Transplant 14(Suppl 5): 1-50, 1999

7. NKF-K/DOQI™ clinical practice guidelines for anemia, update 2000, www.kidney.org/professionals/kdoqi/index/cfm

8. NKF-K/DOQI™ clinical practice guidelines for nutrition update 2000, www.kidney.org/professionals/kdoqi/index/cfm

9. NKF-K/DOQI™ clinical practice guidelines for managing dylipidemias in chronic kidney disease. www.kidney.org/professionals/Kdoqi/index/cfm

10. Ritz E, Bianchi G, London GM, Marcelli D, Massy ZA, Parfrey PS, Passlick-Deetjen J, Rabelink TJ, Wanner Chr: Clinical algorithms on cardiovascular risk factors in renal patients. Nephrol Dial Transplant 15(Suppl. 5): 125-154, 2000

11. The United States data report on chronic renal disease (USRDS), Chapter 10, cardiovascular special studies: 166-176, 2002

12. NKF-K/DOQI™ clinical practice guidelines for bone metabolism and disease in chronic kidney diasease. www.kidney.org/professionals/kdoqi/index/cfm

13. Stenvinkel P, Heimburger O, Paultre F, Diczfalusy U, Wang T, Berglund L, Jogestrand T: Strong association between malnutrition, inflammation, and atherosclerosis in chronic renal failure. Kidney Int 55(5): 1899-1991, 1999

14. Qureshi AR, Alvestrand A, Divino-Filho JC, Gutierrez A, Heimbürger O, Lindholm B, Bergström J: Inflammation, malnutrition, and cardiac disease as predictors of mortality in hemodialysis patients. J Am Soc Nephrol 13: S28-S36, 2002

15. Bloembergen WE, Port FK: Epidemiological perspective on infections in chronic dialysis patients. Adv Ren Replace Ther 3(3): 201-207, 1996

16. Rocco MV, Yan G, Gassman J, Lewis JB, Ornt D, Weiss B, Levey AS, Hemodialysis Study Group: Comparison of causes of death using HEMO study and HCFA end-stage renal disease notification classification systems. The National Institutes of Health-funded Hemodialysis. Health Care Financing Administration. Am J Kidney Dis 39(1): 146-153, 2002

17. Allon M, Depner TA, Radeva M, Bailey J, Beddhu S, Butterly D, Coyne DW, Gassman JJ, Kaufman AM, Kaysen GA, Lewis JA, Schwab SJ; HEMO Study

Group: Impact of dialysis dose and membrane on infection-related hospitalization and death: results of the HEMO Study. J Am Soc Nephrol 14(7): 1863-1870, 2003

18. Sarnak MJ, Jaber BL: Mortality caused by sepsis in patients with end-stage renal disease compared with the general population. Kidney Int 58(4): 1758-1764, 2000

19. Vanholder R, Van Biesen W: Incidence and infectious morbidity and mortality in dialysis patients. Blood Purif 20(5): 477-489, 2002

20. Ma JZ, Ebben J, Xia H, Collins AL: Hematocrit level and associated mortality in hemodialysis patients. J Am Soc Nephrol 10: 610-619, 1999

21. Okechukwu CN, Lopes AA, Stack AG, Feng S, Wolfe RA, Port FK: Impact of years of dialysis therapy on mortality risk and the characteristics of longer term dialysis survivors. Am J Kidney Dis 39(3): 533-538, 2002

22. Ofsthun N, LaBreque J, Lacson E, Keen M, Lazarus JM: The effects of higher hemoglobin levels on mortality and hospitalization in hemodialysis patients. Kidney Int 63: 1908-1914, 2003

23. Lowrie EG, Lew NL: Death risk in hemodialysis patients: the predictive value of commonly measured variables and an evaluation of death rate differences between facilities. Am J Kidney Dis 15(5): 458-482, 1990

24. Owen WF jr, Lew NL, Liu Y, Lowrie EG, Lazarus JM: The urea reduction ratio and serum albumin concentration as predictors of mortality in patients undergoing hemodialysis. N Engl J Med 329(14): 1001-1006, 1993

25. Kopple JD: Effect of nutrition on morbidity and mortality in maintenance dialysis patients. Am J Kidney Dis 24(6): 1002-1009, 1994

26. Bergström J: Nutrition and mortality in hemodialysis. J Am Soc Nephrol 6(5): 1329-1341, 1995

27. Kopple JD: Nutritional status as a predictor of mortality in maintenance dialysis patients. ASAIO Journal: 246-250, 1997

28. Shinzato T, Nakai S, Akiba T, Yamazaki C, Sasaki R, Kitaoka T, Kubo K, Shinoda T, Kurokawa K, Marumo F, Sato T, Maeda K: Survival in long-term haemodialysis patients: results from the annual survey of the Japanese Society for Dialysis Therapy. Nephrol Dial Transplant 12: 884-888, 1997

29. Herselman M, Moosa MR, Kotze TJ, Kritzinger M, Wuister S, Mostert D: Protein-energy malnutrition as a risk factor for increased morbidity in long-term hemodialysis patients. J Ren Nutr 10(1): 7-15, 2000

30. Stenvinkel P, Heimbürger O, Lindholm B, Kaysen GA, Bergström J: Are there two types of malnutrition? Evidence for relationships between malnutrition, inflammation and atherosclerosis (MIA syndrome). Nephrol Dial Transplant 15: 953-960, 2000

31. Combe C, Chauveau P, Laville M, Fouque D, Azar R, Cano N, Canaud B, Roth H, Leverve X, Aparicio M: Influence of nutritional factors and hemodialysis adequacy on the survival of 1.610 French patients. Am J Kidney Dis 37(1 Suppl2): S81-S82, 2001

32. Leavey SF, McCullough K; Hecking E, Goodkin D, Port FK, Young EW: Body mass index and mortality in "healthier" as compared with "sicker" haemodialysis patients: results from the Dialysis Outcomes and Practice Patterns Study (DOPPS). Nephrol Dial Transplant 16: 2386-2394, 2001

33. Stenvinkel P, Barany P, Heimbürger O, Pecoits-Filho R, Lindholm B: Mortality, malnutrition, and atherosclerosis in ESRD: What is the role of interleukin-6? Kidney Int 61(Suppl 80): S103-S108, 2002

34. Port FK, Ashby VB, Dhingra RK, Roys EC, Wolfe RA: Dialysis dose and body mass index are strongly associated with survival in hemodialysis patients. J Am Soc Nephrol 13: 1061-1066, 2002

35. Pifer TB, McCullough KP, Port FK, Goodkin DA, Maroni BJ, Held PJ, Young EW: Mortality risk in hemodialysis patients and changes in nutritional indicators: DOPPS. Kidney Int 62(6): 2238-2245, 2002

36. Eknoyan G, Beck GJ, Cheung AK, Daugirdas JT, Greene T, Kusek JW, Allon M, Bailey J, Delmez JA, Depner TA, Dwyer JT, Levey AS, Levin NW, Milford E, Ornt DB, Rocco MV, Schulman G, Schwab SJ, Teehan BP, Toto R for the Hemodialysis (HEMO) Study Group: Effect of dialysis dose and membrane flux in maintenance hemodialysis. N Engl J Med 347(25): 2010-2019, 2002

37. Kimmel PL, Chawla LS, Amarasinghe A, Peterson RA, Weihs KL, Simens SJ, Alleyne S, Burke HB, Cruz I, Veis JH: Anthropometric measures, cytokines and survival in haemodialysis patients. Nephrol Dial Transplant 18: 326-332, 2003

38. Chauveau P, Nguyen H, Combe C, Azar R, Cano N, Canaud B, Chene G, Foque D, Laville M, Leverve H, Roth H, Aparicio M: Analysis of the influence of nutritional factors and membrane permeability on the survival of French hemodialysis patients. Abstract (SU-PO0830), ASN, 2003

39. Bergström J, Heimbürger O, Lindholm B, Qureshi AR: Elevated C-reactive protein is a strong predictor of increased mortality and low serum albumin in hemodialysis (HD) patients. (Abstract) J Am Soc Nephrol 6: 573, 1995

40. Bologa RM, Levine DM, Parker TS, Cheigh JS, Serur D, Stenzel KH, Rubin AL: Interleukin-6 predicts hypoalbuminemia, hypocholesterolemia, and mortality in hemodialysis patients. Am J Kidney Dis 32(1): 107-114, 1998

41. Kimmel PL, Phillips TM, Simmens SJ, Peterson RA, Weihs KL, Alleyne S, Cruz I, Yanovski JA, Veis JH: Immunologic function and survival in hemodialysis patients. Kidney Int 54: 236-244, 1998

42. Zimmermann J, Herrlinger S, Pruy A, Metzger T, Wanner C: Inflammation enhances cardiovascular risk and mortality in hemodialysis patients. Kidney Int 55(2): 648-658, 1999

43. Yeun JY, Levine RA, Mantadilok V, Kaysen GA: C-reactive protein predicts all-cause and cardiovascular mortality in hemodialysis patients. Am J Kidney Dis 35(3): 469-76, 2000

44. Coresh J, Longenecker JC, Eustace J, Liu Y, Levin N, Tracy RP, Powe NR, Klag MJ: C-reactive protein and mortality among incident dialysis patients the CHOICE study. (Abstract) J Am Soc Nephrol 13(9): 423A, 2002

45. Bayés B, Pastor MC, Bonal J, Juncà J, Hernandez JM, Riutort N, Foraster A, Romero R: Homocysteine, C-reactive protein, lipid peroxidation and mortality in haemodialysis patients. Nephrol Dial Transplant 18: 106-112, 2003

46. Block GA, Hulbert-Shearon TE, Levin NW, Port FK: Association of serum phosphorus and calcium× phosphate product with mortality risk in chronic hemodialysis patients: A national study. Am J Kidney Dis 31(4): 607-617, 1998

47. Block GA, Klassen P, Danese M, Ofsthun N, LaBrecque J, Kim J, Lazarus JM: Association between proposed NKF-K/DOQI bone metabolism and disease guidelines and mortality risk in hemodialysis patients. Abstract (SA-PO801), ASN, 2003

48. Innes A, Charra B, Burden RP, Morgan AG, Laurent G: The effect of long, slow haemodialysis on patient survival. Nephrol Dial Transplant 4(4): 919-922, 1999

49. Lowrie EG, Laird NM, Parker TF, Sargent JA: Effect of the haemodialysis prescription on patient morbidity: report from the National Cooperative Dialysis Study. N Engl J Med 305: 1176-1181, 1981

50. Charra B, Calemard E, Ruffet M, Chazot C, Terrat JC, Vanel T, Laurent G: Survival as an index of adequacy of dialysis. Kidney Int 41: 1286-1291, 1992

51. Kopple JD, Hakim RM, Held PJ, Keane WF, King K, Lazarus JM, Parker III TF, Teehan BP: Recommendations for reducing the high morbidity and mortality of United States maintenance dialysis patients. Am J Kidney Dis 24(6): 968-973, 1994

52. Held PJ, Carrol CE, Liska DW, Turenne MN, Port FK: Hemodialysis Therapy in the United States: What is the dose and what does it matter? Am J Kidney Dis 24(6): 974-980, 1994

53. Parker III TF: Role of dialysis dose on morbidity and mortality in maintenance hemodialysis patients. Am J Kidney Dis 24(6): 981-989, 1994

54. Consensus conference on morbidity and mortality of renal disease: an NIH consensus conference panel. Ann Intern Med 121: 62-70, 1994

55. Held PJ, Port FK, Wolfe RA: The dose of haemodialysis and patient mortality. Kidney Int 50: 550-556, 1996

56. Port FK, Orzol SM, Held PJ, Wolfe RA: Trends in treatment and survival for hemodialysis patients in the United States. Am J Kidney Dis 32(6, Suppl 4): S34-S38, 1998

57. Lowrie EG, Chertow GM, Lew NL, Lazarus JM, Owen WF: the urea (clearance x dialysis time) product (Kt) as an outcome-based measure of haemodialysis dose. Kidney Int 56: 729-737, 1999

58. Wolfe RA, Held PJ, Hulbert-Shearon TE, Ashby VB, Port FK: URR> 75% is associated with lower mortality among females but not among males. (Abstract) J Am Soc Nephrol 13(9): 20A, 2002

59. Bosch JA, Nabut J, Hegbrant J, Alquist M, Walters BA: Increased survival for hemodialysis patients with a dialysis dose above the KDOQI guidelines. (Abstract) J Am Soc Nephrol 13(9): 21A, 2002

60. Depner TA: Prescribing hemodialysis: the role of gender. Adv Ren Replace Ther 10(1): 71-77, 2003

61. Keane WF, Collins AJ: Influence of comorbidity in patients treated with hemodialysis. Am J Kidney Dis 24(6): 1010-1018, 1994

62. Ikizler TA, Wingard RL, Harvell J, Shyr Y, Hakim RM: Association of morbidity with markers of nutrition and inflammation in chronic hemodialysis patients: a prospective study. Kidney Int 55(5): 1945-1951, 1999

63. Longenecker JC, Liu Y, Klag MJ, Marcovina M, Powe NR; Levey AS; Fink NE, Giaculli F, Coresh J: High lipoprotein(a) level and small apolipoprotein(a) size prospectively predict cardiovascular disease events in end-stage renal disease: the CHOICE study. (Abstract) J Am Soc Nephrol 13(9): 423A, 2002

64. Jaar BJ, Astor B, Longenecker JC, Fink N, Klag MJ, Powe NR, Selhub J, Tracy RP, Marcovina S, Coresh J: Lipoprotein(a) and C-reactive protein are predictors of peripheral vascular disease among incident dialysis patients: the CHOICE study. (Abstract) J Am Soc Nephrol13(9): 424A, 2002

65. Foley RN, Parfrey PS, Sarnak: Clinical epidemiology of cardiovascular disease in chronic renal disease. Am J Kidney Dis 32(5, Suppl 3): S112-119, 1998

66. Depner TA: How will the results of the HEMO study impact dialysis practice? Sem Dial 16(1): 8-11, 2003

67. Gotch FA: How will the results of the HEMO study impact dialysis practice? Sem Dial 16(1): 11-13, 2003

68. Port FK, Wolfe RA: How will the results of the HEMO study impact dialysis practice? Sem Dial 16(1): 13-16, 2003

69. Lindsay RM, Blake GB: How will the results of the HEMO study impact dialysis practice? Sem Dial 16(1): 13-19, 2003

70. Locatelli F: How will the results of the HEMO study impact dialysis practice? Sem Dial 16(1): 20-21, 2003

71. Levin N, Greenwood R: Reflections on the HEMO study: the American viewpoint. Nephrol Dial Transplant 18(6): 1059-1060, 2003

72. Locatelli F: Dose of dialysis, convection and haemodialysis patients outcome--what the HEMO study doesn't tell us: the European viewpoint: Nephrol Dial Transplant 18(6): 1061-1065, 2003

73. Locatelli F, Hannedouche T, Jacobson S, La Greca G, Loureiro A, Martin-Malo A, Papadimitriou M, Vanholder R: The effect of membrane permeability on ESRD: design of a prospective randomised multicentre trial. J Nephrol 12(2): 85-88, 1999

74. Greene T, Beck GJ, Gassman JJ, Gotch FA, Kusek JW, Levey AS, Levin NW, Schulman G, Eknoyan G: Design and statistical issues of the hemodialysis (HEMO) study. Control Clin Trials 21(5): 502-525, 2000

75. Daugirdas JT, Depner TA, Gotch FA: Comparison of methods to predict equilibrated Kt/V in the HEMO pilot study. Kidney Int 52: 1395-1405, 1997

76. Daugirdas JT, Depner TA for the HEMO study group: Association of achieved eKt/V with mortality: an example of dose targeting bias. (Abstract) J Am Soc Nephrol 13(9): 613-614A, 2002

77. Levin NW, Zasuwa G, Dumler F: Effect of membrane type on causes of death in hemodialysis patients. (Abstract) J Am Soc Nephrol 2: 335, 1991

78. Hornberger JC, Chernew M, Petersen J, Garber AM: A multivariate analysis of mortality and hospital admissions with high-flux dialysis. J Am Soc Nephrol 3(6):1227-1237, 1992

79. Chandran PK, Liggett R, Kirkpatrick B: Patient survival on PAN/AN69 membrane hemodialysis: a ten-year analysis. (Letter) J Am Soc Nephrol 4(5): 1199-1204, 1993

80. Hakim RM, Stannard D, Port F, Held P: The effect of the dialysis membrane on mortality of chronic hemodialysis patients in the US. (Abstract) J Am Soc Nephrol 5: 451, 1994

81. Bonomini V, Coli L, Scolari MP, Stefoni S: Structure of dialysis membranes and long-term clinical outcome. Am J Nephrol 15(6): 455-462, 1995

82. Hakim RM, Held PJ, Stannard DC, Wolfe RA, Port FK, Daugirdas JT, Agodoa L: Effect of the dialysis membrane on mortality of chronic hemodialysis patients. Kidney Int 50: 566-570, 1996

83. Koda Y, Nishi S, Miyazaki S, Haginoshita S, Sakurabayashi T, Suzuki M, Sakai S, Yuasa Y, Hirasawa Y, Nishi T: Switch from conventional to high-flux membrane reduces the risk of carpal tunnel syndrome and mortality of hemodialysis patients. Kidney Int 52(4): 1096-1101, 1997

84. Bloembergen WE, Hakim RM, Stannard DC, Held PJ, Wolfe RA, Agodoa L, Port FK: Relationship of dialysis membrane and cause specific-mortality. (Special Article) Am J Kidney Dis 33(1): 1-10, 1999

85. Leypold JK, Cheung AK, Carroll CE, Stannard DC, Pereira BIS, Agodoa LY, Port FK: Effect of dialysis membranes and middle molecule removal on chronic hemodialysis patient survival. Am J Kidney Dis 33(2): 349-355, 1999

86. Locatelli F, Marcelli D, Conte F, Limido A, Malberti F, Spotti D: Comparison of mortality in ESRD patients on convective and diffusive extracorporeal treatments. The Registro Lombardo Dialyisi E Trapianto. Kidney Int 55(1): 286-293, 1999

87. Woods HF, Nandakumar M: Improved outcome for haemodialysis patients treated with high-flux membranes. Nephrol Dial Transplant 15(Suppl 1): 36-42, 2000

88. Port FK, Wolfe RA, Hulbert-Shearon TE, Daugirdas JT, Agodoa LY, Jones C, Orzol SM, Held PJ: Mortality risk by hemodialyzer reuse practice and dialyzer membrane characteristics: results from the USRDS dialysis and mortality study. Am J Kidney Dis 37(2): 276-286, 2001

89. Scribner BH, Blagg CR: Effect of dialysis dose and membrane flux in maintenance hemodialysis. (Letter) N Engl J Med 348(15): 1491-1492, 2003

90. Friedman EA: Effect of dialysis dose and membrane flux in maintenance hemodialysis. (Letter) N Engl J Med 348(15): 1492, 2003

91. Hoenich NA: Effect of dialysis dose and membrane flux in maintenance hemodialysis. (Letter) N Engl J Med 348(15): 1492, 2003

92. Locatelli F: Effect of dialysis dose and membrane flux in maintenance hemodialysis. (Letter) N Engl J Med 348(15): 1492-1493, 2003

93. Prichard S: ADEMEX and HEMO trials: Where are we going? Blood Purif 21: 42-45, 2003

94. Chauveau P, Nguyen H, Combe C, Azar R, Cano N, Canaud B, Chene G, Foque D, Laville M, Leverve H, Roth H, Aparicio M: Analysis of the influence of nutritional factors and membrane permeability on the survival of French hemodialysis patients. Abstract (SU-PO0830), ASN, 2003

95. Kleophas W, Haastert B. Backus G, Hilgers P, Westhoff A, van Endert G: Long-term experience with an ultrapure individual dialysis fluid with a batch type machine. Nephrol Dial Transplant 13: 3118-3125, 1998

96. Katzarski KS, Charra B, Luik AJ, Nisell J, Divino Filho JC, Leypoldt JK, Leunissen KM, Laurent G, Bergström J: Fluid state and blood pressure control in patients treated with long and short haemodialysis. Nephrol Dial Transplant 14(2): 369-375, 1999

97. Hornberger JC. The hemodialysis prescription and quality-adjusted life expectancy. Renal Physicians Association. Working Committee on Clinical Guidelines. J Am Soc Nephrol 4(4): 1004-1020, 1993

98. Kimmel PL, Peterson RA, Weihs KL, Simmens SJ, Alleyne S, Cruz I, Veis JH: Psychosocial factors, behavioural compliance and survival in urban hemodialysis patients. Kidney Int 54(1): 245-254, 1998

99. McClellan WM, Soucie JM, Flanders WD: Mortality in end-stage renal disease is associated with facility-to-facility differences in adequacy of hemodialysis. J Am Soc Nephrol 9(10): 1940-1947, 1998

100. Sehgal AR, Leon JB, Siminoff LA, Singer ME, Bunosky LM, Cebul RD: Improving the quality of hemodialysis treatment: a community-based randomized controlled trial to overcome patient-specific barriers. JAMA 287(15): 1961-1967, 2002

101. Plantinga LC, Fink NE, Jaar BG, Sadler JH, Coresh J, Klag MJ, Powe NR: Association of frequency of patient care rounds with mortality and intermediate clinical outcomes in hemodialysis patients: The ESRD Quality (EQUAL) Study. Abstract (F-FC012), ASN, 2003

Section E.
Dialyser reuse

12. Dialyser reuse

Reuse of dialysers is common practice in many countries. In the United States, the tendency to reuse increased from 18% of dialysis centres in 1976 to 82% in 1997, and decreased slightly thereafter to 80% in 1999 and 2000 (**figure 12.1**, [1, 2]). Further decreases have been postulated (e.g. only 60% of all U.S. centres practising reuse by 2003) due to on-going changes away from reuse and towards single-use in many U.S. dialysis clinic chains, such as those run by Fresenius Medical Care and Gambro [3]. Nevertheless, reuse is still common in America. This prevalence is not reflected in other parts of the industrialised world. Values for Europe are difficult to access as they vary from country to country and rarely appear in national registers (insofar as such exist), but the percentage of patients treated with reused dialysers was reported to be under 10% for Europe as a whole in 1990 (ranging from 0% to about 76% for individual countries) [4]. The corresponding values for Australia were about 35%, and no reuse is practised in Japan [4]. Among centres that reuse disposable dialysers in the United States, the overall average number of reuses was 15 in 1997 (average maximum was 30); this also increased from 9 in 1986 (average maximum then was 23) [5].

The necessity of reducing therapy costs due to the rapidly expanding dialysis population and the introduction of expensive treatment modes makes multiple use of dialysers appear attractive (e.g. [6]). Reliable and comparable data on actual costs are difficult to find due to variations in practices from country to country, between types of dialysis centres, and in the cost factors taken into consideration (e.g. personnel salaries and training, capital investment in equipment, hospital services, recurrent treatment expenses, medication, routine investigations etc.) (e.g. [7]). In Australia in 1984, substantial savings were made for up to 6 uses of a dialyser only - thereafter the additional savings were only slight [8]. A much more recent cost analysis conducted in one N. American centre comparing reuse of traditional polysulfone dialysers using heat with single use of the new Optiflux® polysulfone dialyser from Fresenius Medical Care found that a change to a non-reuse program with the Optiflux® membrane would actually result in a cost savings in that particular centre of 15.7% [9]. Costs aside, many fear that dialyser reuse

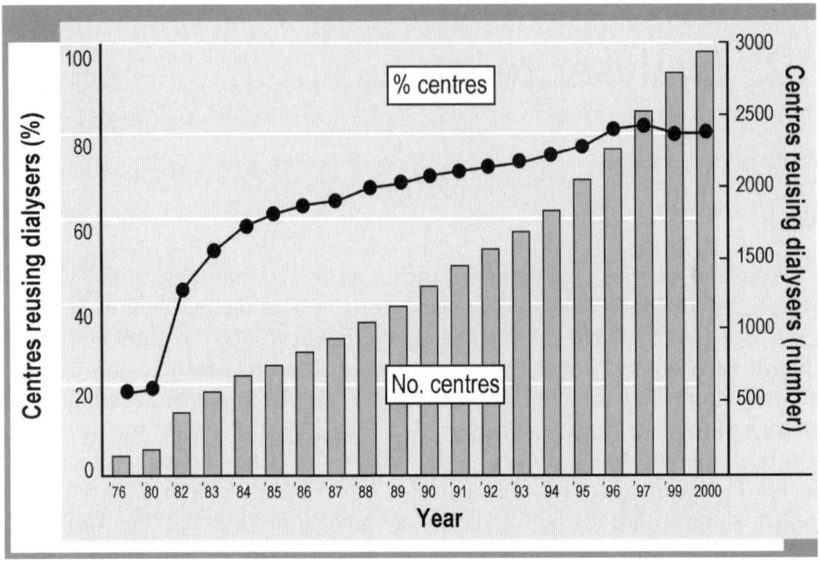

Figure 12.1: Numbers and percentages of centres in the U.S.A. that practised dialyser reuse from 1976 until 2000. *Note: these numbers will decrease in upcoming years as Fresenius Medical Care, Gambro Healthcare and other dialysis providers now promote single use in their U.S. dialysis centres ([3], data from [2]).*

means a reduction in treatment quality and an additional health risk factor. Consequently, reuse of dialysers has been intensely and emotionally discussed in the dialysis community for some time; many of the numerous papers published on this subject are controversial, out-dated (in that they refer to older membranes and procedures) and contradictory.

The performance and biocompatibility of a dialyser which is repeatedly used changes due to (a) its previous use and (b) the reprocessing procedure to which it has been subjected. This chapter offers some insight into the nature and degree of these alterations.

What happens to a dialyser during clinical use?

It is a well-documented fact that the solute removal ability of most dialysers decreases during the course of a treatment session (e.g. ß2-m sieving coefficients decrease significantly in the first 20 minutes of treatment [10, 11]); this phenomenon is commonly termed filter fouling. The usage factor primarily responsible for fouling is the adsorption of blood proteins (especially albumin and fibrinogen, as these are present in high concentrations in the plasma [11]) onto the surface of the dialysis membrane – and indeed into its porous structure. The consequence of this adsorption is a blockage of membrane pores and a lengthening of the diffusive path for blood solutes, which negatively affect performance, and a change in the physico-chemical nature of the membrane surface, which affects membrane biocompatibility (as discussed in chapter 8). Clotting and/or rupture of individual fibres and blood coagulation in the header regions can also occur. For a used dialyser to function as well as a new one, absorbed proteins and clots must be removed, leaks must be ruled out and the sterility of the complete device must be guaranteed.

What happens to a dialyser during reprocessing?

As multiple use of dialysers was practised in about 80% of centres in the United States in 2000 (**figure 12.1**), it is not surprising that the currently accepted standards world-wide (or at least in industrialised nations) for the practice of reprocessing are based on those issued by the American Association for Advancement of Medical Instrumentation (AAMI) [12]. These steps are summarised in **figure 12.2**. Although these recommendations were formulated in the year 1993, they are still valid today – with one exception: the American National Kidney Foundation's DOQI (Dialysis Outcome Quality Initiative) guidelines recommend that the *baseline* performance measurement be done for *each* dialyser prior to its use, rather than taking an average of preprocessing values for about 10 dialysers, as stated in the AAMI recommendations [13]. In practice, variations in the procedure are found at almost all levels in this diagram; the most significant of these are summarised in **table 12.1**.

Use of a cleaning agent is deemed optional by the AAMI, but peracetic acid, bleach (sodium hypochlorite) and hydrogen peroxide are cleaning agents used in many reprocessing procedures. Only bleach was found to be effective at removing protein deposits [4, 15]. However, high concentrations

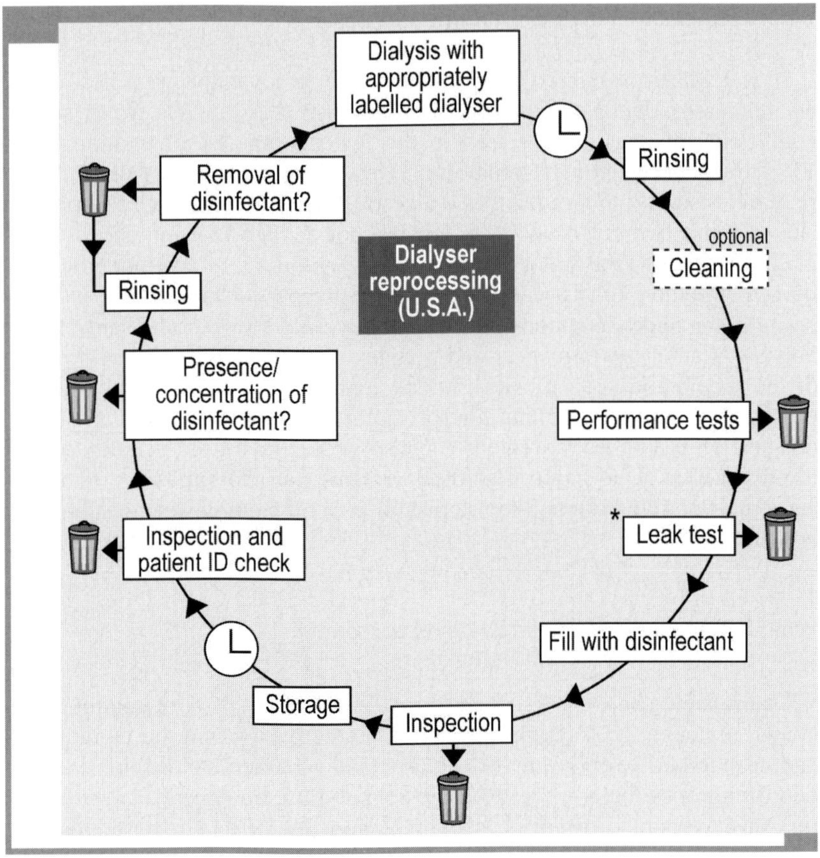

Figure 12.2: Recommended steps for the reprocessing of used dialysers. *Guidelines for conventional methods of dialyser reprocessing as recommended by the AAMI in the USA and adopted as regulations by the Centers of Medicare and Medicaid Services are shown. Critical time factors are indicated by the clock symbol. Cleaning is optional. The cleaning agent bleach (sodium hypochlorite) should be thoroughly rinsed from the dialyser before disinfection with formaldehyde or peracetic acid as interactions between the chemicals produce noxious vapours. *This may be done later but must precede dialysis (adapted from [4] and [12]).*

(e.g. > 2%) and long exposure times (e.g. > 10 minutes) can weaken and even damage the dialyser membranes. For example, bleach reprocessing increased the effective pore size of earlier polysulfone membranes, possibly through the removal of the polysulfone copolymer polyvinylpyrrolidone (PVP), causing a significant loss of blood proteins into the dialysis fluid [16, 17]. Noxious vapours may be produced when residues of bleach come into contact with peroxyacetic acid (a constituent of the disinfectant Renalin®) or formaldehyde, and the compounds can be consequently degraded. Therefore, bleach must be meticulously removed before filling the cleaned dialyser with these disinfectants [4, 12]. The production of gas is also the reason why the bleach-Renalin® combination is not recommended by the AAMI in the USA [12].

Regarding the reprocessing chemicals, disinfectants rather that sterilants are employed in reprocessing procedures. Disinfection is less lethal for micro-organisms than sterilisation, as even high-level disinfection does not destroy bacterial endospores. Sterilisation (i.e. a reduction in the chance of survival of a viable micro-organism to less than one in a million) may, however, be attained if the contact time of the high-level disinfectant is sufficiently long and the concentration of the disinfectant is high enough. The water used to rinse used dialysers and dilute disinfectants in reprocessing procedures should, ideally, be highly purified in order to reduce the risk of reuse-related sepsis and pyrogenic reactions occurring [4, 18]. **Figure 12.3** shows the common disinfecting liquids employed in reprocessing practices in the USA from 1983 to 2000.

Use of formaldehyde as a disinfectant has decreased significantly over the years in the USA, while peracetic acid solutions (e.g. Renalin®) have become much more popular; the latter were used in 59% of centres there in 2000. Formaldehyde was then the second most popular disinfectant and was chosen by 31% of N. American centres. Disinfection/sterilisation by glutaraldehyde and heat were less common, being employed in only 5% and 4% of centres there, respectively (**figure 12.3**). Sterilisation by heat and citric acid was introduced in the early nineties [21-23]: used polysulfone dialysers were cleaned, filled with processed water and sterilised by subjecting them to temperatures of 100 - 105°C for 20 hours in a dry-heat, forced convection oven. Addition of 1.5% citric acid to the water allowed a reduction in the temperature (e.g. to 95°C). So far, this heat reprocessing technique is limited to polysulfone dialysers with heat-resistance polycarbonate casings and polyurethane potting compound [17, 23, 24].

Reprocessing feature	Common variations in clinical practice
Time factor	The rinsing process should, optimally, begin within 10 mins after the patient has been disconnected, but substantial delays can ensue in clinics with large numbers of patients per session. Sometimes the dialysers are refrigerated until reprocessing can begin. Minimum and maximum storage times are generally adhered to.
Rinsing	A variety of rinsing techniques, some involving pre-rinsing and rinsing steps, are used in both automated and manual reprocessing methods. Fluid temperature, rinse time, flow rate, volume, pressure (continuous or pulsatile), fluid composition, use of reverse flushing and reverse ultrafiltration are all variable parameters. Water (tap water, RO-processed water or deionised water) or saline, with or without heparin, are all commonly used rinsing solutions.
Cleaning	Considered optional by the AAMI. It involves the use of a chemical agent to remove any blood protein residue after rinsing. Automated systems generally employ a cleaning agent. The technique of cleaning varies in a manner similar to that of rinsing.
Performance tests	Different reprocessing systems provide different sets of tests. The most common tests in both manual and automated reprocessing systems are the total cell volume (TCV) test, the fibre bundle volume (FBV) test and ultrafiltration coefficient or rate measurements (described in text). In some rare cases, only a leak test is conducted.
Disinfection	The procedures used to disinfect vary not only in the choice of agent but also in the storage time, storage temperature and chemical removal technique.
Final inspection	AAMI recommendations state that there should be no more than a few (e.g. 10 - 15) dark, clotted fibres and that the headers should be free from all but small peripheral clots. Synthetic fibres are not as transparent as cellulosic fibres, labels often hinder the view of the fibres, and not all dialyser headers can be removed to facilitate inspection, so that the degree of visual inspection varies.

Table 12.1: Common variations in the practice of reprocessing compared to the procedure recommended by the American Association for the Advancement of Medical Instrumentation *(AAMI) [4, 14].*

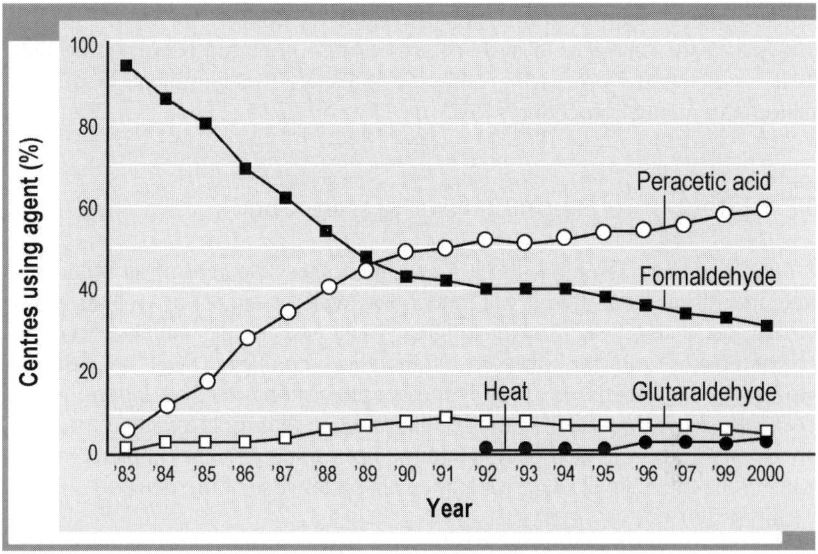

Figure 12.3: Agents used to disinfect/sterilise used dialysers in reprocessing procedures in the U.S.A. between 1983 and 2000*. Various concentrations of formaldehyde were used up to about 1989 (e.g. ≤ 2%, 3%, 4% or ≥ 5%); now 4% formaldehyde or higher concentrations are used due to the recognised inadequacy of lower concentrations regarding the destruction of non-tuberculous mycobacteria [19, 20]. Renalin® is a common peracetic acid solution: it is a mixture of 2% peracetic acid, acetic acid and hydrogen peroxide. Diacide® is a popular glutar(di)aldehyde solution. Up to now, heat has only been employed for reprocessing polysulfone dialysers [4]. (Data from [2]).*

Chloramine is another disinfectant used in reprocessing, albeit not usually in the USA. It is available in three forms depending on the pH: monochloramine (NH_2Cl) at pH > 8, dichloramine ($NHCl_2$) at pHs between 4 and 5, and trichloramine (NCl_3) at pH values under 4. It has a number of short-comings compared to the disinfectants mentioned in **figure 12.3**: it does not penetrate biofilms effectively; repeated dosing with chlorine may result in selection of chlorine-resistant amoebae with an increased virulence; levels above 0.25 mg/l cause side effects; and it is also difficult to remove completely [25]. Furthermore, compounds containing active chlorine caused damage to cellulose and polysulfone dialyser membranes that resulted in blood leaks and outbreaks of pyrogenic reactions and septicaemia [4, 26]. Consequently chloramine is not a popular disinfectant for reprocessing.

Automated reprocessing machines were introduced in 1980-1981. By 1997, 62% of American dialysis centres used automated reprocessing only, 34% used manual processing only and 4-5% used a combination of automated and manual procedures [5].

12.1 Effect of reuse on dialyser performance

It is generally assumed that if a used dialyser is cleaned of all blood residue and disinfected, then it will function as well, or almost as well, as a new device, i.e. at least 90% of the original small and middle molecule removal characteristics and the dialyser ultrafiltration coefficient will be restored. However, exact tests to confirm these assumptions are too laborious and cost-intensive to conduct in the routine clinical setting. In practice, performance tests of reprocessed dialysers range from none at all to simple measures which reflect the small solute clearance characteristics of the device.

How is the performance of used dialysers usually tested?

Dialyser manufacturers must specify the performance of their devices within narrow ranges of values, as stipulated by national and international regulatory commissions (e.g. DIN in Germany, AAMI in the USA, EN in Europe and ISO internationally). Clinics that reprocess dialysers for further treatments and adhere to the AAMI guidelines are only obliged to guarantee that the small solute clearance of the cleaned (not yet disinfected) dialyser should be within 10% of that of the new dialyser.

In America, *in vitro* total cell volume (TCV or, alternatively, fibre bundle volume (FBV)) or ultrafiltration rate measurements are generally employed to test dialyser performance instead of *in vitro* clearance measurements, as clearance measurements are more complicated to conduct. TCV is the volume of aqueous fluid necessary to fully prime the blood compartment of a hollow fibre dialyser; it is actually the sum of the FBV and the header volume, but these two terms are often used interchangeably in practice. TCV is determined by measuring the amount of liquid displaced by an air or nitrogen rinse of the dialyser blood compartment [4]. An acceptable TCV is defined as at least 80% of the original (baseline) TCV [12]. This value was chosen on the basis of correlation analyses between TCV and urea and creatinine clearances conducted by Gotch, where 20% loss in TCV corresponded to a urea or creatinine clearance reduction of 4 - 11% [4, 27].

Use of ultrafiltration coefficient (UF_{coeff}) or ultrafiltration rate (Q_F) measurements to assess dialyser performance is more common in automated procedures than in manual reprocessing, and is frequently employed in addition to TCV measurements. The rationale is that blocked fibres and protein coating reduce the effective dialyser surface area and membrane hydraulic permeability, and so affect the UF_{coeff} and Q_F. The ultrafiltration coefficient is determined on the basis of eqn. 5.2 by measuring the volume of water that passes through the membrane per minute (Q_F) at a given transmembrane pressure (TMP). Dialysers are discarded if the ultrafiltration coefficient or rate falls below 75% of its original value [4].

Theoretically, the chosen test or tests should be shown to correlate with the small solute clearances of the actual dialyser type used and under actual operating conditions. Some units perform only pressure leak tests on used dialysers. While these are certainly inadequate indicators of performance, the importance of conducting such on all reprocessed dialyser prior to reuse has been pointed out [28, 29].

It was recently shown that one of the newer technological advancements could also be employed to test the performance of reprocessed dialysers, namely techniques for the on-line measurement of dialyser clearance (or, more specifically, ionic dialysance) [30]. Such on-line clearance monitors are relatively inexpensive and provide real-time information on the changes in low molecular weight performance characteristics of reused dialysers in a non-invasive manner during dialysis. In future, this technology may well play a more dominant role in the testing of reprocessed dialysers.

What role does the cleaning agent play in performance changes?

Deterioration in dialyser performance during dialysis treatment results from the loss of membrane area and/or porosity due to blood clots and protein deposits. Removal of adsorbed proteins is most effectively achieved with the use of the cleaning agent bleach (sodium hypochlorite). Recent studies have shown that particularly ß2-microglobulin (ß2 m) elimination by most high-flux membranes is sensitive to the removal of adsorbed blood proteins: use of disinfectants alone does not generally restore the original ß2-m removal abilities of high-efficiency/high-flux membranes (e.g. [17, 31, 32]). **Figure 12.4** shows the effect of peracetic acid reprocessing without bleach and formaldehyde/glutaraldehyde reprocessing with bleach on the ß2-m clearance abilities of high-flux cellulose triacetate membranes: the reduction in clearance values when bleach cleaning was not conducted is due to protein adsorption onto the membrane. Consequently, bleach should be employed for reprocessing these high-flux membranes. It should especially be used for reprocessing membranes which remove significantly high amounts of ß2-m by adsorption (e.g. polyacrylonitrile, polymethylmethacrylate and polyamide membranes), as adsorption sites otherwise remain blocked (see **figure 12.5** for an example involving a polyacrylonitrile membrane) [17, 23, 31, 33, 34].

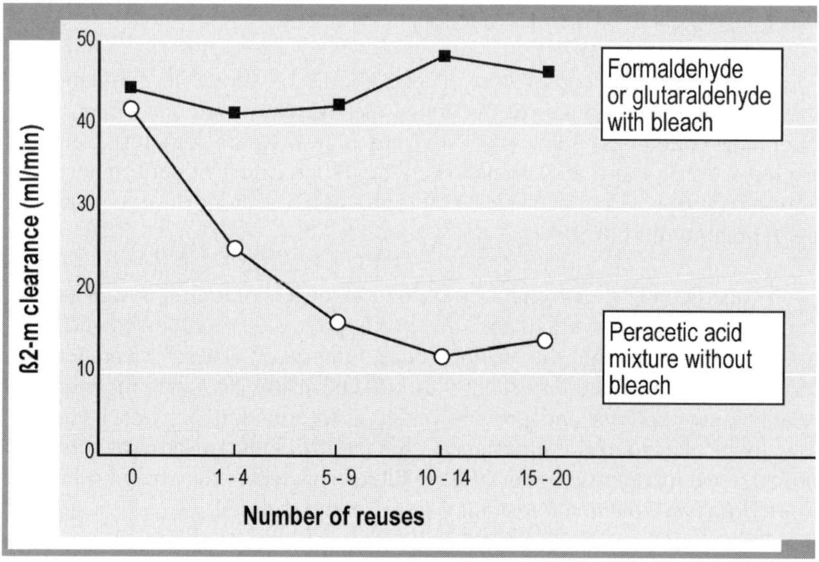

Figure 12.4: Effect of bleach (sodium hypochlorite) on ß2-m clearances by reused cellulose triacetate membranes. *Reprocessing of the high-flux, synthetic cellulose triacetate membrane (Toyobo/Baxter) using a peracetic acid mixture (Renalin®) alone reduced the ability of the dialyser to remove ß2-microglobulin. Even though all dialysers passed the TCV performance tests, the mean ß2-m clearance fell by 67.2 ± 2.7% between the first and the 10th-14th reuses. The numbers of observations for each range of reuse numbers varied between 103 (15-20 range) and 488 (1-4 range). In contrast, reprocessing of the cellulose triacetate dialysers with either formaldehyde or glutar(di)aldehyde (Diacide®) in combination with a bleach cleaning step retained (or even slightly increased) the original ß2-m clearances. Here the number of observations for each range of re-use numbers varied between 38 (15-20 range) and 184 (1-4 range) (adapted from [17]).*

On the other hand, the use of bleach has also been associated with membrane alterations such that the permeability for ß2-microglobulin, amino acids and proteins is increased in cellulose triacetate and polysulfone membranes [16, 17, 35-40]. The increase in ß2-m permeability may be considered a welcome side effect of bleach use in reprocessing these membranes. The data in **figure 12.4** indicate that, although ß2-m clearances for the cellulose triacetate membrane investigated in that study were higher when bleach was used, the total effect in this case was rather a revival of the original ß2-m clearance properties of the membrane. In the case of the polysulfone membrane, use of bleach in combination with formaldehyde or peracetic acid (not glutaraldehyde) was found to significantly increase the membrane's permeability for ß2-m with increasing number of uses [17]. However, care must be taken to ensure that membrane permeability for amino acids and albumin is not also increased to clinically significant levels. This has been reported for cellulose triacetate [39] and the original version of the polysulfone membrane [16, 36]: the permeability of the original F80 polysulfone dialyser was so enhanced during reprocessing involving bleach that the manufactures changed the membrane configuration – the F 80A dialyser was then designed for no reuse

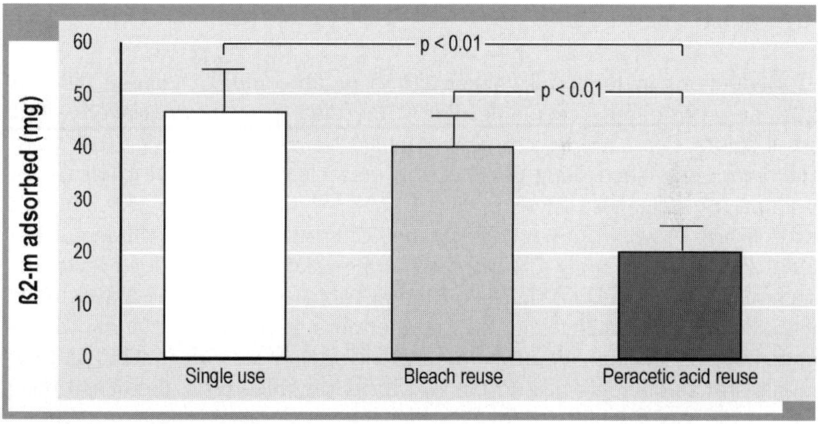

Figure 12.5: Effect of bleach (sodium hypochlorite) on ß2-microglobulin adsorption by reused polyacrylonitrile membranes. *The adsorption capacity of the high-flux AN69® membrane for ß2-microglobulin was more or less maintained after reprocessing with bleach (0.5%), as determined from* in vitro *measurements using uraemic plasma and* ^{125}*I-labelled ß2-microglobulin. However, failure to clean the membrane with bleach and simple use of the commonly employed disinfectant peracetic acid (3%) caused a statistically significant drop in the membrane's adsorptive capacity for ß2-m. N = 5 (adapted from [33]).*

or reuse without bleach, while the F 80B was suitable for reuse with bleach [15, 17, 40-42]. Details on amino acid and albumin losses with reused dialysers are given in section 12.2, as these are generally discussed in association with clinical side effects rather than performance side effects.

Changes in middle molecule membrane permeability due to the effect of bleach clearly fall into the category of "damage incurred to membranes by the reprocessing procedure itself". This problem exemplifies the fact that not all membrane-chemical combinations are compatible in the interest of restoring high-flux dialyser performance to close to its original state.

12.1.1 Main concerns

Although thousands of patients per year are safely treated with reprocessed dialysers worldwide, the standard tests described above cannot absolutely guarantee that a reprocessed dialyser performs as well as a new one. The reasons for this are summarised in **table 12.2**.

Acceptable limits

Reductions in total cell volume (TCV) or fibre bundle volume (FBV) of 20% are considered acceptable due to the once proven association with a small solute clearance decrease of 4 - 11% (as described under *Test basis*). However, even such slight decreases in urea clearance can be clinically important: for delivered dialysis doses of $Kt/V \leq 1.3$, a decrease of 0.1 in urea Kt/V (which is within this accepted range of clearance loss) has been associated with approximately 7% increase in the relative risk of death (see also section 12.2.1 for further details on the possible association of dialysis reuse with increased mortality) [43, 44]. Furthermore, a prospective study of 436 patients revealed that, although the prescribed Kt/V was identical in all treatments and all dialysers passed the AAMI performance tests, the actual delivered dose was significantly lower when the reuse number was on average 13.8 as opposed to only 3.8 [45].

Test feature	Weakness
Definition of acceptable limits	≤ 10% loss in small solute clearance of new device* or ≤ 20% reduction in TCV or FBV of new device* or ≤ 25% reduction in UF_{coeff} or Q_F of new device**
Test timing	Prior to approx. 48 - 72 h contact with aggressive disinfectant/sterilants (which could damage the membrane)
Basis	Tests other than clearance are often not validated in the dialysis unit, or are validated using different membranes and test conditions.
Nature	Tests offer no security regarding middle molecule removal by high-flux membranes. Ambiguity concerning need to remove adsorbed proteins

Table 12.2: Shortcomings of performance tests conducted during dialyser reprocessing. *TCV: total cell volume; FBV: fibre bundle volume; UF_{coeff}: ultrafiltration coefficient; Q_B: blood flow. TCV is the volume of aqueous fluid necessary to fully prime the blood compartment of a hollow fibre dialyser, i.e. the sum of the FBV and the header volume. *USA (AAMI), **not recommended by the AAMI since 1993 due to controversy about validity [12].*

Test timing

Due to the need to disinfect/sterilise the dialyser prior to next use, performance tests must be performed before membrane contact with the appropriate agents. The subsequent, usually long, contact time (typically 48 - 72 hours) with these more-or-less aggressive agents can cause membrane degradation, resulting in leaks [19]. The leak detector on the dialysis machine may not detect some such leaks. For example, in high-flux dialysers, backfiltration of dialysis fluid into the blood occurs in the area proximal to the dialysis fluid inlet port; a leak here allows the undetected passage of high quantities of possibly contaminated dialysis fluid into the blood and alters dialyser performance.

Test basis

The foundation of the tests themselves constitutes a major source of concern. In practice, the validation of using TCV or ultrafiltration measurements is frequently assumed on the basis of measurements conducted over 20 years ago on older dialysers in external clinics under operating conditions which differ from those presently employed. To be more specific, TCV-clearance and ultrafiltration-clearance correlations were originally validated using low blood flows of around 200 ml/min, low molecular weight solutes, low-flux cellulose membranes and manual reprocessing techniques with formaldehyde [27]. Present membrane permeabilities, fluid flows, disinfection techniques and solutes targeted for removal are frequently very different. This can result in a dissociation between TCV and actual small molecule clearance, which can then only be detected during the routine urea kinetic measurements (which are conducted regularly but at intervals of some weeks). Many such dissociation cases have been reported in the literature (e.g. [4, 46-48]). Indeed, a report from the Task Force on Reuse of Dialysers by the American National Kidney Foundation published in 1997 emphasised that small solute clearances can decrease with dialyser reprocessing even though AAMI standards are rigorously adhered to [49].

These standard performance tests are certainly unable to detect changes in dialyser performance due to channelling of dialysis fluid [46] and tend not to detect undesired increases in dialyser permeability due to damage caused by inappropriate reprocessing chemicals (e.g. [1]). Changes in TCV only poorly predict changes in the ultrafiltration characteristics of a membrane, while the ultrafiltration method of assessing performance in reprocessing underestimates the actual *in vivo* performance loss. Close attention must then be paid to expected and actual weight losses during treatment with reprocessed dialysers and machines that do not have automatic ultrafiltration control [4].

The dilemma of reusing high-flux membranes

A particularly critical facet of the "test nature" problem is the widespread use of high-flux dialysis membranes. These are indicated for the removal of middle molecules, especially ß2-microglobulin, but validation of the elimination of such molecules after reprocessing poses an additional, at present insurmountable, problem. Even dialyser manufacturers must conduct extensive tests to define the ß2-m removal capabilities of their filters. A number of studies have demonstrated that dialyser reprocessing can result in a substantial reduction in the ß2-m removal capacities of some dialysers, even when the TCV and the small molecule clearances remain within the AAMI restrictions (e.g. **figure 12.4** and [17, 31-33, 50]). Also enhanced values of ß2-m removal with increasing numbers of dialyser uses have been reported, although the TCV tests were passed, whereby these usually involve the cleaning agent bleach (see [51]). These results prove that the TCV tests used today fail to recognise changes in dialyser middle and large molecule removal properties (e.g. [16, 17, 31-33, 35, 36, 52]).

Only high-flux dialysers are available for reuse in Canada [7], and one oft-quoted reason for reusing dialysers is that the financial savings involved facilitate the procurement of the more expensive high-flux dialysers. This explains why the frequency of use of high-flux dialysers is greater in facilities that reuse compared to facilities that do not in the U.S. (97% versus 65%) [53]. However, the rationale is faulty, at the very least, given the fact that middle molecule removal characteristics of high-flux membranes are unpredictably altered by reuse.

Summary

Although TCV tests tend to reflect small solute performance more or less reliably (e.g. [17, 32, 35, 54, 55]), actual clearance measurements are much more reliable and safer for the patient [4, 17, 31, 37, 45, 47, 48]. Such measurements have revealed that the small solute clearances in reprocessed dialysers tend to be better preserved for low-flux cellulose than for high-flux synthetic membranes [35, 37, 51, 56]. Adherence to TCV limitations usually (not always) means only slight reductions in small solute clearance, which may or may not be clinically relevant. None of the performance tests conducted in reprocessing procedures provide acceptable assurance of middle solute removal or protein retention by high-flux dialysers.

12.2 Effect of reuse on dialyser biocompatibility and clinical behaviour

Recovery of the original dialyser or membrane biocompatibility profiles after use and reprocessing cannot be proven (or tested for) in routine clinical practice. *In vitro* and *in vivo* investigations, mostly conducted over 10 years ago, delivered a spectrum of results regarding the effects of reuse on biocompatibility. **Table 12.3** summaries these without offering a comprehensive analysis of the numerous papers published on this topic over the past decades. The qualifying comments in the table explain that the effects once considered positive are now largely obsolete. The comments also explain that many of the negative effects can be (and often are) caused by less than strict adherence to internationally recognised procedural standards, e.g. inadequate/excessive disinfectant concentration, poor quality of the water used for rinsing and diluting the disinfectants, and non-adherence to reprocessing procedure guidelines. Many undesired phenomena can be avoided by choosing appropriate new dialysers (e.g. steam sterilised dialysers produced by manufacturers with strict quality controls so as to avoid material contaminants), by employing chemical concentrations recommended by manufacturers of reprocessing equipment, and by strict adherence to standards for water quality in dialysis and reprocessing (e.g. [12, 61]). The low number of operational parameters in the new method of reprocessing using heat alone or in combination with citric acid may explain why pyrogenic reactions, sepsis and subjective symptoms are rare with this method [42, 62].

Regarding water quality, in the United States quality requirements for water used in haemodialysis applications were established by the Association for the Advancement of Medical Instrumentation (AAMI), and have been adopted as regulations by the Centers of Medicare and Medicaid Services (CMS) [61, 63]. The Task Force on Reuse of Dialysers appointed by the American National Kidney Foundation reported that some practitioners believe the water standards to be insufficient, and point out that European Pharmacopoeia guidelines are more stringent at present ([49], see [18] for specific guidelines).

"Header sepsis" in **table 12.3** is a term used to describe a particular instigator of bacteraemia and pyrogenic reactions which has to do with the removal of the dialyser headers and O-rings during reprocessing procedures (see [14]). This is common practice in many facilities as it permits the removal of clots formed in the header regions of the dialyser. However, it also allows organisms access to surfaces on or below the O-rings which, due to the tight seal after reassembling, are not exposed to the disinfectant later filled into the dialyser. During reuse, the pulsing of the blood through the dialyser causes the O-rings to move and bacteria that have proliferated in the meantime can enter the patient's blood. Nowadays, many reprocessing machines have extended procedures for disinfection of O-rings, headers and caps before reassembling and reprocessing. Some authors recommend that the headers not be removed at all (e.g. [14]), and indeed some dialyser manufacturers have made this impossible.

12.2.1 Open questions

A number of subjects, some of them referred to in **table 12.3**, are topics of active discussion and research. The most important of these with respect to membranes and dialysers are outlined here.

Should the proteins adsorbed during treatment be removed during reprocessing?

The employment of an effective cleaning agent to remove resistant clots and protein deposits has both advantages and disadvantages regarding the performance (especially middle molecule removal) of individual membranes, as was discussed in a previous section of this chapter. The situation regarding dialyser biocompatibility is less complicated, as only complement-activating membranes (i.e. regenerated cellulose) appear to benefit from not removing the adsorbed proteins. For these membranes, masking of the bioincompatible surfaces with a protein layer appears to retard complement activation and reduce sequelae of leukopenia due to pulmonary sequestration of leukocytes, with resultant hypoxaemia (e.g. [4, 34, 37, 64-66]). Use of an effective cleaning agent to remove the adsorbed proteins was shown to result in a revival of the original biocompatibility profile of dialysis membranes in the early eighties [66, 67]. Also a more recent randomised, double-blind, prospective study of 37 patients conducted by Pereira et al. found that reprocessing of dialysers containing regenerated cellulose membranes with bleach (protein removal) and glutaraldehyde reinstated the inherent bioincompatibility of these membranes (parameters measured were IL-1 Ra, C3a, LBP (lipopolysaccharide binding protein, an acute phase reactant), BPI (bactericidal permeability-increasing protein, a neutrophil primary granule protein) and intradialytic symptoms) [68].

Two explicit bio*in*compatibility aspects of protein adsorption have been revealed in other works (e.g. [20, 23]). These are (A) the postulated detrimental influence of these adsorbed proteins on device sterility, and (B) possible bioincompatibility aspects associated with these proteins after their alteration by the reprocessing chemicals.

Positive effects of dialyser reuse		Negative effects of dialyser reuse	
Effect	**Comment**	**Effect**	**Comment**
Avoidance of "first use" syndrome	Was proven to be mostly an anaphylactic reaction to EtO in the then commonly used EtO sterilised devices.	Allergic reactions and haemolysis	Inadequate rinsing of reprocessed dialysers Failure to dilute disinfectants properly Allergy to formaldehyde (case report)
Improved biocompatibility and less intradialytic symptoms (e.g. complement activation, leukopenia and hypoxaemia) associated with RC membranes.	Effect not relevant for biocompatible membranes or for RC membranes reprocessed with bleach.	Enhanced risk of pyrogenic reactions, bacteraemia and septicaemia	Mostly due to use of inadequate concentrations of disinfectants or use of contaminated water for rinsing or diluting disinfectants Possible contribution of protein layer to chemical degradation Header sepsis Inadequate hygiene during reprocessing
Reduced exposure to plasticisers and small particles in new dialysers	Older reports. Present day good quality production and adequate prerinsing guarantee safety (otherwise market withdrawal of product)	Increased bradykinin release	Only one study (abstract): due to contact activation by denatured proteins after reuse without bleach.
		Significant amino acid and protein loss Significant reduction in ß2-m removal by high-flux membranes	Only observed with some PSu and CTA membranes in association with the use of bleach. Usually observed when bleach is *not* used in reprocessing (see performance section for details)

Table 12.3: Reported effects of reuse on dialyser biocompatibility and clinical symptoms. *EtO: ethylene oxide gas; RC: regenerated cellulose; PSu: polysulfone; CTA: cellulose triacetate. For detailed references, see [1, 4, 17, 18, 49, 57-60].*

(A) Failure to use a cleaning agent or, in fact, the use of cleaning agents other than bleach (hypochlorite), means that proteins and cellular elements deposited on the surface of the membranes are not removed during reprocessing (e.g. [15, 23, 69, 70]). This protein layer can provide a good substrate for bacterial survival after reprocessing, especially if reprocessing solutions are used which are not in themselves sterile or pyrogen free, as is known to frequently be the case [20]. For example, contamination of water used to rinse dialysers and water used to make up the disinfectant was identified as the most likely source of pyrogenic reactions or *Mycobacterium chelonae* infection during treatment with dialysers reprocessed with very diluted formaldehyde, 2.5% Renalin® (peracetic acid) and 4% Renalin® [20, 71, 72]. It was postulated that increased protein disposition on the membrane could provide a better substrate for bacterial survival and/or accelerate disinfectant degradation.

(B) Proteins adsorbed onto the membrane surface are denatured (e.g. oxidised) due to the action of the various chemicals employed in the reprocessing procedure. Adhered, denatured proteins can remain attached during reprocessing, but become detached during the subsequent dialyses and so gain entry to the blood stream [59, 70]. The denatured substances may be sufficiently antigenic to result in an enhanced immunological response that may contribute to antibody formation (such as anti-N-like antibodies, described later). Ng et al. showed this in combined *in vivo - in vitro* investigations of formaldehyde-only reprocessed dialysers [70]. In another study, a strong oxidative modification of such adsorbed proteins due to the interaction with reprocessing chemicals was held responsible for contact phase activation with subsequent significant release of bradykinin. Here the negative charge involved in contact phase activation may originate in the cysteinic acid that results from oxidation of the amino acid cystein [59, 73].

In summary, the positive effects of protein deposition on device biocompatibility are now outdated due to the present widespread use of biocompatible membranes. While strict adherence to stipulations for disinfectant concentration and water quality will minimise the danger associated with the presence of a protein layer, further investigations into possible long-term effects of the denatured proteins on patient welfare are still necessary.

Is the formation of anti-N-like antibodies due to reprocessing with formaldehyde a problem?

A number of factors, mostly relating to the occupational hazards for staff using formaldehyde in reprocessing units, have led to a partial renunciation of this once most popular disinfectant (**figure 12.3**). Nevertheless, formaldehyde was still the second most popular disinfectant in the United States in 2000, being employed in 31% of dialysis centres conducting reuse there, so that any effects on dialyser biocompatibility remain topical. One main aspect of formaldehyde reuse was reviewed in detail in 1996 by Miles and Friedman: the induction of anti-N-like antibodies to the N antigen of the red cell surface MN antigen system by chronic intravenous exposure to small residual amounts of formaldehyde in reprocessed dialysers [4]. Red cell N antigens are altered in a dose-dependent manner, and the altered red cell antigen induces formation of a cold agglutinin that is associated with early renal allograft rejection, reductions in red cell life span (haemolysis) and difficulties in cross-matching blood.

Induction of anti-N-like antibodies was first not believed to occur when residual formaldehyde levels were kept low. This is the basis for the widely accepted standard for residual formaldehyde of ≤ 5 ppm in a reprocessed dialyser before being reused [4, 58] (although even lower levels were recommended by others [74, 75]). Intensive dialyser prerinsing then appeared to provide adequate protection against this adverse effect. However, formaldehyde levels have been observed to rebound by as much as 6 mg/l as formaldehyde diffuses out of the potting compound, and formaldehyde is difficult to rinse out of dialysers due to its binding to the amino groups of proteins deposited onto the membrane and in the headers (see [4, 70, 76] for more details). Furthermore, anti-N-like antibody formation was even detected when residual formaldehyde levels were no greater than 2-3 ppm and 0.5 ppm in two separate studies: in these reports, 10% and 11.1% (statistically significant values) of patients dialysed with such reprocessed dialysers were tested positive for the anti-N-like antibodies [75, 77].

Therefore, should formaldehyde be employed for reprocessing, then care should be taken to ensure optimal removal by very intensive prerinsing and prior removal of adsorbed blood proteins using bleach. Further studies are needed to clarify the actual clinical significance of anti-N-like antibody production: a role in haemolysis was reported in some older studies and not in others (e.g. [78, 79] as opposed to [77]), and the postulated contribution to allograft rejection and blood cross-matching problems also remains unclear.

Is haemolysis more severe with reused dialysers?

There are many possible causes for haemolysis in dialysis patients but a number of studies have reported enhanced signs of haemolysis in dialysers which were reused (e.g. [23, 79]). The use of formaldehyde has been associated with haemolysis in the past by causing red cell ATP depletion and defective red cell metabolism, and was linked with the formation of anti-N-like antibodies [4, 49, 74, 78, 79]. However, even dialysers reprocessed in other ways are affected. For example, more haemoglobin was found on dialysers that had been used 15 times using heat plus citric acid compared with single use dialysers [23]. The presence of haemoglobin on the surface of the dialyser membranes indicates that some destruction of red cells took place during dialysis, probably due to haemodynamic stresses. The authors point out, however, that it remains unclear whether haemolysis is really more severe for reprocessed than for new dialysers, or whether the affinity of the reprocessed surface for haemoglobin increases [23]. Also a more recent study of anti-N-like antibody formation after formaldehyde reprocessing came to the conclusion that, despite antibody induction, haemolysis is rarely a serious consequence of dialyser reuse [77].

Is dialyser reuse associated with enhanced patient mortality?

The possible influence of dialyser reuse on patient mortality has been a topic of discussion for many years. While studies published in the eighties indicated that outcomes were better or equally good in centres practising reuse compared to "single use only" centres [65, 80], later publications found a link between the practice of dialyser reuse and enhanced patient mortality, at least for certain reuse procedures, types of facilities and times of treatment [57, 81-85]. The studies have been criticised for a number of reasons, including lack of randomisation and appropriate controls, inadequate consideration of patient comorbidities, and/or insufficient information on dialysis dose delivered and other patient-specific data. For example, a factor which is favourable for survival in reuse units is that facilities that reuse dialysers tend to deliver a higher dose of dialysis than facilities that do not reuse (e.g. [45, 49, 53]). In fact, the Task Force on Reuse of Dialysers set up by the American National Kidney Foundation recommends that " ..dialysis prescriptions in units practising reuse should be designed to deliver a Kt/V or URR value that exceeds the dose used for patients treated with single-use dialyzers to make allowance for any possible reuse-induced reduction in dialyzer efficiency" [49]. Consequently, the actual dialysis dose received by patients treated with reused dialysers remains unclear. The influence of comorbidity on the results was analysed by Feldman et al. for a small sample of the U.S. ESRD population in free-standing dialysis facilities only for whom comorbidity data were available: the practice of dialyser reuse was still found to be associated with higher death rates [82].

A later general analysis of the 1994 to 1995 USRDS Dialysis Mortality and Morbidity Study which took all the above-mentioned factors into consideration came up with a different picture [57]. With respect to dialyser reuse practice, three interesting results of this prospective investigation of 12,791 haemodialysis patients in 1394 clinics were as follows: (1) The relative risk of death (RR) was not found to differ for patients in reuse versus non-reuse clinics. (2) For reuse without bleach, the RR was found to be marginally greater for peracetic acid compared to formaldehyde in the case of cellulose-based membranes (36%), while differences were not statistically significant for synthetic membranes (**figure 12.6**). (3) Regarding the use of the cleaning agent bleach (sodium hypochlorite), reuse of synthetic high-flux membranes using this was associated with the lowest estimated mortality (shown arbitrarily as the reference group in **figure 12.7**), while the RR was statistically significantly increased for all low-flux membrane types reprocessed without bleach, as well as for cellulose low-flux membranes reprocessed with bleach.

Interpretation of these results is extremely difficult: if we are to accept that removal of middle molecules is effective in reducing patient mortality (as indicated by the lower RR values for high-flux membranes in **figure 12.7**, and as reported by some others, e.g. [42, 86]), and if we take reports on enhanced risk of infection in reuse centres seriously (e.g. [1, 62, 87] - see **table 12.3** for reasons), then practices which may increase survival (e.g. bleach reprocessing of high-flux membranes for enhanced middle molecule removal) are mixed with practices which may negatively affect survival (e.g. infection or albumin loss), leading possibly to false averages and statistics. Further studies are clearly necessary to clarify the situation, especially regarding potentially higher-risk associations with certain common disinfectants. The recent moves towards single-use in some U.S. dialysis centres promises some insight into the effects of reuse versus single-use on patient mortality in the long-term. Preliminary results indicate that the use of new synthetic dialysers for each dialysis session is associated with a survival advantage for patients compared to the use of reprocessed dialysers [88].

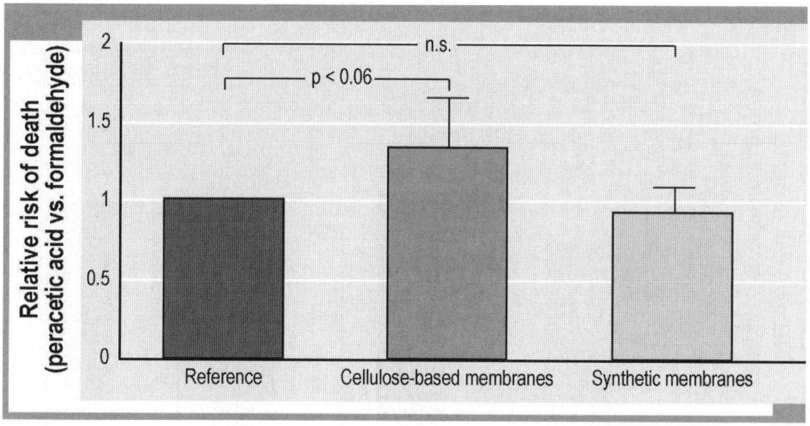

Figure 12.6: Relative risk of death (RR) for dialysers reprocessed with peracetic acid mixture compared to formaldehyde (no bleach). *As peracetic acid mixture is typically used without bleach (> 96% of cases in this study), this analysis was limited to reuse without the cleaning agent bleach. Values of RR > 1 (reference) mean that the risk of death was greater with peracetic acid mixture than with formaldehyde. The data sets were adjusted for demographics, comorbidities, facilities and membrane types. The group "cellulose-based membranes" comprises membranes made from plain regenerated cellulose as well as low- and high-flux membranes made from substituted cellulose. The group "synthetic membranes" contains both low- and high-flux synthetic membranes. Upper 95% confidence intervals are shown (adapted from [57]).*

Is protein and amino acid loss a problem associated with dialyser reuse?

Hypoalbuminemia is a marker of nutritional status and a significant predictor of mortality in patients with ESRD. For example, serum albumin concentrations below 4 g/dl were shown to be associated with a significant increase in the adjusted relative risk of death in 2 large-scale studies involving 12,000 and 13,535 haemodialysis patients [89, 90]. Substantial loss of amino acids and albumin with bleach use in reprocessing has been reported for cellulose triacetate dialysers and for some polysulfone membranes reused in the USA up to 1998, as mentioned in section 12.1 [16, 36, 39]. However, no clinically significant losses were observed when the polysulfone dialysers in question and the new F 80A polysulfone dialysers were reprocessed without bleach, and when the F 80B dialysers (configuration of polysulfone designed for reuse with bleach) were reprocessed with bleach (e.g. maximum losses were 0.3 - 1.5 g after 15 - 20 uses in four separate studies) [10, 15, 16, 35, 37, 39, 40,

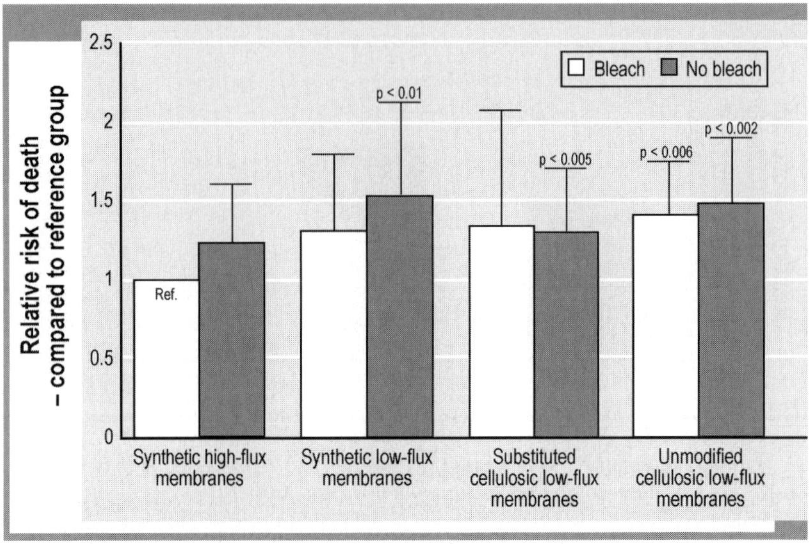

Figure 12.7: Relative risk of death (RR) for various membrane types and use of bleach compared to synthetic, high-flux membranes reprocessed with bleach. *Synthetic, high-flux membranes reprocessed with bleach had the lowest estimated mortality – this was then defined as the reference, i.e. the RR value is one. Values of RR > 1 for other groups indicate a higher risk of death. p values refer to comparisons with the reference group: only the statistically significant or marginally significant p values are shown. Values were adjusted for demographics, comorbidities, facilities and reuse agent. Upper 95% confidence intervals are shown (adapted from [57]).*

50]. There remains some ambiguity concerning cellulose triacetate dialysers: while an *in vitro* study calculated only insignificant albumin loss (maximum 1.1 g after 15 uses), a recently conducted *in vivo* investigation reported significant losses of 4.24 g/dialysis after 20 reuses with bleach [39].

While removal of amino acids and albumin has a negative effect on patient welfare, removal of ß2-m and other middle molecules is targeted for the alleviation of patient morbidity and mortality (e.g. [57, 86]). In general, increases in membrane permeability for amino acid and albumin due to reprocessing can be expected to go hand in hand with increases in middle molecule removal (although exceptions are reported, e.g. [40]). Correspondingly, membrane changes aimed at restricting albumin loss must take care to ensure continued good ß2-m removal [16, 35, 37, 91]. Increases in dialyser permeability for ß2-m have been observed with increasing bleach reuse number, e.g. increases of 40 - 50% and more [17, 37, 40]. In addition to improved ß2-m removal, another possible side effect of very open membranes that could be considered beneficial is the removal of protein-bound uraemic toxins. Ongoing research is striving to define marker molecules for dialysis adequacy which are of more accepted toxicity than urea. One much-favoured representative for the group of protein-bound molecules is p-cresol, a small molecule with a molecular weight of 108 which is 100% and 90% protein-bound in healthy subjects and uraemics, respectively [92]. This has multiple biological side effects and behaves like a number of other protein-bound compounds with pathophysiological effects, such as 3-carboxy-4-methyl-5-propyl-2-furanpropionic acid (CMPF) [92-95]. Removal of such protein-bound compounds has been shown to improve renal anaemia, and has been observed in CAPD and with protein-leaking membranes [96, 97]. However, protein malnutrition remains an item of serious concern, so that albumin losses should be minimised. Regarding upper limits for "acceptable" albumin loss, a recent review came to the conclusion that this is impossible to derive from the data presently available [98]. Two publications mentioned values of 5 g and 8 -10 g per treatment ([99] and [100], respectively), but others reported detrimental clinical effects of albumin losses in excess of 4 g/session [101, 102]. Membrane producers now usually aim for lower values (e.g. ≤ 3 g per treatment). Should future dialysis strategies target removal of protein-bound solutes, or should such protein losses due to extensive reuse of certain dialysers be tolerated, then increased protein supplementation must be given due consideration.

References

1. Roth VR, Jarvis WR: Outbreaks of infection and/or pyrogenic reactions in dialysis patients. Seminars in Dialysis 13(2): 92-96, 2000

2. Tokars JI, Frank M, Alter MJ, Arduino MJ: National surveillance of dialysis-associated diseases in the United States, 2000. Seminars in Dialysis 15(3): 162-171, 2002

3. Burgansky A, Gasteyger S: Growth opportunities in the US – Company Update – Fresenius Medical Care. Credit Suisse First Boston: 1-31, 5th September, 2003

4. Miles AM, Friedman EA: Dialyzer reuse - techniques and controversy in *Replacement of renal function by dialysis*, 4th ed., edited by Jacobs C, Kjellstrand

CM, Koch KM, Winchester JF, Dordrecht, Kluwer Academic Publishers: 454-471, 1996

5. Tokars JI, Miller ER, Alter MJ, Arduino MJ: National surveillance of dialysis-associated diseases in the United States, 1997. Seminars in Dialysis 13(2): 75-85, 2000

6. Powe NR, Thamer M, Hwang W, Fink NE, Bass EB, Sadler JH, Levin NW: Cost-quality trade-offs in dialysis care: A national survey of dialysis facility administrators. Am J Kidney Dis 39(1): 116-126, 2002

7. Manns BJ, Taub K, Richardson RM, Donaldson C: To reuse or not to reuse? An economic evaluation of hemodialyzer reuse versus conventional single-use hemodialysis for chronic hemodialysis patients. Int J Technol Assess Care 18(1): 81-93, 2002

8. Bourke M, Mathew T, Fazzalari R, Thurlwell G, Disny A: Multiple use of dialyzers: six uses is optium. The Medical Journal of Australia: 10-12, 1984

9. Helmandollar AW, Rosner MH, Abdel-Rahman E, Kline Bolton W: Comparative urea and beta-2 microglobulin clearances between Optiflux and heat-citric acid reuse F80A hemodialysis membranes: Is reused still justified? (Abstract) J Am Soc Nephrol 13: 602A, 2002

10. Röckel A, Hertel J, Fiegel P, Abdelhamid S, Panitz N, Walb D: Permeability and secondary membrane formation of a high flux polysulfone hemofilter. Kidney Int 30: 429-432, 1986

11. Clark WR, Gao D: Low-molecular weight proteins in end-stage renal disease: potential toxicity and dialytic removal mechanisms. J Am Soc Nephrol 13: S41-S47, 2002

12. AAMI standards and Recommended Practices; volume 3: Dialysis. Reuse of hemodialyzers, Arlington, VA, ANSI/AAMI RD47, 85-118, 1993

13. National Kidney Dialysis Outcome Quality Initiative (DOQI): Guidelines for hemodialysis adequacy - Update 2000. Available at http://www. kidney.org/professionals/doqi/guidelines. Accessed August 27, 2002

14. Arduino MJ: How should dialyzers be reprocessed? Seminars in Dial 11: 282-284, 1998

15. Cornelius RM, McClung WG, Barre P, Brash JL: Effects of reuse and bleach/formaldehyde reprocessing on polysulfone and polyamide hemodialyzers. ASAIO J 48(3): 300-311, 2002

16. Kaplan AA, Halley SE, Larkin RA, Graeber CW: Dialysate protein losses with bleach processed polysulphone dialyzers. Kidney Int 47: 573-578, 1995

17. Cheung AK, Agodoa LY, Daugirdas JT, Depner TA, Gotch FA, Greene T, Levin NW, Leypoldt JK and the HEMO study group: Effects of hemodialyzer reuse on clearances of urea and $ß_2$-microglobulin. J Am Soc Nephrol 10: 117-127, 1999

18. Bonnie-Schorn E, Grassmann A, Uhlenbusch-Körwer I, Weber C, Vienken J: Water quality in hemodialysis, 1st ed., edited by Vienken J, Lengerich, Pabst Science Publishers, 1998

19. Boland G, Reingold AL, Carson LA, Silcox VA, Woodley CL, Hayes PS, Hightower AW, McFarland L, Brown JW, Petersen NJ, Favero MS, Good RC, Broome CV: Infections with *Mycobacterium chelonei* in patients receiving dialysis and using processed hemodialyzers. J Infect Dis 152(5): 1013-1019, 1985

20. Lowry PW, Beck-Sague CM, Bland LA, Aguero SM, Arduino MJ, Minuth AN, Murray RA, Swenson JM, Jarvis WR: *Mycobacterium chelonae* infection among patients receiving high-flux dialysis in a hemodialysis clinic in California. J Infect Dis 161: 85-90, 1990

21. Kaufman AM, Frinak S, Godmere RO, Levin NW: Clinical experience with heat sterilization for reprocessing dialyzers. Am Soc Artif Int Organs J 38: M338, 1992

22. Levin NW, Parnell SL, Prince HN, Gotch F, Polaschegg HD, Levin R, Alto A, Kaufman AM: The use of heated citric acid for dialyzer reprocessing. J Am Soc Nephrol 6: 1578-1585, 1995

23. Cornelius RM, McClung WG, Richardson RM, Estridge C, Plaskos N, Yip CM, Brash JL: Effects of heat/citric acid reprocessing on high-flux polysulfone dialyzers. ASAIO J 48(1): 45-56, 2002

24. Parker TF: Technical advances in hemodialysis therapy. Seminars in Dialysis 13(6): 372-377, 2000

25. Vienken J: Survey on sterilization methods and associated adverse reactions. (Presentation) Dialysis Academy, Germany, April 1999

26. Center for Disease Control: Bacteremia associated with reuse of disposable hollow-fiber hemodialyzers. MMWR Morb Mortal Wkly Rep 35(25): 417-418, 1986

27. Gotch FA: Mass transport in reused dialyzers. Proc Dial Transplant Forum 10: 81-85, 1980

28. Alter M, Favero M, Miller J, Coleman P, Bland L: Reuse of hemodialyzers: results of nationwide surveillance for adverse effects. JAMA 260: 2073-2077, 1988

29. Bland LA, Favero MS, Oxborrow GS, Aguero SM, Searcy BP, Danielson JW: Effect of chemical germicides on the integrity of hemodialyzer membranes. Trans Am Soc Artif Intern Organs 34: 172-175, 1988

30. Rahmati MA, Rahmati S, Hoenich N, Ronco C, Kaysen GA, Levin R, Levin NW: On-line clearance: a useful tool for monitoring the effectiveness of the reuse procedure. ASAIO Journal 49: 543-546, 2003

31. Leypoldt JK, Cheung AK, Deeter RB: Effect of hemodialyzer reuse: dissociation between clearances of small and large solutes. Am J Kidney Dis 32(2): 295-301, 1998

32. Ouseph R, Smith BP, Ward RA: Maintaining blood compartment volume in dialyzers reprocessed with peracetic acid maintains Kt/V but not $ß_2$-microglobulin removal. Am J Kidney Dis 30(4): 501-506, 1997

33. Goldman M, Lagmiche M, Dhaene M, Amraoui Z, Thayse C, Vanherweghem JL: Adsorption of ß2-microglobulin on dialysis membranes: comparison of different dialyzers and effects of reuse procedures. Int J Artif Org 12(6): 373-378, 1989

34. Westhuyzen J, Foreman K, Battistutta D, Saltissi D, Fleming SJ: Effect of dialyzer reprocessing with Renalin on serum beta-2-microglobulin and complement activation in hemodialysis patients. Am J Nephrol 12(1-2): 29-36, 1992

35. Scott MK, Mueller BA, Sowinski KM, Clark WR: Dialyzer-dependent changes in solute and water permeability with bleach reprocessing. Am J. Kidney Dis 33(1): 87-96, 1999

36. Ikizler TA, Flakoll PJ, Parker RA, Hakim RM: Amino acid and albumin losses during hemodialysis. Kidney Int 46: 830-837, 1994

37. Murthy BV, Sundaram S, Jaber BL, Perrella C, Meyer KB, Pereira BJ: Effect of formaldehyde/bleach reprocessing on *in vivo* performances of high-efficiency cellulose and high-flux polysulfone dialyzers. J Am Soc Nephrol 9(3): 464-472, 1998

38. Diaz RJ, Washburn S, Cauble L, Siskind MS, Van Wyck D: The effect of dialyzer reprocessing on performance and *ß*2-microglobulin removal using polysulfone membranes. Am J Kidney Dis 21(4): 405-410, 1993

39. Kaysen GA, Dubin JA, Müller HG, Mitch WE, Rosales LM, Levin NW, and the HEMO group: Relationships among inflammation nutrition and physiologic mechanisms establishing albumin levels in hemodialysis patients. Kidney Int 61: 2240-2249, 2002

40. Ward RA, Ouseph R: Impact of bleach cleaning on the performance of dialyzers with polysulfone membranes processed for reuse using peracetic acid. Artificial Organs 27(11): 1029-1034, 2003

41. Sargent JA, Gotch FA: Principles and biophysics of dialysis in *Replacement of renal function by dialysis*, 4th ed., edited by Jacobs C, Kjellstrand CM, Koch KM, Winchester JF, Dordrecht, Kluwer Academic Publishers: 188-230, 1996

42. Murthy VB, Pereira BJ: Does reuse have clinically important effects on dialyzer function?. Seminars in Dialysis 13(5): 282-286, 2000

43. National Kidney Dialysis Outcome Quality Initiative (DOQI): Clinical practice guidelines: hemodialysis adequacy and peritoneal dialysis adequacy. Am J Kid Dis 30 (3, Suppl 2): S1-S64, 1997

44. Held PJ, Port FK, Wolfe RA, Stannard DC, Carroll CE, Daugirdas JT, Bolembergen WE, Greer JW, Hakim RM: The dose of hemodialysis and patient mortality. Kidney Int 50: 550-556, 1996

45. Sherman RA, Cody RP, Rogers ME, Solanchick JC: The effect of dialyzer reuse on dialysis delivery. Am J Kidney Dis 24(6): 924-926, 1994

46. Delmez JA, Weerts CA, Hasamear PD, Windus DW: Severe dialyzer dysfunction undetectable by standard reprocessing validation tests. Kidney Int 36: 478-484, 1989

47. Chandran PK, Anderson MJ, Liggett R: Performance of AN69 dialyzers after reprocessing. (Abstract) ASAIO 38th Annual Meeting, 1992

48. Chan JK, Lau N: Optimal reuse of cuprammonium rayon hollow-fibre dialyzers. Int J Artif Organs 12: 223-228, 1989

49. Task force on reuse of dialyzers, Council on dialysis, National Kidney Foundation: National kidney foundation report on dialyzer reuse. Am J Kidney Dis 30(6): 859-871, 1997.

50. Scott MK, Mueller BA, Sowinski KM: The effects of peracetic acid-hydrogen peroxide reprocessing on dialyzer solute and water permeability. Pharmacotherapy 19(9): 1042-1049, 1999

51. Leypoldt JK: Does reuse have clinically important effects on dialyzer function?. Seminars in Dialysis 13(5): 281-282, 2000

52. Vinhas J, dos Santos JP: Haemodialyser reuse: facts and fiction. Nephrol Dial Transplant 15: 5-8, 2000

53. Agodoa LY, Wolfe RA, Port FK: Reuse of dialyzers and clinical outcomes: fact or fiction. Am J Kidney Dis 32 (6 Suppl 4): S88-S92, 1998

54. Sridhar NR, Ferrand K, Reger D, Hayes P, Pinnavaia L, Butts D, Kohli R, Papandenatos G: Urea kinetics with dialyzer reuse - a prospective study. Am J Nephrol 19(6): 668-673, 1999

55. Kerr PG, Argiles A, Canaud B, Flavier JL, Mion C: The effects of reprocessing high-flux polysulfone dialyzers with peroxyacetic acid on β_2-microglobulin removal in hemodiafiltration. Am J Kidney Dis 19(5): 433-438, 1992

56. Vanholder RC, Sys E, DeCubber A, Vermaercke N, Ringoir SM: Performance of cuprophane and polyacrylonitrile dialyzers during multiple use. Kidney Int 24 (Suppl): S55-S56, 1988

57. Port FK, Wolfe RA, Hulbert-Shearon TE, Daugirdas JT, Agodoa LY, Jones C, Orzol SM, Held PJ: Mortality risk by hemodialyzer reuse practice and dialyzer membrane characteristics: Results from the URSDS dialysis morbidity and mortality study. Am J Kidney Dis 37(2): 276-286, 2001

58. Ogden DA: Dialyzer reuse in *Dialysis therapy*, edited by Nissenson AR, Fine RN, Gentile DE, Norwalk, Connecticut, Appleton & Lange: 172-210, 1990

59. Sodemann K, Lubrich-Birker I, Berger O., Mahiout A: Identification of oxidized protein and bradykinin generation in dialyzer-reuse with polysulfone membranes. International Society of Nephrology meeting, Sydney, 1997

60. Salem M, Ivanovich PT, Ing TS, Daugirdas JT: Adverse effects of dialyzers manifesting during the dialysis session. Nephrol Dial Transplant 9 (Suppl 2): 127-137, 1994

61. Ouseph R, Ward RA: Water treatment for hemodialysis: ensuring patient safety. Seminars in Dialysis 15(1): 50-52, 2002

62. Tokars JI, Miller ER, Alter MJ, Arduino MJ: National surveillance of dialysis associated diseases in the United states, 1995. Am Soc Artif Int Org J 44: 98-107, 1998

63. Association for the Advancement of Medical Instrumentation: Water treatment equipment for hemodialysis applications (ANSI/AAMI RD62:2001). Arlington, VA: Association for the Advancement of Medical Instrumentation, 2001

64. Kes P, Reiner Z, Ratkovic-Gusic I: Dialyzer reprocessing with peroxyacetic acid as sole cleansing and sterilizing agent. Acta Med Croatica 51; 87-93, 1997

65. Kant KS, Pollak VE, Cathey M, Goetz D, Berlin R: Multiple use of dialyzers, safety and efficacy. Kidney Int 19(5): 728-738, 1981

66. Hoenich NA, Johnson SR, Buckley P, Harden J, Ward MK, Kerr DN: Haemodialysis reuse: Impact on function and biocompatibility. Int J Artif Organs 6: 261-266, 1983

67. Rancourt M, Senger K, DeOreo P: Cellulose membrane induced leukopenia after reprocessing with sodium hypochlorite. Trans Am Soc Artif Intern Organs 30: 49-51, 1984

68. Pereira BJ, Snodgrass B, Barber G, Perella C, Chopra S, King AJ: Cytokine production during *in vitro* hemodialysis with new and formaldehyde- or renalin-reprocessed cellulose dialyzers. J Am Soc Nephrol 6(4): 1304-1308, 1995

69. Sotonyi P, Jaray J, Padar Z, Woller J, Furedi S, Gal T: Comparative study on reused haemodialysis membranes. Int J Artif Organs 19: 387-392, 1996

70. Ng Y-Y, Yang A-H, Wong K-C, Lan H-Y, Hung T-L, Kerr PG, Huang T-P: Dialyzer reuse: Interaction between dialyzer membrane, disinfectant (formalin), and blood during dialyzer reprocessing. Artificial Organs 20(1): 53-55, 1996

71. Gordon SM, Tipple M, Bland LA, Jarvis WR: Pyrogenic reactions associated with the reuse of disposable hollow-fiber hemodialyzers. JAMA 260: 2077-2081, 1988

72. Rudnick JR, Arduino MJ, Bland LA, Cusick L, McAllister SK, Aguero SM, Jarvis WR: An outbreak of pyrogenic reactions in chronic hemodialysis patients associated with hemodialyzer reuse. Artif Organs 19(4): 289-294, 1995

73. Vienken J, Diamantoglou M, Hahn C, Kamusewitz H, Paul D: Considerations on developmental aspects of biocompatible dialysis membranes. Artif Organs 19(5): 398-406, 1995

74. Lewis KJ, Dewar PJ, Ward MK, Kerr DN: Formation of anti-N-like antibodies in dialysis patients: effect of different methods of dialyzer rinsing to remove formaldehyde. Clin Nephrol 15(1): 39-43, 1981

75. Vanholder R, Noens L, De Smet R, Ringoir S: Development of anti-N-like antibodies during formaldehyde reuse in spite of adequate predialysis rinsing. Am J Kidney Dis 11(6): 477-480, 1988

76. Stragier A, Wenderickx D, Jadoul M: Rinsing time and disinfectant release of reused dialyzers: comparison of formaldehyde, hypochlorite, warexin and renalin. Am J Kidney Dis 26(3): 549-553, 1995

77. Ng Y-Y, Chow M-P, Wu S-C, Lyou J-Y, Harris DC, Huang T-P: Anti-Nform antibody in hemodialysis patients. Am J Nephrol 15(5): 374-378, 1995

78. Koch KM, Frei U, Fassbinder W: Hemolysis and anemia in anti-N-like antibody positive patients. Trans Am Soc Artif Intern Organs 24: 709-713, 1978

79. Orringer EP, Mattern WD: Formaldehyde-induced hemolysis during chronic hemodialysis. N Engl J Med 294: 1416-1420, 1976

80. Held PJ, Pauly MM, Diamond LH: Survival analysis of patients undergoing dialysis. JAMA 247: 645-650, 1987

81. Held PJ, Wolfe RA, Gaylin DS, Port FK, Levin NW, Turenne MN: Analysis of the association of dialyzer reuse practices and patient outcomes. Am J Kidney Dis 23: 692-708, 1994

82. Feldman HI, Bilker WB, Hackett MH, Simmons CW, Holmes JH, Pauly MV, Escarce JJ: Association of dialyzer reuse with hospitalization and survival rates amoung U.S. hemodialysis patients: Do comorbidities matter? J Clin Epidemiol 52(3): 209-217, 1999

83. Feldman HI, Kinosian M, Bilker WB, Simmons C, Holmes JH, Pauly MV, Escarce JJ: Effect of dialyzer reuse on survival of patients treated with hemodialysis. JAMA 276(8): 620-625, 1996

84. Collins AJ, Ma JZ, Constantini EG, Everson SE: Dialysis unit and patient characteristics associated with reuse practices and mortality: 1989-1993. J Am Soc Nephrol 9: 2108-2117, 1998

85. Ebben JP, Dalleska F, Ma JZ, Everson SE, Constantini EG, Collins AJ: Impact of disease severity and hematocrit level on reuse-associated mortality. Am J Kidney Dis 35(2): 244-249, 2000

86. Leypoldt JK, Cheung AK, Carroll CE, Stannard DC, Pereira BJ, Agodoa LY, Port FK: Effect of dialysis membranes and middle molecule removal on chronic hemodialysis patient survival. Am J Kidney Dis 33(2): 349-355, 1999

87. Arduino MJ: CDC investigations of noninfectious outbreaks of adverse events in hemodialysis facilities, 1979-1999. Seminars in Dialysis 13(2): 86-91, 2000

88. Lowrie EG, Li Z, Ofsthun N, Lazarus JM: The reuse of dialyzers: Current death risk relationships for patients. (Abstract) J Am Soc Nephrol 14: 249A, 2003

89. Lowrie EG, Lew NL: Death risk in hemodialysis patients: The predictive value of commonly measured variables and an evaluation of death rate differences between facilities. Am J Kidney Dis 15(5): 458-482, 1990

90. Lowrie EG, Lew NL: Commonly measured laboratory variables in hemodialysis patients: relationships among them and to death risk. Semin Nephrol 12(3): 276-283, 1992

91. Ahrenholz PG, Winkler RE, Michelsen A, Lang DA, Bowry SK: Dialysis membrane-dependent removal of middle molecules during haemodiafiltration: the ß2-microglobulin / albumin relationship. Clinical Nephrology, submitted August 2003.

92. Vanholder R, DeSmet R, Lesaffer G: p-cresol: a toxin revealing many neglected but relevant aspects of uraemic toxicity. Nephrol Dial Transplant 14: 2813-2815, 1999

93. Vanholder R, De Smet R, Vogeleere P, Hsu C, Ringoir S: The uraemic syndrome in *Replacement of renal function by dialysis*, 4th ed., edited by Jacobs C, Kjellstrand CM, Koch KM, Winchester JF, Dordrecht, Kluwer Academic Publishers: 1-33, 1996

94. Vanholder R, DeSmet R, Lesaffer G: Dissociation between dialysis adequacy and Kt/V. Seminars in Dialysis 15(1): 3-7, 2002

95. Vanholder R, DeSmet R, Lameire N: Protein-bound uremic solutes: the forgotten toxins. Kidney Int 59 (Suppl 78): S266-S270, 2001

96. Niwa T, Asada H, Tsutsui S, Miyazaki T: Efficient removal of albumin-bound furancarboxylic acid by protein-leaking hemodialysis. Am J Nephrol 15: 463-467, 1995

97. Niwa T, Yazawa T, Kodama T, Uehara Y, Maeda K, Yamada K: Efficient removal of albumin-bound furancarboxylic acid, an inhibitor of erythropoiesis, by continuous ambulatory peritoneal dialysis. Nephron 56: 241-245, 1990

98. Krieter DH, Canaud B: High permeability of dialysis membranes: what is the limit of albumin loss? Nephrol Dial Transplant 18: 651-654, 2003

99. Combarnous F, Tetta C, Chapuis Cellier C, Wratten ML, Custaud MA, De Catheu T, Fouque D, David S, Carraro G, Laville M: Albumin loss in on-line hemodiafiltration. Int J Artif Organs 25(3): 203-209, 2002

100. Lebedo I: Does convective dialysis therapy applied daily approach renal blood purification?. Kidney Int 59 (Suppl 78): S286-S291, 2001

101. Kaysen GA, Stevenson FT, Depner TA: Determinants of albumin concentration in hemodialysis patients. Am J Kidney Dis 29: 658-668, 1997)

102. Kim ST, Yamamoto C, Asabe H, Sato T, Takamiya T: On-line haemodiafiltration: effective removal of high molecular weight toxins and improvement in clinical manifestations of chronic haemodialysis patients. Nephrology 2: S183-S186, 1996.

Glossary

AAMI (Association for the Advancement of Medical Instrumentation): independent committee of experts recommending standards for medical procedures, including dialysis, for the USA.

Acute phase proteins: proteins (e.g. C-reactive protein, serum amyloid P, mannose-binding protein, haptoglobin, ceroluplasmin, transferrin) secreted by the liver and resulting from the action of TNF, IL-1 and IL-6 on hepatocytes. These proteins are found in blood of patients with systemic illnesses (e.g. infections, burns, rheumatoid diseases, myocardial infarction and cancer).

Acute phase response: the primary response to infection or other inflammatory stimuli triggered by mediators (e.g. IL-6) of immune cell activation. The response consists of systemic effects, such as the production of *acute phase proteins,* and may be accompanied by clinical symptoms, such as fever.

Acute reactions: side effects appearing during and/or shortly after the dialysis session.

Aldehydes (liquid): solutions used in dialyser and haemofilter reprocessing, e.g. glutaraldehyde (e.g. trade name Diacide®) and formaldehyde in concentrations of 2% - 5%.

Allergic reaction: response to innocuous environmental antigens or allergens due to pre-existing antibodies or T-cells. There are various immune mechanisms, the most common being the binding of IgE antibody by mast cells; this causes asthma, hays fever and other common allergic reactions.

Alternative complement pathway: in contrast to the *classical pathway,* this is triggered by the binding of complement factor C3b to a foreign surface, such as that of a pathogen or the artificial surface of dialysis membranes. Products of activation are the *anaphylatoxins* C3a and C5a and the *terminal complement complex C5b-9* (also called the *membrane attack complex).*

Amyloidosis, dialysis-related: long-term complication of haemodialysis related to the accumulation and retention of ß2-microglobulin in combination with its incomplete or atypical proteolysis. Deposition of ß2-m leads to symptoms, such as generalised arthralgia, scapulohumeral periarthritis, bone cysts, pathological fractures and carpal-tunnel syndrome.

Anaphylactic reaction: *hypersensitivity reaction* involving IgE antibodies without the activation of *complement.*

Anaphylactoid reaction: *hypersensitivity reaction* without specific IgE antibodies but with direct *complement activation* or *bradykinin* generation.

Anaphylaxia: *hypersensitivity reaction* of a sensibilised organism after re-exposure to the antigen. Based on the liberation of vasoactive mediators from cells that had an antigen-antibody reaction at their surface.

Anaphylatoxin: small fragment of complement protein released by cleavage during complement activation - namely C5a, C3a or C4a (listed according to decreasing biological potency). It stimulates inflammatory cells to move to sites of infection.

Angiotensin-converting enzyme (ACE) inhibitors: a class of drugs used in the treatment of hypertension and/or cardiac diseases; they reduce peripheral arterial resistance and the pre- and afterload of the heart by blocking the conversion of angiotensin I to angiotensin II. Angiotensin II is a powerful vasoconstrictor and a substance responsible for many vasculopathic states.

Anti-N-like antibodies: antibodies to the N antigen of the red cell surface MN antigen system. These are produced, for example, in response to chronic intravenous exposure to small residual amounts of formaldehyde.

Arylane: high-flux dialysis membrane made of *poly(aryl)ethersulfone* and *polyvinylpyrrolidone* (PVP) produced by Hospal (France).

Asahi Polysulfone®: high-flux dialysis membrane made of *polysulfone* and *polyvinylpyrrolidone* (PVP) produced by Asahi (Japan).

Atopy: condition of increased susceptibility to immediate *hypersensitivity,* usually mediated by IgE antibodies.

Autoclave: high-pressure steriliser. A heatable, double-walled pressure tank with lockable lid, manometer, safety valve, thermometer and control unit, which is used for sterilisation by steam at 1 - 2 atm. negative pressure.

Automated reprocessing: reprocessing of used dialysers with a specially designed machine or set-up that automatically conducts rinsing, filling and performance testing.

Backdiffusion: process by which constituents of dialysis fluid cross dialysis membranes from the dialysis fluid to the blood compartment, driven by a concentration gradient.

Backfiltration: movement of dialysis fluid into the blood compartment due to a pressure gradient (as opposed to a concentration gradient, as in *backdiffusion*).

Backtransport: sum of *backdiffusion* and *backfiltration*

Bactericidal/permeability-increasing protein (BPI): a neutrophil primary granule protein that binds or inhibits lipopolysaccharide (LPS).

Bands: earlier attempt at performance-enhancing dialyser design involving the weaving of small numbers of individual fibres into bands with the help of threads. This technologically complex approach has been largely abandoned in favour of *spacer yarn, fins* or *undulations.*

ß2-microglobulin: in its monomeric form, a 11,818 molecular weight protein (dimeric and polymeric forms as well as different fragments exist). It is the precursor protein of the amyloid found in *dialysis-related amyloidosis* (Aß2-microglobulin-amyloid fibrils).

Biocompatibility: ability of a material, device or system to perform with an appropriate host response in the clinical situation (as defined at the Consensus Conference on Biocompatibility, Königswinter, Germany 1993).

Bleach: *sodium hypochlorite*. Cleaning agent frequently used in dialyser reprocessing.

BUN: blood urea nitrogen

C3/C5 convertase: component of the *complement system* generated on foreign surfaces. Acts as an enzyme to catalyse the formation of the *terminal complement complex,* also termed the *membrane attack complex.*

CD (clusters of differentiation) nomenclature: terminology describing cell-surface molecules that are identified by the same groups of monoclonal antibodies. The cell surface molecule is designated CD (cluster of differentiation) followed by a number (e.g. CD54, CD2).

CD14: myeloid differentiation antigen; major surface receptor for *lipopolysaccharide (LPS), endotoxin* and peptidoglycans on *peripheral blood mononuclear cells.* Also involved in recognition and phagocytosis of apoptotic cells. LPS, together with *LPS binding protein,* upregulates CD14 expression. CD14 is also released from *monocytes* in a soluble form.

Chain scission: splitting of the sugar-phosphate backbone of DNA (by ionising radiation, for example); replication of micro-organisms is subsequently prevented.

Channelling: shunting of fluid, e.g. *dialysis fluid,* in a restricted region within the dialyser, as opposed to homogenous distribution of fluid flow through the complete dialyser interior.

Cimino Brescia shunt: a direct arteriovenous fistula, surgically created, to facilitate blood access for chronic *haemodialysis.*

Classical complement pathway: in contrast to the *alternative pathway,* this is activated by antigen-antibody complexes and involves the complement components C1, C4 and C2 in the generation of *C3/C5 convertase.*

Cleaning: a step in some dialyser reprocessing procedures aimed at removing residual blood clots and, optimally, adsorbed proteins. Special cleaning agents (e.g. *bleach*) are sometimes used.

Clearance: hypothetical amount of blood that is totally cleared of a particular substance in a minute. Usually only solute removal by diffusion (i.e. due to a concentration gradient) is meant, as opposed to *total clearance.* The latter also includes solute removal by *convection* or *solvent drag* due to a hydrostatic pressure gradient across the membrane. The clearance (diffusive) of a given dialyser for a particular substance is calculated from the percent reduction in the blood concentration of the substance multiplied by the blood flow through the dialyser. For example, if the reduction rate for urea is 70% at a blood flow of 300 ml/min, the urea clearance is 0.7 x 300 = 210 ml/min. That means 210 ml of blood are completely cleared of urea per minute. In practice, clearance can be calculated using the following general formula:

$$\text{Clearance} = \text{blood flow} \bullet \frac{C1 - C2}{C1} \text{ ml/min}$$

C1 = concentration in the blood at its entry to the dialyser
C2 = concentration in the blood at its exit from the dialyser

CML: carboxymethyllysine

CMPF: 3-carboxy-4-methyl-5-propyl-2-furanpropionic acid

Coefficient of ultrafiltration (UF_{coeff}): describes the permeability of a dialyser membrane to water. It is defined as the number of millilitres of fluid per hour that are transferred across the membrane per mmHg *TMP* and is a direct function of the membrane surface area (also termed *ultrafiltration coefficient*).

Contact phase activation: activation of the clotting cascade or the kallikrein-kinin system at negatively charged surfaces, such as activated platelets or negatively charged dialysis membranes (e.g. polyacrylonitrile), via clotting factor XII, prekallikrein and high-molecular weight kininogen.

Convection: in renal replacement therapies, this refers to the movement of fluid across the semipermeable dialyser membrane due to the application of a *transmembrane pressure gradient.* Solutes are transported with the fluid by nature of the *solute drag* principle insofar as the membrane is permeable for such.

Complement: enzyme-triggered cascade system consisting of about 30 plasma and membrane-bound factors. Key factors are C3b, which binds - after activation - to the foreign surface and thereby attracts *phagocytes.* C3a and C5a are important *anaphylatoxins.* The *terminal complement complex or "membrane attack complex"* penetrates foreign surfaces, forming a pore that results in cell leakage.

Copolymer: a polymer in which two or more monomers or base units are combined.

C-reactive Protein (CRP): antibacterial agent produced by liver cells in the course of most inflammatory reactions in response to *cytokines,* particularly interleukin 6 (IL-6). In cases of inflammation, CRP-levels can rise as much as 1000 fold in 24 hours. CRP is a pentameric ß-globulin with a MW of 130,000 that attaches to the microbial surface and activates both *complement* and phagocytosis.

Cross-linking: a covalent linkage between two polymers or between two different regions of the same polymer caused, for example, by ionising radiation. Replication of micro-organisms is subsequently prevented.

Crystalline structure: orderly, densely packed orientation of polymer chains. Such structures are less flexible than *amorphous structures.*

Cuprammonium rayon membranes: regenerated cellulose membranes from Japanese manufacturers (Asahi, Terumo, Teijin).

Cuprophan®: see *regenerated cellulose*

Cutting surface: the face of a fibre bundle embedded in potting compound which has to be sliced to allow access of fluid (blood) to the internal cavities of the individual fibres.

CVVH: continuous venovenous haemofiltration

Cytokine-inducing substances (CIS): all substances that activate *monocytes* to synthesise and liberate cytokines. Relevant substances for dialysis include derivatives of bacteria (e.g. *endotoxins,* peptidoglycans, muramyl peptides, exotoxins) and yeast (e.g. 1,3 ß-D-glucans), as well as extracts from dialyser membranes.

Cytokines: regulatory proteins produced by *monocytes* and *macrophages.* Examples of immuno-modulating cytokines are *interleukins, interferons* (IFN α, β, γ) and *tumor necrosis factor* (TNF). Cytokines are synthesised in response to infection, inflammation and immune challenge, and act at even femtomolar (10^{-15}) concentrations on a variety of tissues by changing gene expression and cellular metabolism. Increased production of IL-1, IL-6 and TNF is observed in haemodialysis patients, suggesting monocyte activation.

Diffusion: movement of substances due to a concentration gradient.

Dialysance: amount of a particular substance that can be removed from the blood by diffusion through the dialyser membrane in a particular time span. In general terms:

$$\text{Dialysance} = \text{blood flow} \bullet \frac{C1 - C2}{C1 - D} \text{ ml/min}$$

C1 = concentration in the blood at its entry to the dialyser
C2 = concentration in the blood at its exit from the dialyser
D = concentration in the dialysate

Dialysate: dialysis fluid after its passage through the dialyser, i.e. dialysis fluid containing waste products. See also *dialysis fluid.*

Dialysis fluid: treated water enriched by so-called dialysis fluid concentrates, resulting in either bicarbonate dialysis fluid or acetate dialysis fluid. Fluid entering the dialysate compartment of a dialyser during dialysis is generally termed dialysis fluid, while fluid leaving this compartment and containing waste is termed *dialysate*.

Diffusive clearance: see *clearance*

DIAPES®: dialysis membrane family (low-flux, high-performance, high-flux types) made of poly(aryl)ethersulfone and polyvinylpyrrolidone (PVP) produced by the German manufacturer Membrana.

DIN: Deutsche Industrie Norm. Standards regulatory body in Germany

Disequilibrium syndrome: cerebral reaction to rapid removal of osmotically active substances, such as sodium, from the blood during dialysis. The steep osmotic gradient between the brain and blood leads to the development of oedema in the brain with resulting clinical symptoms, such as headache, vomiting, high blood pressure and seizures.

Disinfection: process for the destruction of micro-organisms. Disinfection reduces the number of micro-organisms without necessarily killing all those present.

Distribution space or volume: the volume throughout which a drug or tracer substance appears to have been evenly distributed, and is calculated by dividing the amount of drug/tracer by its concentration after equilibrium.

DOQI: Kidney Disease Outcome Quality Initiative™ from the National Kidney Foundation in the USA. Formulated guidelines for the treatment of patients with chronic and end-stage renal disease in the USA. www.kidney.org/professionals/kdoqi/index/cfm

Electrolyte: any ion or solution of ions capable of conducting electricity, e.g. bicarbonate buffer, potassium, sodium, magnesium, calcium and chloride ions in dialysis fluids.

eKt/V: see *Kt/V*

EN: European standard (norm)

Endotoxin: a pyrogenic substance, chemically *lipopolysaccharide,* which is released from the outer cell wall of gram-negative bacteria when they grow or die. Endotoxins are biologically active substances and can be detected with the *LAL-assay*.

Ethylene oxide gas (EtO): a fumigant used by many dialysis suppliers for sterilising products, e.g. dialysers.

European Best Practice Guidelines (EBPG) for haemodialysis (part 1): guidelines for when to refer a patient to nephrological care, when to start dialysis, how to conduct dialysis treatment and how to follow up haemodialysis-associated infections, uraemia-related vascular disease and other risk factors. Written by the EBPG expert group on haemodialysis: Kessler M, Canaud B, Pedrini LA, Tattersell J, ter Wee PM, Vanholder R and Wanner C, published by the European Renal Association (Nephrol Dial Transplant 17 (Suppl 7), 2002).

EVAL®: low-flux or high-performance dialysis membrane produced from ethylvinylalcohol polymer by the Japanese manufacturer Kawasumi.

Extracellular (EC) compartment: sum of all transcellular, plasma and interstitial fluids, representing about 40% of total body water and 25% of total body weight.

F 80A: variation of the standard F 80 polysulfone dialyser from Fresenius Medical Care which is suitable for single-use or reuse with chemicals other than bleach.

F 80B: adaptation of the standard F 80 polysulfone dialyser from Fresenius Medical Care which can be safely reprocessed using the cleaning agent bleach.

Fibre bundle volume (FBV) test: performance test carried out on used dialysers during reprocessing. In practice, it is synonymous with the *total cell volume (TCV) test.*

Fick's law: the direction of movement of a solute by diffusion is always from a higher to a lower concentration, and the solute flux is proportional to the concentration gradient and the area of diffusion (see appendix for formula).

Filaments: see *multifilament yarn*

Fins: fin-like constructions at the ends of certain dialyser fibres (cellulose acetate from Teijin), which enhance dialyser performance by improving dialysis fluid flow throughout the fibre bundle.

First use syndrome: collection of symptoms occurring during dialysis that were originally observed when new (unused) dialysers were used.

There are two types, A and B. Type A is an anaphylactic type with symptoms which begin during the first few minutes of treatment; it is now known to be frequently caused by reactions to the sterilant *ethylene oxide*. Type B is non-specific in nature and symptoms may appear within 20 - 30 minutes, but also an hour or longer after start of treatment.

Flow distributor: ring or other construction within a dialyser aimed at ensuring a more homogenous flow of dialysis fluid around and throughout the fibre bundle.

Foam cells: cells that have ingested or accumulated material, especially lipids. These cells are characterised by abundant, pale-staining, vacuolated cytoplasm and are suspected to play a role in the development of atherosclerosis.

Fouling (membrane fouling): loss of dialyser performance due the deposition of blood proteins on the membrane surface or within the membrane pores.

Fresenius Polysulfone®: dialysis membrane family (*low-flux, high-performance, high-flux* types) made from a polymer that consists of sulfone, alkyl or aryl and isopropyliden groups. *Polyvinylpyrrolidone* (PVP) is added in order to make the hydrophobic polymer more hydrophilic. The membrane is produced by the German manufacturer Fresenius Medical Care.

G-O-P DIAFIL®: dialysis membrane made of *regenerated cellulose* by the German manufacturer Renaselect.

Gram-negative bacteria: classification of bacteria using a staining method named after the inventor. Bacteria which loose the initial blue stain and take up the red counterstain under the microscope are defined as Gram-negative, whereby blue-stained bacteria are classified as Gram-positive. The mechanism of differentiation with this method is based on the different structure of the cell wall of the particular bacterial class. Examples of gram-negative bacteria are enterobacteriaceae, like *E.coli*, and Pseudomonads, like *Pseudomonas aeroginosa*.

Granulocytes: group of *leukocytes* containing granula in the cytoplasm. One distinguishes between neutrophilic (= neutrophils), basophilic (containing heparin and histamin) and eosinophylic granulocytes (important in the defence against parasites, in autoimmune diseases and allergic reactions). *Neutrophils* are important in unspecific defence. Once activated, the neutrophils produce *reactive oxygen species* that destroy cell structures and inactivate enzymes. Furthermore, phospholipids are liberated from the cell wall, and these develop into the important tissue hormones *leukotrienes*, thromboxanes, *prostaglandins*, and prostacyclins by enzymatic cleavage. Polymorphonuclear neutrophils liberate elastase, a marker for inflammation.

Haemoconcentration: increase in solute concentration of the blood during the course of dialysis, haemofiltration or haemodiafiltration due to the removal of plasma water.

Haemodiafilter: generally a dialyser of particularly high hydraulic permeability and permeable to *middle molecules*, such as *ß2-microglobulin*.

Haemodiafiltration: renal replacement treatment incorporating the principles of both *diffusion* and *convection*. The procedure resembles that of haemofiltration but with the addition of a dialysis fluid flow.

Hagen-Poiseuille's Law: law defining the drop in pressure along the length of a tube (see appendix for formula).

Header: ends of a dialyser into and from which the blood flows. The header volume is the volume between the *cutting surface* and the end of the device.

Header sepsis: a particular instigator of bacteraemia and *pyrogenic reactions* that has to do with the removal of the dialyser headers and O-rings during reprocessing procedures. Organisms can then gain access to surfaces on or below the O-rings that, due to the tight seal after reassembling, are not exposed to the disinfectant. During reuse, the pulsing of the blood through the dialyser causes the O-rings to move and bacteria, which have proliferated in the meantime, can enter the patient's blood.

Heat sterilisation (steam or dry heat): *see thermal sterilisation*

Helixone®: a polysulfone membrane produced by Fresenius Medical Care using *nanotechnology* to increase mean pore size while simultaneously reducing the variety of pore widths present. The individual fibres have numerous small *undulations*, and the membrane In embedded in the new generation of FX class dialysers and haemofilters with their innovative header designs.

HEMO (Hemodialysis outcome) study: randomised, multicentre, prospective clinical trial in the USA supported by the National Institute of Diabetes, Digestive and Kidney Diseases of the National Institutes of Health. The trial was designed to assess the effects of standard versus higher dialysis dose and low versus high dialysis membrane flux on morbidity and mortality of chronic hemodialysis patients (first published in N Engl J Med 347(25): 2010-2019, 2002).

High-flux (highly permeable) dialysers: dialysers with membranes possessing *ultrafiltration coefficients* higher than 8-10 ml/h/mmHg. Nowadays, higher values are generally expected, e.g. > 14 and > 20 ml/h/mmHg in the USA and Germany, respectively. Many national bodies add the stipulation, at least for haemofilters, that the membranes must also be permeable to *middle molecules*, e.g. *ß2-microglobulin*.

High-performance dialysers: dialysers containing membranes with ultrafiltration coefficients higher than low-flux dialysers but in the lower range of that officially defined as high-flux, e.g. 10 - 20 ml/h/mmHg in Europe or 8 - 14 ml/h/mmHg in the USA.

Highly purified water: dialysis water which (a) has passed a water treatment system to attain a chemical purity in accordance with national standards, and (b) has a total bacterial count of ≤ 100 CFU and an endotoxin level of ≤ 0.25 IU/ml.

Homopolymer: a polymer composed of a series of identical monomers, e.g. polylysine, polyglucose, in contrast to *copolymers*.

Hydraulic permeability: the volumetric flow rate of water per unit area of membrane per unit pressure gradient (ml/min/cm^2/mmHg).

Hydrostatic ultrafiltration: ultrafiltration driven by a hydrostatic pressure gradient across the dialysis membrane from blood to dialysis fluid.

Hyperphosphataemia: serum levels of phosphorous that are above the normal range of 1.0 - 1.4 mmol/l or 3.0 - 4.5 mg/dl.

Hypersensitivity reactions (HR): immune response to innocuous antigens that lead to symptomatic reactions upon re-exposure. In haemodialysis, these side effects occur either immediately or between 5 and 20 - 30 (maximum) minutes after dialysis start. Symptoms range from a feeling of warmth (at the fistula site or throughout the body), itching, urticaria, flushing, nausea, chest tightness and dyspnoe to severe reactions, such as abdominal cramps, laryngeal oedema, respiratory and cardiac arrest. Type A reactions, *first use syndrome, anaphylactic reactions* or *anaphylactoid reactions* are all hypersensitivity reactions. The reaction is mediated by preformed antibodies or primed cells and, depending on the type of HR, involves IgE antibodies, *complement* activation (C5a/C3a), cytotoxic antibodies, immune complexes, T-cells and/or macrophages and kinin (bradykinin) generation.

Hypoalbuminaemia: serum levels of albumin that are below the normal range of 35 - 55 g/l or 3.5 - 5.5 g/dl.

Inflammatory response: non-specific response of the body to foreign structures; involves the activation of the complement and coagulation cascade, capillary dilatation and the accumulation of *phagocytes.*

In-line steam sterilisation: specific steam sterilisation method employed by Fresenius Medical Care for certain polysulfone dialysers. One particular advantage is the automatic rinsing out of all sterilisation by-products and bacterial debris during actual dialyser production.

Innate immune response: defence mechanism of the body against infection; consists of ready available systems, such as those involving lysozymes, *complement,* phagocytic cells, *acute phase proteins* (e.g. *C-reactive protein*) or *interleukins.* As opposed to the *adaptive immune response,* this works non-specifically and without memory effect.

Internal filtration: when high-flux membranes are used, the blood and dialysis fluid pressure profiles along the length of the dialyser are such that fluid will be filtered from the blood to the dialysis fluid compartment and backfiltration of dialysis fluid into the blood compartment always occurs - even when Q_F = 0 ml/min. The blood to dialysis fluid movement here is referred to as "internal filtration".

Interferon (IFN): see *cytokines*

Interleukins: see *cytokines*

Interleukin Hypothesis: formulated by L. Hendersen, K. Koch, C. Dinarello and S. Shaldon in 1983. Exposure of whole blood to cellulosic membranes results in the production of interleukin-1 (see *cytokines).* This cytokine is a powerful mediator of the acute phase response and contributes to the development of symptomatic hypotension during dialysis.

Intracellular (IC) compartment: sum of all fluids in body cells, representing approximately 60% of the total body water and 35% of the total body weight.

Irradiation sterilisation (γ or ß): see *radiation sterilisation*

ISO: international standards organisation

Isotropic: a body is isotropic if its properties are the same in all directions.

Kiil dialyser: a parallel-flow, flat-plate dialyser developed in 1960; it became increasingly popular after the introduction of Cuprophan® in 1966.

K_0A: see *mass transfer area coefficient*

Kt/V: common measure of dialysis dose. K is urea *clearance*, t is dialysis time and V is the urea *distribution volume* in the patient. Kt/V can be expressed as single pool Kt/V (i.e. spKt/V) or equilibrated Kt/V (i.e. eKt/V) (see appendix for detailed formulae). Single pool urea kinetic modelling does not account for the post-dialysis urea rebound that results from intercompartmental solute re-equilibration at the end of the session, or for recirculation through the vascular access. Therefore, sp-based calculations of HD dose (spKt/V) will invariably overestimate the effective delivered or equilibrated dose (eKt/V). The magnitude of urea rebound, measured as the percent increase in urea concentration from HD end to the equilibrated value, varies between 10% and 17% in standard HD, and is around 24% after high-efficiency treatments (whereby values of even 45% have been measured in some patients). A difference between spKt/V and eKt/V of approximately 0.2 U was found in standard dialysis; this difference increases unpredictably in high-flux dialysis. (European Best Practice Guidelines for haemodialysis (Part 1). Nephrol Dial Transplant 17(Suppl 7): 1-107, 2002).

LAL-assay (Limulus Amoebocyte Lysate)-assay: highly specific assay for the detection of *endotoxins;* it works with a lysate of immunocompetent cells (amoebocytes) from the horseshoe crab *Limulus polyphemus.*

Large molecules: in this work, this is term used to describe all molecules of molecular weight in excess of 15,000. No particular definition is universally recognised, but the general trend is to use this term for molecules of size greater than *ß2-microglobulin* (MW 11,818) and including albumin.

Lipopolysaccharides (LPS): chemical term for *endotoxin* referring to the chemical structure of this bacterial cell wall component; consists of lipids and sugars (polysaccharides).

Lipopolysaccharide-binding protein (LBP): serum protein that binds *lipopolysaccharides (LPS).* The complex of LBP and LPS is then bound by the receptor CD14 on the surface of neutrophils, where it is finally phagocytosed.

LPS fragments/subunits/derivatives: degradation products of the whole *LPS* molecule that are biologically active and can, therefore, also be termed *exogenous pyrogens*.

Leak test: air test employed during dialyser *reprocessing* to detect blood and *dialysis fluid* compartment integrity separately. At pressures of +300 mmHg, the test should be capable of detecting an air leak of 1 ml/min.

Leukocytes: group of blood cells containing nuclei, which make a significant contribution to the body's defence mechanism against microbes and viruses. Cell types included in this group are *granulocytes, monocytes* and *lymphocytes*. Leukocytes are amoebic motile and able to leave the blood stream by penetrating the endothelium.

Leukopenia: sub-normal levels of white blood cells; in haemodialysis, this usually occurs 15 – 30 min after start of dialysis.

Low-flux dialysers: dialysers with membranes possessing *ultrafiltration coefficients* up to 8 (USA) or 10 (Europe) ml/h/mmHg, respectively.

Macrophages: phagocytic cells originating from bone marrow cells that develop into circulating blood *monocytes* (one nucleus) and, finally, mature macrophages (widespread throughout tissue, mainly lung, liver, kidney, spleen and lymph nodes). Activated macrophages produce and liberate *leukotrienes, interleukin-1* and *interferons*.

Manual reprocessing: *reprocessing* of dialysers manually, i.e. not using a machine.

Margination: adherence of polymorphonuclear cells to upregulated adhesion molecules (ICAM-I and ELAM-I) on endothelial cells via their upregulated $ß_2$-integrin receptors CD11a/CD18 and CD11b/CD18. Mediators at sites of inflammation induce the upregulation of endothelial as well as polymorphonuclear receptors.

Mass transfer area coefficient (K_0A): a measure of filter performance that is independent of the particular blood and dialysis fluid flows. It enables one to estimate clearances of a dialyser under various flow conditions, and allows easy comparison of the solute removal characteristics of dialysers of different sizes:

K_OA	$=$	$[Q_B/(1 - Q_B/Q_D)]$	$\ln [(1 - K/Q_D)/(1 - K/Q_B)]$
Mass transfer area coefficient		Blood and dialysis fluid factor	Flow-adapted *in vitro* urea clearance factor

Mast cells: round cells with small nuclei in the surrounding of small blood vessels in connective tissue; they contain granules with vascular permeability mediators (histamine, heparin), as well as chemotactic factors which attract granulocytes. Mast cells do not phagocytise.

MDA (4,4'- methylene dianiline): carcinogenic substance released from some *aromatic polyurethanes* in the *potting compounds* of dialysers during their sterilisation by γ *radiation*. The polyurethane in question is that composed of *4,4'- diphenylmethane diisocyanate (MDI)*, and MDA formation is attributed to the fact that radiation cleaves the urethane linkage proximal to terminal free amino groups.

MDI (4,4'- diphenylmethane diisocyanate): basic constituent of certain *potting materials* for dialysers that are made from *aromatic polyurethane*.

Medicare: official US American program paying for ESRD therapy in cases of insufficient insurance coverage.

Membrane attack complex (MAC): synonymous for *terminal complement complex (TCC)*.

Metabolic acidosis: *acidosis* caused by a decrease in the plasma bicarbonate concentration.

Middle molecules: in this work, this is term used to describe all molecules with molecular weights in the range 500 - 15,000. Specifications of lower and upper molecular sizes vary throughout the literature, e.g. a lower limit of 300 and an upper limit of just 2000. However, nowadays ß2-microglobulin is widely considered a classical middle molecule.

MPO (Membrane Permeability and ESRD Patient Outcome) study: European multicentre study investigating the influence of membrane permeability on the outcome of dialysis patients. Designed in 1999 by Locatelli F, Hannedouche T, Jakobson S, La Greca G, Loureiro A, Martin-Malo A, Papadimitriu M and Vanholder R; a maintenance period of 3-5 years is planned.

Moiré structure: see *undulations*; synonymous with *wave structure*.

Monocytes: premature, circulating leukocytes in the blood with the highest phagocytic activity. They contain surface receptors for complement factors (C3b) and immunoglobulins (Fc-receptor). Monocytes are part of the body's cellular defence against invasion by infectious organisms. Monocytes differentiate into *macrophages* in the tissue. Monocytes and macrophages can bind and phagocytise micro-organisms, particularly antigens. In addition, they are involved in both the initiation and the effector phases of the immune response. They secrete a variety of enzymes, plasma proteins, *prostaglandins, leukotrienes* and *cytokines*, such as interferon-α (IFN-α), the proinflammatory cytokines *interleukin-1* (IL-1), *tumor necrosis factor* (TNF) and interleukin-6 (IL-6). These *cytokines* are produced in response to infection, inflammation and immune challenge.

Molecular weight (MW): relative molecular mass. The sum of the atomic weights of all the atoms contained in a molecule. Being a ratio of molecular masses, it is dimensionless, but often erroneously appears with the unit Dalton in the literature.

Multifilament spacer yarn: a type of *spacer yarn* that is dispersed throughout the fibre bundle of some dialysers to optimise dialysis fluid flow and avoid *channelling*.

Nanotechnology: the development and use of devices that have a size of only a few nanometers. Advanced fabrication techniques employed for the *Helixone*® membrane are based upon nanotechnology principles, employing technology which focuses on pore sizes of some few namometers in diameter (e.g. 3 nm).

Neutropenia: transient drop of neutrophils in the blood; normally observed 15-30 min after dialysis start.

Neutrophil: white blood cell type (*granulocyte*) with a multilobed cell nucleus; main phagocyte in the blood and important for engulfing and killing extracellular pathogens. Neutrophils are activated by some dialysis membranes to release reactive oxygen species (ROS).

Oncotic pressure: pressure caused by colloids, like proteins. The oncotic pressure in blood is small because of the low concentration of colloids (24 mmHg for a protein content of 7%). Oncotic pressure is important for the binding of water in tissue.

On-line clearance monitor (OCM): here the direct correlation between urea and sodium *dialysances* is utilised to determine the effective urea *clearance*, the dialysis dose (*Kt/V*) and the plasma sodium concentration on-line during dialysis.

On-line haemodiafiltration: haemodiafiltration procedure involving the production of substitution fluid on-line from ultrapure bicarbonate dialysis fluid and using at least one endotoxin filter.

Opsonins: molecules that make particles they coat more susceptible to engulfment by *phagocytes* (*complement* factor C3b, for example).

Packing density: the compactness of the fibre bundle in dialysers; the ratio of fibre number to internal casing volume.

PAN: polyacrylonitrile

PEPA®: *high-flux* dialysis membrane consisting of a copolymer of polyethersulfone and polyarylate. The membrane is produced by the Japanese manufacturer Nikkiso.

Peracetic acid solutions (e.g. Renalin®): weak solutions of acid containing a peroxide group; commonly employed during dialyser *reprocessing* for *disinfection* and, sometimes, *cleaning*.

Percentage reduction in urea (PRU): synonymous with *urea reduction ratio (URR)*.

Performance-enhancing technology: the application of scientific studies and engineering principles for practical improvements in dialyser performance.

Performance tests: tests conducted on dialysers during *reprocessing* after rinsing and *cleaning*, but prior to *disinfection*. The types of tests range from none at all to simple measures that reflect the small solute *clearance* characteristics or, alternatively, the hydraulic permeability of the device. In the USA, *total cell volume (TCV)* or *fibre bundle volume (FBV)* measurements are generally employed instead of actual clearance measurements, due to the ease of measurement, and acceptable changes are defined on the basis of a clearance loss of • 10%.

Peripheral blood mononuclear cells (PBMC): *leukocytes* circulating in blood; comprises monocytes, natural killer cells and T-lymphocytes.

PES: see *poly(aryl)ethersulfone*

Phagocytes: immunocompetent cells capable of engulfing micro-organisms. Phagocytes are *macrophages* and *polymorphonuclear granulocytes*. After ingestion of the micro-organism, killing proceeds with the help of enzymes and oxygen species.

Pinnacle structure (ends of the polypropylene filter casing): small pointed structures at the ends of the *Helixone®* dialyser cylindrical casings that are finally covered by the device *headers*. They facilitate good *dialysis fluid* distribution during treatment and offer flexibility in *polyurethane* potting.

PMMA: middle and high-flux dialysis membrane made of polymethylmethacrylate by the Japanese manufacturer Toray.

Poly(aryl)ethersulfone: synonymous with polyethersulfone. Polymer consisting of sulfone and alkyl or arylether groups. *PEPA®*, *Arylane, DIAPES®* and *Polyamix™* are all polyarylethersulfone membranes.

Polymer: a substance characterised by long chains of repeated molecule units ("mers") that intertwine. Depending to the polymer chain orientation, the structure can be *amorphous* or *crystalline*.

Polymer alloy, blend: a mixture of various polymer chains to form a distinct polymer substance. It can include additives, reinforcements and fillers.

Polymorphonuclear granulocytes (*syn.* polymorphs, polymorphonuclear leukocytes): cells that develop from the same stem cell as *monocytes* and that have a segmented nucleus and a cytoplasm that is characterised by an array of granules. The granules contain different enzymes, depending on the type of granulocyte in question, i.e. neutrophilic granulocytes contain lysozyme, myeloperoxidase, lactoferrin, acid hydrolases and cationic proteins, while basophilic granulocytes contain histamine, heparin and other substances Neutrophils, eosinophils and basophils can be distinguished by their size and staining patterns.

Polyamide S™: now termed *Polyamix™*

Polyamix™: an alloy of the heat-resistant polymer polyarylethersulfone with small amounts of polyamide produced by Gambro (Sweden) formerly termed as Polyamide S™.

Polyethylene glycol (PEG): condensation polymer of ethylene oxide and water; PEGs are soluble in water and their consistency varies with molecular size.

Polysulfone: group of polymers containing sulfone groups, alkyl or arylether groups and in contrast to polyarylethersulfone isopropyliden groups. Dialysis membranes made of polysulfone are *Fresenius Polysulfone®*, *Helixone®*, *Asahi Polysulfone®*, *Toraysulfone®* and *α Polysulfone*.

Polyurethane: a polymer containing the urethane group prepared by reacting di-isocyanates with appropriate diols and triols. In dialysers, polyurethanes are employed as a *potting compound* for embedding the individual fibres of a bundle in the filter casing. The polyurethane is cut in such a way that blood has access to the fibre lumen.

Polyvinylpyrrolidone (PVP): a synthetic polymer consisting mainly of 1-vinyl-2-pyrrolidone groups. PVPs with mean molecular weights between 20,000 and 40,000 are sometimes used as plasma extenders. In the haemodialysis industry it is used to make hydrophobic membrane polymers more hydrophilic.

Porosity (membrane porosity (ρ)): this is a function of pore number and size, but is particularly sensitive to the latter, being defined as

$$\rho = N \cdot \pi \cdot r_p^2$$

ρ	=	N	·	π	·	r_p^2
membrane porosity		number of pores				pore radius

Post-conditioning: treatment of dialyser fibres immediately following their sterilisation, usually to remove any residue of the *sterilising agent,* e.g. subjection of the fibres to increased temperatures and several air changes to effectively remove residual *ethylene oxide gas.*

Postdilution haemodiafiltration (HDF): haemodiafiltration procedures where the substitution fluid is added to the patient's blood after its passage through the filter.

Potting compound (material): material, usually *polyurethane,* used to embed the fibres of a bundle in the dialyser casing, thereby allowing blood access to the fibre lumen.

Predilution haemodiafiltration (HDF): haemodiafiltration procedures where the substitution fluid is added to the patient's blood prior to its passage through the filter.

Prostaglandins: mediators of inflammation that, like *leukotrienes* and thromboxane, are derived from membrane phospholipids and the precursor molecule arachidonic acid. Prostaglandins (e.g. prostacyclin) are involved in several vital physiological processes, such as thrombocyte aggregation and peripheral and central vasodilation.

Pyrogenic reaction: during dialysis, this is defined as an elevation of body temperature over 37.8°C in an initially afebrile patient who showed no signs or symptoms of infection prior to the initiation of the dialysis treatment. The reaction can be asymptomatic or associated with symptoms of chills, rigors, myalgia, nausea, vomiting, hypotension or even vascular instability.

Radiation sterilisation (γ or ß): sterilisation of medical devices by exposing them to either γ or ß rays. Atoms in the irradiated products are ionised by the high-energy rays and free radicals are formed; the subsequent dimerisation of DNA bases and *chain scission* or *cross-linking* of the sugar-phosphate backbone prevents replication of micro-organisms.

Reactive oxygen species (ROS): oxygen radicals (e.g. NO, H_2O_2, O_2^-) that are unstable in that they readily react with other substances, with deleterious consequences for cell metabolism.

Regenerated cellulose (RC): polymerisation of dissolved raw cotton (mostly linters). The cellulosic polymer chains are rearranged during the production process. Synonymous with cuprammonium rayon, xanthogenat and the brand names *Cuprophan®* and *G-O-P DIAFIL*.

Reprocessing: procedure by which used dialysers are cleaned and disinfected so that they can be used again.

Reuse: multiple use of dialysers.

RO-processed water: water that has been subjected to a membrane separation process that purifies the water by molecular sieving and ionic rejection. It is effective in removing ions and dissolved organic contaminants with molecular weights above 100.

Sieving coefficient (SC): generally defined to be the ratio of the solute concentration in the *ultrafiltrate* to the mean solute concentration in the plasma, i.e.

SC	=	$2\,C_F$	/	$(C_{Pi}$	+	$C_{Po})$
sieving coefficient		concentration in filtrate		concentration in incoming plasma		concentration in outgoing plasma

A SC of one for a given substance represents unhindered transport through the membrane, while a value of zero means that the membrane is impermeable for this substance.

Small molecules: low molecular weight solutes that are capable of penetrating both *low-flux* and *high-flux* dialysis membranes. In this work, they are defined as those having a molecular weight below 500.

Sodium hypochlorite: synonymous with *bleach*. Cleaning agent frequently used in dialyser *reprocessing*.

Solvent drag: movement of solutes through dialyser membranes by means of *convection* along with the ultrafiltered water.

Spacer yarn: yarn threaded throughout a fibre bundle to enhance dialysis fluid movement along and between the individual fibres. The presence of the thread also reduces *channelling* of *dialysis fluid*.

Spiral access: term used to describe the blood port of the new generation of dialysers produced by Fresenius Medical Care, for example (i.e. the FX class). A helicoidal distributor built into the header region forces the inflowing blood to turn around a cylindrical helix, thereby maximising radial blood velocity and increasing homogenous access to all hollow fibres.

spKt/V: see *Kt/V*

S protein: natural occurring inhibitor of terminal complement complexes C5b67, C5b-678, C5b-6789; soluble in plasma and identical to vitronectin.

Sterility: expressed as a statistic, a device is termed sterile when the chance of survival of a viable micro-organism is less than one in a million or, in other words, at most one device per million may theoretically contain one viable germ after sterilisation.

Sterilisation: the reduction of the number of micro-organisms to a safe, predetermined level. Total killing of all organisms is virtually impossible.

Subjective global assessment: judgement of individual nutritional state based on several markers and the results of physical examinations (e.g. weight loss, anorexia, subcutaneous fat and muscle mass). Subjective weightings made by the examiner reflect the nutritional status and finally lead, via a scoring system, to a classification of the individual nutritional state into normal, mild to moderate malnutrition or severe malnutrition.

TDI (toluene diisocyanate): component of some *polyurethanes* used as *potting materials*; an alternative to *4,4'-diphenylmethane diisocyanate (MDI)* (which has the disadvantage of *MDA* formation upon radiation sterilisation). It is itself also a toxic and mutagenic compound.

Terminal complement complex (TCC): synonymous with *membrane attack complex (MAC)*. Terminal product of *complement* activation via both classical and alternative pathways. TCC consists of varying amounts of the complement factors C5, C6, C7, C8 and C9, which assemble to generate a pore in a bilayer membrane. The result is membrane damage with subsequent leakage of the cell.

Thrombocytopenia: decrease in the number of platelets in the blood, normally from 130,000 - 400,000 platelets per µl blood to less then 60,000 platelets per µl. Results in an increased tendency of bleeding.

Thrombogenicity: ability to induce the formation of a *thrombus*.

Thrombus: solid or semi-solid mass of cross-linked fibrin with trapped cells and platelets, resulting from activation of the coagulation cascade.

TMP (transmembrane pressure): total pressure difference across the dialyser membrane, calculated as the average pressure in the blood compartment minus the average pressure in the dialysis fluid compartment.

Total cell volume (TCV) test: performance test carried out on used and washed dialysers targeted for reuse. The total cell volume is the volume of aqueous fluid necessary to fully prime the blood compartment of a hollow fibre dialyser or haemofilter; it is actually the sum of the *fibre bundle volume (FBV)* and the *header* volume, but the terms FBV and TCV are often used interchangeably in practice. TCV is determined by measuring the amount of liquid displaced by an air or nitrogen rinse of the dialyser blood compartment.

Total clearance: hypothetical amount of blood that is totally cleared of a particular substance in a minute, irrespective of the driving force. As opposed to simple diffusive clearance (generally just called *clearance*), total clearance also takes solute removal by *convection* or *solvent drag* into consideration.

Tumor necrosis factor (TNF): see *cytokines*

Ultrafilter: filter device containing membranes with a pore size less than 0.1 µm. Separation is based on molecular sieving exclusion, whereby micro-organisms, colloids and dissolved high molecular weight organic contaminants are eliminated from the incoming fluid. Ultrafilters are employed to remove microbial contaminants from *dialysis fluid* in the post-treatment section of a water treatment system or, more commonly, from dialysis fluid.

Ultrafiltrate: plasma water which has passed through a dialyser or haemofilter membrane; it contains all plasma solutes which were capable of passing through the membrane.

Ultrafiltration: the convective transport of solutes by *solute drag* across dialyser or haemofilter membranes due to a hydrostatic pressure gradient.

Ultrafiltration coefficient (UF_{coeff}): see *coefficient of ultrafiltration*

Ultrafiltration rate (Q_F): rate of filtrate flow

Ultrapure dialysis fluid: dialysis fluid produced from highly purified dialysis water and pure dialysis fluid concentrate and which has passed through an *ultrafilter* shortly before entering the dialyser. The bacterial count is ≤ 1 CFU/ml and the *endotoxin* concentration is ≤ 0.03 EU/ml.

Undulations: synonymous with *wave structure* or *moiré structure*; a wavy or undulated design of the individual hollow fibres which discourages the formation of a stagnant dialysis fluid layer at the membrane outer surface, thus reducing dialysis fluid-side mass transfer resistance; the shape also hinders too close an aligning of the fibres, which would hinder inter-fibre dialysis fluid flow.

Urea reduction ratio (URR): a measure of the effectiveness of a dialysis treatment based on changes in patient blood levels of urea. Sometimes called *percentage reduction in urea (PRU)*; see formula in appendix.

USRDS: abbreviation for the United States Renal Data System, a data system which collects, analyses and distributes information on ESRD in the USA. The USRDS is funded directly by the National Institute of Diabetes and Digestive and Kidney Diseases (NIDDK) in conjunction with Centers for Medicare and Medicaid Services (CMS). The USRDS coordinating Center is operated under contract with the Minneapolis Medical Research Foundation.

Wave structure: see *undulations*; synonymous with *moiré structure*

Appendix 1 – Relevant formulae

1. Clearance

$$K = Q_{Bi}\,((C_{Bi} - C_{Bo})/C_{Bi}) \quad + \quad Q_F\,(C_{Bo}/C_{Bi})$$

or

$$K = Q_{Di}\,((C_{DFi} - C_{DFo})/C_{Bi}) \quad + \quad Q_F\,(C_{DFo}/C_{Bi})$$

Clearance = Diffusive term + Convective term

In the absence of adsorption, the ultrafiltration rate (Q_F) is given by

$$Q_F = Q_{Bi} - Q_{Bo}$$

K stands for clearance, Q for flow, C for concentration, subscripts B, DF and F for blood, dialysis fluid and filtrate, respectively; and subscripts i and o for fluids flowing into and out of the dialyser, respectively. The equations for clearance are reduced to their first parts in the absence of filtrate flow. Clearance of a dialyser is mostly characterised by its diffusive clearance values alone (i.e. is measured in the absence of filtration).

2. Dialysance

$$D = Q_{Bi}\,((C_{Bi} - C_{Bo})/(C_{Bi} - C_{DFi})) \quad + \quad Q_F\,(C_{Bo}/(C_{Bi} - C_{DFi}))$$

or

$$= Q_{DFi}\,((C_{DFi} - C_{DFo})/(C_{Bi} - C_{DFi})) \quad + \quad Q_F\,(C_{DFo}/(C_{Bi} - C_{DFi}))$$

Dialysance = Diffusive term + Convective term

Dialysance exceeds clearance: for blood values [1],

$$K = ((C_{Bi} - C_{DFi})/\,C_{Bi}) \cdot D$$

Clearance = Concentration factor · Dialysance

Nomenclature as above.

3. Fick's First Law:

$$J = -D \cdot A \cdot (dc/dx)$$

J: Solute flux; D: Solute diffusivity; A: Area; (dc/dx): Concentration gradient

4. Hagen-Poiseuille's Law:

$$\Delta p = p_{in} - p_{out}$$

Δp: Transmembrane pressure difference; $p_{in} - p_{out}$: Pressure inside minus pressure outside

$$= (8\eta \cdot Q_B \cdot \Delta l) / (N \cdot r^4 \cdot \pi)$$

η: Blood viscosity; Q_B: Blood flow; Δl: Fibre length; N: Number of fibres; r: Fibre radius

5. Kt/V:

$$(K \cdot t) / V = \text{Index for dialysis efficiency}$$

K: Real urea clearance of dialyser *in vivo*; t: Dialysis time (minus time lost due to interruptions); V: Urea distribution volume in the patient (usually measured anthropometrically according to Watson or Hume-Weyer)

<u>V according to Watson:</u>

Male: $V = 2.447 - (0.09156 \cdot \text{age}) + (0.1074 \cdot \text{height}) + (0.3362 \cdot \text{weight})$

Female: $V = -2.097 + (0.1069 \cdot \text{height}) + (0.2466 \cdot \text{weight})$

with age in years, height in cm and weight in kilograms [2].

<u>V according to Hume-Weyer:</u>

Male: $V = (0.194786 \cdot \text{height}) + (0.296785 \cdot \text{weight}) - 14.012934$

Female: $V = (0.34454 \cdot \text{height}) + (0.183809 \cdot \text{weight}) - 35.270121$

with age in years, height in cm and weight in kilograms [2].

Kt/V can be expressed as single-pool Kt/V (spKt/V) or equilibrated Kt/V (eKt/V). The value for spKt/V should be derived from the formal single-pool variable volume urea kinetic model [3]. As an alternative, the natural logarithm formula provides an adequate estimate of spKt/V [4, 5], i.e.

$$spKt/V = -\ln (R - 0.008 \cdot T) + (4 - 3.5 \cdot R) \cdot (dBW/BW)$$

$$\text{where } R = C_{postdialysis} / C_{predialysis}$$

where $C_{postdialysis}$: Postdialysis blood urea concentration; $C_{predialysis}$: Predialysis blood urea concentration

ln is the natural logarithm, T is the dialysis length in hours, BW is the patient's body weight postdialysis in kg, and dBW is patient's weight loss during dialysis in kg.

Single-pool urea kinetic modelling does not account for post-dialysis urea rebound resulting from intercompartmental solute re-equilibration at the end of the session, or for recirculation through the vascular access. Therefore, sp-based calculation of dialysis dose (spKt/V) will invariably overestimate the effective delivered or equilibrated dose (eKt/V). The mathematical relationship between the equilibrated and the single-pool Kt/V will vary depending upon the location of the angioaccess and the site from which the postdialysis blood urea sample was obtained. spKt/V, calculated using an arterial postdialysis urea sample from an arteriovenous angioaccess, will be greater than that calculated from a mixed venous postdialysis blood urea measurement, drawn through a venovenous angioaccess. The corresponding eKt/V values are calculated by:

$$eKt/V = spKt/V - (0.6 \times spKt/V/T) + 0.03$$ (for an arteriovenous access)

or

$$eKt/V = spKt/V - (0.47 \times spKt/V/T) + 0.02$$ (for a venovenous access, i.e. in the absence of cardiopulmonary recirculation)

As above, T is the dialysis treatment time in hours and t is the dialysis time in minutes [5, 6]. Alternatively, the eKt/V value can also be obtained by using blood urea measurements made 30 minutes after the end of the session instead of $C_{postdialysis}$ in the spKt/V equation [5].

6. Mass transfer area coefficient (K_OA):

K_OA	=	$[Q_B/(1 - Q_B/Q_D)]$	$\ln [(1 - K/Q_D)/(1 - K/Q_B)]$
Mass transfer area coefficient factor		Blood and dialysis fluid flow	Flow-adapted *in vitro* urea clearance factor

7. Membrane porosity (ρ):

ρ	=	N	$\cdot$	π	$\cdot$	r_p^2
Membrane porosity		Number of pores				Pore radius

8. Membrane surface area:

A	=	2	$\cdot$	π	$\cdot$	r	$\cdot$	Δl	$\cdot$	N
Surface area						Fibre radius		Fibre length		Fibre number

9. Sieving coefficient (SC):

SC	=	$2\,C_F$	/	$(C_{Pi}$	+	$C_{Po})$
Sieving coefficient		Concentration in ultrafiltrate		Concentration in incoming plasma		Concentration in outgoing plasma

The plasma concentrations of $ß_2$-m measured at any time "t" after start of treatment can be corrected for haemoconcentration due to ultrafiltration, assuming that all plasma proteins are confined to the vascular space (see next section for correction factors).

10. Urea reduction ratio (URR):

URR	=	$((C_{predialysis}$	-	$C_{postdialysis})$	/	$C_{predialysis})$	$\cdot$	100
Index for dialysis efficiency		Predialysis blood urea concentration		Postdialysis blood urea concentration		Predialysis blood urea concentration		

Here postdialysis plasma concentrations must be corrected for haemoconcentration resulting from ultrafiltration. Different correction factors appear in the literature, for example the popular correction for ß2-microglobulin supplied by Bergström and Wehle [7]:

Corrected C_{post}	= Measured C_{post}	/ [1 +	$(BW_{pre} - BW_{post})$	/ $(0.2 \cdot BW_{post})$]
Postdialysis plasma conc. corrected for haemoconcentration	Measured postdialysis plasma ß2-m concentration		Change in body weight	Postdialysis body weight during dialysis

or that given by Lesaffer et al. [8], Floege et al. [9] and others:

Corrected $C_P(t)$	=	$Cp(t)$	$\cdot$	$(TP(t_0)$ / $TP(t))$
		Measured plasma concentration at time "t"		Ratio of total plasma protein at start of dialysis (t0) and at time "t"

References

1. Hoenich NA, Woffindin C, Ronco C: Haemodialysers and associated devices in *Replacement of renal function by dialysis*, 4th ed., edited by Jacobs C, Kjellstrand CM, Koch KM, Winchester JF, Dordrecht, Kluwer Academic Publishers: 188-230, 1996

2. National Kidney Dialysis Outcome Quality Initiative (DOQI): Clinical practice guidelines. hemodialysis adequacy and peritoneal dialysis adequacy. Am J Kid Dis 30 (3, Suppl 2): S1-S64, 1997

3. Sargent JA, Gotch FA: Mathematic modelling of dialysis therapy. Kidney Int 18(Suppl 10): S2-S10, 1980

4. Daugirdas JT: Second generation logarithmic estimates of single-pool variable volume Kt/V: an analysis of error. Am J Soc Nephrol 4: 1205-1213, 1993

5. Kessler M, Canaud B, Pedrini LA, Tattersell J, ter Wee PM, Vanholder R Wanner C: European Best Practice Quidelines: Section II. Haemodialysis adequacy. Nephrol Dial Transplant 17(Suppl 7): 16-31, 2002

6. National Kidney Dialysis Outcome Quality Initiative (DOQI): Guidelines for hemodialysis adequacy - Update 2000. Available at http://www. kidney.org/professionals/doqi/guidelines. Accessed February, 2003

7. Bergström J, Wehle B: No change in corrected $ß_2$-microglobulin concentration after Cuprophane haemodialysis. Lancet 1: 628-629, 1987

8. Lesaffer G, De Smet R, Lameire N, Dhondt A, Duym P, Vanholder R: Intradialytic removal of protein-bound uraemic toxins: role of solute characteristics and of dialyser membrane. Nephrol Dial Transplant 15: 50-57, 2000

9. Floege J, Granolleras C, Deschodt G, Heck M, Baudin G, Branger B, Tournier O, Reinhard B, Eisenbach GM, Smeby LC, Koch KM, Shaldon S: High-flux synthetic versus cellulosic membranes for $ß_2$-microglobulin removal during hemodialysis, hemodiafiltration and hemofiltration. Nephrol Dial Transplant 4: 653-657, 1989

Appendix 2 – List of dialysers and membranes available on the market

All data was taken from manufacturer's brochures and summarised by Fresenius Medical Care, St. Wendel.

Conditions if not specified: clearances at Q_B=200ml/min, Q_D=500ml/min, Q_F=0; KUF with blood Hct. 32%, protein 6%.

Abbreviations:

KUF : Coefficient of ultrafiltration
Crea. : Creatinine
Phos. : Phosphate
V. B_{12} : Vitamin B_{12}
Steri. : Sterilisation mode
Vol. : Priming volume
Lum. : Fibre lumen
Surf. : Surface area
Appl. : Application
HD : Haemodialysis
HDF : Haemodiafiltration
HF : Haemofiltration

	Performance Data					Technical Data							
Dialyser	**KUF** ml/hmmHg	**Urea** ml/min	**Crea.** ml/min	**Phos.** ml/min	**V. B_{12}** ml/min	**Steri.**	**Vol.** ml	**Membrane material**	**Wall** µm	**Lum.** µm	**Surf.** m²	**Appl.**	**Notes**
Allmed													
OPAL 110 S	5,8	170	136	131	48	heat	54	Cellulose (Hemophan®)	8	200	1,1	HD	
130 S	6,8	178	146	136	54		62				1,3		
160 S	8,2	187	154	141	62		74				1,6		
180 S	8,8	191	183	164	75		94				1,8		
200 S	9,7	193	186	169	81		105				2,0		
220 S	10,8	195	189	174	86		115				2,2		
QUARTZ 100 S	8,4	171	155	134	91	heat	65	Polyethersulfone Low-Flux	35	200	1,0	HD	Clearances at TMP=50 mmHg; Spacer yarns (P.E.T.®)
130 S	10,4	181	169	149	108		80				1,3		
160 S	12,1	188	178	158	117		99				1,6		
180 S	13,7	191	183	163	124		112				1,8		
TOPAZ 100 S	27,4	180	165	155	98	heat	65	Polyethersulfone Medium-Flux	35	200	1,0	HD	
130 S	36,7	188	177	169	114		80				1,3		
160 S	50,7	193	184	178	128		99				1,6		
180 S	59,2	195	187	182	135		112				1,8		
RUBY 130 S	56	190	182	177	137	heat	80	Polyethersulfone High-Flux	30	200	1,3	HD / HDF	
160 S	69	194	185	182	144		99				1,6		
180 S	85	196	188	187	154		112				1,8		
Amicon													
Minifilter						ETO	6	Polysulfone (Minntech)		1100	0,01	acute	for babies
Minifilter Plus							15			570	0,08	acute	for children
Diafilter D-20						ETO	38	Polysulfone (Minntech)		200	0,4	acute / HF	
Diafilter D-30							58			250	0,7		
Asahi													KUF with saline
AM-BIO-HX- 650	24,0	187	167	150	92	γ (wet)	88	Cellulose (Cuprammonium Rayon with Poly-ethylenglycol layer)	15	180	1,3	HD	
AM-BIO-HX- 750	27,8	191	174	158	101		100				1,5		
AM-BIO-HX-1000	37,0	194	185	169	119		128				2,0		
AM-BIO UP-650	19	179	162	144	86	γ (wet)	88		15	180	1,3	HD	KUF with saline
AM-BIO UP-750	22	189	173	154	98		100				1,5		
AM-BIO- 500 Wet	5,7	175	153	127	54	γ (wet)	63		10	180	1,0	HD	Clearances at TMP=100mmHg
AM-BIO- 650 Wet	7,8	184	166	142	66		78				1,3		
AM-BIO- 750 Wet	8,8	188	172	150	74		94				1,5		
AM-BIO-1000 Wet	12,0	195	180	163	89		123				2,0		KUF with saline

PAN HFD 160	25	180	145		95	ETO	85	PAN	55	200	1,25	HDF	
PAN- 65 DX	29	181	167	156	117	ETO	100	Polyacrylonitrile	35	250	1,3	HDF/	
PAN- 85 DX	38	190	176	168	134		124	(PAN)			1,7	HF	
PAN-110 DX	49	193	183	176	144		161				2,2		
PAN- 650 SF	30	194	189	174	146	ETO	96	PAN	35	250	1,3	HD/	Fibre bundle with
PAN- 900 SF	41	198	194	187	165		127				1,8	HF/	Polyester filaments
PAN-1000 SF	46	199	195	188	172		139				2,0	HDF	
PAN-50 P	15	128	112		63	ETO	50	PAN	55	200		acute	
PAN-150	23	162	137		86		70				1,0	"/HF	
PAN-200	27	170	145		103		85				1,4	HF	
PAN-250	30	174	174		115		120				1,8	HF	
PAN-03	16	136	104	97	53	ETO	33	PAN	35	250	0,3	acute/	Clearances at
PAN-06	25	178	160	149	85		63				0,6	HF	TMP= 100mmHg;
PAN-10	29	185	172	159	97		87				1,0		KUF with saline
APS-550 S	50	180	172	155	117	γ	66	Polysulfone	45	200	1,1	HD/	KUF at
APS-650 S	57	186	176	170	130	(wet)	80	Asahi PS			1,3	HDF	TMP=50 mmHg
APS-900 S	68	192	181	178	148		105	(APS™)			1,8		
APS-1050 S	75	193	189	183	158		114				2,1		
APS-650 MD	48	183	172	164	126	γ	80	Polysulfone	45	200	1,3	HD/	KUF at
APS-900 MD	56	190	181	178	145	(wet)	105	Asahi PS			1,8	HDF	TMP=50mmHg
APS-1050 MD	58	192	188	183	156		114	ALBRANE			2,1		
Baxter													
CF 12	3,0	162	134	118	34	ETO	54	Cellulose	8	200	0,7	HD	Clearances at
CF 15	3,7	168	142	124	41		63	(Cuprophan®)			0,9		TMP=100 mmHg
CF 23	5,2	176	156	139	55		91				1,25		
CF 25	6,5	191	170	159	62		112				1,6		
HAT 80	3,2	160	134	129	43	ETO	50	Cellulose	8	200	0,8	HD	
HAT 100	4,0	170	146	139	52		69	(Hemophan®)			1,0		
HAT 130	5,6	182	163	159	63		85				1,3		
HAT 170	6,7	188	173	167	76		109				1,7		
PSN 120	6,7	180	159	140	61	ETO	75	Cellulose	9	200	1,2	HD	Spacer yarns
PSN 140	7,6	184	166	149	67		84	(Polysynthane™			1,4		(P.E.T.®)

	Performance Data					Technical Data							
Dialyser	**KUF** ml/hmmHg	**Urea** ml/min	**Crea.** ml/min	**Phos.** ml/min	**V. B_{12}** ml/min	**Steri.**	**Vol.** ml	**Membrane material**	**Wall** µm	**Lum.** µm	**Surf.** m^2	**Appl.**	**Notes**
CA 50	2,4	128	88	53	26	ETO	38	Cellulose	15	200	0,5	HD	Manufacturer:
CA 70	3,4	153	112	70	34	G=γ	51	Acetate			0,7		Nipro;
CA 90	4,3	169	132	86	42		64				0,9		Clearances at
CA 110	5,3	176	144	103	52		74				1,1		TMP=100 mmHg
CA 130	5,6	179	148	101	53		85				1,3		
CA 150	7,2	185	162	132	66		98				1,5		
CA 170	7,6	194	172	151	66		110				1,7		
CA 210	10,1	198	178	158	77		133				2,1		
CA 50 G	2,6	129	97	62	27	ETO	35	Cellulose	15	200	0,5	HD	Manufacturer:
CA 70 G	3,5	148	117	75	35	G=γ	45	Acetate			0,7		Nipro;
CA 90 G	4,2	163	133	89	42		60				0,9		KUF at
CA 110 G	4,9	173	146	101	52		70				1,1		TMP=100 mmHg
CA 130 G	5,7	180	154	111	58		80				1,3		
CA 150 G	7,1	184	162	120	64		95				1,5		
CA 170 G	8,2	188	168	129	70		105				1,7		
CA 210 G	9,8	192	176	139	82		125				2,1		
CA-HP 90	7,3	172	146	115	60	ETO	60	Cellulose	15	200	0,9	HD	Manufacturer:
CA-HP 110	7,7	177	156	126	70		70	Diacetate			1,1		Nipro
CA-HP 130	9,1	186	165	138	79		80				1,3		
CA-HP 150	10,2	187	174	147	88		95				1,5		
CA-HP 170	10,0	192	181	156	94		105				1,7		
CA-HP 210	13,2	194	184	165	106		125				2,1		
DICEA 90 G	6,8	173	148	116	60	γ /	60	Cellulose	15	200	0,9	HD	Manufacturer:
110 G	8,4	179	159	128	69	ETO	70	Diacetate			1,1		Nipro;
130 G	10,0	186	167	139	79		80				1,3		KUF at
150 G	11,4	189	175	148	90		95				1,5		TMP=150 mmHg
170 G	12,5	191	179	156	95		105				1,7		
210 G	15,5	196	185	165	105		125				2,1		
CT 90 G	19	181	158	147	87	γ	58	Cellulose	15	200	0,9	HD	Manufacturer:
CT 110 G	22	185	168	166	109		70	Triacatate			1,1		Nipro;
CT 150 G	29	190	175	170	118		91	(CTA)			1,5		Clearances at
CT 190 G	36	192	182	182	137		114				1,9		UF=7 ml/min
TRICEA 110 G	25	188	177	161	119	γ	65	Cellulose	15	200	1,1	HD/	Manufacturer:
150 G	29	197	189	179	142		90	Triacetate			1,5	HF/	Nipro;
190 G	37	198	194	182	151		115	(CTA)			1,9	HDF	KUF at
210 G	39	199	198	191	164		125				2,1		TMP=100 mmHg

EXELTRA™ 150	31	193	186	179	132	γ	95	Cellulose	15	200	1,5	HD/	Labelled for
170	34	196	190	179	138		105	Triacetate			1,7	HF/	Single Use
190	36	197	190	186	143		115	(CTA)			1,9	HDF	
Plus 210	47	199	198	191	164		125				2,1		
SYNTRA™ 120	58	185	173	167	127	γ	87	Polyethersulfone	30	200	1,2	HD	Clearances
160	73	190	180	173	139		117	(DIAPES®)			1,6	HDF	at UF=10 ml/min;
													Spacers (P.E.T.®)
Renaflow II													
HF 400						ETO	28	Polysulfone	40	200	0,3	acute	Manufacturer:
HF 700							53	(Minntech)			0,71		Minntech
HF 1200							83				1,25		
HF 2000							132				1,98		
Minifilter Plus							14		100	620	0,07		for babies,childr.
Bellco / Sorin													
Spiraflo													
NT 1175	4,5	215	166	137	48	ETO	52	Cellulose	7,5	200	1,08	HD	Clearances at
NT 1375	5,9	237	187	156	59		67	(Cuprophan®)			1,35		Q_B=300ml/min,
NT 1675	7,4	251	213	173	69		83				1,64		UF=10ml/min
NT 1975	8,6	266	223	191	77		96				1,95		
NT 1375 S	5,5	208	175	150	51	heat	73		7,5	200	1,35	HD	
NT 1675 S	7,0	226	194	160	63	(wet)	90				1,64		
NT 1208 H	5,9	229	186	152	59	ETO	67	Cellulose	8	200	1,15	HD	
NT 1408 H	7,4	247	208	169	69		83	(Hemophan®)	8		1,36		
NT 1808 H	8,6	258	222	182	77		96		8		1,72		
NT 1265 H	7,3	231	192	176	66		70		6,5		1,20		
NT 1665 H	9,2	254	218	199	77		88		6,5		1,60		
NT 1208 HG	3,1	211	174	148	44	γ	67		8	200	1,15	HD	
NT 1408 HG	4,0	238	198	163	48		83		8		1,36		
NT 1808 HG	4,5	253	213	175	53		96		8		1,72		
NT 1265 HG	3,9	231	192	176	51		70		6,5		1,20		
NT 1665 HG	5,2	254	218	199	60		88		6,5		1,60		
NT 1208 HS	5,5	208	175	150	51	heat	73		8	200	1,35	HD	
NT 1408 HS	7,0	226	194	160	63		90				1,64		
NC 0985 G	2,9	164	127	108	36	γ	58	Cellulose	8,5	200	0,90	HD	Spacer yarns
NC 1285 G	3,8	179	148	128	45		73	(SMC®)			1,15		(P.E.T.®)
NC 1485 G	4,9	184	153	136	53		91				1,45		
NC 1785 G	5,6	189	165	147	58		103				1,70		

	Performance Data					Technical Data							
Dialyser	**KUF** ml/hmmHg	**Urea** ml/min	**Crea.** ml/min	**Phos.** ml/min	**V. B_{12}** ml/min	**Steri.**	**Vol.** ml	**Membrane material**	**Wall** µm	**Lum.** µm	**Surf.** m²	**Appl.**	**Notes**
NC 0985	4,7	164	127	108	37	ETO	58		8,5	200	0,90	HD	Spacer yarns (P.E.T.®)
NC 1285	6,2	179	148	128	46		73				1,15		
NC 1485	7,9	184	153	136	56		91				1,45		
NC 1785	9,0	189	165	147	63		103				1,70		
NC 2085	10,3	192	171	154	70		117				1,95		
NC 1285 SD	6,2	226	175	146	58	heat	65		8,5	200	1,15	HD	
NC 1485 SD	7,9	237	182	157	66		76				1,45		
NC 1785 SD	9,0	249	201	173	72		84				1,70		
NC 2085 SD	10,3	257	211	184	80		98				1,95		
BLS 642	9,0	213	179	134	54	ETO	63	Polysulfone LF	40	200	1,09	HD	Clearances at Q_B=300ml/min
BLS 643	11,2	228	194	146	65		78				1,36		
BLS 621	29	201	163	142	80	ETO	41	Polysulfone HF	40	200	0,68	HD / HF / HDF	
BLS 624	34	233	199	185	110		63				1,09		
BLS 627	47	251	215	201	126		78				1,36		
BLS 632	56	266	228	213	143		105				1,89		
BLS 812 G (SD)	51	241	216	205	160	γ (G) heat (SD)	73	Polyethersulfone (DIAPES® HF)	30	200	1,2	HD / HF / HDF	Clearances at Q_B=300ml/min, Q_F= 10ml/min; KUF at 50mmHg
BLS 814 G (SD)	61	246	223	213	166		85				1,4		
BLS 816 G (SD)	68	250	227	218	170		94				1,6		
BLS 819 G (SD)	80	255	234	226	177		109				1,9		
BLS 512 G (SD)	10	226	207	177	119	γ (G) heat (SD)	77	Polyethersulfone (DIAPES® LF)	35	200	1,27	HD	Spacer yarns (P.E.T.®)
BLS 514 G (SD)	12	229	210	183	126		85				1,41		
BLS 517 G (SD)	17	234	216	193	137		99				1,68		
SG 2		228	205	160	86	ETO	98	Polysulfone HF / Hemophan	40 8	200	0,55/ 1,15	HDF	Paired Filtration Dialysis (PFD) System; Clearances at Q_B=300ml/min; Polysulfone from Fresenius. In SG 8 Plus: PS=DIAPES®
SG 3		255	227	187	107	ETO	118	Polysulfone HF / Hemophan	40 8		0,55/ 1,36		
SG 5		265	232	218	111	ETO	129	Polysulfone HF / Hemophan	40 6,5		0,55/ 1,60		
SG 6		259	230	200	109	ETO	124	Polysulfone HF / Hemophan	40 8		0,68/ 1,36		
SG 8		270	235	220	122	ETO	149	Polysulfone HF / SMC	40 8,5		0,55/ 1,95		
SG 8 Plus		274	241	221	132	γ	149	Polysulfone HF / SMC	30 8,5		0,70/ 1,95		
SG 30		250	219	174	121	ETO	118	Polysulfone HF / Polysulfone LF	40 40		0,55/ 1,36		

PHF 0719	80	244	241	220	185	γ	54 109	Polysulfone (DIAPES® HF)	30	200	0,7 1,9	HDF	On-line Paired Hemodiafiltration; Clearances at Q_B=300ml/min, Q_F= 10ml/min; KUF at 50mmHg
Braun/Schiwa													
Diacap CE 1100	4,5	173	142	121	35	ETO	52	Cellulose (Cuprophan®)	7,5	200	1,1	HD	
CE 1400	5,9	184	156	135	45		67				1,4		
CE 1600	7,4	190	172	147	55		83				1,6		
CE 2000	8,6	195	177	159	60		96				2,0		
HE 1200	5,9	178	152	129	38	ETO	67	Cellulose (Hemophan®)	7,5	200	1,2	HD	
HE 1400	7,4	185	165	139	47		83				1,4		
HE 1700	8,6	192	175	150	55		96				1,7		
HE1200G	3,0	170	145	125	34	γ	67	Cellulose (Hemophan®)	8	200	1,15	HD	
HE1400G	3,7	180	158	135	38		83				1,36		
HE1700G	4,2	190	170	145	43		96				1,72		
SMC 1,0	6,0	179	148	128	46	ETO	71	Cellulose (SMC®)	8,5	200	1,04	HD	Spacer yarns (P.E.T.®)
SMC 1,2	7,7	184	153	136	56		89				1,24		
SMC 1,5	8,8	189	165	147	63		101				1,54		
SMC 1,8	10,2	192	171	154	70		115				1,84		
SMC 1,0 SD	6,2	176	144	123	47	heat	63		8,5	200	1,0	HD	
SMC 1,2 SD	7,9	182	148	130	52		74				1,2		
SMC 1,5 SD	9,0	187	160	141	56		82				1,5		
SMC 1,8 SD	10,3	190	166	147	62		95				1,8		
LO PS 10	6,8	176	157	126	68	γ	58	Polysulfone-PVP blend (á Polysulfone LF)	40	200	1,0	HD	Manufacturer: Saxonia
LO PS 12	7,9	183	166	139	77		68				1,2		
LO PS 15	9,8	189	173	146	83		90				1,5		
LO PS 18	12,3	192	180	157	100		104				1,8		
LO PS 20	13,7	194	183	164	110		113				2,0		
HI PS 8	22	170	148	140	86	γ	48	Polysulfone-PVP blend (á Polysulfone HF)	40	200	0,8	HD / HDF	
HI PS 10	34	180	162	160	100		58				1,0		
HI PS 12	42	186	173	171	115		68				1,2		
HI PS 15	50	190	178	176	127		90				1,5		
HI PS 18	55	192	182	180	137		110				1,8		
HI PS 20	58	194	184	183	143		121				2,0		
Diacap Acute S							48	Polysulfone	40	200	0,8	Acute	
Acute M							90				1,5		
Acute L							113				2,0		

	Performance Data					Technical Data							
Dialyser	KUF ml/hmmHg	Urea ml/min	Crea. ml/min	Phos. ml/min	V. B_{12} ml/min	Steri.	Vol. ml	Membrane material	Wall µm	Lum. µm	Surf. m²	Appl.	Notes
Dynamic													
DS-190	59	189	181	170	130	ETO	135	Polysulfone			1,9	HD/HDF	
El Nasr													
A1	2,9	155	120	100	35	ETO	45	Cellulose (Cuprophan®)	8	200	0,7	HD	
A2	4,3	173	148	130	48		60				1,0		
A3	5,8	178	158	140	56		80				1,2		
B2	5,8	178	155	135	60	ETO	60	Cellulose (Hemophan®)	8	200	1,0	HD	
B3	6,2	182	163	149	62		80				1,2		
FIDIA													Modern Realization Group Clearances at TMP=100 mmHg; KUF with saline
EVEN 110 H	5,2	174	144	110	56	ETO	72	Cellulose (Hemophan®)	8	200	1,1	HD	
130 H	6,2	176	157	115	61		83				1,3		
150 H	7,1	182	161	119	64		95				1,5		
180 H	8,7	186	166	124	69		115				1,8		
200 H	9,5	191	171	130	72		128				2,0		
DIADEMA 110 MF	12,4	178	156	116	60	γ	63	Cellulose Diacetate	30	200	1,1	HD	
130 MF	13,6	182	162	123	66		76				1,3		
150 MF	17	188	168	127	71		90				1,5		
170 MF	19,2	191	172	136	79		104				1,7		
190 MF	21,4	193	177	142	84		116				1,9		
210 MF	23,8	195	182	147	91		120				2,1		
DIADEMA 110 HF	18,6	188	176	163	109	γ	58	Cellulose Triacetate	18,5	200	1,1	HD	
130 HF	22	191	182	169	118		62				1,3		
150 HF	27,2	194	186	174	127		73				1,5		
170 HF	29,4	196	190	179	134		79				1,7		
190 HF	32,4	197	193	184	143		91				1,9		
210 HF	37	198	196	188	147		114				2,1		
Syntex 110 S	13,6	210	190	168	100	γ	63	Cellulose (SMC®)	8,5	200	1,1		
130 S	15,0	242	201	184	103		76				1,3		
150 S	18,7	255	225	207	110		90				1,5		
170 S	21,0	267	230	210	115		104				1,7		
190 S	23,4	272	235	219	120		116				1,9		
210 S	26,0	280	246	223	136		120				2,1		

Fresenius Medical Care													
Hemoflow													
F 3	1,7	125	95	50	20	ETO	28	Fresenius Polysulfone® (Low-Flux)	40	200	0,4	HD	F 3 pediatric
F 4	2,8	155	128	78	32		42				0,7		
F 5	4,0	170	149	103	45		63				1,0		
F 6	5,5	180	164	123	60		82				1,3		
F 7	6,4	184	169	132	68		98				1,6		
F 8	7,5	186	172	138	76		110				1,8		
F 4 HPS	8	170	149	123	75	inline steam	51	Fresenius Polysulfone® (Low-Flux)	40	200	0,8	HD	Clearances for F8/10 HPS at Q_B=300ml/min
F 5 HPS	10	179	162	139	84		63				1,0		
F 6 HPS	13	186	173	148	92		78				1,3		
F 7 HPS	16	188	175	155	102		96				1,6		
F 8 HPS	18	252	224	193	118		113				1,8		
F 10 HPS	21	259	230	208	131		132				2,2		
F 40 (S)	20	165	140	138	80	ETO S = inline steam	42	Fresenius Polysulfone® (High-Flux)	40	200	0,7	HD / HDF	
F 50 (S)	30	178	160	158	100		63				1,0		
F 60 (S)	40	185	172	170	118		82				1,3		
F 70 (S)	50	190	177	174	127		98				1,6		
HF 80 (S)	55	265	245	240	180	inline steam	110		40	200	1,8	HF / HDF	Clearances at Q_B=300, Q_F=60
HdF 100 S	60	285	272	260	215		138		35	185	2,4		
FX 40	20	170	144	138	84	inline steam	32	Polysulfone (Helixone®)	35	185	0,6	HD / HDF / HF	Clearances for FX80/100 at Q_B=300 ml/min
FX 50	33	189	170	165	115		53				1,0		
FX 60	46	193	182	177	135		74				1,4		
FX 80	59	276	250	239	175		95				1,8		
FX 100	73	278	261	248	192		116				2,2		
AV 400 S						inline steam	52	Fresenius Polysulfone®	35	220	0,7	acute	
AV 600 S							100				1,4		
AV 1000 S							130				1,8		
Gambro													
Alwall													
GFE 12	6,0	177	151	140	51	ETO	65	Cellulose (Cuprophan®)	8	200	1,3	HD	
GFE 15	6,4	182	162	145	56		75				1,5		
GFE 18	8,3	190	170	155	70		95				1,8		
GFS 12	6,5	177	151	140	51	heat	65		8	200	1,3	HD	
GFS 16	8,2	189	171	157	59		90				1,6		

	Performance Data					Technical Data							
Dialyser	**KUF** ml/hmmHg	**Urea** ml/min	**Crea** ml/min	**Phos.** ml/min	**V. B_{12}** ml/min	**Steri.**	**Vol.** ml	**Membrane material**	**Wall** µm	**Lum.** µm	**Surf.** m²	**Appl.**	**Notes**
GFS Plus 11	5,5	171	144	148	48	heat	60	Cellulose	8	210	1,1	HD	Clearances for
GFS Plus 12	6,8	180	156	160	60		70	(Hemophan®)	8		1,3		Vit. B_{12} at
GFS Plus 16	9,4	190	170	171	72		95		8		1,7		TMP=100mmHg,
GFS Plus 20	11,4	192	173	176	84		100		6,5	200	1,8		GF16;20 Q_B=300
Lundia													
Alpha 400	4,8	158	129	113	44	ETO	53	Cellulose	8	Plate	0,9	HD	
Alpha 500	6,1	173	146	131	55		62	(Cuprophan®)	8		1,2		
Alpha 600	8,3	179	155	145	74		83		8		1,6		
Alpha 700	11,2	186	167	152	83		99		6,5		1,6		
Aria 550								Cellulose		Plate	1,0	HD	
Aria 700								(Hemophan®)			1,3		
Pro 100	2,2	71	58	49	24	ETO	25	Polycarbonate	15	Plate	0,3	HD	Clearances at
Pro 200	3,5	114	94	78	45		49	(Gambrane®)			0,5		TMP=100mmHg
Pro 500	7,5	162	138	122	72		70				1,0		
Pro 600	9,8	174	154	134	82		90				1,3		
Pro 800	12,0	184	168	146	98		110				1,6		
Polyflux 6 S	34	147	125	121	71	heat	57	Polyamide S™ =	50	215	0,6	HD /	Pediatric
Polyflux 11 S	53	177	160	156	110		81	Polyamide /			1,1	HDF	Clearances for
Polyflux 14 S	62	186	172	168	125		102	Polyarylether-			1,4		Pf 24S at
Polyflux 17 S	71	191	179	176	136		121	sulfone / PVP			1,7		Q_B =300ml/min
Polyflux 21 S	83	195	187	185	149		152	blend			2,1		
Polyflux 24 S		274	255	249	192		165		40	190	2,4		
Polyflux 140 H	52	193	180	174	127	heat	75	Polyamix =	50	200	1,4	HD /	Clearances for
170 H	65	195	184	178	134		94	Polyarylethersulfone/			1,7	HDF /	Pfl. 210 H at
210 H	78	282	259	252	185		120	PVP/Polyamide			2,1	HF	Q_B =300ml/min
Polyflux 14 L	9,5	190	174	157	92	heat	77	Polyamide S™	50	200	1,4	HD	
17 L	12,5	192	178	162	99		103				1,7		
21 L													
Hemoflux 14						ETO	90	Polyamide	60	215	1,4	HF	
Hemoflux 20							130				2,0		
FH 22 H						ETO	13	Polyamide	50	220	0,20	HF /	
FH 66 D							55		50	220	0,60	acute	
FH 77 H							90		60	215	1,40		
FH 88 H							137		60	215	2,00		

Haidylena													
HL 90	5,0	158	138	123	41	ETO / γ / heat	52	Cellulose (Cuprophan®)	8	200	0,9	HD	
HL 100	5,5	164	139	125	44		53				1,0		
HL 110	6,0	169	146	126	52		54				1,1		
HL 120	6,3	172	150	129	54		60				1,2		
HL 130 S	7,0	177	152	134	56		66				1,3		
HL 160	8,7	185	161	140	60		80				1,6		
HL 100 H	5,0	175	149	130	48	ETO / γ / heat	57	Cellulose (Hemophan®)	8	200	1,0	HD	KUF at TMP=150mmHg, Hct. 25%
HL 110 H	5,5	178	154	138	50		61				1,1		
HL 120 H	6,0	181	159	144	55		63				1,2		
HL 130 H	6,6	184	164	148	59		70				1,3		
HL 140 H	7,0	186	168	153	62		76				1,4		
HL 160 H	8,0	189	174	159	67		84				1,6		
HL 180 H	8,8	192	179	187	75		94				1,8		
HL 200 H	9,7	195	184	172	81		105				2,0		
HL 220 H	10,8	197	188	177	86		115				2,2		
HL 100 B	8,7	175	151	135	72	ETO / γ	57	Cellulose (Bioflux®)	18,5	200	1,0	HD	Spacer yarns (P.E.T.®)
HL 130 B	12,0	185	165	148	97		68				1,3		
HL 160 B	16,0	189	170	154	109		84				1,6		
HP H 130 S	52	243	221	208	164	ETO / γ / heat	80	Polyethersulfone Plus HF	30	200	1,3	HD / HDF	Clearances at Q_B =300 ml/min+ TMP=50 mmHg
HP H 160 S	67	250	227	218	171		99				1,6		
HP H 180 S	78	253	231	224	176		112				1,8		
HP M 100 S	27,4	180	165	155	98	ETO / γ / heat	65	Polyethersulfone Plus MF	35	200	1,0	HD	Clearances at TMP=50 mmHg; Spacer yarns (P.E.T.®)
HP M 130 S	36,7	188	177	169	114		80				1,3		
HP M 160 S	50,7	193	184	178	128		99				1,6		
HP M 180 S	59,2	195	187	182	135		112				1,8		
HP 100 S	8,4	171	155	134	91	ETO / γ / heat	65	Polyethersulfone Plus LF	35	200	1,0	HD	Clearances at TMP=50 mmHg; Spacer yarns (P.E.T.®)
HP 130 S	10,4	181	169	149	108		80				1,3		
HP 160 S	12,1	188	178	158	117		99				1,6		
HP 180 S	13,7	191	183	163	124		112				1,8		
Helbio													
Ac 10	3,8	180	145	126	55	ß/γ	60	Cellulose Acetate	30	195	1,0	HD	Modern Realization Group Clearances at Q_B =300 ml/min
Ac 13	5,2	194	170	151	57		75				1,3		
Ac 15	6,7	210	191	166	61		90				1,5		
Ac 18	7,2	223	209	178	61		110				1,8		
Ac 22	8,6	238	215	189	88		125				2,2		
Dia 10	9,6	190	173	150	89	ß/γ	60	Cellulose Diacetate (Middle-Flux)	30	195	1,0	HD	
Dia 13	12,9	224	188	171	95		75				1,3		
Dia 15	16,7	236	207	189	103		90				1,5		
Dia 18	18,5	248	215	197	109		110				1,8		
Dia 22	21,4	259	224	206	129		125				2,2		

	Performance Data					Technical Data							
Dialyser	**KUF** ml/hmmHg	**Urea** ml/min	**Crea.** ml/min	**Phos.** ml/min	**V. B_{12}** ml/min	**Steri.**	**Vol.** ml	**Membrane material**	**Wall** µm	**Lum.** µm	**Surf.** m²	**Appl.**	**Notes**
Dia 100	12,5	205	183	158	110	ß/γ	60	Cellulose	30	195	1,0	HD	Clearances at
Dia 130	16,8	235	200	179	125		75	Diacetate			1,3		Q_B =300 ml/min
Dia 150	21,7	247	223	196	129		90	(High-Flux)			1,5		
Dia 180	23,4	253	231	204	141		110				1,8		
Dia 220	27,8	262	240	223	170		125				2,2		
Tria 130	11,3	206	192	169	98	ß/γ	75	Cellulose	15	195	1,3	HD	
Tria 150	15,2	230	214	187	105		90	Triacetate			1,5		
Tria 180	19,5	247	230	203	112		110	(Middle-Flux)			1,8		
Tria 210	25,2	263	242	218	137		125				2,1		
Tria 1300	17	230	201	179	136	ß/γ	75	Cellulose	15	195	1,3	HD /	
Tria 1500	22,8	241	218	198	155		90	Triacetate			1,5	HDF	
Tria 1800	35,6	259	234	210	174		110	(High-Flux)			1,8		
Tria 2100	42,0	282	258	229	193		125				2,1		
Bio 100	6,5	175	157	135	65	ß	60	Polysulfone LF	40	200	1,0	HD	
Bio 120	7,7	182	165	140	75		71				1,2		
Bio 140	8,8	188	170	147	92		83				1,4		
Bio 160	9,9	192	178	152	100		90				1,6		
Bio 180	11,0	195	182	158	102		104				1,8		
Bio 200	12,2	198	187	165	109		112				2,0		
Bio 1000	36	180	165	161	108	ß	60	Polysulfone HF	40	200	1,0	HD /	
Bio 1200	43	186	169	164	120		71				1,2	HF /	
Bio 1400	51	190	174	171	132		83				1,4	HDF	
Bio 1600	58	195	180	177	140		90				1,6		
Bio 1800	65	197	185	183	151		104				1,8		
Bio 2000	72	198	188	185	160		112				2,0		
Hospal / Cobe													
Hospal													
Disscap 120 SE	4,2	172	148	123	47	ETO	57	Cellulose	8	200	1,1	HD	
150 SE	5,2	176	159	135	57		70	(Cuprophan®)			1,3		
180 SE	6,8	186	171	147	65		90				1,7		
210 SE	8,2	189	177	158	76		110				2,1		
Filtral 6	15	139	117	92	53	ETO	48	Polyacrylonitrile	50	240	0,60	HD /	Clearances at
Filtral 8	22	157	134	110	68	G = γ	56	AN 69® HF			0,75	HF /	UF=10 ml/min
Filtral 10	26	167	143	118	72		65				0,90	HDF	
Filtral 12 (G)	35	175	160	139	88		89				1,30		
Filtral 16 (G)	48	188	174	151	101		112				1,70		
Filtral 20	62	195	182	163	116		142				2,05		

Crystal 2800	31	203	168	136	75	γ	93	AN 69® ST		Plate	1,0	HD /	Clearances at
Crystal 3400	36	218	184	154	90		116	(surface treated)			1,2	HF /	Q_B =300 ml/min
Crystal 4000	46	230	201	170	104		140				1,5	HDF	
Nephral ST 200	33	173	156	135	85	γ	64	AN 69® ST	42	210	1,05	HD /	
Nephral ST 300	40	181	166	146	96	(wet)	81				1,30	HF /	
Nephral ST 400	50	189	176	156	111		98				1,65	HDF	
Nephral ST 500	65	195	184	168	126		126				2,15		
Hemospal						ETO	64	AN 69® S	23	Plate	0,43	acute	
Multiflow 60							48	AN 69® HF	50	240	0,6		
Multiflow100							65		50	240	0,9		
Acepal 1100	7,0	160	134	106	53	ETO /	61	Cellulose	14	200	1,0	HD	Fibers with FINs
Acepal 1300	8,0	167	142	114	59	γ	70	Diacetate			1,2		
Acepal 1500	10	177	156	132	74		92				1,5		
Acepal 1700	13	184	165	142	83		107				1,7		
Diacepal 12	9,2	179	158	131	71	γ	63	Cellulose	15	200	1,2	HD	
Diacepal 14	12,3	187	170	150	85		77	Diacetate			1,4		
Diacepal 16	13,7	190	174	154	89		88				1,6		
Diacepal 20	17,7	194	183	166	103		113				2,0		
Cobe													
200	3,0	145	116	112	33	ETO	34	Cellulose	11	200	0,7	HD	
300	4,3	160	130	125	35		42	(Cuprophan®)	8		0,9		
400	5,5	175	156	140	50		46		6,5		1,0		
700	8,3	190	170	155	70		95		8		1,8		
108 G	4,9	168	143	122	48	γ	45	Cellulose	6,5	200	0,8	HD	Vit.B_{12} at
110 G	5,0	174	149	132	50		60	(Cuprophan®)	8		1,0		TMP=100mmHg
112 G	5,4	180	156	138	55		63		8		1,2		
HG 100	1,6	72	62	57	19	γ	18	Cellulose	6,5	200	0,22	HD	Spacer yarns;
HG 400	4,5	169	148	140	52		47	(Hemophan®)			0,9		Clear. HG 100 at
HG 500	6,4	182	164	151	64		58				1,1		Q_B =100 ml/min
HG 600	7,4	187	178	160	82		88				1,6		
HG 700	11,0	193	183	172	97		113				2,0		

	Performance Data					Technical Data							
Dialyser	**KUF** ml/hmmHg	**Urea** ml/min	**Crea.** ml/min	**Phos.** ml/min	**V. B_{12}** ml/min	**Steri.**	**Vol.** ml	**Membrane material**	**Wall** µm	**Lum.** µm	**Surf.** m²	**Appl.**	**Notes**
450 HS	4,2	180	156	160	60	heat	70	Cellulose	8	200	1,3	HD	
700 HS	5,9	190	170	171	72		95	(Hemophan®)			1,7		
9-CA	4,7	175	145	117	67	ETO	47	Cellulose	15	200	0,9	HD	Spacer yarns
11-CA	7,0	185	162	137	81		54	Acetate			1,1		
15-CA	10,4	192	179	147	102		83				1,5		
19-CA	13,1	197	191	166	121		104				1,9		
H 1	58	179	167	158	114	γ	77	Polyarylether-	50	215	1,04	HD /	H 1:fiber bundle
H 4	62	185	175	167	124		95	sulfone / PVP			1,35	HDF	with spacer yarns
H 6	69	190	181	174	132		108	blend			1,57		
H 9	88	194	187	182	148		139	(ARYLANE)			2,01		
M 4	15,4	185	173	151	101	γ	95		50	215	1,35	HD	
M 6	18,5	189	178	159	109		108				1,62		
M 9	23,0	194	187	179	128		139				2,01		
IDEMSA													Modern
12	4,0	160	143	109	44	ETO /	55	Cellulose	8	200	0,8	HD	Realization Group
15	4,2	169	152	117	48	γ	60	(Cuprophan®)			0,9		
20	4,7	172	155	121	50		63				0,95		Clearances at
23	5,0	178	161	129	53		72				1,1		TMP=100 mmHg;
25	6,0	184	167	139	58		83				1,3		KUF with saline
28	7,0	189	172	147	61		95				1,5		
30	8,4	192	175	154	66		115				1,8		
32	9,2	195	178	159	69		128				2,0		
34	11,2	197	185	166	76		147				2,3		
36	12,3	198	188	168	78		158				2,6		
12 H	4,2	161	145	111	47	ETO /	55	Cellulose	8	200	0,8	HD	
15 H	4,4	170	154	119	51	γ	60	(Hemophan®)			0,9		
20 H	4,7	173	157	123	53		63				0,95		
23 H	5,2	179	163	131	56		72				1,1		
25 H	6,2	185	169	141	61		83				1,3		
28 H	7,2	190	174	149	64		95				1,5		
30 H	8,6	193	177	156	69		115				1,8		
32 H	9,4	196	180	161	72		128				2,0		
34 H	11,4	198	187	168	78		147				2,3		
36 H	12,5	199	190	170	79		158				2,6		

100	12	170	152	137	91	ETO / γ	47	Cellulose (Bioflux®)	12,0	200	1,0	HD	Spacer yarns (P.E.T.®)
120	15,2	176	161	142	94		57				1,2		
140	18,4	183	166	151	100		63				1,4		
160	21,6	185	172	157	107		70				1,6		
180	24	188	176	161	114		84				1,8		
200	27,2	190	179	165	120		91				2,0		
H 900	16,0	170	155	142	98	ETO / γ	46	Cellulose (Bioflux®)	18,5	200	0,9	HD	Spacer yarns (P.E.T.®)
H 1100	19,2	175	164	147	101		58				1,1		
H 1300	22,4	182	169	158	110		77				1,3		
H 1500	28,0	185	175	165	116		90				1,6		
H 1800	35,2	188	182	174	128		113				2,0		
H 2000	40,0	190	183	177	130		127				2,2		
P 100	12	175	165	143	104	γ (wet)	62	Polyethersulfone	40	200	1,0	HD	Clearances at UF=10 ml/min
P 120	14	179	170	149	113		71				1,2		
P 140	17	181	175	153	122		81				1,4		
P 160	20	185	179	157	132		88				1,6		
P 180	23	192	184	165	138		104				1,8		
P 200	26	194	188	173	141		112				2,0		
1.000	57	178	170	150	134	γ (wet)	62	Polyethersulfone	40	200	1,0	HD / HDF / HF	Clearances at UF=10 ml/min
1.200	63	183	175	158	139		71				1,2		
1.400	73	185	180	165	149		81				1,4		
1.600	83	191	185	170	154		88				1,6		
1.800	93	196	195	178	176		104				1,8		
2.000	103	197	194	182	184		112				2,0		
100 MHP	26	176	166	145	121	γ (wet)	62	Polyethersulfone	40	200	1,0	HD / HDF / HF	Clearances at UF=10 ml/min
120 MHP	29	180	171	151	127		71				1,2		
140 MHP	33	182	176	154	134		81				1,4		
160 MHP	37	186	180	158	142		88				1,6		
180 MHP	44	193	185	166	159		104				1,8		
200 MHP	50	195	189	174	161		112				2,0		
JMS													
JC 1080	5,5	164	142	126	44	ETO	50	Cellulose (Cuprophan®)	8	200	1,0	HD	
JC 1280	6,5	173	149	132	50		58				1,2		
JC 1480	7,5	180	155	136	54		66				1,4		
JC 1680	8,7	185	161	140	58		74				1,6		
JH 1080	5,5	164	142	128	44	ETO	50	Cellulose (Hemophan®)	8	200	1,0	HD	
JH 1280	6,5	174	150	133	51		58				1,2		
JH 1480	7,4	181	157	138	57		66				1,4		
JH 1680	8,2	187	158	141	65		74				1,6		

	Performance Data					Technical Data							
Dialyser	KUF ml/hmmHg	Urea ml/min	Crea. ml/min	Phos. ml/min	V. B_{12} ml/min	Steri.	Vol. ml	Membrane material	Wall µm	Lum. µm	Surf. m²	Appl.	Notes
Kawasumi / Kuraray													
Renak													
RE-08 H	3,4	160	136	114	39	ETO	46	Cellulose	8	200	0,8	HD	
RE-08 U	4,5	163	139	117	45		46	(Cuprophan®)	6,5		0,8		
RE-10 H	4,4	170	148	126	46		55		8		1,0		
RE-10 U	5,4	174	152	131	54		55		6,5		1,0		
RE-12 H	5,2	177	156	136	52		63		8		1,2		
RE-12 U	6,4	180	161	141	61		63		6,5		1,2		
RE-15 H	7,2	185	168	149	61		82		8		1,5		
RE-15 U	9,4	188	172	154	72		82		6,5		1,5		
RE-18 H	8,3	189	174	157	68		101		8		1,8		
RE-18 U	10,2	192	179	163	80		101		6,5		1,8		
RA-08 H	3,4	158	133	111	38	heat	46	Cellulose	8	200	0,8	HD	
RA-08 U	4,5	163	139	117	45	(wet)	46	(Cuprophan®)	6,5		0,8		
RA-10 H	4,4	168	145	123	44		55		8		1,0		
RA-10 U	5,4	173	151	130	53		55		6,5		1,0		
RA-12 H	5,2	174	153	132	49		63		8		1,2		
RA-12 U	6,4	179	160	140	60		63		6,5		1,2		
RA-15 H	7,2	183	164	145	58		82		8		1,5		
RA-15 U	9,4	187	171	153	71		82		6,5		1,5		
RA-18 H	8,3	187	171	152	64		101		8		1,8		
RA-18 U	10,2	191	178	161	78		101		6,5		1,8		
ME-08 H	3,7	160	136	117	39	ETO	46	Cellulose	8	200	0,8	HD	
ME-08 U	4,6	163	139	120	45		46	(Hemophan®)	6,5		0,8		
ME-10 H	4,6	170	148	130	46		55		8		1,0		
ME-10 U	5,4	174	152	134	54		55		6,5		1,0		
ME-12 H	5,5	177	156	139	52		63		8		1,2		
ME-12 U	6,5	180	161	144	61		63		6,5		1,2		
ME-15 H	7,7	185	168	152	61		82		8		1,5		
ME-15 U	8,7	188	172	157	72		82		6,5		1,5		
ME-18 H	8,0	189	174	159	68		101		8		1,8		
ME-18 U	9,1	192	179	165	80		101		6,5		1,8		

MA-08 H	3,6	158	133	115	38	heat	46	Cellulose	8	200	0,8	HD	
MA-08 U	4,4	163	139	120	45	(wet)	46	(Hemophan®)	6,5		0,8		
MA-10 H	4,2	168	145	126	44		55		8		1,0		
MA-10 U	5,1	173	151	133	53		55		6,5		1,0		
MA-12 H	5,2	174	153	135	49		63		8		1,2		
MA-12 U	6,2	179	160	143	60		63		6,5		1,2		
MA-15 H	7,2	183	164	148	58		82		8		1,5		
MA-15 U	8,4	187	171	156	71		82		6,5		1,5		
MA-18 H	7,8	187	171	155	64		101		8		1,8		
MA-18 U	8,8	191	178	164	78		101		6,5		1,8		
KF 101 0,8 D5	4,5	155	127	100	52	ETO	73	Ethylvinylalcohol	25	175	0,8	HD	Clearances at
KF 201 0,8 D5	5,8	161	134	107	60	γ(wet)		(EVAL® D)					TMP=100 mmHg
KF 101 1,0 D5	5,5	164	138	111	60	ETO	85				1,0		
KF 201 1,0 D5	7,0	171	144	118	69	γ(wet)							
KF 101 1,3 D5	6,8	172	150	125	71	ETO	107				1,3		
KF 201 1,3 D5	8,7	179	159	133	80	γ(wet)							
KF 101 1,6 D5	8,2	177	159	136	81	ETO	128				1,6		
KF 201 1,6 D5	10,4	184	166	146	89	γ(wet)							
KF 101 0,8 C5	6,3	161	134	110	60	ETO	73	Ethylvinylalcohol	25	175	0,8	HD	
KF 201 0,8 C5	7,4	167	143	119	71	γ(wet)		(EVAL® C)					
KF 101 1,0 C5	7,5	168	144	121	70	ETO	85				1,0		
KF 201 1,0 C5	8,9	174	153	130	81	γ(wet)							
KF 101 1,3 C5	9,4	174	155	134	82	ETO	107				1,3		
KF 201 1,3 C5	11,1	181	165	143	93	γ(wet)							
KF 101 1,6 C5	11,3	177	162	144	92	ETO	128				1,6		
KF 201 1,6 C5	13,3	186	173	154	103	γ(wet)							
KF 201 1,0 M5	9,2	167	143	115	68	γ	85	Ethylvinylalcohol	25	175	1,0	HD	Clearances at
KF 201 1,3 M5	11,5	175	155	133	85	(wet)	107	(EVAL® M)			1,3		UF=10ml/min/m²
KF 201 1,6 M5	13,8	181	164	142	95		128				1,6		
KF 201 1,8 M5	15,3	185	169	146	100		139				1,8		
RA-1.0 SH	9,0	166	151	132	70	heat	58	Cellulose	18,5	200	1,0	HD	Spacer yarns
RA-1.2 SH	11,0	175	161	145	80	(wet)	70	(Bioflux®)			1,2		(P.E.T. ®)
RA-1.5 SH	13,5	182	170	155	90		84				1,5		
SMC R 10	5,0	169	144	134	50	γ	60	Cellulose	9	200	1,0	HD	Spacers(P.E.T.®);
SMC R 13	6,5	181	159	150	62		76	(SMC®)			1,3		UF at 100mmHg
SMC R 16	8,0	188	170	162	72		94				1,6		
DIAPES R 12	35	177	161	166	113	γ	63	Polyethersulfone	30	220	1,2	HD/	Spacers(P.E.T.®);
DIAPES R 15	40	185	171	177	129		82	(DIAPES®)			1,5	HDF	KUF at 100mmHg
DIAPES R 18	45	190	174	184	138		101				1,8		

	Performance Data					Technical Data							
Dialyser	**KUF** ml/hmmHg	**Urea** ml/min	**Crea.** ml/min	**Phos.** ml/min	**V. B_{12}** ml/min	**Steri.**	**Vol.** ml	**Membrane material**	**Wall** µm	**Lum.** µm	**Surf.** m²	**Appl.**	**Notes**
Kimal													
KF 1000	57	180	164	161	115	γ	62	Polyethersulfone	40	200	1,0	HD/	
KF 1200	63	186	169	166	122		71				1,2	HF/	
KF 1400	73	190	175	172	135		81				1,4	HDF	
KF 1600	83	195	181	178	141		88				1,6		
KF 1800	93	197	186	183	152		104				1,8		
KF 2000	103	198	189	186	161		112				2,0		
Medica													
D 100						ETO	16	Polysulfone	125	500	0,1	acute	for neonatal
D 150							18	(MediSulfone®)	50	250	0,25		for pediatric
D 200							51		50	250	0,6		for adult
D 300							76		50	250	1,0		for adult
D 400							115		50	250	1,5		for adult
D 500							146		50	250	2,0		for adult
Meditech													
NP 08	4,0	165	130	112	41	β	49	Cellulose	8	200	0,8	HD	
NP 10	4,9	169	138	120	45		58	(Cuprophan®)			1,0		
NP 12	5,5	178	148	131	47		68				1,2		
NP 15	7,0	185	167	142	57		81				1,5		
NP 18	7,4	191	170	152	61		89				1,8		
NP-08	4,5	167	131	115	42	ETO	49	Cellulose	8	200	0,8	HD	
NP-10	5,4	171	140	126	47		58	(Cuprophan®)			1,0		
NP-12	6,3	179	150	135	49		68				1,2		
NP-15	7,7	191	169	143	59		81				1,5		
NP-18	8,0	192	171	148	62		89				1,8		
MO 08	4,1	166	131	115	42	γ	49	Cellulose	8	200	0,8	HD	
MO 10	5,0	171	141	126	47		56	(Hemophan®)			1,0		
MO 12	5,7	179	150	136	52		66				1,2		
MO 16	7,2	189	170	155	62		80				1,5		
MO 18	7,6	193	173	158	65		88				1,8		
MO 20	8,0	194	175	160	67		90				2,0		
MO 08	4,7	168	132	116	44	ETO	49	Cellulose	8	200	0,8	HD	
MO 10	5,5	173	143	127	49		58	(Hemophan®)			1,0		
MO 12	6,3	180	152	136	53		68				1,2		
MO 16	7,7	190	172	157	63		81				1,5		
MO 18	8,1	193	174	159	66		89				1,8		
MO 20	8,5	195	177	161	68		90				2,0		

BioF 10	12	171	153	143	79	γ	55	Cellulose (Bioflux®)	18,5	200	1,0	HD	Spacer yarns (P.E.T.®)
BioF 13	14	180	165	155	84		68				1,3		
BioF 16	17	186	180	166	93		78				1,6		
BioF 10	13	173	155	146	80	ETO	55	Cellulose (Bioflux®)	18,5	200	1,0	HD	
BioF 13	15	182	168	158	86		68				1,3		
BioF 16	18	188	182	169	95		78				1,6		
MF 4	6,0	170	155	144	45	β	72	Polyethersulfone	40	200	1,0	HD	
MF 6	8,0	188	165	163	55		83				1,3		
MF 40	22	172	161	151	119		72				1,0		
MF 60	29	190	172	173	142		83				1,3		
Minntech													
Diafilter D-20 NR	31					ETO	38	Polysulfone (Minntech PS)	70	260	0,26	HF/ HC	
D-30 NR	48						65				0,66		
Renaflow® II													
HF 400						ETO	28	Polysulfone (Minntech PS)	40	200	0,3	acute	
HF 700							53				0,71		
HF 1200							83				1,25		
HF 2000							132				1,98		
Minifilter Plus							14		100	620	0,07		for babies,childr.
Primus 1350	34	177	167	154	106		92	Polysulfone, Minntech PS (Polyphen®)	40	200	1,35	HD/ HF/ HDF	recommended for multiple use
Primus 2000	41	184	177	166	122		137				1,98		
Nephros													
OLpur MD 190	90					γ / ETO	140	Polyethersulfone (DIAPES®)	30	200	1,9	HDF	Mid-dilution HDF
Nikkiso													
BLF-12 G	5,2	172	150	130	44	γ	67	Cellulose (Hemophan®)	8	200	1,2	HD	Clearances at UF=10 ml/min
BLF-14 G	6,3	186	165	141	48		83				1,4		
BLF-18 G	7,1	193	173	150	53		96				1,8		
FLX- 8 GWS	24	176	164	150	109	γ (wet)	50	Polyethersulfone + Polyarylate (PEPA® = Polyester – Polymer Alloy)	30	210	0,8	HD/ HDF	Clearances at UF=10 ml/min
FLX-10 GWS	40	177	168	154	116		60				1,0		
FLX-12 GWS	45	183	174	168	131		76				1,2		
FLX-15 GWS	50	190	179	175	143		92				1,5		
FLX-18 GW S	57	191	184	178	149		108				1,8		
FLX-21 GWS	63	193	187	181	159		135				2,1		

	Performance Data					Technical Data							
Dialyser	**KUF** ml/hmmHg	**Urea** ml/min	**Crea.** ml/min	**Phos.** ml/min	**V. B_{12}** ml/min	**Steri.**	**Vol.** ml	**Membrane material**	**Wall** µm	**Lum.** µm	**Surf.** m²	**Appl.**	**Notes**
FLY 10 GWS	41	179	170	155	120	γ (wet)	60	PEPA®	30		1,0	HD/ HDF	Clearances at UF=10 ml/min
FLY 12 GWS	46	185	175	169	136		76				1,2		
FLY 15 GWS	51	191	181	176	147		92				1,5		
FLY 18 GWS	59	192	186	180	155		108				1,8		
FLY 21 GWS	63	194	189	183	162		135				2,1		
BL 130 GW	8,9	189	166	153	71	γ (wet)	180	Cellulose + Poly-ethylenglycol (Poly-EG-Membr)	10		1,3	HD	Clearance Vit.B_{12} TMP=100 mmHg
BL 150 GW	11,4	191	174	168	87		180				1,5		
NM-12 G	15,8	172	166	156	115	γ	79	Polyethersulfone	35		1,2	HD	Clearances at UF=10 ml/min
NM-15 G	19,8	183	175	164	124		96				1,5		
Nipro													
FB- 50 T	2,1	141	115	81	34	γ	35	Cellulose Diacetate	15	200	0,5	HD	Clearances at UF=10 ml/min
FB- 70 T	3,0	159	134	97	43		45				0,7		
FB- 90 T	3,9	170	147	109	51		55				0,9		
FB-110 T	4,7	177	155	116	58		65				1,1		
FB-130 T	5,6	182	161	122	64		75				1,3		
FB-150 T	6,4	186	166	125	70		90				1,5		
FB-170 T	7,3	190	172	133	77		105				1,7		
FB-190 T	8,1	192	176	140	82		115				1,9		
FB-210 T	9,0	194	180	146	88		125				2,1		
FB- 50 H / A	4,1	146	119	93	43	γ	35	Cellulose Diacetate	15	200	0,5	HD	Clearances at UF=10 ml/min
FB- 70 H / A	5,8	165	141	114	57		45				0,7		
FB- 90 H / A	7,5	176	153	126	68		55				0,9		
FB-110 H / A	9,1	182	161	135	77		65				1,1		
FB-130 H / A	10,8	187	168	142	85		75				1,3		
FB-150 H / A	12,4	190	172	147	93		90				1,5		
FB-170 H / A	14,1	193	178	154	101		105				1,7		
FB-190 H / A	15,7	195	182	160	107		115				1,9		
FB-210 H / A	17,4	196	185	165	113		125				2,1		

FB- 50 U	9,9	160	142	130	71	γ	35	Cellulose Triacetate (CTA)	15	200	0,5	HD / HDF	Clearances at UF=10 ml/min
FB- 70 U	13,9	176	161	150	89		45				0,7		
FB- 90 U	17,9	185	172	163	103		55				0,9		
FB-110 U	21,8	190	179	171	114		65				1,1		
FB-130 U	25,8	194	184	177	125		75				1,3		
FB-150 U	29,8	196	188	182	133		90				1,5		
FB-170 U	33,7	198	192	186	141		105				1,7		
FB-190 U	37,7	198	193	189	147		115				1,9		
FB-210 U	41,7	199	195	192	153		125				2,1		
SUREFLUX-P													
50 P	8,5	153	136	118	65	γ	35	Cellulose Triacetate (CTA)	15	200	0,5	HD	Clearances at UF=10 ml/min
70 P	11,9	170	154	138	82		45				0,7		
90 P	15,3	180	167	151	96		55				0,9		
110 P	18,6	186	174	160	107		65				1,1		
130 P	22,0	190	180	167	117		75				1,3		
150 P	25,4	193	184	172	125		90				1,5		
170 P	28,8	196	188	178	133		105				1,7		
190 P	32,2	197	190	182	140		115				1,9		
210 P	35,6	198	193	185	146		125				2,1		
SUREFLUX-E													
50 E	6,9	150	132	115	62	γ	35	Cellulose Triacetate (CTA)	15	200	0,5	HD	Clearances at UF=10 ml/min
70 E	9,6	167	151	134	78		45				0,7		
90 E	12,3	178	163	148	92		55				0,9		
110 E	15,1	184	171	157	102		65				1,1		
130 E	17,8	188	176	164	112		75				1,3		
150 E	20,5	191	181	169	121		90				1,5		
170 E	23,3	195	186	175	129		105				1,7		
190 E	26,0	196	188	179	135		115				1,9		
210 E	28,8	197	191	183	141		125				2,1		
SUREFLUX-G													
50 G	5,9	149	130	111	58	γ	35	Cellulose Triacetate (CTA)	15	200	0,5	HD	Clearances at UF=10 ml/min
70 G	8,3	167	149	131	74		45				0,7		
90 G	10,6	177	162	144	88		55				0,9		
110 G	13,0	183	169	153	98		65				1,1		
130 G	15,3	188	175	160	108		75				1,3		
150 G	17,7	191	180	166	116		90				1,5		
170 G	20,0	194	185	172	124		105				1,7		
190 G	22,4	195	187	176	130		115				1,9		
210 G	24,7	197	190	180	137		125				2,1		

	Performance Data					Technical Data							
Dialyser	**KUF** ml/hmmHg	**Urea** ml/min	**Crea.** ml/min	**Phos.** ml/min	**V. B_{12}** ml/min	**Steri.**	**Vol.** ml	**Membrane material**	**Wall** µm	**Lum.** µm	**Surf.** m²	**Appl.**	**Notes**
SUREFLUX-L													
30 L	3,1	115	97	80	30	γ	25	Cellulose	15	200	0,3	HD	Clearances at
50 L	4,3	149	130	111	50		35	Triacetate			0,5		UF=10 ml/min
70 L	6,0	167	149	131	64		45	(CTA)			0,7		
90 L	7,7	177	162	144	77		55				0,9		
110 L	9,4	183	169	153	87		65				1,1		
130 L	11,1	188	175	160	92		75				1,3		
150 L	12,8	191	180	166	100		90				1,5		
170 L	14,5	194	185	172	108		105				1,7		
190 L	16,2	195	187	176	115		115				1,9		
210 L	17,9	197	190	180	122		125				2,1		
SUREFLUX-FH													
110 FH	49	194	186	183	136	γ	60	Cellulose	15	185	1,1	HD /	Clearances at
150 FH	67	198	194	193	155		85	Triacetate			1,5	HDF	UF=10 ml/min
190 FH	84	199	197	197	168		110	(CTA)			1,9		
210 FH	93	200	198	198	173		120				2,1		
SURELYZER													
PES-110 DH	32	187	174	166	128	γ	68	Polyethersulfone	30	200	1,1	HD /	Clearances at
PES-150 DH	43	195	187	181	148		93				1,5	HDF	UF=10 ml/min;
PES-190 DH	55	198	193	188	162		118				1,9		spacers P.E.T.®
UF 203	34	196	188	184	145	γ	105	Cellulose	15	200	1,7	HF	
UF 205	39	197	190	189	149		115	Triacetate (CTA)			1,9		
RenaSelect													
Altair 10	5,3	174	149	130	48	ETO /	57	Cellulose	8	200	1,0	HD	
Altair 12	6,3	178	161	140	55	γ	63	(Hemophan®)			1,2		
Altair 14	7,4	183	165	147	59		72				1,4		
Altair 16	8,5	188	167	151	61		84				1,6		
Nouvelle 10	8,4	178	155	136	54	ETO /	62	Cellulose	11	210	1,0	HD	
Nouvelle 12	10,2	180	161	140	61	γ	73	(G-O-P DIAFIL®)			1,2		
Nouvelle 14	12,2	184	166	145	75		84				1,4		
Nouvelle 16	13,8	188	169	148	84		95				1,6		
Saxonia													
Saxon													
1080 C	5,5	164	142	126	44	ETO /	50	Cellulose	8	200	1,0	HD	Performances for
1280 C	6,5	173	149	132	50	γ /	58	(Cuprophan®)			1,2		heat: 10% lower
1480 C	7,5	180	155	136	54	heat	66				1,4		
1680 C	8,7	185	161	140	58		74				1,6		

1080 H	5,5	165	142	128	44	ETO / γ / heat	50	Cellulose (Hemophan®)	8	200	1,0	HD	
1280 H	6,5	174	150	133	51		58				1,2		
1480 H	7,5	181	157	138	57		66				1,4		
1680 H	8,7	187	163	141	62		74				1,6		
1018 B	11	155	141	132	65	γ	58	Cellulose (Bioflux®)	18,5	200	1,0	HD	Spacer yarns (P.E.T.®)
1318 B	16	163	150	140	78		75				1,3		
LF 10 PS	7,0	164	152	127	62	γ	52	Polysulfone	40	200	1,0	HD	
LF 12 PS	8,5	175	165	138	75		68				1,2		
LF 15 PS	10,5	187	174	142	82		90				1,5		
1230 D	47	182	177	171	135	ETO/ γ/heat	68	Polyethersulfone (DiaPES)	30	200	1,2	HD / HDF	Spacer yarns (P.E.T.®)
Terumo													
Clirans													
E 12 NL	9,0	178	156	142	66	heat (wet)	79	Cellulose (Excebrane)	23	200	1,2	HD	Clearances at UF=10 ml/min
E 15 NL	10,2	183	164	148	74		90				1,5		
E 18 NL	13,4	184	169	152	87		106				1,8		
EE 12 NL	15,0	185	160	149	80	heat (wet)	79		26	200	1,2	HD	
EE 15 NL	16,7	188	164	156	89		90				1,5		
EE 18 NL	20,4	196	173	166	94		106				1,8		
Toray													
Filtryzer													
B1-1,0	7,2	164	139	115	66	γ (wet)		Polymethyl-methacrylate (PMMA)	20	200		HD	Clearances at TMP=100 mmHg
B1-1,0 H	9,0	169	141	123	73								
B1-1,3 H	12	180	156	140	86								
B1-1,6 H	14	187	167	155	98								
B1-1,6 U	30	187	167	152	105	γ (wet)		PMMA	30	200		HD / HDF	Clearances at UF=10 ml/min
B1-2,1 U	39	192	177	168	119								
B2-1,0 H	4,1	165	137	88	56	y (wet)		PMMA	20	200		HD	Clearances at TMP=100 mmHg
B2-1,2 H	4,9	174	147	97	62								
B2-1,5 H	6,0	183	159	112	72								
B2-2,0	6,4	189	169	117	79								
B3-0,5 A	3,8	137	106	68	45	γ (wet)	35	PMMA	20	200	0,5	HD	pediatric
B3-0,8 A	5,9	163	134	92	61		49				0,8		pediatric
B3-1,0 A	7,0	175	146	105	70		61				1,0		
B3-1,3 A	8,8	184	160	121	81		76				1,3		Clearances at TMP=100 mmHg
B3-1,6 A	8,7	188	167	128	88		95				1,6		
B3-2,0 A	11	193	177	142	101		118				2,0		

	Performance Data					Technical Data							
Dialyser	KUF ml/hmmHg	Urea ml/min	Crea. ml/min	Phos. ml/min	V. B_{12} ml/min	Steri.	Vol. ml	Membrane material	Wall µm	Lum. µm	Surf. m²	Appl.	Notes
BK-1,0 F	13	172	146	127	83	γ (wet)	58	PMMA	30	200	1,0	HD	Clearances at UF=10 ml/min
BK-1,3 F	16	183	160	144	99		76				1,3		
BK-1,6 F	20	190	172	157	111		94				1,6		
BK-2,1 F	26	195	181	171	128		126				2,1		
BK-1,0 U	21	169	143	123	82	γ (wet)	58	PMMA	30	200	1,0	HD / HDF	
BK-1,3 U	26	180	157	140	96		76				1,3		
BK-1,6 U	31	187	169	153	108		94				1,6		
BK-2,1 U	40	193	179	168	125		126				2,1		
BK-1,0 P	21	171	145	123	82	γ (wet)	58	PMMA	30	200	1,0	HD / HDF	
BK-1,3 P	26	182	159	140	98		76				1,3		
BK-1,6 P	33	189	171	152	110		94				1,6		
BK-2,1 P	41	194	180	168	127		126				2,1		
BS-1.3	47	193	181	180	136	γ (wet)	81	Polysulfone (Toraysulfone®)	40	200	1,3	HD / HDF / HF	Clearances at UF=10ml/min KUF at TMP=100 Subst. Vol. max. 20 liter
BS-1.6	50	195	184	183	143		102				1,6		
BS-1.8	52	198	189	188	151		116				1,8		
BS-1,3 U	47	192	180	179	135	γ (wet)	81	Polysulfone (Toraysulfone®)	40	200	1,3	HD / HDF / HF	
BS-1,6 U	50	194	183	182	142		102				1,6		
BS-1,8 U	52	197	188	187	150		116				1,8		
VMP													
AHF 10	36	180	165	161	106	γ	60	Polysulfone (Synphan HF600)	35	220	1,0	acute	Clearances at TMP=100 mmHg;
AHF 14	51	190	174	171	132		83				1,4		
AHF 20	72	198	188	185	160		112				2,0		
CDF 100	6,5	175	157	135	65	γ	60	Polysulfone (Synphan LF100)	35	220	1,0	HD	
CDF 120	7,7	182	165	140	75		71				1,2		
CDF 140	8,8	188	170	147	92		83				1,4		
CDF 160	9,9	192	178	152	100		90				1,6		
CDF 180	11,0	195	182	158	102		104				1,8		
CDF 200	12,2	198	187	165	109		112				2,0		

Index

C

D

M

P

R

T

U

V

W

X

Z